AN OCCUPATIONAL THERAPIST'S GUIDE TO HOME MODIFICATION PRACTICE

SECOND EDITION

AN OCCUPATIONAL THERAPIST'S GUIDE TO HOME MODIFICATION PRACTICE

SECOND EDITION

Elizabeth Ainsworth, MOccThy, Grad Cert Health Sci
Private Practice Occupational Therapist and Access Consultant
Home Design for Living
Coorparoo, Australia

Desleigh de Jonge, MPhil (OccThy), Grad Cert Soc Sci
Adjunct Research Fellow
School of Health and Rehabilitation Sciences
The University of Queensland
St Lucia, Australia

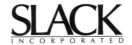

SLACK
INCORPORATED

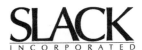

SLACK Incorporated
6900 Grove Road
Thorofare, NJ 08086 USA
856-848-1000   Fax: 856-848-6091
www.Healio.com/books
© 2019 by SLACK Incorporated

Senior Vice President: Stephanie Arasim Portnoy
Vice President, Editorial: Jennifer Kilpatrick
Vice President, Marketing: Michelle Gatt
Acquisitions Editor: Tony Schiavo
Managing Editor: Allegra Tiver
Creative Director: Thomas Cavallaro
Cover Artist: Stacy Marek
Project Editor: Dani Malady

An Occupational Therapist's Guide to Home Modification Practice, Second Edition includes ancillary materials specifically available for faculty use. Please visit http://www.efacultylounge.com to obtain access.

Library of Congress Cataloging-in-Publication Data

Names: Ainsworth, Elizabeth, author. | De Jonge, Desleigh, author.
Title: An occupational therapist's guide to home modification practice /
   Elizabeth Ainsworth, MOccThy, Grad Cert Health Sci,   Private Practice
   Occupational Therapist and Access Consultant, Home Design for Living,
   Coorparoo, Australia, Desleigh de Jonge, MPhil (OccThy), Grad Cert Soc
   Sci, Adjunct Research Fellow, School of Health and Rehabilitation
   Sciences, The University of Queensland, St Lucia, Australia.
Description: Second edition. | Thorofare : Slack Incorporated, [2018] |
   Includes bibliographical references and index.
Identifiers: LCCN 2018035903 (print) | LCCN 2018037252 (ebook) | ISBN
   9781630912192 (epub) | ISBN 9781630912208 (web) | ISBN 9781630912185
   (hardback)
Subjects: LCSH: Occupational therapy. | Home care services. | People with
   disabilities--Housing--Design and construction. | BISAC: MEDICAL / Allied
   Health Services / Occupational Therapy.
Classification: LCC RM735 (ebook) | LCC RM735 .A635 2018 (print) | DDC
   615.8/515--dc23
LC record available at https://lccn.loc.gov/2018035903

Dedication

Dedicated to our families and friends, who have loved and supported us during this project, and to our clients, who provide inspiration and wisdom to expand our thinking and our practice and who challenge us to make a real difference in their lives. We would also like to dedicate this book to our colleagues who continue to embrace the complexities within the home environment to achieve quality outcomes for older people and people with disabilities.

CONTENTS

An Occupational Therapist's Guide to Home Modification Practice, Second Edition includes ancillary materials specifically available for faculty use. Please visit http://www.efacultylounge.com to obtain access.

ACKNOWLEDGMENTS

We would like to thank Brien Cummings and staff at SLACK Incorporated for providing us with the opportunity to showcase occupational therapy research and practice, and for supporting and promoting our work.

We are grateful for the generous support and assistance of the various knowledgeable writers and others who contributed to the first edition of the book, and to those who reviewed and contributed new material for this second edition.

We thank our clients and colleagues around the world who have read and used the first edition, and provided us with invaluable feedback to further refine the book.

We are indebted to our colleagues at The University of Queensland who have provided us with encouragement and support to continue refining the material gathered from our home modification research and practice.

Finally, we would like to thank our partners and families for providing us with support and encouragement as we have worked on this project for our profession and for older people and people with disabilities over the last decade.

ABOUT THE AUTHORS

Elizabeth Ainsworth, MOccThy, Grad Cert Health Sci graduated in 1989 with a bachelor of occupational therapy (honors) degree and completed a master's in occupational therapy (contemporary clinical practice at the University of Queensland) and a graduate certificate in health science (environmental modifications at the University of Sydney) in 2000. She is a private practice occupational therapist, accredited and qualified access consultant, and PhD candidate at The University of Queensland.

Elizabeth has had over 20 years' experience aiding older people and people with disabilities who require home modifications or alternative housing. She has a history of working in government and non-government agencies that assist people living in a range of housing tenures such as private and social housing and private rental accommodation. Elizabeth provides consultancy services to clients and their families, and to organizations, about housing and home modification solutions. She also completes medico legal work, providing information to the courts in Australia and overseas about the housing and home modification needs of people who have had complex or catastrophic injuries. She provides home modification and universal design education and training to occupational therapy university undergraduate and postgraduate students and to occupational therapy clinicians working in a range of settings in the community, both in Australia and overseas. She is a member of the Australian Network for Universal Housing Design (ANUHD), Universal Design Australia, the Australian Access Consultants Association (ACAA), the Australian Rehabilitation and Assistive Technology Association (ARATA), and Values in Action.

Desleigh de Jonge, MPhil (OccThy), Grad Cert Soc Sci graduated in 1978 with a bachelor of occupational therapy from The University of Queensland, completed a master's in philosophy in 2001, and is currently completing a PhD at this university. She has over 35 years' clinical experience as an occupational therapist and 12 years teaching and research at the School of Health and Rehabilitation Sciences at The University of Queensland, where she currently holds an honorary research title. Her teaching and research is focused on interventions and outcome measures that recognize client goals and priorities. Desleigh's national and international reputation in client-oriented analysis of assistive technologies, environmental design, and home modifications has earned her invitations to present at international conferences on assistive technology and home modification services and outcomes in the United States and Australia, and she has been published extensively in national and international journals. Desleigh was on the editorial board of *Disability and Rehabilitation: Assistive Technology* from 2006 to 2012 and regularly reviews articles for national and international journals.

Elizabeth and Desleigh have worked together for at least 18 years to provide training to occupational therapy students and practitioners. They have presented at national and international conferences on home modifications and universal design to a broad range of people from various backgrounds. The second edition of this book is testament to their dedication to equipping occupational therapists to achieve quality home modification outcomes for older people and people with disabilities internationally.

Contributing Authors

Tammy Aplin, PhD, BOccThy (Hons) (Chapters 1, 14)
Lecturer
Division of Occupational Therapy
School of Health and Rehabilitation Sciences
The University of Queensland
St Lucia, Brisbane, Queensland, Australia

*Kathleen Baigent, Dip COT, Dip Health Prom
   (Chapter 15)*
Occupational Therapist
Housing and Homelessness Services
Queensland Department of Housing and Public
   Works
Brisbane, Queensland, Australia

*Ruth Cordiner, Dip COT, Grad Cert Occ Thy
   (Chapter 15)*
Occupational Therapist
Housing and Homelessness Services
Queensland Department of Communities
Brisbane, Queensland, Australia

Shirley Darlison, BOccThy (Chapter 15)
Senior Occupational Therapist
Housing and Homelessness Services
Queensland Department of Housing and Public
   Works
Brisbane, Queensland, Australia

May Eade, BOccThy (Chapter 15)
Former Senior Occupational Therapist
Queensland Department of Housing and Public
   Works
Brisbane, Queensland, Australia

Louise Gustafsson, PhD, BOccThy (Hons) (Chapter 14)
Associate Professor
Division of Occupational Therapy
School of Health and Rehabilitation Sciences
The University of Queensland
St Lucia, Brisbane, Queensland, Australia

*Melanie Hoyle, BSc (Psych), MOccThySt, Grad Dip
   Health Sci, Post Grad Dip Psych (Chapters 6, 9,
   10, 13)*
Honorary Associate Lecturer/PhD Candidate
School of Health and Rehabilitation Sciences
The University of Queensland
St Lucia, Brisbane, Queensland, Australia

Andrew Jones, BA, MSW, GCE (Chapter 2)
Emeritus Professor
The University of Queensland
St Lucia, Brisbane, Queensland, Australia

*Barbara Kornblau, JD, OTR/L, FAOTA, FNAP, DASPE,
   CDMS, CCM, CPE (Chapter 12)*
Adjunct Professor
Florida Agricultural and Mechanical University
Tallahassee, Florida

Rhonda Phillips, MPhil, BA, Grad Dip (Chapter 2)
Adjunct Research Fellow
Institute of Social Science Research
The University of Queensland
St Lucia, Brisbane, Queensland, Australia

Jon Pynoos, MCP, PhD (Chapter 2)
UPS Foundation Professor of Gerontology, Policy
   and Planning
Andrus Gerontology Center
Director, National Resource Center on Supportive
   Housing and Home Modification
Co-Director, Fall Prevention Center of Excellence
University of Southern California
Los Angeles, California

Jon Sanford, MArch, BS (Chapter 4)
Professor, School of Industrial Design
Director, Center for Assistive Technology and
   Environmental Access (CATEA)
Georgia Institute of Technology
Atlanta, Georgia

*Bronwyn Tanner, BOccThy, Grad Cert Occ Thy, Grad
   Cert Soc Planning, MPhil (Chapters 1, 2, 11)*
College of Healthcare Sciences
James Cook University
Queensland, Australia

*Merrill Turpin, PhD, Grad Dip Counsel, BOccThy
   (Chapter 3)*
Senior Lecturer, Occupational Therapy
School of Health and Rehabilitation Sciences
The University of Queensland
St Lucia, Brisbane, Queensland, Australia

General Contributors to the Book

Catherine Bridge, PhD, Arch, BAppSc, MCogSci
Director, Home Modification Information Clearinghouse
Research Leader, Community Engagement CRC LCL—
  Faculty Leadership
Associate Dean of Research, ADR Unit
Architectural Studies
Architecture, Enabling Environments Program
Smart Cities
University of New South Wales
Sydney, Australia

Diane Bright, OTR, MSc ID
Director, Alliance Therapy/Access Answers
Troy, Michigan

Ben Burton, PG Dip Surv, LLB
idapt planner 3D (part of the idapt Group)
Bristol, England

Nigel Burton, CIOB, MAPM, MAPS, MCMI
idapt planner 3D (part of the idapt Group)
Bristol, England

Paul Coonan, BDesSt, BArch
Registered Architect (Queensland)
Director, Queensland Government Accommodation Office
Queensland Department of Housing and Public Works
Brisbane, Queensland, Australia

Richard Duncan, BA, MRP
Executive Director, Universal Design Institute
Better Living Design Institute
Asheville, North Carolina

Alan Healey, BOccThy
Occupational Therapist, Housing and Homelessness
  Services
Queensland Department of Housing and Public Works
Brisbane, Queensland, Australia

Mitch Hubbard, BOccThy
Director, OT Draw
Sales and Support
Insighted Pty Ltd
New South Wales, Australia

Rodney Hunter, FDip, Arch RMIT, Architect (Retired)
Managing Director, Rod A Hunter and Associates Pty
  Ltd
T/A Hunarch Consulting
Balwyn, Victoria, Australia

Rob Imrie
Visiting Professor
Goldsmiths, University of London
London, England

Richard Kirk, BDesSt, BArch
Registered Architect (Qld)
Director, Richard Kirk Architect
Brisbane, Queensland, Australia

Kate Kirkness BOccThy
Occupational Therapist
Scope Home Access
New England Region, New South Wales, Australia

Trish Lapsley, BOccThy
Private Practice Occupational Therapist
Brisbane, Queensland, Australia

Mary Law, PhD, FCAOT, FCAHS
Professor Emeritus, School of Rehabilitation Science
Co-Founder, CanChild Centre for Childhood Disability
  Research
McMaster University
Hamilton, Ontario, Canada

Danise Levine, March, AIA, CAPS
Architect and Assistant Director, IDeA Center
School of Architecture and Planning
University at Buffalo
Buffalo, New York

Rachel Russell, PhD
Occupational Therapist
Salford University
Salford, England

Dory Sabata, OTD, OTR/L, SCEM, FAOTA
Clinical Assistant Professor
University of Kansas Medical Centre
Department of Occupational Therapy Education
Kansas City, Kansas

John P. S. Salmen, FAIA, CAE
President of Universal Designers & Consultants, Inc.
Silver Spring, Maryland

Bevin Shard, Assoc Dip App Sc Building
Former Superintendent Representative in Queensland
  Government
Builder
North Ipswich, Queensland, Australia

Nicholas Smith,
Occupational Therapist
Housing and Homelessness Services
Queensland Department of Housing and Public Works
Brisbane, Queensland, Australia

Jonathan Ward, BDesSt
Architect
Australia

Amy Wagenfeld, PhD, OTR/L, SCEM, CAPS, FAOTA
Assistant Professor
Department of Occupational Therapy
Western Michigan University
Kalamazoo, Michigan

PREFACE

With the integration of people with disabilities into society, there has been increasing interest in modifying homes to enable them to live independently in the community. The aging population has also raised concerns about how well homes can support people's health and safety as they age. Occupational therapists have been identified as having the skills and knowledge to assess the modification needs of these clients, including consideration of their current and future requirements and the nature and use of the home environment. However, to be effective, therapists also need to understand the technical aspects of the built environment, design approaches, and the application of a range of products and finishes to determine appropriate modification solutions. This book aims to provide therapists with all the knowledge and skills they need to effectively provide home modification recommendations.

In this book, we use a transactional approach to examine the person-occupation-environment interaction and provide therapists with a detailed understanding of the various dimensions of the home environment that impact on home modification decisions. We also examine the context of home modification services and the impact of various demographic, legislative, policy, and service delivery traditions on the development and delivery of home modification services. In particular, we explore the roles and perspectives of each stakeholder in the home modification process, and we present a range of strategies to assist occupational therapists to achieve effective and positive service delivery outcomes. Additionally, we review the current legislative environment and the funding schemes that facilitate service delivery. We examine, in detail, the home modification process, including a review of approaches to evaluating, measuring, and drawing the environment; identifying and evaluating interventions; applying design standards; and reporting and legal issues. To assist the reader in identifying bases for evidence-based practice and topics for future research and theory development, we provide an overview of the literature on evaluating home modification outcomes and review the evidence for home modification interventions. The book concludes with a series of case studies that highlight the application of the home modification process in developing effective solutions for a range of client groups.

Our challenge in developing this text has been to provide a textbook that not only presents the theory relating to the person-occupation-environment transaction, but also one that provides therapists with the information they need to examine and influence this transaction. This knowledge has been acquired through years of extensive clinical, educational, and research experience in home modification practice and in training undergraduate, graduate, and postgraduate occupational therapy students as well as novice and experienced practitioners. This book provides us with an opportunity to share our expertise and years of experience of working with older people and people with disabilities to identify their home modification requirements. In addition, our experience as supervising practitioners working in the field has enabled us to identify the essential learning needs of occupational therapists providing home modification services. To date, the small amount of the literature in this field has been based solely on expert opinion. This book emerges from a solid theoretical foundation to provide practical real-life applications and strategies. It also provides a framework for examining the efficacy of home modification practice, shaping future research using evidence in practice.

Home modification practice is of interest in many countries around the world today. This book capitalizes on this international interest by focusing on the theory, knowledge, and skills that cross borders. People who require modifications to their homes face similar issues across the world. Similarly, occupational therapists worldwide are concerned with optimizing occupational performance and ensuring that people can live safely, independently, and comfortably in their own homes. This book seeks to address these universal issues while acknowledging the legislative and funding contexts that shape service delivery in respective countries.

We have written this book to meet the needs of students and clinicians from a range of settings. It is often challenging for students when translating general theoretical principles, which are outlined in generic occupational therapy texts, into practice. Particularly difficult is balancing the many complexities when working in the home environment—how to work collaboratively with the client to develop a mutually acceptable outcome and how to utilize scientific, narrative, pragmatic, ethical and interactive reasoning to develop an effective intervention. In this text, we discuss how to consider the physical, personal, social, temporal, occupational, and societal dimensions of the home in decision making and provide students with a systematic process for identifying and evaluating home-based interventions. The practical application of theory, legislation, and standards is a strong focus of the information presented and will equip student occupational therapists to work with people with a broad range of disabilities and to implement an occupational therapy process in the home environment. It takes them systematically through the process in a detailed and practical way, which is often not provided in generic occupational therapy texts. This book also supports students on clinical placement and those new graduates who find themselves in practice with foundation knowledge and skills but who are keen to acquire a deeper understanding of how to deal with the complexities they face in various settings. Although students are provided with an overview of knowledge required for practice during university training, it is not until they are faced with real-world practice situations that they understand the importance of the information presented in class and are ready to integrate the detail that is provided in this text.

This text also provides practitioners with tools and resources for home modification practice. We have provided several comprehensive case studies to assist novice therapists to understand the range of issues they need to consider conceptualizing solutions. For experienced therapists, we have provided theory and practical detail that draws on research and international literature to affirm and refine their practice. The depth of this book also supports practicing therapists by providing a rich and detailed description of the issues they encounter in day-to-day practice. It draws on the expertise of clinicians with extensive experience in providing interventions in the home and reviews international legislative and service systems, research, and literature to support practice. The text also encourages experienced therapists to develop structures to systematically gather information on the outcomes of home modification practice to ensure good outcomes for clients, to refine occupational therapy intervention, and to build a body of evidence to support this field of practice. This information will assist them in continuous improvement of service delivery and in advocating for the systemic change required to achieve good home modification outcomes for individuals, groups and populations.

This book provides a range of resources and tools, and it can be used as a teaching aid to support students, interns, and novice therapists or as a manual for more experienced home modification practitioners. The case studies also expose therapists to scenarios that they may not have encountered and broaden their knowledge base to inform future practice with a range of client groups. The book is unique in that it strongly focuses on the practical application of theory and research in day-to-day practice, working toward enabling people to stay in their homes and communities.

In identifying contributors for the book, one of our goals was to draw on the views of experts practicing in the field to bring a breadth of perspectives to the discussion about how to undertake home modification practice. Although occupational therapists might experience limitations in their home modification practice because of a lack of funding or the requirements of the service in which they work, we hope that the theory presented in this book will stimulate interesting and lively thinking and promote discussion about future research and practice in the field. An Instructor's Manual and a series of presentations, based on the content of this book, has been developed for use by students and clinicians to enable them to further reflect on and learn from their practice.

Home modification practice is a dynamic and evolving area of practice, and we see this book as a starting point for the future development of occupational therapy knowledge and skill. We welcome comments and contributions to further inform this area of practice.

Elizabeth Ainsworth, MOccThy, Grad Cert Health Sci
Desleigh de Jonge, MPhil (OccThy), Grad Cert Soc Sci

FOREWORD

As our population ages and the number of people with chronic disease and disability increases, the occupational therapist has a major role in creating livable environments that support the everyday lives of people and support those who provide care for individuals that have experienced occupational performance problems. We are very fortunate that the team of Elizabeth Ainsworth and Desleigh de Jonge have again joined forces to edit a second edition of *An Occupational Therapist's Guide to Home Modification Practice.*

All of us have created living environments that support our daily lives. Many people's lives have been interrupted by disease, trauma, or disability, and those interruptions need knowledgeable occupational therapists to help them develop strategies and alter their environments so they can care for themselves and engage with their friends and families, work, and engage in their communities.

This is the book that employs an occupational therapist's lens and very specific information to prepare the occupational therapist for assessing client and family needs to create the best possible environments to support independence and participation. The information in this book will be valuable to practitioners who need information to work with families prior to hospital or rehabilitation discharge. The depth of the book will prepare clinicians to work with architectural and engineering firms as a consultant to address the design issues that will support the needs of their client. The book will also prepare the practitioner who wants to work with community planners to work at a population level as more emphasis is placed on universal design and preparation for a normative environment for older adults who will need their mobility, sensory, and cognitive needs addressed without obvious alterations.

I am excited that knowledge is evolving in this area of occupational therapy practice that requires a second edition of the book. I want to repeat a reference and comment I made when I wrote the foreword for the first edition 8 years ago. Stegner (1992) asked us to consider space as a container of experiences and remind us that no space is a place until that which happens in it is remembered. Occupational therapists are the enablers that help clients maximize their experiences in their space to move in it, function in it, be safe in it, and, when there are problems, identify and remove barriers that compromise it.

The editors and authors of chapters in this book fit the qualifications of extreme excellence. When we look for guidance, we look to people with both knowledge and experience. Occupational therapists in Australia have worked for the Department of Housing serving the Queensland State Government for well over a decade. Many of them are the authors of chapters in this book. As more and more policy worldwide is focused on health, safety, and well-being, occupational therapists bring the unique perspective of fostering social participation to this initiative. Actually, occupational therapists are leaders in this work, and this book gives us the tools to lead in this movement.

Reference

Stegner, W. (1992). The sense of place. In W. Stegner (Ed.), *Where the bluebird sings to the lemonade springs* (pp. 199-206). New York, NY: Random House

Carolyn Baum, PhD, OTR/L, FAOTA
Elias Michael Director and Professor
Occupational Therapy, Neurology and Social Work
Program in Occupational Therapy
Washington University School of Medicine
St. Louis, Missouri

1

The Home Environment

Tammy Aplin, PhD, BOccThy (Hons) and
Bronwyn Tanner, BOccThy, Grad Cert Occ Thy, Grad Cert Soc Planning, MPhil

Occupational therapists play a key role in recommending modifications to the physical home environment, usually to enhance a person's occupational performance, health, safety, independence, and well-being. Yet as a profession, we have given little consideration to the meaning that this unique context has for our clients or to the impact that these changes may have on their experience of home. Drawing from recent occupational therapy literature and the disciplines of environmental psychology and gerontology, this chapter explores the nature of home and then presents a framework for considering the experience of home, describing the physical, personal, occupational, social, temporal, cultural, and societal dimensions that occur when one engages with or occupies the home environment. The relationship between a person and their dwelling is unique and complex, and it is important that therapists understand and acknowledge the nature of this relationship if they are to successfully negotiate changes.

CHAPTER OBJECTIVES

By the end of this chapter the reader will be able to:

+ Explain how home environments become places of significance and meaning

+ Describe the role of person-environment transactions in the creation of home as a place of being, doing, becoming, and belonging

+ Describe his or her own personal experience of home, including values and beliefs about home and how this may affect home assessments

+ Outline the various dimensions of the experience of home

+ Utilize these dimensions of experience when exploring client needs, concerns, and requests during the home modification process

+ Interpret how the experience of home may affect occupational therapy practice, in particular, decisions made about changes to the home environment

INTRODUCTION: DEFINING HOME

"The ache for home lives in all of us, the safe place where we can go as we are and not be questioned." Maya Angelou (1986).

Ainsworth, E., & de Jonge, D. *An Occupational Therapist's Guide to Home Modification Practice, Second Edition (pp. 1-15).*
© 2019 SLACK Incorporated.

The use of the word *home* in our general vocabulary is so commonplace and unconscious that it almost defies definition. In a sense, it is an archetype—a concept that seems to represent something universal to human nature, as indicated in the quote from Maya Angelou. For centuries poets and songwriters have utilized the nostalgic and emotional response that this one word evokes. If you were asked to write a list of words that reflected what "home" means to you, your response may include comfort, support, intimacy, belonging, family, and safety. Although many of us may have similar responses, the experience of home is a deeply personal experience and concept. "Home" is used to denote a range of places and meanings. It can evoke images of the home we currently live in, a childhood home, a hometown, or a home country.

Historically the concept of home has been widely researched, and a proliferation of writing exists within the areas of sociology, anthropology, psychology, human geography, architecture, and philosophy. The concept of home and its meaning in theoretical, social, and cultural contexts has also been the focus of several decades of research in the fields of environmental psychology and gerontology. Although there exists within the literature "pronounced conceptual and empirical diversity" about the meaning of home (Oswald & Wahl, 2005, p. 21), many researchers argue that, in essence, home is a relationship created between an individual and his or her environment in which the individual attaches psychological, social, and cultural significance and meaning to objects and spaces (Dovey, 1985; Hasselkus, 2011; Moore, 2000; Werner, Altman, & Oxley, 1985). In other words, when we talk about a "house" we are speaking of a dwelling place, but when we talk of "home" we are often speaking of a relationship between an individual and a setting (Felix, De Haan, Vaandrager, & Koelen, 2015). Rowles and Bernard (2013) emphasize this critical distinction between physical living spaces such as houses and apartments and home. They propose that a dwelling place is an empty space or location without meaning that only becomes a home when the space is claimed and afforded meaning by an individual or a group through habitation. It is this understanding of home that will be the focus of this chapter.

Home as Place

Within environmental psychology and gerontology literature, much of the writing about the concept of home is based on the premise that people live in worlds of meaning. An example of this is the idea of space and place. Space is a neutral physical dimension that lacks meaning, whereas places are spaces that have been shaped and transformed by human events and interaction into places of meaning (Hasselkus, 2011; Mayes, Cant & Clemson, 2011; Rowles & Bernard, 2013). Places hold the memories of personal experiences and have personal meaning in the context of ongoing life (Hasselkus, 2011; Rowles & Bernard, 2013). Throughout life, people interact with their social and physical environments and create "meaningful representations of the self within the environment" (Oswald & Wahl, 2005, p. 23). Frankel (1978, as cited in Hasselkus, 2011) suggested that the search for and creation of meaning is an essentially human characteristic. The meanings that individuals give to experiences and contexts are influenced by their own unique needs, goals, histories, and experiences, as well as shared social and cultural understandings and knowledge. In attributing such meaning, people make sense of their life experiences (Hasselkus, 2011; Rubinstein, 1989).

The creation of place as a context of personal meaning usually comes about through action. Rowles and Bernard (2013) outline three key elements in the process of transforming space into place. First, there is the use of an environment—usually through repeated patterns of habitual behavior, such as daily routines that make up everyday life. Through the repeated routine use of a physical space, people develop an intimacy with the physical aspects of the home environment—a "physical insideness" (Dovey, 1985, p. 362). Rowles and Bernard (2013) refer to this "insideness" as a cognitive awareness of the physical home environment, and this is the second element in the process of creating place. This "profound sense of familiarity" is often unconscious and only becomes apparent when threatened or destroyed (Dovey, 1985, p. 362). The final element in the process of place-making is the emotional attachment and sense of ownership that develop for the individual through the use and awareness of familiar and known spaces (Rowles & Bernard, 2013).

This transformation of space into place can occur across a range of frequently used settings such as a regular table in a frequented café or restaurant or a favorite chair in the local library. However, the home environment is likely to be the strongest experience of place as it involves an "intimate interweaving of person and location over time" (Rowles & Bernard, 2013, p. 11). For many people, the creation of home and emotional attachment to a dwelling occur because of some action on the physical environment, such as personalizing a space by putting up objects of personal value, or creating new spaces, such as a garden. In acting on the environment, a person establishes a history of being "in place" and spaces take on a significance that they previously did not have for the individual. Home, as a relationship, is created through the transactions that occur between individuals and the environment where action results in the creation of meaning (Dovey, 1985). This idea of acting on and being acted upon is at the heart of a transactional approach to people and environments.

Person-Environment Transactions: The Heart of Home

A transactional view of people and their contexts has been explored by philosophers such as John Dewey (Bunting, 2016) and was adopted by environmental psychologists to explain the relationship between people and their contexts. As outlined in environmental psychology, a transactional approach interprets the interaction between a person and their environment or context as something that is dynamic and always changing. The person and context can only be understood when examined together as a unified system (Werner et al., 1985). Trying to gain knowledge or understanding about the person as separate from the context in which they live and act is a meaningless exercise because the two elements (person and context) are interwoven and interdependent (Altmann, Brown, Staples, & Werner, 1992). Within a transactional approach, the term *context* refers to much more than just the physical surroundings and encompasses personal, social, cultural, and political aspects.

To illustrate this, consider the case of an older woman in a hospital who is being considered for discharge to her home following a stroke. In therapy, she can manage three to four steps easily with the assistance of one person. A pre-discharge visit to the home reveals an entrance with two to three steps. As part of her discharge plan, education is provided to her husband regarding how to aid her when using steps in the hospital. Based on her performance in the hospital, she is deemed to be safe to manage the steps at home and is discharged. When the community health team visits a few weeks after discharge, however, they find that she has not been able to leave the house, as she is unable to use the two to three steps. Why is her performance at home different from what she was doing in the hospital? She has not deteriorated physically, but the context has changed. In the first place, the steps of her home have a slightly higher rise than those in the hospital, creating a greater level of difficulty. This, however, was not the only reason. In the hospital, she was either assisted or supervised by a trained aide or therapist who provided her with encouragement and confidence when undertaking the task of climbing stairs. In her home context, her husband did not feel

comfortable assisting her, partly because of a lack of experience but also because assisting his wife was not in line with his cultural expectations. Both husband and wife came from a cultural background where the wife was the one who gave assistance, and this had been her role up until her stroke. He therefore was neither comfortable nor willing to take on the role of her assistant, and she was unable to use the steps without his help. The approach taken in discharging this woman was to assume that her performance (managing two to three stairs) in the hospital would be the same in the home context. A transactional approach would not assume that a person's performance or behavior would be the same if the environment or context changed. A different context is highly likely to result in a different outcome as the nature of person-environment transactions are dynamic and interdependent.

In addition to seeing people and contexts as interrelated and interwoven, a key defining feature of a transactional perspective is the realization that person-environment transactions are both observable and unobservable. Transactions occur at the level of observable actions (activities, tasks, routines, rituals) and through unobservable psychosocial processes by which people evaluate, interpret, and ascribe meaning to their experiences (Werner et al., 1985).

This understanding of person-environment transactions has formed the basis of many occupational therapy frameworks that focus on occupational performance such as the Person-Environment-Occupational Model (Law et al., 1996), the Model of Human Occupation (Keilhofner, 2002), the Ecological Model of Occupation (Dunn, Brown, & Youngstrom, 2003), the Person-Environment Occupational Performance Model (Baum, Christiansen, & Bass, 2015), and the Canadian Model of Occupational Performance and Engagement (Polatajko, Townsend, & Craik, 2007; Polatajko et al., 2013). Although these frameworks acknowledge the dynamic nature of person-context interactions as well as the "subjective (emotional or psychological) and objective (physically observable) aspects of performance" (American Occupational Therapy Association, 2008, p. 628), in day-to-day practice, occupational therapists are often so focused on the observable, measurable aspects of people acting in their environments that they are at risk of giving little consideration to the unobservable meaning-making processes that occur within the home context.

The focus on observable activity is historically embedded within the occupational therapy profession (Hasselkus, 2011). Although finding a universally agreed definition is difficult, occupation has often been "categorized as everything people do to occupy themselves, including looking after themselves (self-care), enjoying life (leisure), and contributing to the social and economic fabric of their communities (productivity)" (Canadian Association of Occupational Therapy, 2002, p. 34). This focus on "doing" has been "inadequate to address issues of meaning in people's lives" (Hammel, 2004, p. 296), and recent theorists have challenged traditional understandings of occupation.

Occupation: Doing, Being, Belonging, Becoming

Wilcock and Hocking (2015) present a conceptual model of occupation in relation to health comprising four elements: doing, being, belonging, and becoming. *Doing* relates to the observable elements of occupation and is a central and familiar aspect of our professional practice (Hitch, Peppin, & Stagnitti, 2014). *Being* is the sense of personal existence, supported by beliefs and values. It is the personal aspect of occupation and is often experienced as a quiet time of thinking and reflection (Wilcock & Hocking, 2015). Although linked to doing, being can be independent of occupational engagement, a time to sit with emotions or simply exist (Hitch et al., 2014). *Belonging* pertains to the social aspects of occupation—being a part of groups, communities, and places. It relates to the idea of being a part of something bigger than oneself, of friendship, affirmation, and mutual support (Hitch et al., 2014). *Becoming* relates to the notions of change, development, and transformation over time. For some people (e.g., those with a chronic illness) becoming may not always mean improvement; it can also mean maintaining or even managing over time as a condition progresses.

Although only briefly outlined here, this view of occupation aligns well with the perspective that views transactions as both observable and unobservable meaning-making processes. As occupational therapists, we observe and assess the day-to-day routines and habits that people "do" as part of their daily occupations in their home environments. It is important to realize that even the most mundane "doing" has elements of "being." How we structure our daily routines—the way we make the bed, clean our teeth, when we shower—all have some connection to our sense of who we are, or the "being" side of occupation. Even small changes to these elements of "doing" can dramatically affect "being," "belonging," and even "becoming."

Within the context of home, a focus on the observable, doing elements of person-environment transactions alone can significantly affect the relationship that exists between a person and his or her home and can detract from the meaning of home to an individual (Aplin, de Jonge, & Gustafsson, 2015; Hawkins & Stewart, 2002; Heywood, 2005; Tanner, Tilse, & de Jonge, 2008). It is therefore essential that occupational therapists working within the home environment and those engaged in recommending alterations to that environment understand the place that is home and the possible impact that they may have on this domain of significant personal meaning.

UNDERSTANDING THE EXPERIENCE OF HOME: THE DIMENSIONS OF THE HOME FRAMEWORK

For many occupational therapists, their place of work and the focus of their intervention is the client's home environment. This is particularly true of therapists working in the field of home modifications; however, to date, there has been limited information in our professional literature about this particular context and the impact our interventions have on a person's experience of his or her home environment. When the home environment has been examined, researchers have referred to the experience of home as occurring across various domains (Hayward, 1975; Sixsmith, 1986; Smith, 1994). Recent work, involving a review of the literature base, and a substantive qualitative study aimed to build upon this earlier work to provide a comprehensive framework for understanding the experience of home. The physical, personal, social, temporal, occupational, and societal dimensions were identified to contribute to the experience of home (Figure 1-1; Aplin, de Jonge & Gustafsson, 2013, 2015). The physical, personal, and social dimensions were previously well-established core dimensions of the home environment (Oswald & Wahl, 2005; Sixsmith, 1986; Tanner et al., 2008). The temporal and occupational dimensions, although not as well described, were also previously defined in occupational therapy, architecture, gerontology and environmental psychology literature as contributing to the experience of home (de Jonge, Jones, Phillips, & Chung, 2011; Despres, 1991; Haak, Dahlin-Ivanoff, Fänge, Sixsmith, & Iwarsson, 2007; Hayward, 1977; Sixsmith, 1986; Tanner et al., 2008). The societal dimension had not been previously clearly described in the literature. This dimension acknowledges the macro environment and its influence on the meaning of home (Aplin et al., 2015) and is a context that the literature had previously been critiqued for its bias in ignoring (Despres, 1991).

Figure 1-1. Six dimensions of home.

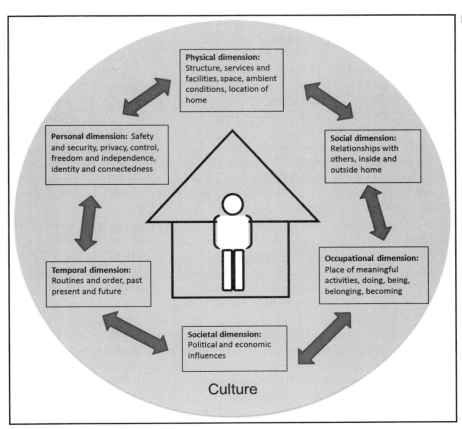

The Dimensions of Home Framework was developed to provide a way to understand each person's unique experience of home and the various dimensions that contribute to this experience. It seeks to make explicit the various aspects of person-environment transactions by describing unobservable as well as observable aspects of the home environment so that therapists might develop a deeper understanding of each client's unique and personal experience of home. The relative importance of each of these dimensions will differ from individual to individual and is influenced by the cultural context. Individual priorities will also change over time as life circumstance, values, and roles change. When considering the experience of home for our clients, it is important to understand the dimensions of home that are most important now, how this might change in the future, and what compromises and trade-offs are acceptable.

The Physical Dimension

The physical home is concerned with the idea of real space—the raw material from which the dweller builds a home. Professional education and training alert occupational therapists to the physical environment, and it is therefore the dimension with which occupational therapists are most familiar. Literature outside of occupational therapy, from gerontology and psychology examining the home environment and its meaning, also identify the physical dimension as important in understanding the experience of home (Despres, 1991; Oswald & Wahl, 2005; Sixsmith, 1986; Smith, 1994).

The interconnected nature of the dimensions of home is demonstrated by the physical dimension, as it both influences and is influenced by the other dimensions. Consider the changes that people might make to their home, such as a new kitchen, an extra bedroom, or a deck or patio. While these are physical changes, the motivations for and the considerations required when making these changes reflect the wider dimensions. The addition of another room, for example, may be important to create a study area (occupational dimension) or a room for friends and family to be able to stay overnight (social dimension). A deck may be added to provide an entertaining area to socialize (social dimension).

The importance of the physical dimension and its influence on the experience of home is illustrated by the fact that when people describe negative experiences of home, it is most commonly in relation to the physical aspects (Smith, 1994). To illustrate this, consider the case of Janice. Janice lived in a small social housing studio unit and had previously been close to homelessness. Her experience of her current home, however, was one of discomfort that affected her well-being. The small space meant she was unable to have friends or family over for dinner and unable to have her granddaughter visit and stay overnight. These were dearly missed occupations. At times, she found the ambience of the house unbearable. She felt closeted in the small space. It was dark, and the smell of cigarette smoke had seeped into the brick walls from a previous tenant, affecting her sleep. She described her home as a "big dark coffin." Janice's story demonstrates that the physical aspects of home are powerful, influencing our day-to-day comfort and well-being. Most people are aware of this impact, as evidenced by the simple changes many of us make to our homes, such as painting a room, adding new furniture, tidying up, or adding a garden, which often enhances our experience of home.

The physical dimension has been conceptualized as having four elements (Aplin et al., 2013, 2015). These are (1) the structure, services, and facilities; (2) space; (3) ambient conditions; and (4) the location of home.

Structure, Services, and Facilities

The structure of the home refers to the raw structural elements such as the roof, floor, and walls, and the materials and finishes such as flooring and paint. This element of the physical dimension also includes the fittings and fixtures such as taps, sinks, and cupboards (de Jonge, 2011; Sanford & Bruce, 2010). The services and facilities of home include those that make the home comfortable and usable, such as wiring, plumbing, air conditioning, and ventilation (de Jonge, 2011). Other examples of services and facilities include internet access, rubbish removal, and sewage. Seemingly "nonessential" features might include a pool or smart technology features such as automated lights, doors, and blinds.

Space

The space in and around the home influences what we do and our comfort at home. If you have ever lived in a small home with many people, you will know that it can be difficult to find a quiet or private space. The amount of space is determined by the layout and orientation of structures and furniture within the home (Hayward, 1975; Sanford & Bruce, 2010). For example, a room with windows and doors on every wall affects the usability of the space, making it difficult to fit in all the furniture. Our need for space changes over time. The space required for a single person compared to couple or a family of five or six is different. This need for more or less space is often a driving factor in relocating.

For example, a larger home is needed when a family grows or a smaller home is needed when older adults are wanting to downsize.

Storage space is another important factor. A lack of storage space often means the usable space in rooms and walkways is reduced to accommodate extra pieces of furniture, equipment, and belongings. Storage space can often be overlooked when considering renovation or modification. Yet, for many people, it is critical, as insufficient storage space often results in clutter that affects the experience of home and subjective well-being (Roster, Ferrari, & Jurkat, 2016).

The space needed to store and maneuver equipment can require significant modification and frequently makes relocating necessary. This is often the case for families of children with disabilities, who speak of the arduous decision of whether to modify their existing home or move to something more accessible. If they choose to modify, however, the enhanced space can make important changes to daily life in the home, enabling freedom of movement, enhancing privacy, or facilitating relationships that may have been harmed by a lack of space (Heywood, 2005).

Ambient Conditions

The ambient conditions include those aspects of the home that can bring comfort and enjoyment, creating our favorite places where we sit in the morning sun or enjoy the view out of a window. Occupations like these of rest and relaxation in an enjoyed place reflect the "being" aspects of occupation that are important in creating a positive experience of home. Ambient conditions include lighting, airflow and breezes, shade, a view, sound, and the weather or the climatic impact on the temperature and comfort of the home (Aplin et al., 2013; Sanford & Bruce, 2010). In the earlier description of Janice's experience of home, her poor experience was in part due to the darkness and smell of her home. For a number of people, noise can also be a significant barrier to their enjoyment of home, such as noise from a busy road. The significance of the ambient aspects of our homes is often highlighted only when they are lost or negatively experienced. Before I moved into my current home, I lived in a unit that overlooked a vacant large block of land. My view was of trees and birdlife. While I was living there, it was cleared for a unit development. I had not realized how much I enjoyed my view until it was gone. My view was replaced with overcrowded back decks used to store items such as washing lines, bikes, and boxes that did not fit into the small flats. The sounds also changed, from birds and running water to the private conversations of neighbors, children, and cars.

Location of Home

The location of home relates to its position within the neighborhood, in the street, and on the site. Location is a particularly important physical aspect of home and is often a key priority when we are looking to rent or purchase an existing home or build a new home. Location considerations such as the climate; the topography or lay of the land; and the proximity to family, friends, local services and facilities such as shops, doctors, recreational activities, and transport contribute to our quality of life (Dahlin-Ivanoff, Haak, Fänge, & Iwarsson, 2007; Despres, 1991). Where we live with regard to the climate influences our day-to-day activities and the design, services, and facilities in our homes. When living in a cold climate, heating and insulation are a priority. In warmer climates, ventilation and air conditioning are important, along with outdoor living spaces for socializing. The topography of the area may also influence the activities that can be undertaken. For example, older adults who live in hilly areas may experience limitations to participation if they are unable to walk to the local shop, doctor, or bus stop. Consider the significant impact location would have on your daily life if you had no control or choice over where you lived. In a research interview, Joan and Greg expressed their disappointment over the location of their dwelling. As social housing tenants, they were given little choice in their location, and their house was a great distance from their family and grandchildren whom they had been supporting and visiting regularly prior to the move. The move to a new location resulted in a loss of important social roles and reduced family engagement.

The Personal Dimension

The personal dimension assumes an emotionally based, meaningful relationship exists between an individual and his or her dwelling place (Dovey, 1985; Moore, 2000). This dimension captures those aspects that transform a physical dwelling place into a home where we experience security, comfort, and a place to belong. Our emotional relationship with home is complex, individual, and linked to our history and values. Four aspects to the personal dimension of home have been identified in the literature and home modification research, including (1) safety and security; (2) privacy; (3) control, freedom, and independence; and (4) identity and connectedness (Aplin et al., 2013).

Safety and Security

Home should be where we feel most safe; it is a haven from the outside world, a place of security and comfort. For this "safe haven" to exist, a place for retreat, refreshment, and relaxation, we must have control over the home to keep intrusions from the public or "outside" separate to the private or "inside" domain. Our sense of safety and security at home is both physical and emotional. The physical aspects, which contribute to the sense of safety and security, include the physical structure of the home, the functionality and ease of use of the home amenities, and living in a familiar neighborhood with help at hand if needed (Dahlin-Ivanoff et al., 2007; Smith, 1994). For example, some people feel more secure or safe in a brick home compared to a timber home. For others, having security screens and being high off the ground can feel safer. The presence of supportive neighbors, or having neighbors who will "keep an eye on things," can also make a big difference to how secure we feel in our home and neighborhood.

Emotionally, feeling secure in our home is associated with the sense of permanence and familiarity that home can bring (Dahlin-Ivanoff et al., 2007; Sebba & Churchman, 1986; Sixsmith, 1986). Home ownership is a goal for many and reflects the sense of security that comes from having a permanent home—a home that you have control over and where you can make plans for the future. In contrast, many people who rent experience poor security of tenure, requiring them to move if the owner chooses to sell, for example. This lack of secure tenure is recognized as a cause of stress and threat to a renter's well-being (Lewis, 2006).

Continuity and the memories associated with the home are also important in contributing to the sense of security (Dahlin-Ivanoff et al., 2007; Sebba & Churman, 1986; Smith, 1994). Living in one place for many years, feeling a part of the place, and growing old in one place create security and comfort in daily life. Compare this to when you move to a new location, the sense of familiarity and security can be initially lost and daily stress might increase due to the simple things being difficult (e.g., not knowing how to get to the local shop or how to use public transport).

Privacy

Privacy has been described as having an important contribution to the experience of home (Smith, 1994; Tognali, 1987; Zingmark, Norberg & Sandman, 1995). Home is our most private space, and it is only when we are able to control the access of others, our social interactions, and space that privacy is afforded to us (Gifford, 2002). In our homes, there are both public and private spaces, which can differ for each household and different family members (Sebba & Churchman, 1986). For example, the bathroom may be a shared space, but private for all at certain times.

In some households, bedrooms are private for parents and caregivers but not for children.

The significance of privacy within the home is most strongly felt when it is not present, with negative experiences of home associated with a lack of privacy and freedom (Smith, 1994). These include, for example, a lack of control over social interactions, having intrusive flat mates or guests, lacking a space of one's own, or lacking privacy from the street (Smith, 1994). These experiences are common and illustrate the importance of privacy to achieve a positive experience of home. For adults receiving formal caregiver support in the home, privacy can often be lost, with the home no longer being a private space, but a workplace for staff (Lund & Nygard, 2004). There may be a loss of control over not only who is in the home, but also the control of private spaces and activities, such as bathing and toileting. The impact of support workers on the experience of home can be dramatic. Craig and Susan's experience reflects this. They were a couple who lived together and had daily paid workers coming into their home to assist Craig with his self-care activities. They described their experience of having paid support workers in the home as feeling like their home had been invaded. They felt their home had become institutionalized and their privacy was continually compromised by the presence of support workers. Additionally, workplace health and safety requirements of the service provider had reduced Craig's independence, requiring him to use more equipment. Overall, Craig felt as though his home had become more of a workplace than a home. Craig and Susan's story demonstrates the significance of privacy in the home, as their loss of privacy and control significantly altered their relationship with their home. This loss was keenly felt by Craig, who had lived in his home for over 18 years and which had previously been a symbol of his independence.

Control, Freedom, and Independence

Privacy is closely linked to our sense of control and freedom at home, as we need control to have the privacy we desire (Gifford, 2002). As a refuge from the outside world, our home is where we should have control and independence, free to make our own choices and actions (Despres, 1991). Control has been described as an important aspect of the experience of home (Oswald and Wahl, 2005; Sixsmith, 1986; Tanner et al., 2008). It is central to our experience, as control over our home and access to ourselves creates privacy, facilitates a sense of security, permits routines and order to develop, and allows us to personalize and create a home that is our own (Despres, 1991; Smith, 1994; Zingmark et al., 1995). For many, the first move out of the family home into your own home brings a sense of control and freedom. You have far greater control and choice over your daily routines, such as when you have dinner, what you eat, and who you invite into your home. You are able to choose your own furniture and decorate and use your home space as you choose. Having a space that you can truly make your own, a place for yourself, is a freedom that many are unable to obtain.

For both older adults and people with a disability, home can facilitate independence by providing control over what they do and when they want to do it (de Jonge et al., 2011; Heywood, 2005). It is this presence of control that distinguishes home from other living situations, specifically institutions. Loss of control is what people most fear about living in an institution. In considering the experience of living in an aged care facility for example, control over many aspects of life is lost. The choice of location may be limited, and you may be required to move to an area not familiar to you. You usually can only bring limited personal items and have limited choice in the setup of the room, furniture, or style. It is likely that you will have no choice over your neighbors or roommates, or even who sits with you at dinner. Your daily routine is usually structured by others, including when you shower, when and what you eat, and when you can have visitors. Your activity and mood are recorded, and your life becomes medicalized and monitored. This loss of control in such an institutional setting is in sharp contrast to what most of us experience in our home environment and highlights the important role that control plays in our experience of home.

Identity and Connectedness

Home as a place of identity and connection is the most personal aspect of home as it is associated with our sense of self. There is a deepening relationship with home that begins with how we personalize our homes through self-expression and extends to the deeper connections of identity and belonging. We express our style, interests, and values through our home; it is a reflection of how we want to see ourselves and how we want others to see us (Despres, 1991; Hayward, 1977; Sixsmith, 1986). Our identity is often reflected in how we decorate and organize our homes. When we first move into a home, we organize our personal items, decorate, paint, or renovate. It is through this process of self-expression that the physical space of a house or apartment begins to become a home (Tognali, 1987). Home as a place of identity represents who we are and is an extension or embodiment of ourselves (Hayward, 1975, 1977;

Sixsmith, 1986). This identity is not only associated with the physical home and its reflection of our values and style, but also our routines and the history and memories associated with home (Sixsmith, 1986).

Our home connects us to our past. When memories are found in each room and on each corner of the neighborhood, we form an emotional attachment to our home, and our sense of identity becomes connected to place, particularly if we have lived there for some time (Dovey, 1985). This identification with place over time is particularly important for older adults. Rowles (1983) describes this identity connected to place as "autobiographical insideness," or "being a part of the places of one's life and of the places being a part of oneself" (Rowles, 2000, p. 531).

The connection we feel to our homes is also related to the sense of rootedness and continuity of home (Hayward, 1975, 1977; Heywood, 2005; Oswald & Wahl, 2005; Smith, 1994; Tognali, 1987; Zingmark et al., 1995). Having control over one's home, a sense of ownership and permanency, and of knowing it is your place in the world leads to continuity (Hayward, 1977). It is only over time that this sense of continuity and rootedness, where home is the center point for life and a place to return to, can develop (Despres, 1991). Home can therefore lead to a strong sense of belonging. The story of my grandfather illustrates this deep connection to home. He lived and worked on the family farm his entire life. He watched his children and grandchildren play in the same places where he grew up. His connection to place extended to the local town, where he had a house to be close to services when his wife was unwell. This deep sense of rootedness to place appeared to create a contentedness in life, the sense of knowing oneself in the world. There was no uncertainty of where to be or what to do, he was sure of who he was and where he belonged. He was grounded and demonstrated a confidence and calmness in life from his connection to place.

The introduction of modifications or equipment can be challenging for many reasons, but some of the key concerns can be associated with identity and connection to home. Changes to the home may be affronting because they look "clinical" or "disabled" for example, and this is not how the person sees him- or herself. There can also be important connections and memories associated with furniture, objects, and the design or fixtures and fittings in a room that may lead people to be resistant to suggested changes. For example, a colleague told the story of an older client who needed access to her home. The most important consideration for the client was that the front steps were not altered. Her father had built the stairs and, because of this, they retained strong personal meaning. These concerns related to aspects of the personal dimension can be difficult for people to articulate and reflect those unobservable meaningful aspects of home. It is important that we consider these unobservable aspects when gathering information about the home and in discussions about recommendations as modifications can change these deeply personal aspects that contribute to the experience of home.

The Social Dimension

The social dimension refers to the emotional environment created by relationships with others. First of all, the social home involves those relationships most significant to the individual, such as a spouse or family who may live in the same dwelling. The social dimension also expands beyond this to include those who enter or occasionally may influence the home, such as relatives, neighbors, friends, and community networks. These relationships and connections within the home are central to the meaning of home (Despres, 1991; Hayward, 1977).

Home is often described as the center of family life, a place where children grow, learn, and explore (Somerville, 1997). The childhood home can be a place with strong emotional connections (Mallet, 2004). The social dimension recognizes that home is often where our closest relationships occur. It is the place where these relationships are strengthened and developed, with feelings of love, caring, and intimacy associated with home (Despres, 1991; Hayward, 1977). In our homes, we spend time with family and pets and entertain and socialize with friends. The importance of good social relationships, both within and external to the home, is highlighted when there are negative relationships at home. This can create an atmosphere of unease, where the home is no longer the warm and comfortable place one expects (Sixsmith, 1986).

For older adults, living close to friends, helpful neighbors, and family is important for a positive experience of home (de Jonge et al., 2011). For many people, being close to others, especially those who are important in their lives, and fulfilling valued social roles are reasons they stay in their home. Consequently, it can be the most important aspect of home for older adults (Tanner, 2011). An example of this is Betty, reported by Tanner and colleagues (2008). Betty was in her late 60s and lived in a larger, older house. She had great difficulty accessing her home environment, including the front steps and bathroom. Minor modifications had been made; however, due to her functional limitations, she was unable to properly access the bath area and washed using a basin. When offered new accommodation that was fully accessible within the same suburb less than 1 km away from her current home, she chose to remain in an inconvenient and ill-suited physical dwelling. The reason for this was to maintain her ongoing involvement with the local children who gathered in her front yard each morning to get on the school bus. As she said,

> By them (the children) being here the bus comes along up the road here, they walk across to catch it and I know they're safe … It makes you feel you're doing something even though I'm not really doing anything … to most of the neighborhood children, I'm Nana. It doesn't matter whether they are related or not. I'm Nana. Even the 18- and 19-year-olds still refer to me as Nana. I've got a very large family! (Tanner et al., 2008, p. 203)

This valued social role and important social network would have been lost by the move because the new accommodation was not on the school bus route (Tanner et al., 2008). This type of social relationship and connection with others is an integral part of the experience of home, particularly as one ages. Being able to contribute and do things for others has been found to be important in strengthening personal identity and the sense of being a valued part of society (Haak et al., 2007). An absence of relationships with others, however, can result in loneliness and isolation for older people, and home can be experienced as "a prison" (Haak et al., 2007, p. 99). Thus, the location of home with regard to its ability to facilitate and sustain social networks and support valued social roles is an important aspect of the social dimension and consideration for occupational therapists. It is these meaningful aspects of the social dimension of home—having family close, grandchildren being able to visit, being able to provide care for others, and being able to pop in to see a neighbor for a cup of tea and chat—that are essential to the meaning of home for many and contribute to the sense of belonging.

The Temporal Dimension

The temporal dimension highlights the dynamic and changing nature of home, where occupants' needs and wants change over time. There are both cyclical and linear aspects to the temporal dimension of home (Werner et al., 1985). The cyclical nature of home describes the familiarity, routines, and order of home, whereas the linear aspects refer to home in the past, present, and future.

Home as Routine and Order

The home moves through daily, weekly, and annually occurring events and activities. These routines of life and the order of our homes are personal and have cultural and social influences (Dovey, 1985). With these unique influences, each home has its own order and routine, developed from childhood, and changing over time as circumstances and preferences change. This influences the placement, storage, and use of household goods and furniture and the activities that occur in our homes. For example, cooking may occur indoors or outdoors; food may be eaten at the table or on the couch. Further, the routines of home life prescribe the timing and responsibility of household chores and unique family traditions, such as Christmas, Sunday morning breakfasts, and birthdays, which can be markedly different across households. These everyday routines and order of life are most markedly noticed when a change occurs, such as a new resident in the house or physical changes to the home as a result of renovations or a home modification. For some, particularly older adults who have lived in their home for decades, the idea of changing a bath to a level access shower, moving a piece of furniture, or moving to a different bedroom would be unthinkable. So strong is their sense of order and familiarity with what is in place that they often cannot explain why the suggestion is a problem, just that this is the way things have always been and should not change. There is a comfort in familiarity, and when these familiar aspects of the home are combined with an enjoyed ambience and aesthetic, they can have even more significance, making change more difficult.

This order to home or the familiarity with the home environment was described by Rowles (1983) as *physical insideness*, where habitual routines and a familiarity with the home develop over time. This explains how a home environment, which may seem unsafe, is easily navigated and compensated for by older people. Knowing the home environment inside and out is also described by Rubinstein's (1989) first aspect of a person-centered process: accounting. This physical order of home, as known only by its occupants, is how people can navigate in the dark and know where those little-used items are, such as a flashlight or spare light bulbs.

Sociocultural influences affect the routines and order of everyday life. For example, traditionally in Western cultures, men of the household performed outdoor household chores such as mowing and repairs, whereas women undertook cleaning and cooking. There can also be shared norms and social roles within a neighborhood or community. For example, within a neighborhood, there may be shared expectations about garden maintenance or the appearance of homes. These routines and order develop over time and therefore can have more significance to older adults, who have a stronger attachment to homes they have lived in for some time (Rowles, 1983).

Home as the Past, Present, and Future

Home is not static but rather constantly adapting with the changing needs and preferences of its occupants, as well as external societal influences. Sixsmith (1986) described the home as occurring within a temporal framework, where the meaning and needs of home change through different stages of life, such as childhood, early adulthood, having a family of one's own, and retirement. This can sometimes mean a change in home, such as relocating to a larger home when having more children or downsizing in later life. Sometimes this can be outside of our control. We may need to move for work or to provide support for a family member. For many older adults and people with a disability, this may be a decision that is forced upon them due to the poor accessibility of their home, a lack of housing, or support services being close by.

The temporal nature of home is closely related to the personal dimension, providing a connection to the past through history and memories (Dovey, 1985). The past events of home provide the story of the home, the significance of objects, features, and places within the home that are often invisible to the visitor. The future is also an important consideration as we often imagine future possibilities through the lens of our homes or where and how we are living (Dovey, 1985). Our future plans often include improvements to the home or a move to a new home. For example, we may move to be closer to friends or family, to have more space, or to live at the beach or in the country. In these moves, we aim to facilitate a more positive experience of home.

The Occupational Dimension

The occupational dimension recognizes the home as a place of doing, where many of the everyday activities of life occur and where some of our most meaningful occupations take place. Literature outside and within occupational therapy highlights the significance of occupation to home and the importance of activities performed within the home contributing to the meaning and value of life at home and "being" in the home (Rowles, 1991). Home has been described as a "center" or "base" of activities supporting work, hobbies, leisure, eating, sleeping, and recreation (Despres, 1991; Hayward, 1977).

In occupational therapy literature, the relationship between occupation and home has been examined closely, with home being identified as a place for valued and meaningful occupations (de Jonge et al., 2011; Haak et al., 2007; Heywood, 2005). When we first consider the home from the perspective of "doing," we can understand the home as a hub of activity. It is where the day-to-day "doing" of our life occurs, such as getting ready for work or school, making meals, cleaning, gardening, relaxation, and rest. This "doing" of the everyday activities of life (e.g., moving from room to room, getting in and out of the house, making a meal, using the toilet and shower, and taking out the trash) should be easily completed without hassle, fear, or frustration. When the "doing" at home is easy, the home is a place of comfort and ease. It is often when we experience difficulties that the value of this dimension of home is highlighted. When a home is being renovated, for example, there is often mud and dirt in the yard, and planks of timber may be put down so you can access the house. A camping kitchen may be set up, and a family of four uses the en suite bathroom while the main bathroom is not available. "Doing" in this environment becomes stressful, may create tension in a family, and may negatively affect the comfort and well-being of those living in the home.

Home modifications have been reported to positively affect the ease of "doing" within the home environment for older adults, people with a disability, and their family members (Aplin et al., 2015). The value of this ease to everyday life cannot be underestimated as difficulty in daily activity can create a negative experience of home and affect important aspects of "being." Consider the story of Bec. Bec lives in a home with her two adult children. She had an above-knee amputation and mainly used a wheelchair for mobility rather than her prosthesis. Her home had three steps, and her children had built her a homemade ramp over the steps. Using this ramp was difficult because it was not fixed, and Bec required the assistance of both her children when using it to leave the house. Because of this difficulty, Bec rarely left her house, mostly staying indoors. Bec spoke of missing the simple enjoyment of sitting in the garden, which was her favorite place to spend time and reflect. Because of the difficulty in daily "doing," Bec missed the opportunity to just "be" in her favorite part of her home. Bec's story reflects the importance of both "doing" and "being" and demonstrates that, although being able to do activities in and around the home is important, feeling "at home" or simply "being" at home is equally valuable.

The activities performed within the home are unique and personal and contribute to a sense of "being." Whether sitting in the garden, reading a book in a favorite room, or reflecting on life as you hang out the washing in the sun, everyone seeks to find a place of reflection or to simply be with oneself. These activities are key to creating meaning and connection and enriching our home life, which contribute to our sense of well-being.

We engage in some of our most enjoyable and valued occupations at home. Leisure activities, hobbies, or activities that are important to our well-being and valued roles contribute to our sense of self as we fulfill and experience our identity (Christiansen, 1999). The story of Andrew reflects the need for our homes to enable these meaningful occupations. Andrew worked in music production and used his home as his office with clients frequently visiting. Andrew's bathroom housed a range of mobility and transfer equipment, which he felt identified him as having a disability and did not reflect his identity as a professional. He modified his home to have an additional accessible en suite bathroom that was able to house his equipment, leaving a bathroom for the use of his clients that was free of disability-related clutter.

Occupations also provide a means by which we engage with others within the home (e.g., preparing food and eating together), or even being a contributing member of the household through tidying up, taking the bins out, and working in the garden. These activities build relationships and connections with others at home and create a sense of belonging. People with a disability, who are often unable to access spaces or participate in and contribute to household activities, can find themselves isolated within the home, thus limiting their opportunities to belong. For example, if the kitchen, deck, or family room are inaccessible, people are unable to participate in the daily activities that are part of the fabric of home life.

The home is also a place of change and growth, providing opportunities for development, transformation, and, ultimately, "becoming." People often seek a home to support their idea of their future selves, such as buying a home with additional space for a growing family, a private space for study, enough land to raise animals, or a basement for retirement activities. The home, in this realm of change and growth, can be an important place for recovery; for example, participants recovering from stroke found engaging in everyday activities at home to be important in creating a new sense of fulfillment and "becoming" (Hodson, Aplin, & Gustfasson, 2016). Parents of children with a disability also seek to provide opportunities for "becoming" within the home by creating spaces for the child to grow, explore, develop, and enjoy life (Aplin, Thornton & Gustafsson, 2017). Parents may modify a bathroom to allow the child to develop independence in self-care activities or provide access to the kitchen to allow the child to make his or her own lunch, building self-reliance and mastery.

The home as a place of occupation is complex, and it is difficult to observe the meaning and value that activities have for the individual. As occupational therapists, we are often restricted to focusing on a limited range of "doing" occupations in the home, prioritizing self-care, domestic activities, and community access without a full appreciation of how these contribute to being, belonging, and becoming. Occupational therapists have a responsibility to recognize the activities that are meaningful to their clients and the potential these offer for being, belonging, and becoming.

The Societal Dimension

Our homes and their meaning in our lives do not occur in a vacuum. Many external factors influence the experience of home, such as rental policies, government housing policies, and the resources we have available to change our homes. The societal dimension has emerged in the literature as an important dimension influencing the experience of home (Aplin et al., 2013, 2015).

The societal dimension recognizes the impact of political and economic conditions on the resources and control that people have over their homes (Aplin et al., 2015). For example, the affordability of homes is dictated by a range of external factors that influences where and what type of home we live in. Our home design, and the changes we can make to our homes, is also determined by a range of building codes and government guidelines. The impact of the societal dimension is deeply felt by people who rent. For renters, the continuity of home life is influenced by the length of a lease agreement, and control over the home environment is dictated by the landlord. The experiences of residents living in social housing in the United States who were forced to relocate due to urban renewal policies demonstrate the influence of the societal dimension. Residents described the experience of relocation as traumatic due to loss of community, social networks, and attachment to place (Fullilove, 2004). Societal factors also affect older private renters, who often experience difficulty accessing home modifications, as home modification services are reluctant to invest in rental homes, and landlords may oppose the completion of modifications (Jones, de Jonge, & Phillips, 2008).

Government policies significantly impact the experience of home, influencing funding for modifications, the resources available in a local area, and the planned infrastructure and services to the home. Government policies also dictate whether your local area will have suitable community services available to provide in-home support. Further, national standards such as fire safety or electrical and plumbing codes that are prescribed by government influence the design of housing, as does the availability of services involved in modifying, maintaining, and renovating.

UNDERSTANDING THE EXPERIENCE OF HOME: CULTURE

The dimensions of home described earlier highlight the dynamic and complex nature of it. Within the literature, culture is not identified as a separate dimension or influence; rather, that the experience of home is tied to its cultural context (Lloyd, 2012), with culture shaping each dimension. For example, when considering the physical dimension, the design, layout, space, furnishings, and all aspects of the architecture of the home are influenced by the prevailing culture, which changes over time. Modern home design has changed from a segregated design where the kitchen was a separate workspace and children shared bedrooms to a more communal open floor plan with individual bedrooms (Madigan, Munro, & Smith, 1990). This highlights the cultural changes of the roles of women and children within the home over the last century. The routines and order of the temporal dimension are also largely culturally influenced. Where we place items in our home, the type of furniture we have, and how and when we complete activities in our home are all culturally defined. Culture also influences the societal dimension. For example, home modifications tend to have a lower priority than other social and health service funding, and the funding focus results in interventions that target activities of daily living and safety. This is a reflection of Western culture, where people with a disability and older adults are viewed from a medical model, which prioritizes basic care needs over social and psychological needs. This cultural view of disability also affects the personal dimension of home, with many modifications having a clinical appearance with minimal acknowledgment of aesthetics.

The influence of culture can be seen in the literature describing the experience of home and home modifications. The descriptions of home have evolved over time with associated economic, ideological, and cultural changes (Madigan et al., 1990). A large proportion of this body of work is older and has been widely criticized for its White, Western, owner-occupier, family focus, with diverse perspectives lacking (Despres, 1991; Mallet, 2004; Zuffery, 2015). Consequently, it has had a largely positive perspective of home, with meanings focused on family, safety, and belonging (Mallet, 2004). Varying experiences do exist, and although not widely discussed in the literature, home can be a place of fear and abuse (Mallett, 2004). A recent study examining how the lived experience of class, gender, ethnicity, and age constituted meanings of home for men and women in Australia found differing experiences for different cultural groups (Zufferey, 2015). For refugees and migrants, although they felt safe in Australia, there was not the sense of cultural and familial belonging that they associated with home, and that feeling "at home" occurred when ethnicity and cultural backgrounds were not in question (Zufferey, 2015). In contrast, experiences described by middle-class Australians with no recent family history of migration focused on improving housing circumstances, renovations, descriptions of the ideal home, and living in good school zones (Zufferey, 2015). This highlights the importance of the cultural context of home and the need to understand varying experiences of what makes one feel at home. Understandings of home have also been criticized for their lack of viewpoints from Indigenous peoples. For example, it has been highlighted that the Western view of home being a single-family dwelling place and a physical structure is inappropriate for Indigenous Australians and does not recognize Indigenous mobility or land as home (Zufferey & Chung, 2015).

It is important that occupational therapists have an understanding of the influence of culture on the dimensions of home as it will enable them to practice in a culturally responsive way. Therapists should value and prioritize their client's experiences of home and participate in collaborative decision making that responds to the needs of those from a different cultural background than their own.

CONCLUSION

In this chapter, we have explored the meaning and experience of home drawing from environmental psychology, gerontology, and occupational therapy literature. The aim in doing so was to provide a better understanding of the complex, dynamic, and unique relationship that is "home" and within which the process of home modification assessment and intervention takes place.

People live in worlds of meaning and, as such, change neutral spaces such as a house or apartment into places of significant personal meaning, shaping and transforming them into homes. This transformation occurs through transactions between people and their environments that are both observable actions (activities, tasks, routines, rituals) and unobservable psychosocial processes by which people evaluate, interpret, and ascribe meaning to their experiences.

The Dimensions of Home Framework provides a way to capture the elements of the experience of home as a place of significant and unique meaning. These dimensions provide a clear picture of the dynamic, complex, and personal environment of home within which the home modification process occurs.

Home modifications have the potential to enhance the experience of home, to provide a place that is comfortable, enjoyable, and facilitates the unique way in which we live in our homes. The potential also exists for home modifications to undermine the meaning and experience of home for an individual or family. When the dimensions of home are not valued or understood in the home modification process, negative outcomes can arise, where clients feel out of control, frustrated, and live in homes that do not meet their needs, making day-to-day activities more difficult or unsafe. This can occur if the physical aspects of accessibility and functionality are emphasized and the personal and social meanings of home held by the home dweller are neglected or disregarded.

The challenge for occupational therapists is to first be aware of the complexity of experience that exists in the relationship between a person and their environment and to understand that the meaning of home is not only unique and changing, but also unobservable, not self-conscious, and often taken for granted until threatened. Having an understanding of the dimensions that contribute to the experience of home enables therapists to move beyond a simplistic, functionalist view of person-environment fit to one that embraces the complexity of what home means to an individual and, as such, provide modifications and solutions that benefit the client and enhance their experience of home.

REFERENCES

Altman, I., Brown, B. B., Staples, B., & Werner, C. M. (1992). A transactional approach to close relationships: Courtship, weddings and place making. In W. B. Walsh, K. H. Craik, & R. H. Price (Eds.). *Person-environment psychology: Models and perspectives* (pp. 193-204). Hillsdale, NJ: Lawrence Erlbaum Associates.

American Occupational Therapy Association. (2008). Occupational therapy practice framework: Domain and process (2nd ed.). *American Journal of Occupational Therapy, 62,* 625-683.

Angelou, M. (1986). *All God's children need travelling shoes.* New York: Random House.

Aplin, T., de Jonge, D., & Gustafsson, L. (2013). Understanding the dimensions of home that impact on home modification decision making. *Australian Occupational Therapy Journal, 60*(2), 101-109.

Aplin, T., de Jonge, D. & Gustafsson, L. (2015). Understanding home modifications impact on clients and their family's experience of home: A qualitative study. *Australian Occupational Therapy Journal, 62*(2), 123-131.

Aplin, T., Thornton, H., & Gustafsson, L. (2017). The unique experience of home for parents and carers of children with disabilities. *Scandinavian Journal of Occupational Therapy.* 2017:1-10. doi: 10.1080/11038128.2017.1280079. [Epub ahead of print]

Baum, C. M., Christiansen, C. H., & Bass, J. D. (2015). The person-environment-occupational performance (PEOP) model. In C. H. Christiansen, C. M. Baum, & J. D. Bass (Eds.), *Occupational therapy: Performance, participation and well-being* (4th ed., pp. 49-55). Thorofare, NJ: SLACK Incorporated.

Bunting, K. L. (2016). A transactional perspective on occupation: A critical reflection. *Scandinavian Journal of Occupational Therapy, 23*(5), 327-336.

Canadian Association of Occupational Therapists. (2002). *Enabling occupation. An occupational therapy perspective* (Rev. ed.). Ottawa, ON: CAOT Publications ACE.

Christiansen, C, H. (1999). Defining lives: Occupation as identity: An essay on competence, coherence, and the creation of meaning. *The American Journal of Occupational Therapy, 53,* 547-558.

Dahlin-Ivanoff, S., Haak, M., Fänge, A., & Iwarsson, S. (2007). The multiple meaning of home as experienced by very old Swedish people. *Scandinavian Journal of Occupational Therapy, 14*(1), 25-32.

de Jonge, D. (2011). Developing and tailoring interventions. In E. Ainsworth & D. de Jonge (Eds.), *An occupational therapist's guide to home modification practice* (pp. 189-212). Thorofare, NJ: SLACK Incorporated.

de Jonge, D., Jones, A., Phillips, R., & Chung, M. (2011). Understanding the essence of home: Older people's experience of home in Australia. *Occupational Therapy International, 18*(1), 39-47.

Despres, C. (1991). The meaning of home: Literature review and directions for future research and theoretical development. *The Journal of Architectural and Planning Research, 8*(2), 96-115.

Dovey, K. (1985). Home and homelessness. In I. Altman & C. Werner (Eds.), *Home environments* (pp. 33-64). New York: Plenum.

Dunn, W., Brown, C., & Youngstrom, M. J. (2003). Ecological model of occupation. In P. Kramer, J. Hinojosa, & C. B. Royeen (Eds.), *Perspectives in human occupation: Participation in life.* (pp. 222-263). Baltimore, MD: Lippincott, Williams & Wilkins.

Felix, E., De Haan, H., Vaandrager, L., & Koelen, M. (2015). Beyond thresholds: The everyday lived experience of the house by older people. *Journal of Housing for the Elderly, 29*(4), 329-347.

Fullilove, M. T. (2004). *Root shock: How tearing up city neighborhoods hurts America, and what we can do about it.* New York: One World Ballantine Books.

Gifford, R. (2002). *Environmental psychology: Principles and practice.* Colville, WA: Optimal Books.

Haak, M., Dahlin-Ivanoff, S. D., Fänge, A., Sixsmith, J., & Iwarsson, S. (2007). Home as the locus and origin for participation: Experiences among very old Swedish people. *OTJR: Occupation, Participation and Health, 27*(3), 95-103.

Hammell, K. W. (2004). Dimensions of meaning in the occupations of daily life. *Canadian Journal of Occupational Therapy, 71*(5), 296-305. https://doi.org/10.1177/000841740407100509

Hasselkus, B, R. (2011). *The meaning of everyday occupation.* Thorofare, NJ: SLACK Incorporated.

Hawkins, R., & Stewart, S. (2002). Changing rooms: The impact of adaptations on the meaning of home for a disabled person and the role of occupational therapists in the process. *The British Journal of Occupational Therapy, 65*(2), 81-87.

Hayward, D. G. (1975). Home as an environmental and psychological concept. *Landscape, 20,* 2-9.

Hayward, D. G. (1977). Psychological concepts of 'home'. *HUD Challenge,* February, 10-13.

Heywood, F. (2005). Adaptation: Altering the house to restore the home. *Housing Studies, 20*(4), 531-547.

Hitch, D., Peppin G., & Stagnitti, K. (2014). In the footsteps of Wilcock, Part One: The evolution of doing, being, becoming, and belonging. *Occupational Therapy in Health Care, 28*(3), 231-246.

Hodson, T., Aplin, T., & Gustafsson, L. (2016). Understanding the dimensions of home for people returning home post stroke rehabilitation. *British Journal of Occupational Therapy, 79*(7), 427-433.

Jones, A., de Jonge, D., & Phillips, R. (2008). The role of home maintenance and modification services in achieving health. Community care and housing outcomes in later life. Melbourne: Australian Housing and Urban Research Institute. Retrieved from https://www.ahuri.edu.au/research/final-reports/123

Keilhofner, G. (2002). *A model of human occupation: Theory and application* (3rd ed.). Baltimore, MD: Lippincott, Williams & Wilkins.

Law, M., Cooper, B., Strong, S., Stewart, D., Rigby, P., & Letts, L. (1996). The Person-Environment-Occupation model: A transactive approach to occupational performance. *Canadian Journal of Occupational Therapy, 63*(1), 9-23.

Lewis, J. (2006). How does security of tenure impact on public housing tenants? *AHURI Research and Policy Bulletin, 78.* Melbourne: Australian Housing and Urban Research Institute. Retrieved from https://www.ahuri.edu.au/research/research-and-policy-bulletins/78

Lloyd, J. (2012). Meanings of home in popular culture. In S. J. Smith, M. Elsinga, L. Fox-O'Mahony, S. E. Ong, & S. Wachter (Eds.), *The international encyclopaedia of housing and home* (pp. 258-261). Amsterdam, Netherlands: Elsevier.

Lund, M. L., & Nygard, L. (2004). Occupational life in the home environment: The experiences of people with disabilities. *The Canadian Journal of Occupational Therapy, 71*(4), 243-251.

Madigan, R., Munro, M., & Smith, S. (1990). Gender and the meaning of home. *International Journal of Urban and Regional Research, 14*(4), 625-647.

Mallet, S. (2004). Understanding home: A critical review. *The Sociological Review, 52*(1), 62-89.

Mayes, R., Cant, R., & Clemson, L. (2011). The home and caregiving: Rethinking space and its meaning. *OTJR: Occupation, Participation and Health, 31*(1), 15-22.

Moore, J. (2000). Placing home in context. *Environmental Psychology, 20,* 207-217.

Oswald, F., & Wahl, H. W. (2005). Dimensions of the meaning of home in later life. In G. D. Rowles & H. Chaudhury (Eds.), *Home and identity in late life international perspectives* (pp. 21-45). New York: Springer.

Polatajko, H. J., Davis, J., Stewart, D., Cantin, N., Amoroso, B., Purdie, L., & Zimmerman, D. (2013). Specifying the domain of concern: Occupation as core. In E. A. Townsend & H. J. Polatajko (Eds.), *Enabling occupation II: Advancing an occupational therapy vision for health, well-being & justice through occupation* (2nd ed., pp. 13-36). Ottawa, ON: Canadian Association of Occupational Therapists.

Polatajko, H. J., Townsend, E. A., & Craik, J. (2007). Canadian model of occupational performance and engagement (CMOP-E). In E. A. Townsend & H. J. Polatajko (Eds.), *Enabling occupation II: Advancing an occupational therapy vision of health, well-being & justice through occupation* (p. 23). Ottawa, ON: Canadian Association of Occupational Therapists.

Roster, C. A., Ferrari, J. R., & Jurkat, M. P. (2016). The dark side of home: Assessing possession 'clutter' on subjective well-being. *Journal of Environmental Psychology, 46,* 32-41.

Rowles, G. (1983). Place and personal identity in old age: Observations from Appalachia. *Journal of Environmental Psychology, 3*(4), 299-313.

Rowles, G. (1991). Beyond performance: Being in place as a component of occupational therapy. *American Journal of Occupational Therapy, 45,* 265-271.

Rowles, G. (2000). Habituation and being in place. *Occupational Therapy Journal of Research, 20*(Suppl 1), 525-675.

Rowles G. D., & Bernard M. A. (2013). The meaning and significance of place in old age. In G. D. Rowles and M. A. Bernard (Eds.), *Environmental gerontology: Making meaningful places in old age* (pp. 3-24). New York: Springer Publishing.

Rubinstein, R. L. (1989). The home environments of older people: A description of the psychosocial processes linking person to place. *Journal of Gerontology, 44*(2), 545-553.

Sanford, J. A., & Bruce, C. (2010). Measuring the physical environment. In E. Mpofu & T. Oakland (Eds.), *Rehabilitation and health assessment: Applying ICF guidelines* (pp. 207-228). New York: Springer.

Sebba, R., & Churchman, A. (1986). The uniqueness of home. *Architecture and Behaviour, 3*(1), 7-24.

Sixsmith, J. (1986). The meaning of home: An exploratory study of environmental experience. *Journal of Environmental Psychology, 6,* 281-298.

Smith, S. G. (1994). The essential qualities of a home. *Journal of Environmental Psychology, 14*(1), 31-46.

Sommerville, P. (1997). The social construction of home. *Journal of Architectural Planning Research, 14*(3), 226-245.

Tanner, B. (2011). The home environment. In E. Ainsworth & D. de Jonge (Eds.), *An occupational therapist's guide to home modification practice* (pp. 3-16). Thorofare, NJ: SLACK Incorporated.

Tanner, B., Tilse, C., & de Jonge, D. (2008). Restoring and sustaining home: The impact of home modifications on the meaning of home for older people. *Journal of Housing for the Elderly, 22*(3), 195-215.

Tognali, J. (1987). Residential environmentals. In D. Stokols & I. Altman (Eds.), *Handbook of environmental psychology* (pp. 655-690). New York: Wiley.

Werner, C. M., Altman, I., & Oxley, D. (1985). Temporal aspects of homes: A transactive perspective. In I. Altman & C. M. Werner (Eds.). *Home environments* (vol. 8, pp. 1-32).

Wilcock, A., & Hocking, C. (2015). *An occupational perspective of health* (3rd ed.). Thorofare, NJ: SLACK Incorporated.

Zingmark, K., Norberg, A., & Sandman, P. O. (1995). The experience of being at home throughout the lifespan. Investigation of persons aged from 2 to 102. *International Journal of Aging and Human Development, 41,* 47-62.

Zufferey, C. (2015). Diverse meanings of home in multicultural Australia. *The International Journal of Diverse Identities, 13*(2), 13-21.

Zufferey, C., & Chung, D. (2015). 'Red dust homelessness': Housing, home and homelessness in remote Australia. *Journal of Rural Studies, 41,* 13-22.

Approaches to Service Delivery

Bronwyn Tanner, BOccThy, Grad Cert Occ Thy, Grad Cert Soc Planning, MPhil;
Desleigh de Jonge, MPhil (OccThy), Grad Cert Soc Sci; Andrew Jones, BA, MSW, GCE;
Rhonda Phillips, MPhil, BA, Grad Dip; and Jon Pynoos, MCP, PhD

Occupational therapists have long been interested in helping people to live well in their home environment and have become key stakeholders in the delivery of home modification services. Toward the end of the 20th century, a range of home modification services and resources were developed that enabled occupational therapists to access a selection of public and private services to address those needs. A number of factors have influenced the development and delivery of home modification services. This chapter aims to provide therapists with an understanding of the various demographic, legislative, policy, and service delivery traditions that have influenced, and will continue to influence, the development and delivery of home modification services. The chapter will also examine the roles, perspectives, and responsibilities of key stakeholders in the home modification process and provide a range of strategies to assist occupational therapists achieve effective and positive service delivery outcomes.

CHAPTER OBJECTIVES

By the end of this chapter, the reader will be able to:

✦ Describe various demographic, legislative, policy, and service delivery traditions that have influenced the development and provision of home modification services

✦ Describe the impact of health, community care, and housing service systems on the way home modification services are delivered and the associated implications for occupational therapists and clients of home modification services

INTRODUCTION

As the demographics of societies change, governments and service providers seek to plan for and respond to the changing needs of the community. Advances in health care have resulted in increasing numbers of people surviving significant injuries and poor health conditions and living into old age. The soaring costs of health care and the aging population have impelled governments to establish strategic directions that allow older people and people with disabilities to continue to live in their own homes and communities. Policies such as deinstitutionalization meant that people with disabilities were integrated back into the community in the latter part of the 20th century, and "aging-in-place" policies

Ainsworth, E., & de Jonge, D. *An Occupational Therapist's*
Guide to Home Modification Practice, Second Edition (pp. 17-40).
© 2019 SLACK Incorporated.

reflect a commitment to helping older people, as well as people with disabilities who are living longer, to remain in their communities. Developments in directed care within the disability and aged care sectors in a number of countries have also resulted in people determining where and how money is spent, thus shifting service provision to priorities. Recent demographic changes and policy developments have affected how funding is allocated across a number of service systems—health, community care, and housing—to enable older people and people with disabilities to live safely and independently in the community. Funding allocation and choice and control have also stimulated the development of a range of home modification services. These developments have had a significant impact on the work opportunities for occupational therapists, and while they have traditionally worked within the health system, they are now finding themselves increasingly in demand across a wide range of sectors.

Models of health and disability have also had an influence on how health and disability are conceived and funded and, subsequently, how services are delivered. Disability was viewed traditionally as an attribute of the person, which meant that services were primarily focused on treating the person's disease or disorder. More recently, the social model of disability, which views disability as the inability of society to accommodate the diverse abilities in the community, has shifted the focus from addressing the limitations of the individual to addressing barriers in the environment. Furthermore, antidiscrimination and civil rights legislation, which acknowledges the rights of all people in the community, has led to the development of policies that aim to provide everyone equitable access to community facilities and services. Consequently, revised building standards now ensure that people with disabilities can access public buildings. A growing interest in the design of residential buildings—to enable people to function well in their home environments across their life span—has also led to residential design standards and legislation being developed.

DEMOGRAPHICS

Increased life expectancy, improved child mortality rates, falling fertility rates, and unprecedented socioeconomic development over the last 50 years have resulted in populations aging in almost all countries of the world, with most people worldwide expected to live beyond 60 years of age for the first time in history (United Nations, 2015; World Health Organization [WHO], 2015). Existing evidence shows that older people contribute to society in many ways, despite existing and misleading stereotypes of frailty and dependence (WHO, 2015). The contribution of older people is, however, significantly dependent upon their health, and although poor health does not need to dominate old age, disability is part of the human condition. At some point, almost everyone will experience temporary or permanent difficulties in functioning, and those who live into old age are at increasing risk of acquiring impairments (WHO, 2015). In 2004, it was estimated that over 1 billion people in the world have a disability, approximately 15% of the world's population. Between 110 and 190 million adults worldwide had significant difficulty in daily functioning (WHO, 2011). Lower-income countries had a higher percentage of people with a disability than did higher-income countries; however, in all countries, older people had higher rates of disability (WHO, 2011).

Data from the U.S. Centers for Disease Control and Prevention reported that in 2013, over 50 million U.S. adults (22.2%) reported having a disability, with mobility impairment being most frequently reported, followed by cognitive impairment (Courtney-Long et al., 2015). In the United Kingdom, there are 11.9 million people with a disability, with 67% of people over the age of 75 years reporting a long-standing illness or disability (Papworth Trust, 2016). In Australia, 18.5% of the population has reported having a disability (over 4 million people), with 14.9% (3,412,500) of the Australian population reporting a core activity limitation (limitation in self-care, mobility, and/or communication; Australian Bureau of Statistics [ABS], 2013). Over half (50.7%) of people over age 65 years report having one or more impairments (ABS, 2015).

The incidence of disability is growing worldwide due to both an aging population and an increase in chronic diseases. Population aging has emerged as a key issue for governments globally as the proportion and number of older people in populations around the world increase dramatically as a result of increases in life expectancy and a steady decline in fertility rates (WHO, 2015). In many developed countries, the rise in the birth rate between 1946 and 1964 means that a large number of people are in or approaching retirement. This "wave" of baby boomers is expected to have an enduring impact on Western societies for many decades to come (Freedman, 2007).

In 1950, when baby boomers were first counted in the U.S. Census, people aged 65 years and older made up just 8% of the population. In 2010, people aged 65 years and older were projected to represent 13% of the total U.S. population, and by 2030, this figure is expected to reach 19% (Vincent & Velkoff,

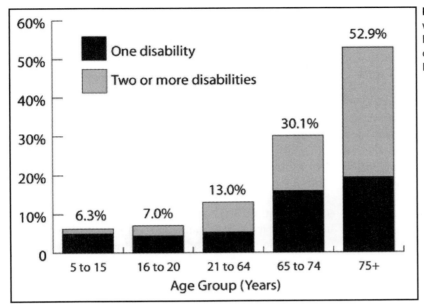

Figure 2-1. Disability and aging. (Reprinted with permission from Bernard Steinman, MS, Research Assistant at the Fall Prevention Center of Excellence, Andrus Gerontology Center USC. Data Source.)

2010). Globally in 2015, people over age 60 years made up 12% of the world's population. This is projected to rise to 22% by 2050, resulting in significant challenges to the economic, health, and social systems (WHO, 2015).

Although there is great diversity in function and health in older individuals, aging is associated with a general decline in physical function, an increased vulnerability to environmental challenges, and a growing risk of disease (WHO, 2015). Aging is frequently associated with loss of sensory function, reduced mobility, declining immune function, and some cognitive changes (WHO, 2015). Older people are also likely to experience more than one chronic condition at the same time (multimorbidity), as well as health conditions that are usually only experienced in old age such as frailty, continence issues, and high risk of falls (WHO, 2015). As a result, daily functional ability and levels of activity may decline.

In the United States, for the population of people 65 years and older, 26% reported activity restrictions as a result of disability (Johnson & Wiener, 2006). Although the incidence of activity limitations is not significantly rising for this population in the United States, there is an increasing incidence of activity limitation for people 55 to 64 years since 2000 (Freedman et al., 2013). Figure 2-1 displays the growing rate of disability that occurs when people age.

The capacity of people to engage in daily activities and remain living in the community as they age or acquire a disability is not only influenced by individual physical and mental capacities, but also by the quality and nature of their living environment,

including social, political, physical, and built environments (WHO, 2015). Relocation in old age is usually the result of a number of interacting aspects of housing and health, including level of dependency in daily activities and the usability or accessibility of the home environment (Granbom, L fqvist, Horstmann, Haak, & Iwarsson, 2014). In 2007, a survey of housing in England identified that only 3.4% of homes had features that made them "visitable" for people with mobility problems, with particular problems associated with older-style housing (Communities & Local Government, 2009). In Australia, many people live in detached houses in the suburbs that are designed for young families with private transport. These dwellings have features that create hazards and barriers for occupants with disabilities or who are aging (Bridge, Parsons, Quine, & Kendig, 2002; Faulkner & Bennett, 2002). Existing housing that is targeted for older people in Australia is also problematic as it often fails to meet accessible design and livability standards (Aged and Community Services Australia [ACSA], 2015). Lack of housing accessibility has been identified as a key indicator for relocating older people to special housing in European countries such as Sweden (Granbom et al., 2014).

Housing is generally designed and constructed with little thought to the access, safety, independence, and location needs of the residents, and the need for accessible housing far exceeds supply in most countries (Imrie & Hall, 2001; Liebermann, 2013). Most housing in the United States is inaccessible, and policy priorities in some states can impede the production of accessible housing (Liebermann, 2013; Steinfeld, Levine, & Shea, 1998). Houses with stairs, narrow doorways and corridors, inaccessible toilets and bathrooms, and limited space "create" disability (Heywood, 2004a; Oldman & Beresford, 2000) and can compromise the safety (Stone, 1998; Trickey, Maltais, Gosslein, & Robitaille, 1993), independence (Frain & Carr, 1996), and well-being (Heywood, 2004a) of older residents and those with disabilities. These design features are costly to modify (Tabbarah, Silverstein, & Seeman, 2000) and can contribute to early institutionalization (Rojo-Perez, Fernandez-Mayoralas, Pozo-Rivera, & Rojo-Abuin, 2001). Because activity limitations are likely to increase as people age, it is not surprising that governments throughout the world are actively engaged in social and health reforms to ensure the ongoing health and well-being of older people and people with disabilities living in aging and unaccommodating homes in the community.

LEGISLATIVE AND POLICY DEVELOPMENTS AND DIRECTIONS

The emergence of the civil rights movement and antidiscrimination legislation in the 1960s and 1970s resulted in many governments committing to ensuring the acceptance and inclusion of people with disabilities in society. More than 40 nations adopted disability discrimination legislation during the 1990s (WHO, 2011). Legislation such as the Americans With Disabilities Act (1990), Australian Disability Discrimination Act (1992), U.K. Equality Act (2010), and the proposed European Accessibility Act all provide provision for the development of accessibility standards for public buildings, recognizing the role of the built environment in affording people access to community facilities. In the residential sector, the movement toward deinstitutionalization contributed to the emphasis on also creating housing environments that could accommodate people with disabilities, as indicated in the United States by the Fair Housing Amendments Act (1968) and in the United Kingdom by the Lifetimes Home Standard (2010). Deinstitutionalization shifted the focus from providing care in specialized settings to supporting people in their own communities. These policy initiatives have stimulated the development of other policies and services dedicated to building and modifying home environments to move people from congregate care to independent community living. In the United States, the 1999 Olmstead Decision requires that states provide services to older people and people with disabilities in the "most integrated setting appropriate," resulting in an increase in demand for community-based services and housing (Pynoos, Nishita, Cicero, & Caraviello, 2008, p. 85). The creation of the United Nations Convention on the Rights of Persons with Disabilities (2006) and the ongoing implementation of disability discrimination or antidiscrimination legislation continue to influence policy relating to the provision of accessible housing within various countries.

The concern around the world about the aging population and its impact on health and social services has resulted in a number of policy initiatives being proposed and implemented. In the United States, the role of housing in supporting older people in the community is gaining recognition from policymakers (Lipman, Lubell, & Salomon, 2012; Pynoos, Liebig, Alley, & Nishita, 2004). Older Americans have been exerting political pressure through organizations such as the American Association of Retired Persons and are increasingly recognized as having significant voting power (National Institute on Aging, 2006). These demographic, social, and policy changes have stimulated a rapid expansion in industries providing services for older people, including health care, aged care, financial services, and housing. These service industries have also become increasingly vocal, organized, and politically influential (Jones, de Jonge, & Phillips, 2008).

Although policy has concentrated on the need for more inclusively designed residential environment, for the most part, the U.S. regulations have applied to multi-unit developments, omitting the vast array of single-family and smaller complexes where older people live. In the United States, there have been attempts to rectify this problem by concentrating on designing existing units and building housing to suit a diversity of users, including older people and people with disabilities in the first instance. The Eleanor Smith Inclusive Home Design legislation has been created to ensure new homes are built with visitable features (to allow someone to visit the home using the no-step entry, sit in the living room, and access the toilet in the bathroom) but has yet to be passed by the U.S. Senate.

There are ongoing efforts to make accessible, adaptable, and universal design part of new home design construction through groups lobbying the government's national construction codes (e.g., Australian Network of Universal Housing Design) and trying to institute voluntary programs with the building sector (e.g., Better Living Design in the United States [http://betterlivingdesign.org/], Livable Housing Australia [http://www.livablehousingaustralia.org.au/], Lifemark Homes in New Zealand [http://www.lifemark.co.nz/home.aspx], and Lifetime Homes in the United Kingdom [http://www.lifetimehomes.

org.uk/]. Although there has been a lack of take-up in the new construction arena of the design guidelines created by these organizations, the guidelines are being used by occupational therapists as a major reference when recommending home modifications to residential dwellings.

However, the reliance on new building development to meet the needs of older people or people with a disability is tenuous, considering it is widely acknowledged that "development, design and building processes are inattentive to the needs of disabled people" (Imrie & Hall, 2001, p. 3).

Of the more than 60 countries that have accessibility legislation worldwide, very few of these consider accessibility to new private residences part of the legislative framework. Even in countries where the concept of "visitability" (basic accessibility features in newly constructed residential homes) is legislated, provisions have been "beset by problems of vagueness and ambiguity and rarely used to their full potential" (Imrie, 2006, p. 15), and it is acknowledged that there is a "long way to go in increasing the number of homes that are accessible and supportive" (Nishita, Liebig, Pynoos, Perelman, & Spegal, 2007, p. 13).

Given this situation, there is a clear role for modification of existing housing as a strategy to support community living for older people and people with a disability. In the United Kingdom, a housing condition survey found that only minor works were needed to increase the number of existing accessible houses from 110,000 to 920,000 (Communities & Local Government, 2009). However, in many developed countries, home modification services, although on the increase, continue to lack appropriate recognition at a legislative and policy level (Jones et al., 2008). Home modifications are starting to be considered in policy development as they can make a general contribution to the implementation of aging policy and, more specifically, to health, community care, and housing policy for older people.

Home modifications can reduce the need for hospitalization of older people and the demand for expensive in-home and residential aged-care services (Kim, Ahn, Steinhoff, & Lee, 2014; Mann, Ottenbacher, Fraas, Tomita, & Granger, 1999). Home modification can also play an important role in preventive health by reducing the incidence of accidents and falls among older people, reducing the costs associated with home injuries, and reducing the mental and physical strain on caregivers (Heywood, 2005; Keall et al., 2015, Newman, 2003). Modifying the homes of older people can also reduce expenditure on social housing because it constitutes a less expensive form of housing assistance than direct social housing provision (Jones et al., 2008). Home modifications can also help caregivers who form the backbone of personal care assistance for disabled people of all ages. There is even some preliminary evidence that home modifications, in conjunction with occupational and physical therapy, can reduce mortality (Gitlin, 2003).

In terms of promoting positive aging, home modification provides a means of facilitating healthy and independent living and allowing older people to continue to participate actively in home and community life. Appropriate housing is fundamental to an individual's well-being and social participation (Jones et al., 2008), and modifications can play an important role in enabling people to live independently and safely, to actively participate in household activities, and to maintain involvement with family and friends (Aplin, de Jonge, & Gustafsson, 2015). When people choose to remain living in their own home for as long as possible, modifications, along with other community care services, can enable them to age in place. If people choose to relocate, they will have access to more suitable housing and locations, where the homes might be designed or adapted to better suit their requirements.

The establishment, design, and delivery of a home modification service varies between countries and, like accessibility in the built environment, is influenced by the type, nature, and direction of legislation and policy in existence in a particular country. Legislation and flow on policy directly affect the way home modification services are resourced, including the amount of funding available, eligibility criteria, and the type and level of modification that is provided (Jones et al., 2008). In many non-Western or developing countries, minimal legislative and policy frameworks are in place and there is minimal welfare support for people with a disability. This lack of legislative support results in few resources or limited infrastructure to support modification of home environments for older people or people with a disability (Imrie, 2006).

Though many developed countries have legislation and policy in place that support full participation and equity for people with disabilities and aging in place for older people, the outworking of these principles is complex, and there is often no overarching framework that legislates the provision of home modification services (ACSA, 2015). In countries such as the United States, New Zealand, and Australia, disability issues are considered within a human rights legislative framework rather than a rehabilitative or health framework as in Sweden.

Sweden provides a clear example of how legislative and policy frameworks support consistent and comprehensive home modification service development. Sweden's legislation in relation to older people and people with a disability establishes a framework for the development of support services, including provision of personal care and home modification services (Anderberg, 2009; Lilja, Mansson, Jahlenius, & Sacco-Peterson, 2003). The Home Modification Law (1992) in Sweden mandates that local authorities provide grants for housing modification services to anyone who has a disability, irrespective of financial or housing situation (Anderberg, 2009; Petersson, Lilja, Hammel, & Kottorp, 2008). Policy arising from the legislation ensures that people with a disability do not bear the cost of reducing environmental barriers to their activities of daily living. Under this legislative framework, home modifications are considered essential elements of health care, and consistent provision of home modifications is supported through policy and practice frameworks (Petersson et al., 2008).

As outlined in Chapter 4, human rights legislation, such as the Americans With Disability Act (1990) and the Fair Housing Amendments Act (1968; housing-specific amendments to the Civil Rights Act of 1968; U.S. Department of Housing and Urban Development, 2007), enshrines the right of people with a disability to equitable and nondiscriminatory access to housing and housing services. However, supporting a person with care needs to live in the community very often requires a diverse array of services, including home help, home maintenance, personal care and assistance, assistive technology, and home modifications. Many of these services vie for the same funding, and home modification service does not always receive distinctive treatment (Lilja et al., 2003; Pynoos, Nishita, & Perelman, 2003).

In many countries such as the United States, the United Kingdom, and Australia, there is a historic fragmentation of housing, health, and community care in policy areas, with the result that there is a lack of coordinated policy development and consequent service provision to support community-based living (Faulkner & Bennett, 2002; Heywood & Turner, 2007). This lack of specific acknowledgment of home modification services within policy and the associated poor integration of related areas at a policy level significantly affect the development and funding of home modification services, with public funding for home modification services being limited. In the United States and Australia, home modification service delivery has been frequently described as being less than ideal, with lack of sufficient funding, poor coordination of services, and lack of geographic coverage of services cited as some of the main barriers to effective service delivery (ACSA, 2015; Duncan, 1998a; Jones et al., 2008; Pynoos, 2001; Sorensen, 2012; Tabbarah et al., 2000).

Funding and Home Modification Services

As indicated previously, funding arrangements for home modification services are directly linked to provisions within the legislation of a particular country. Both Sweden and the United Kingdom have legislation that ensures a specific allocation of funds for home modification services. Within the United Kingdom, the mandatory Disabled Facilities Grant requires local authorities to fund a range of modifications to the homes of eligible people with a disability. However, even within countries that legislate for funding for home modifications, problems exist. Within the United Kingdom, the Disabled Facilities Grant is criticized as being poorly publicized, and the grant is distributed in a reactive rather than proactive way, resulting in poor uptake and less-than-effective administration and outcomes (Awang, 2002; Heywood, 2005). Unlike Sweden, where funds are available irrespective of individual financial circumstance, in the United Kingdom, funding is limited to people on pensions and with low incomes, and there are differing levels of service across different geographical areas. In both the United Kingdom and Sweden, concerns exist as to the impact of an aging population on the viability of the current schemes, with an increasing gap existing between need and available resources.

In contrast, although funding is available for home modifications in both the United States and Australia, it is not mandated by legislation and is generally considered to be difficult to access and insufficient to meet existing needs (ACSA, 2015; Smith, Rayer, & Smith, 2008). Both countries have described the organization and provision of home modification services as a complex "patchwork" of programs (ACSA, 2015; Jones et al., 2008; Pynoos, 2001). Programs are often funded from a variety of diverse sources (federal, state, local, and community), resulting in fragmentation, inflexibility, and administrative burden, and there is an absence of integrated information systems about home modification services (Jones et al., 2008; Smith et al., 2008; Sorensen, 2012). Without a legislative mandate for funding, the cost of home modifications is often borne by the individual (The Scan Foundation, 2010).

In both the United States and Australia, even federally funded programs differ from state to state with regard to requirements and resources available, and funding is often in a block grant with a range of other essential services related to community care vying for priority (Duncan, 1998b; Jones et al., 2008; Sorensen, 2012). In many countries, such as Australia, the United Kingdom, and the United States, there has been a call to reconsider the current approach to the organization and provision of home modification services. There is a clearly identified need to establish specific policy goals and benchmarks for service delivery to address the great disparity that exists in levels of service provision within various countries (ACSA, 2015; Duncan, 1998b; Jones et al., 2008; Pynoos & Nishita, 2003; Sorensen, 2012).

SERVICE DELIVERY SYSTEMS

As identified previously, home modification services in many countries have not developed as a planned and cohesive strategy. Various types of services have been developed and delivered through different service systems, each with their own particular goals, approaches, and interventions. This is largely because modification services in many developed countries have been developed and funded through a variety of programs and provided through an assortment of services with various aims. Occupational therapists generally work across different programs in an effort to stitch together a suitable modification solution for each client. It is often difficult for both therapists and their clients to comprehend the range of services available and what each can offer any given individual. Much of this complexity of home modification services is a result of being at the intersection of health, community care, and housing services and policies. Each of these has a different perspective on the goal of home modifications and tends to shape home modification practice through different policies and funding regimes. As a consequence, the roles of stakeholders involved in home modification practice also vary. Although the role, level, and nature of involvement of each key stakeholder differ between perspectives, there is a general consistency in the type of people (stakeholders) who are usually involved in the delivery of a home modification service (Pynoos, Sanford, & Rosenfelt, 2002). The key people involved in the delivery of home modifications commonly include the person (home dweller) and his or her significant others (this can be family, friends, or caregivers); the referring agency; the organization managing and/or providing funding for the service; construction and building professionals; design professionals; and the health professional, most often an occupational therapist.

Commonly, home modification programs use a combination of employed staff (such as a program coordinator and employed tradesmen/handymen to carry out minor work) and subcontractors, who are usually licensed professionals (including occupational therapists) operating under contract. The challenge for occupational therapists is to operate effectively within and across programs to develop an approach to home modifications that transcends one particular program. In order to appreciate the impact of the service context on practice and to develop a holistic approach to home modification, each of these service environments needs to be examined.

HEALTH PERSPECTIVE

Home modifications and home adaptations are widely defined in health care contexts as "any permanent alteration to a building carried out with the intention of making [it] more suitable for a disabled person" (Heywood, 2004a, p. 134). In this context, changes are made to the home environment "in order to accommodate a particular set of human abilities" (Bridge, 2005, p. 2). Like many interventions within health and rehabilitation settings, home modifications are viewed as a means of addressing or correcting problems specific to an individual (Wylde, 1998). Home modifications are provided as part of discharge planning following hospitalization (Auriemma, Faust, Sibrian, & Jimenez, 1999; Lannin, Clemson, & McCluskey, 2011) or within a community health or health-funded in-home service.

Within a health context, home modifications are generally recommended by professionals to ensure that an individual with a particular impairment or health condition is safe and independent in his or her home (Auriemma et al., 1999) or to decrease the likelihood of admission to a hospital or care facility (Auriemma et al., 1999; Gitlin, Miller, & Boyce, 1999). Health conditions, which are generally viewed as having a standard presentation and predictable pathology, are managed using practice guidelines or protocols of care. This can result in recommendations focusing on a specific health problem, with less consideration being given to other difficulties, impairments, or aspirations the person might have (Tinker et al., 2004). The primary focus of interventions within the health context is often on remediation or correction of the health condition, with medications and interventions that remediate the condition taking precedence over other interventions. Home modifications, assistive devices, and an array of other interventions that promote the safety and independence of people with chronic conditions or long-term disabilities are frequently less of a priority within the health system. This factor is often reflected in the priority these services are given, along with the budget allocated for them.

Focus of the Health Perspective

Within a health perspective, the home environment is typically conceptualized as a discrete physical entity where modifications can be routinely recommended to accommodate specific functional impairments or health-related limitations. Although pre-discharge home visits are acknowledged as important in preventing readmission to hospital, increasing trends toward early discharge have contributed to reduced discharge preparation and decreased numbers of home visits within some health services (Lannin et al., 2011). Frequently, an individual's functional ability is assessed in a clinical setting, and recommendations for modifications to the home environment can be made without undertaking an on-site visit (Lannin et al., 2011; Pynoos, Tabbarah, Angelelli, & Demiere, 1998). When a home visit is undertaken, the focus is often on potential safety hazards or physical barriers to performing self-care activities. Consequently, the inside of the home—in particular, the bathroom and bedroom, as well as an access point in and out of the home—receives most attention. Typically, modification recommendations in health-based services tend toward nonstructural changes, such as grab rails, shower seats, and other assistive devices (Pynoos et al., 1998; Renforth, Yapa, & Forster, 2004). Although funding programs for major modifications involving structural changes such as widening doorways, modifying bathrooms, and installing ramps, do exist in many developed countries, such modifications are less common because of the design and construction time involved, the financial cost, and the expertise and resources required in attaining these modifications (Auriemma et al., 1999; Pynoos et al., 1998; Tabbarah et al., 2000). Moreover, because of regulatory and budget constraints, there is often little follow-up to ensure that modifications are working effectively (e.g., there might be a problem with faulty equipment or poor installation, or the resident or caregiver might need training in how to use them).

With health-based services focused on ensuring that people with health conditions, injuries, or impairments are able to return home from the hospital and be safe and independent when performing self-care tasks in their home, practice and client outcomes are constrained in a number of ways. When function is defined in terms of impairments resulting from a specific injury or health condition, care protocols are developed for each of these. Consequently, the unique needs of the individual are often not well addressed. When people have similar injuries or conditions, the functional limitations—and the impact of these—can vary from one person to another. This generally necessitates a targeted assessment of each individual to assess his or her abilities and the performance of various activities. Furthermore, the particular priorities and preferences of individuals, their personal resources, and the strategies they use to address activity restrictions combine to influence the nature of difficulties identified and how these might be best addressed. With a focus on individual function, less attention is likely to fall on the environment—the challenges it presents when undertaking various activities or how it might be modified to promote further activity engagement. In addition, if performance is evaluated in the hospital environment, this does not acknowledge the interaction between the individual, his or her activities, and the home environment. Consequently, the ability of a person to function on returning home can be either under- or overestimated because the familiarity of, or challenges within, the home environment have not been recognized.

Recent concerns about the prevalence of falls among older people living in the community and the resultant costs to the health system have directed attention to addressing hazards in the home environment. With approximately half of falls occurring inside the home (Rogers, Rogers, Takeshima, & Mohammod, 2004), home modifications have been identified as one of a number of risk-management strategies to reduce the number of falls among the elderly (Gillespie, Gillespie, Cumming, Lamb, & Rower, 2001; Keall et al., 2015; Petersson et al., 2008). A number of potential environmental hazards have been identified, including clutter, obstacles, loose rugs, lack of supports, and poor lighting (Clemson, Roland, & Cumming, 1997; Keall, Baker, Howden-Chapman, & Cunningham, 2008), and interventions are focused on removing these to promote safety. Falls risk and hazard identification have provided the foundation for many health-funded initiatives, and there is some evidence that broadly targeted programs aimed at removing environmental hazards in the homes of older people in the community reduce the incidence of falls (Keall et al., 2015). Success has been achieved with tailored programs targeted at the specific needs of people with increased falls risk, such as the frail elderly (Cumming et al., 1999) and those who have fallen previously (Close et al., 1999; Nikolaus & Bach, 2003). This suggests that the individualized and holistic approach to environmental interventions favored by occupational therapists is likely to be more effective in reducing falls than those focused on hazard reduction alone (Gillespie et al., 2012). A meta-analysis of fall prevention interventions also indicates that multifactorial interventions including medical risk assessment and management, physical activity, and home assessment and modification are likely to produce the largest reduction in falls among those at moderate to high risk (Gillespie et al., 2012; Rubenstein & Josephson, 2006). In this scenario, occupational therapists play a role as members of an interdisciplinary team. Regardless, as a profession, occupational therapists need to provide more evidence of the efficacy of their unique approach if their services expect to benefit from the funding being made available to reduce the incidence of falls among the elderly.

Traditionally, home modification services within health systems have largely focused on physical impairments. This has resulted in well-developed assessments, designs, resources, and services aimed at addressing physical impairments. Somewhat less attention has been given to addressing the sensory, cognitive, emotional, and social changes associated with aging. With the high prevalence of vision and hearing impairment among older people, there is a growing interest in making the home environment more manageable and safe for those with sensory impairments (e.g., using modifications such as enlarged fittings, enhanced lighting, amplification devices, auditory signals, and contrasting colors; Auriemma et al., 1999; Rooney et al., 2016). Although it is important to address existing impairments through environmental interventions, further attention also needs to be directed to creating emotionally and socially supportive home environments that make it easier to carry out daily activities in the home. This would help to promote older people's self-confidence and self-esteem (Pynoos et al., 1998), and it would ensure that they maximize their engagement in daily activities, thus optimizing their general health and well-being. As a result of our less well-developed understanding of sensory, cognitive, emotional, and social issues in the home and associated environmental interventions, there are fewer assessments, designs, resources, and services dedicated to addressing these concerns within the health arena. Consequently, therapists can struggle to adequately address these needs with their clients, who, as a result, continue to struggle to manage in their home environment.

With the aging population and the rising incidence of dementia (Plassman et al., 2007), there is a growing interest in supporting older people with cognitive changes to remain living safely and independently in the community (Giovannetti et al., 2007; Struckmeyer & Pickens, 2015). The focus of health interventions is also to assist the caregivers, who are often responsible for supervising and assisting people in daily activities and managing those who are difficult or dangerous (Colombo, Vitali, Molla, Gioia, & Milani, 1998; Gitlin & Corcoran, 2000; Silverstein & Hyde, 1997). Home modifications might include nonstructural changes, such as reassigning rooms, installing fencing and gates, fitting safety locks on doors and cupboards, adding outlet covers and night lights, and improving lighting. A range of electronic devices has also been used, such as smoke detectors and movement monitoring and alarm systems (Silverstein, Hyde, & Ohta, 1993). Occasionally, structural changes such as an additional bathroom or bedroom are undertaken.

Key Stakeholder Roles and Perspectives

Within the health perspective, the role of the occupational therapist and associated outcomes for clients can be constrained through the health service/organization's policies and funding systems. The role of the occupational therapist within home modification service delivery has been promoted as one of understanding and meeting the individual's goals so that the individual is enabled, enhanced, and empowered to make choices, solve problems, and maintain control (Pickering & Pain, 2003; Pynoos et al., 2003). However, the immediate focus on discharging the person from the hospital into a safe environment can mean that the long-term suitability of the home environment is not adequately addressed (Lannin et al., 2011). Minimizing safety concerns and maximizing independence in self-care activities can often divert therapists' attention from determining the real extent of risk and maximizing engagement in meaningful occupations in the home. A focus on mobility and access into and within the home can result in inadequate attention being paid to access to the yard, neighborhood, and community. In addition, issues of personal concern, such as security, managing the ongoing maintenance of the home and garden (Jones et al., 2008), the social acceptability of the modifications, or the impact of the modifications on the meaning or value of the home (Heywood, 2004b), tend to not be acknowledged or are undervalued.

Within the health perspective, the home dweller may be in the role of "patient" and as such is seen as a passive recipient of services rather than as an active participant in decision making. Inclusion of the home dweller and significant others in decision making about changes to the physical environment is of paramount importance. The issue of participation and control over the modification process is one that has been identified as a key area in the literature (Heywood, 2004b, 2005; Johansson, Borell, & Lilja, 2009; Pickering & Pain, 2003; Tanner, Tilse, & de Jonge, 2008). Poor outcomes in home modification services have been identified as being related to poor understanding of the individual's need and limiting assessment to a functional understanding of the person without consideration of issues of control, participation, or the needs of significant others (Heywood, 2004b).

It is essential that the occupational therapist be committed to a participatory decision-making process. The occupational therapist needs to ensure that the home dweller is actively engaged in the decision making around the intervention planned. Communication needs to be clear and choices around options provided (Heywood, 2004b). This approach will help reinforce the meaning of home as a primary territory with a perceived degree of personal control (Smith, 1994; Tanner et al., 2008).

If the person is accustomed to a passive role with health care or other professionals, the home dweller may not feel confident to voice his or her opinion or to take an active role in decision making. The occupational therapist needs to be sensitive to this dynamic and support the person to give his or her views and opinions, not only in his or her own interactions but in interactions between the person and other stakeholders, including other health professionals, discharge planners, and building professionals. Because the occupational therapist is the person who gathers assessment information about the individual, he or she is often well placed to negotiate better outcomes for an individual.

In summary, health care systems, policies, and programs are key contextual elements in developing and providing home modification services. Within this context, modifications largely have been associated with discharge planning following hospitalization, with care of people with disabilities or chronic health conditions in the home environment (including the older people with dementia and their caregivers), and with fall prevention. Though practices vary widely from one service to another, there are a number of prevailing characteristics of the health approach to home modifications. The primary focus is often on a particular health problem or condition, with home modification perceived as one of a suite of interventions designed to remediate the problem or address dysfunction. Key concerns center on safety and the capacity to independently perform self-care activities. Environmental interventions are generally minor, nonstructural modifications, and structural changes are used infrequently. With a focus on individual function, health-based services are less concerned with the long-term suitability of a residence; the social acceptability of modifications; and issues of identity, meaning, and lifestyle. The occupational therapist's role may involve promoting the home dweller as an active rather than passive participant in decision making, ensuring optimal home modification outcomes for the individual and their significant others. Although there is a growing appreciation of sensory, cognitive, emotional, and social issues and associated environmental interventions, assessments, designs, resources, and services aimed at addressing physical impairments are more highly developed. New technologies present increasing opportunities to assist, as well as manage and monitor, people in their homes; however, these need to be used judiciously to ensure they do not encroach on the rights and autonomy of the householder.

COMMUNITY CARE PERSPECTIVE

In recent decades, home modifications have emerged as one of a range of services provided by community care agencies. Others include home nursing, delivered meals, home help, transport, shopping assistance, allied health services, and respite care. Community care services are designed to directly assist older people and people with disabilities to remain living in their own homes and communities, as well as support their families and caregivers in providing care (Steinfeld & Shea, 1993) and reduce admissions to residential care (Duncan, 1998a; Stone, 1998). Modifications and associated services are seen as being essential in delaying reliance on personal assistance and avoiding an unwanted move (Gitlin et al., 1999). Within this service environment, home modifications have been defined as "adaptations to living environments intended to increase ease of use, safety, security and independence" (Pynoos et al., 1998, p. 3). Although the main focus of health contexts is on home modifications to ensure safety and independence, the community care sector also provides maintenance and security services, acknowledging that older people and people with disabilities also need to maintain the dwelling and be safe and secure in their homes in addition to managing activities in and around the home. The way in which these services are delivered varies considerably from one location to another. However, modification assessments are generally undertaken by professionals working in either health or social services (Klein, Rosage, & Shaw, 1999), whereas maintenance and security assessments can be undertaken by a wide variety of individuals, including handymen, tradespeople, building contractors, social service organizations, and families themselves (Pynoos et al., 1998). Although the modification work is primarily contracted out to builders and other tradespeople, some service providers employ their own trade staff. Some of these providers might be familiar with making modifications; however, many are untrained, thereby requiring specific instructions from the occupational therapist regarding what and where to install them.

A range of strategies is used in the community care context to enable people to remain living in their own homes. These strategies have been classified as being additive, subtractive, transformative, and behavioral (Pynoos, Steinman, Nguyen, & Bressette, 2012; Steinman, Nguyen, & Do, 2011). Additive modifications are those in which supports and structures are added to the home environment. These can be major changes such as ramps, lifts, and stepless showers or minor ones such as additional lighting, grab rails, or special equipment or assistive devices. Subtractive modifications are where items are removed from the environment to improve safety, such as the removal of clutter or hazards. Transformative modifications change or reconfigure existing structures and spaces in the home such as the reorganization of kitchen utensils and rearranging lounge furniture to improve access, as well as structural changes such as widening existing doorways or lowering countertops. Behavioral adjustments alter the way in which activities are carried out in the home environment such as using a shower recess instead of a plunge bath to improve safety (Pynoos et al., 1998).

In the United Kingdom, housing modifications or adaptations are classified as an assistive technology, defined as "any device or system that allows an individual to perform a task that they would otherwise be unable to do, or increases the ease and safety with which the task can be performed" (Cowan & Turner-Smith, 1999, p. 235). However, assistive devices are typically mobile and are not attached to the structure of the house (Pynoos et al., 1998), whereas home modifications are generally permanent, secure, and fixed in place. Assistive devices are sometimes preferred by clients and professionals, especially when they are uncertain about how to undertake structural changes (Pynoos et al., 1998; Steinfeld et al., 1998), when they are reluctant to commit to a permanent or costly modification (Pynoos & Nishita, 2003), or if they are renting and are uneasy about making changes to which a landlord might object or require them to remove if they leave.

Focus of the Community Care Perspective

In community care, the focus shifts from the specific performance limitations of the person to an analysis of the fit between the person and his or her home environment. Lawton and Nahemow (1973) were the first to recognize the challenges, or "press," provided by the environment and proposed that these were unique for each individual. Subsequently, practice models developed over the past decade have highlighted the limitations of focusing on either the person or his or her impairments or on the barriers in the environment, promoting the value of examining the interaction between the person and the environment (Rousseau, Potvin, Dutil, & Falta, 2001). The use of these models in the community sector also encouraged a shift from assessing narrowly defined self-care activities to examining an individual's capacity to manage in the home and the community (Peace & Holland, 2001). The focus is on establishing balance between environmental demands and individual competencies and adapting the home environment to match the capabilities of the person (Gosselin, Robitaille, Trickey, & Maltais, 1993; Rousseau, Potvin, Dutil, & Falta, 2002). In this approach, difficulties experienced by the person in the home are observed and analyzed, and identified environmental challenges are then addressed using environmental interventions tailored to meet the particular needs of the individual.

The role of the environment in supporting competence or creating incapacity is also reflected in the way in which the global view of disability has altered in recent decades. Rather than simply viewing disability as a problem with an individual, disability is now seen as "a dynamic interaction between health conditions and contextual factors, both personal and environmental" (WHO, 2011, p. 4). This "biopsychosocial model" of disability is presented as a "workable compromise" between medical models that focus on the person as disabled and social models that focus on society as the cause of disability (WHO, 2011, p. 4).

Problems in the home result from an inability of the home environment to accommodate the changing capacities of the person (Cowan & Turner-Smith, 1999; Tinker et al., 2004). Older people have been described as being "architecturally disabled" by inadequate design (Hanson, 2001), leading to an emphasis on reducing environmental barriers in the homes of older people and in residential design generally. However, the biopsychosocial model of disability does not restrict its view to purely physical aspects of the individual's immediate environment.

It also acknowledges the impact of society on an individual's capacity to engage in activities identifying "support, relationships, attitudes, services, systems and policies" as environmental factors that can facilitate or hinder an individual's participation (WHO, 2011, p. 5).

Independence is a central concept in community care, both generally and with respect to home modification services (Clapham, 2005). It is commonly understood in this context to mean that the person is able to live at home rather than in residential care. Occupational therapists generally conceive independence to be the ability to perform a task without assistance; therefore, they seek to provide training or a device or to modify the environment in order to remove the person's reliance on others. However, for many people, independence holds a more nuanced association, including "being able to look after oneself," "not being indebted to anyone," and "the capacity for self-direction" (Clough, Leamy, Miller, & Bright, 2004, pp. 119-120). Independence reflects a "sense of being in control with respect to family, friends and formal caregivers" (Heywood, Oldman, & Means, 2002, pp. 55-57). It is possible, then, that some people might consider their independence enhanced by the assistance of others, a home modification, or a move to residential care where they have ready access to caregiving, providing they retain control of when and how assistance is provided. In reality, this paradigm acknowledges the interdependence of people.

Place of Home Modification Services in Community Care

Although home modification services have been established within community care systems in many countries, these services tend to be underdeveloped relative to other community care services as a result of limited funding and scarcity of trained providers (Pynoos et al., 1998). Because community care systems tend to prioritize those at risk of being institutionalized, services are prioritized and directed toward those defined by the service as having the fewest resources and the greatest level of need (Clapham, 2005). Consequently, health and safety concerns take precedence over independence and quality-of-life issues (Mann, Hurren, Tomita, Bengali, & Steinfeld, 1994), leaving home modification services fighting for resources in a system that provides so many essential and costly support services.

Although modifications are seen as part of the range of interventions with the potential to ensure safety and independence and assist people to remain in their homes and community, in reality, it is less developed than the other services in the community care sector where providers are more familiar with the use of formal supports. The use of modifications is also hampered by a lack of understanding of the benefits of environmental interventions, restricted access to services and personnel with appropriate expertise, and the limited budgets available for such interventions (Sorenson, 2012). Balancing priorities and funding across maintenance, security, and modification services is also problematic when these services are competing for their share of inadequate budgets.

Key Stakeholder Roles and Perspectives

Within the community care sector, a key stakeholder is the administrating or funding organization that is often responsible for the coordination of a range of community services, including home modifications. Many organizations that administer home modification services are by nature bureaucracies; that is, organizations based on rationalism, hierarchy, and impersonal rules. Such organizations tend to have a centralized system of policy and procedures that reflect a response to a "typical," situation, and this approach to meeting individual need can result in negative outcomes (Crozier, 1964, cited in Dovey, 1985, p. 56; Heywood, 2004a; Sakellariou, 2015; Tanner et al., 2008). As well as being limited in their response to individual need, the bureaucratic organization model is nonparticipatory by nature, with little scope for service users or recipients to shape or determine service delivery (Awang, 2002).

The majority of service organizations have policies and practices regarding eligibility criteria, which also define the population they are able to serve and the limit of their service. For example, an organization may decide to use allocated funds for minor modifications only and in this way provide service to a larger number of people than if they did major, more costly modifications. This, however, will place limits on the amount and type of modification that can be recommended.

For the home dweller or householder, dealing with a bureaucratic organization can be overwhelming, often due to the complexity of forms, people, and processes that need to be negotiated to get an outcome (Awang, 2002). The "typical situation" approach of bureaucracies also means that, in the application of rules and regulations, the individual becomes invisible and may not be granted power to influence outcomes (Sakellariou, 2015). There is an inherent tension between the bureaucratic organization delivering the home modification service and the service recipient around the issues of power and control. Culturally, a bureaucracy is service-oriented and inflexible, with little scope to allow users or recipients of the service control or power in decision making (Awang, 2002). These negative experiences of organizational service delivery can undermine the experience of home for the person and be profoundly disempowering for him or her, resulting in negative health effects (Dovey, 1985; Heywood, 2004a; Sakellariou, 2015).

Coordinating the variety of services and service providers required for the successful implementation of home modifications remains a prevailing issue (Pynoos, 2004; Steinfeld et al., 1998). Modification services require health and social service providers to work with tradespeople, which can be complex given the differences in roles, knowledge, language, expertise, and expectations. Miscommunication and mistrust prevail if the various stakeholders are not afforded an opportunity to share knowledge and develop an understanding of each other's roles, language, expertise, and expectations. Community care services, which have invested in the development of trained home modification personnel, knowledge, and resources, are well placed to achieve good client outcomes. Services that require health and social service providers to contract out modifications to the private building sector are likely to experience difficulties in delivering high-quality services and outcomes. This is because of the difficulties in locating contractors with the necessary expertise, communicating requirements, and overseeing the work being undertaken.

In the community care sector, occupational therapists have access to a range of services and interventions to assist their clients to remain in their homes and communities. However, the ease with which these resources can be accessed depends largely on the structure of the funding and service system. The development of modification services over the past decade has resulted in a growing body of knowledge and an increasing number of designs and products being available. Recognition of the role of the environment in "disabling" people has resulted in the development of occupational therapy models and practice approaches that address the complexity of the interaction between the person, activities, and environment. Occupational therapists are unique in their understanding of the activity engagement and the role of the environment and stand out among other health professionals in their capacity to provide home modification services. An understanding of environmental fit allows therapists to move from addressing problems to creating enabling homes and communities that recognize the uniqueness of each person and his or her environment. However, restricted funding and service policies often constrain practice in addressing essential issues and make it difficult for therapists to promote activity engagement within the home and community. For example, often the priority in hospital discharge is getting a person out as quickly as possible. As pointed out earlier, even though an occupational therapist assessment and home modification might be essential, these often do not occur, if at all, until the person is already back in his or her home, struggling with both his or her own limitations and that of the environment.

It is important that, wherever possible, the organization's restrictions and limitations do not, in turn, compromise the assessment process for the occupational therapist (Heywood, 2004a). The occupational therapy assessment should reflect as much as possible a full understanding of the needs of the home dweller rather than being restricted to what the organization will or will not fund or what organizational processes typically promote. Because of their focus on the individual, therapists are well placed to speak up for the individual and promote a full understanding of his or her needs within the organizational framework. If necessary, the occupational therapist should push the boundaries of bureaucratic administration if it is important to address the needs of the individual. It is also important that the home dweller be fully aware of the options that are available to him or her and be informed of ways his or her needs can be met through other systems or services.

Use of Technologies

Increasingly, the potential of a range of new technologies is being recognized to help older people and people with disabilities to live safely in their homes and to assist in monitoring and managing people with complex health conditions in the community (Colombo et al., 1998). Mainstream technologies such as mobile phones, sensors, passive alarms, and security cameras are being used to enhance the safety and independence of older people (Tinker, 1999), and dedicated environmental controls, robotics, and communication and security technologies are being developed and integrated into the design of "smart homes" (Cowan & Turner-Smith, 1999; Tinker et al., 2004). Increasingly, smart technologies are being used to help people remain living safely and independently in their own homes. Smart technologies have the potential to decrease adverse incidents in the home and to allow health conditions to be managed at home rather than in a health setting. These technologies support people in their home environment, and the potential to save overall health care costs makes them attractive to those who fund services.

Security and home automation systems such as security cameras, automatic door openers, keyless entry, remote window and curtain opening, automated lighting sensors, etc. afford older people and people with disabilities safety and security and provide them with a means to manage services, devices, and appliances within the home environment. People can regulate the temperature, lighting, electrical outlets, air conditioning, and security of homes, and answer and open front doors through connection with intercoms via an app on their smart phone. Alarms, automated detectors (e.g., falls and seizure), and emergency call devices/systems provide people with access to assistance as required. People with complex health conditions can use devices, sensors, administration aids, and apps at home to monitor vital signs, identify changes in performance and/or behavior, and work with remote health care teams to prevent an adverse event. Medication management devices can also ensure people take their medications regularly and send alerts if medication is not taken. Reminder and scheduling technologies can also be used to prompt people through scheduled activities and specific tasks such as their self-care routine in the bathroom, cooking, and collecting the mail. A range of high- and low-technology assistive devices can also assist people in daily activities by reducing the impact of impairments and conditions/symptoms and enabling greater participation.

However, these technologies can often be costly to purchase and support. Without a significant injection of funding into the already strained reserves of in-home services, they are likely to be overshadowed by low-technology options or remain a wonderful resource that is difficult to access. When budgets are allocated and prioritized, how will intangible and client-related benefits of environmental modifications hold up against the tangible financial benefits of in-home monitoring? These technologies also raise several ethical dilemmas (Tinker, 1999). Whose needs are being met through these technologies? What is their effectiveness in reducing the cost of health care delivery? What impact will they have on the concerns of well-meaning relatives who want assurance that their elderly relative is safe? What role will they play in enabling people to stay safely in their home environment? Homes are a place of privacy, and intrusive technologies could be resented by residents and negatively affect the meaning of home (Heywood, 2004a). Furthermore, there is the possibility that people would be at risk of increased isolation if they are managed and monitored remotely. On the positive side, new communication technologies could increase compliance with drug regimens and summon help quickly if a person has fallen. They can also put older people and people with disabilities in touch with people who otherwise may be unavailable to them and provide reassurance that problems will be relayed quickly to family members or service providers who can respond. Although there are many complexities to consider with the advent of these technologies, occupational therapists are well placed to implement them effectively and balance the other needs of the householder with the potential benefits of ongoing monitoring.

In summary, a key value underpinning community care and occupational therapy services is promoting independence. However, although these services define independence as enabling people to remain living in their own homes or reducing reliance on others for daily tasks, older people and people with disabilities generally think of it in terms of personal control. Recent developments in the community care sector have provided significant impetus for the development of home modification services. Although home modification services remain relatively underdeveloped when compared with other community care services, they have been established as being a legitimate part of the repertoire of community care services designed to enable people to remain living in the community. In community care, additive, subtractive, transformative, and behavioral modifications are closely associated with maintenance and security services. Administration and coordination difficulties persist in working across health, social, and construction sectors, and good intersectoral collaboration is likely to enhance the development of high-quality modification services. An understanding of the interaction between people and their living environment allows modification interventions to be tailored to the individual's unique individual circumstances and promote his or her active participation in the home and the community.

HOUSING PERSPECTIVE

Many people make changes to their home environments quite independent of health and community care systems. It is therefore useful to examine how people use generic services to make changes to their housing, commonly known as *housing adjustments*, to meet their changing needs and preferences. Throughout life, people encounter changes that necessitate them relocating or altering their existing housing—whether it is the composition of their family and household, their health and employment status, or their interests and lifestyle. Consequently, people access a range of housing services that thrive on assisting people to accommodate changes in their circumstances. Occupational therapists often need to work with these services or work with people who use these services to address their ongoing housing needs. In addition, therapists are increasingly recognizing a role for themselves within a diversity of housing services. Consequently, developing a broader view of housing adjustments can assist therapists in understanding home modifications as part of a continuum of housing arrangements and anticipating where occupational therapy can contribute to the delivery and further development of housing services.

From a housing perspective, people alter their housing or relocate when their existing home no longer meets their changed circumstances or lifestyle or no longer reflects their tastes or projected image or identity. Though this view encompasses the notion of "accommodating a particular set of human abilities" (the health perspective; Bridge, 2005, p. 2) or "adapting living environments to increase ease of use, safety, security and independence" (the community care perspective; Pynoos et al., 1998, p. 3), it is more universal in scope in that it recognizes that people make many different types of changes to their housing throughout their lives. These changes are referred to in the housing literature as *housing adjustments* (Howe, 2003; Masnick, Will, & Baker, 2011), *housing careers* (Beer & Faulkner, 2008; Kendig, 1984), *housing pathways* (Clapham, 2005), or *housing transitions* (Beer & Faulkner, 2011). Housing decisions made in response to a health condition or changing capacities are unlikely to be made in isolation and are likely to incorporate a range of goals.

Housing adjustments were first described by Peace and Holland (2001) as the actual changes that individuals and households make to their housing in response to their particular needs, circumstances, and preferences at any point in time. *Housing careers* is a term that is used to describe the sequence of housing adjustments that an individual or household makes over a lifetime. It is recognized that widespread societal changes, including demographic changes and improvements in the standard of living, are transforming established patterns of housing careers in many countries (Beer, Faulkner, & Gabriel, 2006). Housing pathways describe the "patterns of interaction … concerning house and home, over time and space" (Clapham, 2005, p. 27). The concept of housing careers primarily focuses on changes in the consumption of housing related to factors such as age, household structure, income and wealth, employment, and disability, whereas the notion of housing pathways places emphasis on the social meanings and relationships associated with housing

(Jones et al., 2008). The pathways perspective views housing as being more than a set of physical characteristics (i.e., space, layout, condition, access, etc). It recognizes the meaning that a house might hold for the occupants, the patterns of interactions contained within it, and the lifestyle and identity the house affords its residents (Clapham, 2005). More recently, the term *housing transitions* (Beer & Faulkner, 2011) has been used to capture the fluid and complex relationship between individuals and their housing, reflecting the dynamic change that occurs throughout life and placing equal importance on patterns of housing and the subjective experience of housing.

In addition to providing shelter, home has personal, social, physical, temporal, occupational, and societal dimensions that contribute to its meaning and overall experience for individuals (Aplin, de Jonge, & Gustafsson, 2013). It should be a safe place, a refuge, and where we have autonomy and control over the use of space and time (Peace & Holland, 2001). This autonomy allows privacy and the freedom to express oneself. Central to the meaning of home are the relationships with family, friends, neighbors, and the community. It is the presence of these important people and relationships that contribute to the feeling of home (Sixsmith, 1986). It is well recognized that housing contributes significantly to quality of life (Pynoos & Regnier, 1997). The significance of the home is even greater if people have lived there for many years (Pynoos & Regnier, 1997) or if they spend a considerable amount of time at home (Newman, 2003). Increasingly, people are not just interested in finding a house. For many, the home is both emotionally and financially the single biggest investment they make in their lives (Hanson, 2001). Consequently, many seek a community that offers them a distinctive mode of living or a particular lifestyle that enables them to express and define their identity (Clapham, 2005).

Focus of the Housing Perspective

The housing perspective provides a number of distinctive insights into housing decisions that have implications for development and delivery of home modification services. First, people use a broad range of strategies when addressing housing concerns. When making housing adjustments, some have a strong preference to remain living in their own home (Peace & Holland, 2001) and current community (Wiles, Leibing, Guberman, Reeve, & Allen, 2012), whereas others are willing to relocate in response to changes in their needs and preferences (Heywood et al., 2002; Perry, 2012; Stone, 1998). Although home modification services are recognized as assisting people to adapt their homes to their changed circumstances (Tinker, 1999), there are some who are clearly better served by relocating to more suitable accommodations. It is important to recognize that housing adjustment, although common in the general community, is not widely recognized or supported in health and community care services except in determining when someone needs to move into supported accommodations. Many modification services tend to assume that people intend to or should remain in the current home and leave people to make decisions themselves about relocating and downsizing. Many people live in homes that constantly challenge their safety and independence and require a great deal of upkeep (Tinker, 1999). A home that was once a "castle" and a reflection of a person's identity and status in the community can become a "cage" or millstone, undermining identity and restricting freedom and lifestyle (Heywood et al., 2002). Little support is offered to people with the often overwhelming and complex task of making a housing adjustment, and the emotional component of relocation is often neglected (Perry, 2012). Although people who have made many moves during their lives are well placed to deal with the financial, legal, and real estate complexities they are likely to encounter, many are not sufficiently experienced or informed to successfully navigate these systems. Services with a housing perspective could provide an important way of enhancing the range of options available to people to make housing adjustments and "enable people to take control of their pathway through the ability to make choices" (Clapham, 2005, p. 234). These services could also manage the complex systems involved in moving house for people with low incomes or limited skills or capacities.

Second, the housing perspective has also highlighted that people seek housing that reflects their identity and lifestyle aspirations. Very few people consider themselves to be "old" (Wylde, 1998), and even fewer regard themselves as "disabled" (Heywood et al., 2002; Wylde, 1998). Consequently, housing decisions are likely to be shaped by identity and lifestyle choice rather than perceptions of functional need. The health and community care approaches tend to favor professionally defined concepts of functional need, where services are provided to people; consequently, they are unlikely to acknowledge people's lifestyle and identity aspirations (Clapham, 2005). Concern has been raised about the negative impacts of home modifications on the meaning of home and the lack of attention to this dimension by home modification services (Messecar, Archbold, Stewart, & Kirschling, 2002). Adaptations to the home can have a negative

impact on routines, self-image, connection with the home, and a sense of heritage (Heywood, 2005). Modifications can result in people being viewed as different and, of greater concern, can make them vulnerable to ridicule or violence (Fisher, 1998). For example, a person may be willing to put a grab bar in his or her own private bathroom adjoining the bedroom but not in another bathroom that might be used by guests, where it would bring attention to the disability and change the decor of their living space. This underscores the importance not only of choice, but also of identifying home modifications that are attractive and acceptable. When making changes in the home, it is essential that all aspects of the home environment be considered rather than focusing solely on the performance of specific self-care tasks (Heywood, 2005). Acceptance of interventions, such as assistive devices, has been shown repeatedly to be influenced by whether they support or undermine the older person's sense of personal identity (Harrison, 2004). Householders have been found to reject modification services if their perspectives and priorities differ from that of service providers (Gitlin, Luborsky, & Schemm, 1998) or if they anticipate that the changes will affect their sense of independence and autonomy (Messecar et al., 2002).

Third, when building or remodeling housing, there are opportunities to plan ahead to pay particular attention to areas such as entrances, pathways, lighting, kitchens, and bathrooms. This is an ideal time to bring together occupational therapists, remodelers, architects, and interior designers to work as a team to help people plan ahead in terms of thinking about aging in place and adding features that might help them stay in their homes. For example, when remodeling, a resident could install a zero-step entrance, install a walk-in or roll-in shower instead of a conventional bath or shower/bath combination, and fit cabinets in the kitchen that are within easy reach or provide somewhere to sit down to prepare food. These types of features might be found in a universally designed house but can be incorporated into existing homes as well. In addition, rather than considering the dwelling's suitability solely for the resident, it should be seen as a place where others of varying abilities visit. This aspect incorporates the communal nature of housing and underlies the charter of the visitability movement, which has made advances in both England and, to a lesser extent, the United States.

Key Stakeholder Roles and Perspectives

Although involved in both health and community care approaches to home modifications, building and design professionals are central to the housing perspective. Their services are essential when considering the remodeling of a home, undertaking major renovations, or constructing a new dwelling. It is important when working with building or design professionals that occupational therapists understand that all professions have an embedded culture, which includes the norms, values, beliefs, traditional knowledge, skills, and core practices that guide and shape professional behavior and identity (Watson, 2006). It is into this culture that new professionals are socialized through education, training, and work experiences. Understanding the cultural orientation of a profession is important in understanding how professional reasoning and decision making occur.

The building profession has a culture that is strongly embedded in a regulatory environment. It is an industry that is prescribed, regulated, and inspected—and rightly so, given the issues of safety that are involved. This perspective is extremely valuable to home modification services delivery because the building professional is able to advise what is possible and not possible in accordance with various codes and regulations within a home environment. The downside of this, however, is that standard responses to an individual's needs can become entrenched, and documents such as public access standards can be given a higher priority than is practicable or advisable in a unique and dynamic individual situation (Pynoos et al., 2002).

Accessibility codes are typically designed to determine minimal legal guidelines for public access and have a stereotypical view of the end user (e.g., a user of a wheelchair). They have very little to do with the needs, aspirations, desires, and uniqueness of a particular individual and do not cater to the many variations of individual functioning of people who have a disability (Danford & Steinfeld, 1999; Imrie & Hall, 2001). For example, current public access standards in many countries are not based on research for older people, and the assumption that designing for wheelchair use will also meet the needs of an older person with a range of mobility requirements is an untested hypothesis that has not been evidenced in research. In fact, research in the United States has shown that some modifications to the existing accessible standards "may promote more disability among older adults than it ameliorates" (Pynoos et al., 2002, p. 16).

Architectural or technical aspects are emphasized by building professionals, with the home dwelling considered a "piece of hardware" and the personal and social aspects of home disregarded (Imrie, 2006, p. 14). In this way, technical knowledge dominates the construction professional's decision making and actions. Many building professionals have time and money constraints and can be financially vulnerable, particularly if they are subcontractors. Tradition also plays a strong role in the builders' work, with many being resistant to changing the way they do their work (Burns, 2004).

Current literature suggests that the construction industry in many countries does not respond well to the needs of people with a disability and that formal education of building professionals on the needs of people with a disability is "more or less non-existent" (Burns, 2004; Imrie, 2006; Imrie & Hall, 2001, p. 6). Imrie and Hall assert that "inattentiveness to and exclusion of the needs (of people with a disability) are evident at all stages of the design and development of the built environment" (2001, p. 6). The house building industry has been characterized by a lack of innovation and a "poorly developed sense of customer focus when compared to other service sectors" (Burns, 2004, p. 768). This lack of interest or willingness to be innovative has resulted in a standardization of house design where "certain household types and certain bodies are targeted" (Burns, 2004, p. 769). The drive for standardization has been linked to the rise of large-scale corporate property development in which standardized fittings and fixtures are commonplace and the construction "revolves around industry standards, which are inattentive to bodily diversity or differences" (Imrie & Hall, 2006, p. 9). Older people and people with a disability often have requirements that are not met by standard housing designs and thus provide builders with challenges to their traditional designs and techniques (Burns, 2004).

Within the professional culture of the design professions, such as architecture or interior design, designing for the needs of people with a disability has not been a significant feature of design theory or a major part of the design and development process (Goldsmith, 1997; Imrie & Hall, 2001; Liebermann, 2013). The focus of the design process tends to be aesthetics and technical cleverness more than the user or functionality of the building (Goldsmith, 1997), with "the concern of the decorative and the ornamental" remaining a "powerful part of the design professions" (Imrie & Hall, 2001, p. 12). Where the needs of people with a disability have been incorporated into a project, "there is the tendency to reduce disability to a singular form of mobility impairment, that of the wheelchair user" (Imrie & Hall, p. 10; Liebermann, 2013).

Within the architectural profession, there have been, and continue to be, challenges to the dominant design culture. Imrie and Hall (2001) use the terms *social architecture* and *social design* to describe a trend that proposed to "recognize the multiplicity of needs of building users" and the need to accommodate them in building projects (p. 12). This movement has sought to recenter the design process on the user of the building and to incorporate a broader and more holistic understanding of the needs of users of the buildings. The core values of social design align with environmental and social justice and human rights; however, Imrie and Hall report that the movement has had little impact on the thinking of the design professions in relation to people with a disability.

Inclusive design and universal design are similarly social movements that have gained prominence in both the United Kingdom and the United States. Inclusive design, like the social design movement, is concerned with the "sustainability, flexibility and adaptability" of buildings to accommodate the diversity of building users, placing the user of the building in the center of the design process (Milner & Madigan, 2004, p. 734). Universal design is concerned with making products and environments as usable as possible to the broadest range of users. Applied to housing, universal design far exceeds the minimum specification of access standards, seeking to create homes that are "useable by and marketable to people of all ages and abilities" (Mace, 1998, p. 22). This type of design process is in contrast to the compensatory approach in which elements of accessibility are added on to previously inaccessible or standard designs (Imrie & Hall, 2001). Although universal design has been widely accepted and is endorsed by global agencies such as the WHO and United Nations (Imrie, 2012), it is "yet to make an impact on mainstream architectural practice" (Liebermann, 2013, p. 14).

Though professional orientation and culture differ between building and health professionals, they are complementary, and consideration of each stakeholder's perspective is important in establishing good communication, understanding, and effective outcomes. Clear and ongoing communication is the best strategy to facilitate a good working arrangement. It is helpful for the therapist to have a basic understanding of building terminology to be able to understand to some extent the construction issues involved with the modification process. Asking questions and getting clarification are important. Often, therapists need to work through alternative solutions on site with the building professional so that they can fully understand the regulatory requirements and engage in problem solving to explore how performance requirements might be met differently. Therapists also need to communicate their recommendations clearly, both when speaking and writing.

The therapist also has a responsibility to ensure that the individual and his or her needs remain the focus of the work carried out. The therapist needs to ensure that the individual, as the expert of his or her life, is recognized and that his or her thoughts, ideas, and wishes are not overwhelmed by the technical discourse of the building and design professional.

Although there is excellent scope for collaboration, differences in professional culture can also lead to situations of conflict, and good conflict resolution skills are an important part of the occupational therapist's repertoire. Assertive communication that provides, in plain language, the professional reasoning that informs the opinions and decisions regarding occupational therapist recommendations is essential to ensure good understanding and communication.

In summary, from a housing perspective, people make adjustments to their housing throughout life in response to their changing circumstances. These adjustments can include making changes to the current dwelling or seeking alternative living environments. Increasingly, housing decisions are shaped by a quest for a particular lifestyle that allows people to express and define their identity. This perspective alerts occupational therapists to the need to consider people's housing concerns more broadly, to ensure that they are afforded adequate choice, and to ensure that they are provided with sufficient information and support that reflects their housing needs and preferences into the future. Furthermore, it reminds the profession to recognize people's aspirations and the personal nature of the home environment when undertaking modifications.

FUTURE CHALLENGES FOR HOME MODIFICATION SERVICE DELIVERY

Strategic Policy Direction

Awareness of the benefits of home modifications has been increasing; however, there are still significant challenges to the viability and usefulness of home modification service delivery. Emphasis at a legislative and strategic policy level is on implementing change in new construction, as seen by the increase in visibility legislation in most developed countries. Although moves toward inclusive and universal design are gaining momentum at an international level, significant issues still face those living in existing inaccessible and unsafe housing.

At a strategic policy level, there is a need for greater recognition of the importance of home modification to community living for people with a disability and for our increasingly aging population. In many countries, home modification services are intrinsically linked to health and community care policy areas. A report from the Office for Disability Issues in the United Kingdom (Heywood & Turner, 2007) highlighted four main ways in which the provision of housing modifications and equipment produces savings to health and social care budgets. These were savings in the cost of residential care through enabling people to remain in their homes and reducing the cost and need for in-home care services; savings through the prevention of accidents with associated high costs of hospital and residential care admissions; savings through prevention of waste brought about because of underfunding of modification services, which resulted in delays in implementation and provision of inadequate or ineffectual solutions; and, finally, savings through achieving better outcomes for the same expenditure by improving the quality of life of recipients and caregivers and family members (Heywood & Turner, 2007). Though the report found evidence of the preventive and therapeutic role of home modifications, it also highlighted the ongoing issue of underfunding for home modifications and increasingly restrictive eligibility criteria related to this, reducing the availability of home modifications to many people who would benefit (Heywood & Turner, 2007).

As indicated previously, Jones et al. (2008) believe that there is a strong case for reconsidering the current approach to the organization of home modification services and suggest that the future of home modification service delivery may lie in the recognition that home modification services are a major contributor to the housing policy area, rather than being seen primarily under the banner of health and community care policy areas. Aligning home modification services with strategic housing policy links the home modification service to the areas of accessible and inclusive housing and national strategies for housing, while still maintaining links to the health and community sectors (Jones et al., 2008). In this way, strategic policy direction that provides a coordinated funded service delivery response across public and private housing and also links housing into health and aged care services may be more achievable.

Service Design and Delivery Direction

At a service level in the United States and Australia, many of the issues facing home modification service delivery today were being raised more than a decade ago. First, although there is an increase in the organizations and programs funded to provide home modification services, there is a lack of a systematic approach to the organization of such services, with limited policy development, few benchmarks for service delivery, and great disparities in the level of service provision (Jones et al., 2008; Pynoos et al., 1998; Sorenson, 2012). Resourcing is considered to be insufficient to meet demand, and lack of funding results in delays in work being carried out (Jones et al., 2008; Pynoos et al., 1998). Services and service recipients are often overwhelmed by the cumulative impact of numerous building, health, disability, and legal requirements (Awang, 2002; Jones et al., 2008; Sakellariou, 2015), which are in themselves barriers to accessing and delivering an effective home modification service.

Although levels of expertise have developed over the past decade, there are still shortages in skilled professionals from both the health and construction sectors that contribute to delays in service provision (Sorenson, 2012). A lack of awareness about the advantages of home modification continues to exist within both the community and service sectors, resulting in unreliable referral processes (Jones et al., 2008; Pynoos et al., 1998).

Though many issues exist, research has shown overwhelmingly that home modification services are well received, and positive outcomes such as improved independence, heightened confidence and well-being, greater security, prevention of accidents, and improved quality of life are generally reported (Heywood & Turner, 2007; Jones et al., 2008; Keall et al., 2015; Petersson et al., 2008). There is, however, a clear need for the continued development of a research evidence base to underpin home modification services development and delivery, particularly in the areas of the need and demand for home modification services; the outcome and cost-effectiveness of home modification as an intervention; and the identification of particular factors that affect service provision and outcomes, including the supply of expert professionals (Heywood & Turner, 2007; Jones et al., 2008).

Implications for the Occupational Therapist

Involvement with home modification services delivery presents new challenges to occupational therapists, both in the knowledge base they need to acquire and in the professional sectors with whom they collaborate. Effective home modification service delivery relies on ensuring that the individual and his or her unique and particular needs remain central to the assessment and decision-making process, and the occupational therapist has a key role in ensuring that this occurs.

Although the focus of occupational therapy has traditionally been on the individual receiving his or her service, therapists are increasingly being challenged to step outside of their conventional clinical roles and become involved in home modification service delivery as agents of change. First and foremost, occupational therapists are well placed to observe the effect of policy and procedural issues on individual service delivery. Poor communication and information about home modification service delivery and complex application procedures and forms are key barriers to effective home modification service delivery against which therapists can advocate for change. Establishing and undertaking formal evaluation processes, seeking and recording individual client feedback, and providing reports of concerns to the relevant people within organizational structures are all strategies that can be undertaken by individual therapists.

A lack of awareness of the benefits of home modifications is another identified barrier that occupational therapists can assist in addressing. Therapists can play a key role in the education of both community and service sectors regarding the benefits of home modification through both formal presentations about the home modification service to client and referral agencies and through informal professional networking.

Building an evidence base for intervention in this area is also an important role for the profession. Quality research into the outcomes of home modifications from the perspective of the home dweller and evaluating the effectiveness of home modification service delivery are areas that occupational therapists are well equipped to address. Engaging in formal evaluation of environmental interventions can yield important data that can be formulated into reports, publications, or professional presentations. Linking with agencies or institutions that may be interested in undertaking formal research, such as universities, is also advantageous for therapists in terms of professional development, as well as building a much-needed evidence base for practice.

CONCLUSION

Recent demographic, legislative, policy, and service developments have resulted in a range of services being created to promote people's safety, health, independence, and well-being in the home environment. Occupational therapists have an important contribution to make in enabling people to live well in the home and community and need to work effectively within and across health, community care, and housing systems to achieve good outcomes for their clients. Home modification services developed in the health care system are primarily concerned with ensuring safety and enabling independence through the use of minor or nonstructural modifications. Health-based services perceive the home as a physical entity that needs to be modified to accommodate functional deficits, and in so doing, therapists can overlook the long-term suitability of a residence; the social acceptability of modifications; and issues of identity, meaning, and lifestyle when designing interventions. Therapists working in this context need to be mindful of the personal, temporal, social, and cultural nature of the home environment when addressing physical aspects of the environment.

Within community care services, behavioral, nonstructural, and structural modifications are used in conjunction with a range of other services to support people to live safely and independently in the community. An understanding of the interaction between the person and his or her living environment allows modification interventions to be tailored to the individual's unique circumstances and promote his or her active participation in the home and the community. Therapists working in community care settings need to work across health, social, and construction sectors to develop good intersectoral collaboration and enhance the development of quality modification services.

Services developed within the housing sector acknowledge that people make adjustments to their housing throughout life in response to their changing circumstances. Within this sector, modifications are seen as part of a continuum of adjustments, which can also include seeking an alternative living environment that better suits the individual's identity and lifestyle aspirations. Within this perspective, occupational therapists are encouraged to consider people's broader housing concerns, to provide clients with sufficient information and support when making adjustments, and to help clients think ahead in terms of the suitability of modifications to help them age in place.

Clients are likely to be seeking to maintain their safety, health, and well-being as well as their identity and lifestyle within the home and community, regardless of where they access home modification services. Therapists need to be aware of the context in which they work, the way this can shape their service delivery, and the importance of extending their service to acknowledge clients' broader needs or referring them to a service that is better suited to addressing their needs. Furthermore, professionals such as occupational therapists and the organizations that represent them have an important role to play in improving the policies that affect their practice and the lives of the clients they serve.

REFERENCES

Aged and Community Services Australia. (2015). The future of housing for older Australians: Position paper, January 2015. Retrieved from http://www.acsa.asn.au/getattachment/Publications-Submissions/Submissions/2015-submissions/ACSA-Housing-Position-Paper-January-2015-1.pdf.aspx?lang=en-AU

Americans With Disabilities Act. (1990). ADA home page. Retrieved from http://www.usdoj.gov/crt/ada/adahom1.htm

Anderberg, P. (2009). Academic Network of European Disability experts (ANED) country report on the implementation of policies supporting independent living for disabled people: Sweden. Retrieved from http://www.disability-europe.net/content/aned/media/SE-6-Request-07%20ANED%20Task%205%20Independent%20Living%20Report%20Sweden_to%20publish_to%20EC.pdf

Aplin, T., de Jonge D., & Gustafsson, L. (2013). Understanding the dimensions of home that impact on home modification decision making. *Australian Occupational Therapy Journal, 60*, 101-109.

Aplin, T., de Jonge D., & Gustafsson, L. (2015). Understanding home modifications impact on clients and their family's experience of home: A qualitative study. *Australian Occupational Therapy Journal, 62*, 123-131.

Auriemma, D., Faust, S., Sibrian, K., & Jimenez, J. (1999). Home modifications for the elderly: Implications for the occupational therapist. *Physical and Occupational Therapy in Geriatrics, 16*(2-4), 135-144.

Australian Bureau of Statistics. (2013). Disability, ageing and carers, Australia: Summary of findings, 2012. (Cat. No. 4430.0). Retrieved from http://www.abs.gov.au/ausstats/abs@.nsf/Lookup/4430.0main+features12012

Australian Bureau of Statistics. (2015). Disability, ageing and carers, Australia: First results. Retrieved from http://www.abs.gov.au/ausstats/abs@.nsf/productsbytopic/56C41FE7A67110C8CA257FA3001D080B?OpenDocument

Awang, D. (2002). Older people and participation within disabled facilities grant processes. *British Journal of Occupational Therapy, 65*(6), 261-268.

Beer, A., & Faulkner, D. R. (2008). The housing careers of people with a disability and carers of people with a disability. Australian Housing and Urban Research Institute. Retrieved from www.ahuri.edu.au/research/research-papers/the-housing-careers-of-people-with-a-disability-and-carers-of-people-with-a-disability

Beer, A., & Faulkner, D. (2011). *Housing transitions through the life course: Aspirations, needs and policy.* Bristol, UK: Policy Press.

Beer, A., Faulkner, D., & Gabriel, M. (2006). *21st century housing careers and Australia's housing future: Literature review.* Melbourne, Australia: Australian Housing and Urban Research Institute. Retrieved from https://www.ahuri.edu.au/research/final-reports/128

Bridge, C. (2005). Retrofitting, a response to lack of diversity: An analysis of community provider data. Paper presented at National Housing Conference October 2005, Perth, Western Australia.

Bridge, C., Parsons, A., Quine, S., & Kendig, H. (2002). *Housing and care for older and younger adults with disabilities: Positioning paper.* Melbourne, Australia: Australian Housing and Urban Research Institute. Retrieved from https://www.ahuri.edu.au/research/position-papers/23

Burns, N. (2004). Negotiating difference: Disabled people's experiences of house builders. *Housing Studies, 19*(5), 765-780.

Clapham, D. (2005). *The meaning of housing.* Bristol, UK: Policy Press.

Clemson, L., Roland, M., & Cumming, R. G. (1997). Types of hazards in the homes of elderly people. *Occupational Therapy Journal of Research, 17*(3), 200-213.

Close, J., Ellis, M., Hooper, R., Glucksman, E., Jackson, S., & Swift, C. (1999). Prevention of falls in the elderly trial (PROFET): A randomised controlled trial. *Lancet, 353*(9147), 93-97.

Clough, R., Leamy, M., Miller, V., & Bright, L. (2004). *Housing decisions in later life.* New York: Palgrave Macmillan.

Colombo, M., Vitali, S., Molla, G., Gioia, P., & Milani, M. (1998). The home environment modification program in the care of demented elderly: Some examples. *Archives of Gerontology and Geriatrics, 27*(6), 83-90.

Communities & Local Government. (2009). English housing condition survey: 2007. UK Data Archive Study No: 6449. Retrieved from www.communities.gov.uk

Courtney-Long, E., Carroll, D., Zhang, Q, Stevens, A., Griffin-Blake, S., Armour, B. & Campbell, V. (2015). Prevalence of disability and disability types among adults—United States, 2013. *MMWR, 64*(29),776-783. Retrieved from https://www.cdc.gov/mmWR/preview/mmwrhtml/mm6429a2.htm

Cowan, D., & Turner-Smith, A. (1999). *The role of assistive technology in alternative models of care for older people.* London: The Royal Commission on Long Term Care.

Cumming, R. G., Thomas, M., Szonyi, G., Salkeld, G., O' Neill, E., & Westbury, C. (1999). Home visits by an occupational therapist for assessment and modification of environmental hazards: A randomized trial of falls prevention. *Journal of American Geriatric Society, 47*(12), 1397-1402.

Danford, G. S., & Steinfeld, E. (1999). Measuring the influences of physical environments on the behaviours of people with impairments. In E. Steinfeld & G. S. Danford (Eds.), *Enabling environments: Measuring the impact of environment on disability and rehabilitation* (pp. 111-137). New York: Plenum Publishers.

Dovey, K. (1985). Home and homelessness. In I. Altman & C. M. Werner (Eds.), *Home environments* (vol. 8, pp. 33-61). New York: Plenum Press.

Duncan, R. (1998a). Blueprint for action: The National Home Modifications Action Coalition. *Technology and Disability, 8*(1-2), 85-89.

Duncan, R. (1998b). Funding, financing and other resources for home modifications. *Technology and Disability, 8*, 37-50.

Fair Housing Amendments Act. (1968). FHEO programs. Retrieved from http://www.hud.gov/offices/fheo/progdesc/title8.cfm

Faulkner, D., & Bennett, K. (2002). *Linkages among housing assistance, residential (Re), location and the use of community health and social care by old-old adults: Shelter and non-shelter implications for housing policy development.* Melbourne, Australia: Australian Housing and Urban Research Institute. Retrieved from https://www.ahuri.edu.au/research/final-reports/13

Fisher, A. G. (1998). Uniting practice and theory in an occupational framework. *American Journal of Occupational Therapy, 52*(7), 509-520.

Frain, J. P., & Carr, P. H. (1996). Is the typical modern house designed for future adaptation for disabled older people? *Age and Ageing, 25*(5), 398.

Freedman, V. A. (2007). Demographic reflections on the aging baby boom and its implications for health care (commentary). In K. Warner Schaie & P. Uhlenberg (Eds.), *Social structures: Demographic changes and the well-being of older persons* (pp. 80-90). New York: Springer Publishing Company.

Freedman, V. A., Spillman, B. C., Andreski, P. M., Cornman, J. C., Crimmins, E. M., Kramarow, E., . . . Waidmann, T. A. (2013). Trends in late like activity limitations in the United States: An update from five national surveys. *Demography, 50*(2), 661-671.

Gillespie, L. D., Gillespie, W. J., Cumming, R. G., Lamb, S. H., & Rower, B. H. (2001). Interventions for preventing falls in the elderly. *Cochrane Database Systematic Review, 3*, CD000340.

Gillespie, L. D., Robertson, M. C., Gillespie, W. J., Sherrington, C., Gates, S., Clemson, L. M., & Lamb, S. E. (2012). Interventions for preventing falls in older people living in the community. *Cochrane Database Systematic Review, 9*, CD007146.

Giovannetti, T., Magouirk-Bettcher, B., Libon, D., Brennan, L., Sestito, N., & Kessler, R. (2007). Environmental adaptations improve everyday action performance in Alzheimer's disease: Empirical support from performance-based assessment. *Neuropsychology, 21*(4), 448-457.

Gitlin, L. N. (2003). Next steps in home modifications and assistive technology research. In N. Charness & K. W. Schaie (Eds.), *Impact of technology on successful aging* (pp. 188-202). New York: Springer.

Gitlin, L. N., & Corcoran, M. (2000). Making home safer: Environmental adaptations for people with dementia. *Alzheimer Care Quarterly, 1*(1), 50-58.

Gitlin, L. N., Luborsky, M. R., & Schemm, R. L. (1998). Emerging concerns of older stroke patients about assistive devices. *The Gerontologist, 38*(2), 169-180.

Gitlin, L. N., Miller, K. S., & Boyce, A. (1999). Bathroom modifications for frail elderly renters: Outcomes of a community-based program. *Technology and Disability, 10*(3), 141-149.

Goldsmith, S. (1997). *Designing for the disabled: The new paradigm*. London: Architectural Press.

Gosselin, C., Robitaille, Y., Trickey, F., & Maltais, D. (1993). Factors predicting the implementation of home modifications among elderly people with loss of independence. *Physical and Occupational Therapy in Geriatrics, 12*(1), 15-27.

Granbom, M., Löfqvist, C., Horstmann, M., Haak, M., & Iwarsson, S. (2014). Relocation to ordinary or special housing in very old age: Aspects of housing and health. *European Journal of Ageing, 11*, 55-65.

Hanson, J. (2001). From "special needs" to "lifestyle choices": Articulating the demand for "third age" housing. In S. Peace & C. Holland (Eds.), *Inclusive housing in an ageing society* (pp. 29-54). Bristol, UK: Policy Press.

Harrison, M. (2004). Defining housing quality and environment: Disability, standards and social factors. *Housing Studies, 19*(5), 691-708.

Heywood, F. (2004a). The health outcomes of housing adaptations. *Disability and Society, 19*(2), 129-143.

Heywood, F. (2004b). Understanding needs: A starting point for quality. *Housing Studies, 19*(5), 709-726.

Heywood, F. (2005). Adaptation: Altering the house to restore the home. *Housing Studies, 20*(4), 531-547.

Heywood, F., Oldman, C., & Means, R. (2002). *Housing and home in later life*. Buckingham, UK: Open University Press.

Heywood, F., & Turner, L. (2007). *Better outcomes, lower costs: Implications for health and social care budgets of investment in housing adaptations, improvements and equipment: A review of the evidence*. Norwich, UK: Office of Disability Issues, Department for Work and Pensions. Retrieved from http://www.wohnenimalter.ch/img/pdf/better_outcomes_report.pdf

Howe, A. (2003). *Housing an older Australia: More of the same or something different? Keynote address*. Melbourne, Australia: Australian Housing and Urban Research Institute. Retrieved from http://ahuri.ddsn.net/downloads/2003_Events/HFAA/Anna_Howe_keynote.pdf

Imrie, R. (2006). *Accessible housing: Quality, disability and design*. London: Routledge.

Imrie, R. (2012). Universalism, universal design and equitable access to the built environment. *Disability and Rehabilitation, 34*(10), 873-882.

Imrie, R., & Hall P. (2001). *Inclusive design: Designing and developing accessible environments*. London, UK: Spon Press.

Johansson, K., Borell, L., & Lilja, M. (2009). Older persons' navigation through the service system towards home modification resources. *Scandinavian Journal of Occupational Therapy, 16*, 227-237.

Johnson, R., & Wiener, J. (2006). *Profile of frail older Americans and their caregivers (The Retirement Project, Occasional Paper Number 8)*. Washington, DC: The Urban Institute. Retrieved from http:// www.urban.org/UploadedPDF/311284_older_americans.pdf

Jones, A., de Jonge, D., & Phillips, R. (2008). *The impact of home maintenance and modification services on health, community care and housing outcomes in later life: Positioning paper*. Melbourne, Australia: Australian Housing and Urban Research Institute. Retrieved from https://www.ahuri.edu.au/__data/assets/pdf_file/0022/2893/AHURI_Positioning_Paper_No103-The-impact-of-home-maintenance-and-modification-services-on-health.pdf

Keall, M., Baker, M., Howden-Chapman, P., & Cunningham, M. (2008). Association between the number of home injury hazards and home injury. *Accident Analysis and Prevention, 40*, 887-893.

Keall, M., Pierse, N., Howden-Chapman, P., Cunningham, C., Cunningham, M., Guria, J., & Baker, M. (2015). Home modifications to reduce injuries from falls in the Home Injury Prevention Intervention (HIPI) study: A cluster-randomised controlled trial. *Lancet, 385*, 231-238.

Kendig, H. (1984). Housing careers, life cycle and residential mobility: Implications for the housing market. *Urban Studies, 21*(3), 271-283.

Kim, H., Ahn, Y., Steinhoff, A., & Lee, K. (2014). Home modification by older adults and their informal caregivers. *Archives of Gerontology and Geriatrics, 59*, 648-656.

Klein, S. I., Rosage, L., & Shaw, G. (1999). The role of occupational therapists in home modification programs at an area agency on aging. *Physical and Occupational Therapy in Geriatrics, 16*(3-4), 19-37.

Lannin, N., Clemson, L., & McCluskey, A. (2011). Survey of current pre-discharge home visiting practices of occupational therapists. *Australian Occupational Therapy Journal, 58*, 172-177.

Lawton, M. P., & Nahemow, L. (1973). Ecology and the aging process. In C. Eisdorfer & M. P. Lawton (Eds.), *Psychology of adult development and aging* (pp. 619-674). Washington, DC: American Psychological Association.

Liebermann, W. (2013). Crossing the threshold: Problems and prospects for accessible design. *Joint Centre for Housing Studies, Harvard University*. Retrieved from http://www.jchs.harvard.edu/research/publications/crossing-threshold-problems-and-prospects-accessible-housing-design

Lilja, M., Mansson, I., Jahlenius, L., & Sacco-Peterson, M. (2003). Disability policy in Sweden: Policies concerning assistive technology and home modification services. *Journal of Disability Policy Studies, 14*(3), 130-135.

Lipman B., Lubell J., & Salomon E. (2012). *Housing an aging population: Are we prepared?* Washington DC: Center for Housing Policy. Retrieved from http://www.nhc.org/media/files/AgingReport2012.pdf

Mace, R. L. (1998). Universal design in housing. *Assistive Technology, 10*, 21-28.

Mann, W. C., Hurren, D., Tomita, M., Bengali, M., & Steinfeld, E. (1994). Environmental problems in homes of elders with disabilities. *The Occupational Therapy Journal of Research, 14*(3), 191-211.

Mann, W. C., Ottenbacher, K. J., Fraas, L., Tomita, M., & Granger, C. V. (1999). Effectiveness of assistive technology and environmental interventions in maintaining and reducing home care costs for the frail elderly: A randomized control trial. *Archives of Family Medicine, 8*, 210-217.

Masnick, G. S., Will, A., & Baker, K. (2011). *Housing turnover by older owners: Implications for home improvement spending as baby boomers age into retirement.* Cambridge, MA: Joint Center for Housing Studies of Harvard University.

Messecar, D. C., Archbold, P. G., Stewart, B. J., & Kirschling, J. (2002). Home environmental modification strategies used by caregivers of elders. *Research in Nursing and Health, 25*, 357-370.

Milner, J. & Madigan, R. (2004). Regulation and innovation: rethinking 'inclusive' housing design. *Housing Studies, 19*(5), 727-744.

National Institute on Aging. (2006). Dramatic changes in U.S. aging highlighted in new census, NIH report: Impact of baby boomers anticipated. Retrieved from http://www.nia.nih.gov/NewsAndEvents/PressReleases/PR2006030965PlusReport.htm

Newman, S. (2003). The living conditions of elderly Americans. *The Gerontologist, 43*(1), 99-109.

Nikolaus, T., & Bach, M. (2003). Preventing falls in community-dwelling frail older people using a home intervention team. *Journal of the American Geriatric Society, 51*, 300-305.

Nishita, C. M., Liebig, P. S., Pynoos, J., Perelman, L., & Spegal, K. (2007). Promoting basic accessibility in the home: Analysing patterns in the diffusion of visibility legislation. *Journal of Disability Policy Studies, 18*(1), 2-13.

Oldman, C., & Beresford, B. (2000). Home sick home: Using housing experiences of disabled children to suggest a new theoretical framework. *Housing Studies, 15*(3), 429-442.

Papworth Trust. (2016). Disability in the United Kingdom: 2016. Retrieved from http://www.papworthtrust.org.uk/

Peace, S. M., & Holland, C. (2001). *Inclusive housing in an ageing society: Innovative approaches.* Bristol, UK: Policy Press.

Perry, T. (2012). Leaving home later in life: Voluntary housing transitions of older adults as gift giving practices in the Midwestern United States (Doctoral dissertation). Retrieved from https://deepblue.lib.umich.edu/bitstream/handle/2027.42/96022/teperry_1.pdf?sequence=1&isAllowed=y

Petersson, I., Lilja, M., Hammel, J., & Kottorp, A. (2008). Impact of home modifications on ability in everyday life for people ageing with disabilities. *Journal of Rehabilitation Medicine, 40*, 253-260.

Pickering, C., & Pain, H. (2003). Home adaptations: User perspectives on the role of professionals. *British Journal of Occupational Therapy, 66*(1), 2-8.

Plassman, B. L., Langa, K. M., Fisher, G. G., Heeringa, S. G., Weir, D. R., Ofstedal, M. B., . . . Wallace, R. B. (2007). Prevalence of dementia in the United States: The aging, demographics, and memory study. *Neuroepidemiology, 29*, 125-132.

Pynoos, J. (2001). *Meeting the needs of older people to age in place: Findings and recommendations for action.* San Diego, CA: The National Resource Center for Supportive Housing and Home Modification.

Pynoos, J. (2004). On the forefront of the ever-changing field of home modification. *Rehabilitation Management, 17*(3), 34, 35, 50.

Pynoos, J., Liebig, P., Alley, D., & Nishita, C. M. (2004). Homes of choice: Towards more effective linkages between housing and services. *Journal of Housing for the Elderly, 18*(3-4), 5-39.

Pynoos, J., & Nishita, C. M. (2003). The cost and financing of home modifications in the United States. *Journal of Disability Policy Studies, 14*(2), 68-73.

Pynoos, J., Nishita, C. M., Cicero, C., & Caraviello, R. (2008). Aging in place, housing and the law. *The Elder Law Journal, 16*(1), 77-105.

Pynoos, J., Nishita, C., & Perelman, L. (2003). Advancements in the home modification field: A tribute to M. Powell Lawton. *Journal of Housing for the Elderly, 17*(1&2), 105-116.

Pynoos, J., & Regnier, V. (1997). Design directives in home adaptation. In S. Lanspery & J. Hyde (Eds.), *Staying put: Adapting the places instead of the people* (pp. 41-54). Amityville, NY: Baywood.

Pynoos, J., Sanford, J. A., & Rosenfelt, T. (2002). A team approach to home modifications. *OT Practice, 8*, 15-19.

Pynoos, J., Steinman, B., Nguyen, A., & Bressette, M. (2012). Assessing and adapting the home environment to reduce falls and meet the changing capacity of older adults. *Journal of Housing for the Elderly, 26*(1-3), 137-155.

Pynoos, J., Tabbarah, M., Angelelli, J., & Demiere, M. (1998). Improving the delivery of home modifications. *Technology and Disability, 8*, 3-14.

Renforth, P., Yapa, R. S., & Forster, D. P. (2004). Occupational therapy predischarge home visits: A study from a community hospital. *British Journal of Occupational Therapy, 67*(11), 488-494.

Rogers, M. E., Rogers, N. L., Takeshima, N., & Mohammod, M. I. (2004). Reducing the risk for falls in the homes of older adults. *Journal of Housing for the Elderly, 18*(2), 29-39.

Rojo-Perez, F., Fernandez-Mayoralas, G., Pozo-Rivera, F. E., & Rojo-Abuin, J. M. (2001). Ageing in place: Predictors of the residential satisfaction of the elderly. *Social Indicators Research, 54*(2), 173-208.

Rooney, C., Hadjri, K., Rooney, M., Faith, V., McAllister, K., & Craig C. (2016). Meeting the needs of visually impaired people living in Lifetime Homes. *Journal of Housing for the Elderly, 30*(2), 123-140.

Rousseau, J., Potvin, L., Dutil, E., & Falta, P. (2001). A critical review of assessment tools related to home adaptation issues. *Occupational Therapy in Health Care, 14*(3-4), 93-104.

Rousseau, J., Potvin, L., Dutil, E., & Falta, P. (2002). Model of competence: A conceptual framework for understanding the person-environment interaction for persons with motor disabilities. *Occupational Therapy in Health Care, 16*(1), 15-36.

Rubenstein, L. Z., & Josephson, K. R. (2006). Falls and their prevention in elderly people: What does the evidence show? *Medical Clinics of North America, 90*(5), 807-824.

Sakellariou, D. (2015). Home modifications and ways of living well. *Medical Anthropology, 34*(5), 456-469.

The Scan Foundation (2010). Home modifications. DataBrief Series December 2010 No. 7. Retrieved from http://www.thescanfoundation.org/home-modifications

Silverstein, N. M., & Hyde, J. (1997). The importance of a perspective in home adaptation of Alzheimer's households. In S. Lanspery & J. Hyde (Eds.), *Staying put: Adapting places instead of people* (pp. 91-111). Amityville, NY: Baywood.

Silverstein, N. M., Hyde, J., & Ohta, R. (1993). Home adaptation for Alzheimer's households: Factors related to implementation and outcomes of recommendations. *Technology and Disability, 2*(4), 58-68.

Sixsmith, J. (1986). The meaning of home: An exploratory study of environmental experience. *Journal of Environmental Psychology, 6*, 281-298.

Smith, S. G. (1994). The essential qualities of a home. *Journal of Environmental Psychology, 14,* 31-46.

Smith, S. K., Rayer, S., & Smith, E. A. (2008). Aging and disability: Implications for the housing industry and housing policy in the United States. *Journal of the American Planning Association, 74*(3), 289-306.

Sorensen, G. (2012). Home modifications: A national perspective. Facilitator's report from the National Stream Inaugural National Conference. Retrieved from http://www.naca.asn.au/Working_Groups/HomeSup/Service%20Group%205%20-%20Sub%20Group/Item%204%20Attachmnet%20B.pdf

Steinfeld, E., Levine, D., & Shea, S. (1998). Home modifications and the fair housing law. *Technology and Disability, 8,* 15-35.

Steinfeld, E., & Shea, S. (1993). Enabling home environments: Identifying barriers to independence. *Technology and Disability, 2*(4), 69-79.

Steinman, B., Nguyen, A., & Do, Q. (2011). Outcome analysis of the InSTEP home modification component. *Gerontologist, 51,* 378-378.

Stone, J. H. (1998). Housing for older persons: An international overview. *Technology and Disability, 8*(1-2), 91-97.

Struckmeyer, L., & Pickens, N. (2015). Home modifications for people with Alzheimer's disease: A scoping review. *American Journal of Occupational Therapy, 70*(1), 7001270020p1-9.

Tabbarah, M., Silverstein, M., & Seeman, T. (2000). A health and demographic profile of non-institutionalized older Americans residing in environments with home modifications. *Journal of Aging and Health, 12*(2), 204-228.

Tanner, B., Tilse, C., & de Jonge, D. (2008). Restoring and sustaining home: The impact of home modifications on the meaning of home for older people. *Journal of Housing for the Elderly, 22*(3), 195-215.

Tinker, A. (1999). *Ageing in place: What can we learn from each other?* The Sixth F. Oswald Barnett Oration, September 9, 1999, Melbourne, Australia.

Tinker, A., McCreadie, C., Stuchbury, R., Turner-Smith, A., Cowan, D., Bialokoz, A., . . . Holmans, A. (2004). *At Home with AT: Introducing assistive technology into the existing homes of older people: Feasibility, acceptability, costs and outcomes.* London: King's College London and University of Reading.

Trickey, F., Maltais, D., Gosslein, C., & Robitaille, Y. (1993). Adapting older persons' homes to promote independence. *Physical and Occupational Therapy in Geriatrics, 12*(1), 1-14.

United Nations, Department of Economic and Social Affairs, Population Division. (2015). World population ageing 2015. Retrieved from http://www.un.org/en/development/desa/population/publications/pdf/ageing/WPA2015_Report.pdf

U.S. Department of Housing and Urban Development. (2007). FHEO programs. Retrieved from http://www.hud.gov/offices/fheo/progdesc/title8.cfm

Vincent, G. K., & Velkoff, V. A. (2010). The next four decades—The older population in the United States: 2010 to 2050. Retrieved from http://www.census.gov/prod/2010pubs/p25-1138.pdf

Watson, R. M. (2006). Being before doing: The cultural identity (essence) of occupational therapy. *Australian Occupational Therapy Journal, 53,* 151-158.

Wiles, J. L., Leibing, A., Guberman, N., Reeve, J., & Allen, R. E. (2012). The meaning of "ageing in place" to older people. *The Gerontologist, 52*(3), 357-366.

World Health Organization. (2011). *World report on disability.* Geneva, Switzerland: Author.

World Health Organization. (2015). *World report on ageing and health.* Geneva, Switzerland: Author.

Wylde, M. A. (1998). Knowledge of home modifications. *Technology and Disability, 8*(1-2), 51-68.

3

Models of Occupational Therapy

Desleigh de Jonge, MPhil (OccThy), Grad Cert Soc Sci
and Merrill Turpin, PhD, Grad Dip Counsel, BOccThy

Models provide a framework for thinking and clinical decision making. They make explicit the profession's scope of concern (and, therefore, role) and how it identifies and understands issues and problems, and they provide a structure for systematic and comprehensive practice (Turpin & Iwama, 2011) that guides notions of appropriate evaluation and intervention strategies and ways of evaluating outcomes. A number of occupational therapy models of practice have been developed over the years that assist occupational therapists in understanding the difficulties individuals are experiencing and the factors that contribute to them. Each model of practice conceptualizes the person, occupation or performance, environment, and interaction between these in different ways, all of which have an impact on how occupational therapists engage with issues and implement occupational and environmental interventions. This chapter reviews four key approaches used by occupational therapists when undertaking home modifications and examines how each shapes home modification practice and outcomes. The chapter describes the rehabilitation model, Canadian Model of Occupational Performance and Enablement (CMOP-E), ecological occupational therapy models, and Kawa model and examines how each contributes to our understanding of how people engage in meaningful occupations in the home and community. Also

examined is the evolution of occupational therapy practice models and their relevance and integrity in light of politico-sociocultural trends, such as the shift to a social model of disability and the development of client-driven services.

CHAPTER OBJECTIVES

By the end of this chapter, the reader will be able to:

+ Describe how models have shaped occupational therapy practice in the area of home modifications
+ Describe how the rehabilitation model, CMOP-E, ecological models, and Kawa Model structure practice
+ Identify the strengths and limitations of each of these models with respect to home modification practice

INTRODUCTION

As a profession, occupational therapy continues to evolve in response to scientific advancements,

Ainsworth, E., & de Jonge, D. *An Occupational Therapist's Guide to Home Modification Practice, Second Edition (pp. 41-61).*
© 2019 SLACK Incorporated.

as well as philosophical shifts in society and within particular service contexts. Changes in the scope and focus of the profession are clearly evident in the successive models of practice developed to guide and describe occupational therapy practice. Models reflect our thinking and shape our practice (Duncan, 2011) and can be described as being conceptual or procedural in nature. Conceptual models are usually presented in a graphic form, overviewing concepts and describing the relationships between the identified elements. This type of model defines the domain of concern of a profession and assists a professional to think about and interpret situations (Turpin & Iwama, 2011). In contrast, procedural models specify a procedure for attending to issues and elements, directing the process at a very practical level. To illustrate the function of each of these models, imagine you were to plan a trip using a map. A map is like a conceptual model, outlining the boundaries of the geographical area to be explored, various places of interest, their spatial relationships, and their means of connection. Because many of us travel with a finite amount of time and financial resources in mind, we also need to develop a travel schedule (procedural model) so that we can visit all of the important landmarks and plan a methodical and efficient route of travel. Although you might be able to undertake your trip using only one of these approaches, using both a map and a schedule enhances your understanding of the destination and use of relevant resources.

The same is true when using models in practice. Occupational therapists need both conceptual and procedural models to practice effectively. Many occupational therapy models are predominantly conceptual, requiring therapists to develop their own plan of action. Other models are largely procedural, requiring occupational therapists to bring their own understandings of the broader picture, elements of concern, and inter-relationships. Many frames of reference and service models provide this structure. Effective practice relies on having an understanding of all of the areas of concern and their interactions as well as a plan of operation. It is also essential that both the procedural and conceptual models align with and are relevant to each other. There is little point in having a map of the whole of Europe if you confine your trip to Italy. Also, it would be difficult to convince people you have seen Europe if you have traveled only from Rome to Florence, and it would be challenging to navigate between and within small villages if your map only has the major highways marked. Without an appropriate map, your travel experience would not reflect your intentions, nor would it live up to your expectations. Equally, occupational therapists need to ensure that

their actions echo their stated focus and goals. This requires that they have sufficient understanding of the issues they are dealing with (conceptual model) and that these are reflected in an appropriate plan of action (procedural model).

Occupational therapists tend to use different models of practice, either implicitly or explicitly, depending on their primary area of practice, where and when they were trained, and the models they relate to personally. Additionally, service environments and reimbursement schedules have their own procedures, which can affect the focus and scope of practice and can influence occupational therapists' choices of model or shape the way they are operationalized. Consequently, they need conceptual models to help them maintain their discipline focus and embed the philosophy and values of the profession.

Many occupational therapists are not aware of the models or other influences shaping their practice. They generally operate intuitively on internalized understandings (Owen, Adams, & Franszen, 2014; Reed, 1998) or use well-practiced and routine approaches to address issues. As a result, they select and use assessment tools and interventions without necessarily being aware of the beliefs and attitudes directing these decisions. Regardless of whether they are conscious of the models directing their actions, they hold their own views about people and have particular understandings of the cause and impact of impairment or disability. These views delineate their scope of concern; determine the nature of services they offer; and dictate how they work with clients, define and evaluate needs, and focus their interventions. Without a clearly identified model to define the scope of practice and provide a systematic approach, practice is reliant on personal experience, habits, and routines that may not be comprehensive (Turpin & Iwama, 2011). This can make it much more difficult to individualize solutions and negotiate good client outcomes. Models can maximize learning from experience by alerting therapists to the limitations of their current understandings and prompting them to extend their knowledge and skills.

Occupational therapists who are conscious of their conceptual model can explain their unique contribution to the team, describing their expertise or justifying their approach. When they find themselves in conflict with clients or other service providers who might have different understandings or expectations, they can consider the situation and are able to explore the other person's perspective, articulate their own perspective, and identify common goals. Therapists who acknowledge or reflect on their model of practice remain alert to the scope of concern of the profession and select assessment and intervention approaches that address these concerns. With a clear and well-articulated conceptual model of practice, therapists are able to prioritize clients' specific needs over service imperatives and processes. These therapists are also able to recognize and respond to conceptual developments and new knowledge in an area of practice. There is harmony between what they say they do and what they actually do because their procedures are well aligned with their conceptual model.

It is therefore important that therapists be aware of the concepts shaping their practices and driving their decision making. To illustrate the impact of models on the nature of services provided and the outcomes achieved, this chapter examines each model of practice in turn, using the following case study of Mrs. Hume. The way in which each model of practice shapes service delivery and determines outcomes will be described and analyzed with particular reference to their capacity to respond to client concerns and to deal with important aspects of the home environment.

Mrs. Hume is an 82-year-old woman who lives in a four-bedroom detached house in an older outer-city suburb. She has lived in this neighborhood for 60 years, having raised her family in the two-story house her husband built soon after they were married. When her husband died 5 years ago, her previously widowed sister (now 80 years old) moved in. Mrs. Hume has three children—a daughter who lives 10 miles away in the same city, a son who lives in a nearby city, and another son who has moved interstate. She has rheumatoid arthritis and has been admitted to the hospital following a recent flare-up of her condition. Medication has been re-evaluated, and her condition has settled. She has been referred to occupational therapy to assist in her return home.

Before reading any further, take a few moments to reflect, as her occupational therapist, on this case and write down what you would offer Mrs. Hume. Consider the following questions:

+ What would be your main focus?
+ How would you determine need?
+ How would you address needs?
+ How would you work with Mrs. Hume?
+ How do you view the home environment?
+ What outcomes are you expecting from your interventions?

The way occupational therapists regard Mrs. Hume, relate to her and her home environment, and define and address her needs reveals much about the model of practice from which they work. As you read through this chapter, you may recognize aspects of models evident in the approach you identified in relation to Mrs. Hume. Through the discussion of each of these models, you should come to appreciate the impact of your current conceptualizations on the nature of the services you would provide, how you would go about providing them, and the subsequent outcomes you could achieve for Mrs. Hume. In addition, you will be able to reflect on contemporary views of disability and illness, the environment, and person-centered practice, as well as how well these understandings are reflected in your current practice.

REHABILITATION MODEL

Occupational therapy, originally embedded in a humanistic tradition (Schwartz, 2003), has been strongly influenced by medical science and biomedical models of practice. Following World War II and the emergence of rehabilitation medicine, occupational therapy joined other allied health professionals in providing medical care to returning soldiers. By the 1970s, with the proliferation of scientific knowledge and expansion of the health care industry, and as a result of the Rehabilitation Act of 1954, occupational therapy was well established in rehabilitation services (Schwartz, 2003).

The rehabilitation model is founded on extensive knowledge of the structure and function of the human body and the impact of injury and disease. This model has had an enduring influence on the way people with disabilities and illnesses are viewed and their needs defined within rehabilitation services. Within this model, people are considered human organisms consisting of a series of complex systems, with underlying structures and functions that are common to all humans. Traditionally, medical specialists and rehabilitation professionals have defined their scope of concern or responsibilities in terms of particular body systems (e.g., cardiologists are responsible for matters concerning the circulatory system and neurologists focus on the neural system). Similarly, allied health professionals tend to define their roles in terms of functional systems: physiotherapists are primarily concerned with neuromuscular function, psychologists with mental function, and speech-language pathologists with voice and speech function (Seidel, 1998). The initial focus of rehabilitation was to restore an individual's function when his or her capacity had been altered or limited by a physical or mental impairment that could not be remediated by surgery or medical intervention (Seidel, 1998). However, this model has continued to evolve in response to social changes, such as deinstitutionalization and the Independent Living Movement (Schwartz, 2003), resulting in a shift to promoting independence. Consequently, occupational therapists have focused on restoring the individual's ability to function independently in daily activities.

Within this model, the primary challenge to occupational performance is impairment, which is defined as the "loss or abnormality of psychological, physiological or anatomical structure or function" (World Health Organization [WHO], 1980, p. 47). Disability is understood as a restriction or lack of ability to perform an activity in a manner or within the range considered "normal" (Seidel, 1998). Assessment is therefore focused on identifying specific symptoms and signs of abnormality and quantifying the person's functional capacities in various areas, such as neuromuscular, mental, or cardiovascular, as well as independence in daily activities. The rehabilitation model requires the combined and coordinated use of medical, social, educational, and vocational measures to train or retrain an individual to the highest possible levels of function (WHO, 1980). Interventions involve retraining and the use of remedial activities to restore function, compensatory techniques to support the completion of tasks and activities (when restoring function is not possible), and assistive devices and environmental adaptations to accommodate lost function.

In a rehabilitation model, the degree to which maximum function and independence can be achieved is believed to be largely dependent on the individual's level of motivation. The therapist is conceptualized as an expert who brings specialist knowledge about the physiology and pathology of impairment to the process and educates the individual about appropriate remediation and adaptive strategies (Dewsbury, Clarke, Randall, Rouncefield, & Sommerville, 2004). Occupational therapists intervene to regain lost function and prescribe suitable compensatory techniques, assistive devices, or environmental adaptations to promote independence. Typically, assistive devices are recommended more frequently than environmental adaptations because these interventions are both less costly and less complex to implement (Auriemma, Faust, Sibrian, & Jimenez, 1999; Pynoos, Tabbarah, Angelelli, & Demiere, 1998; Tabbarah, Silverstein, & Seeman, 2000). Within this model, the environment is seen as a static physical entity that can be modified to accommodate an individual's identified functional impairments. When considering the environment, the focus is largely on aspects that create barriers to independence in specific self-care activities, such as mobility, bathing, and toileting. The outcomes generally sought by therapists and services using a rehabilitation approach are for the person to regain maximum function and independence. Consequently, outcome measures focus on evaluating the extent of the person's independence and change in functions believed to underpin independence (often measured by comparing the same assessments at baseline and therapy end). Because independence is defined as being able to complete tasks without assistance (Tamaru, McColl, & Yamasaki, 2007), many outcome measures seek to determine the extent to which individuals can complete tasks on their own.

Addressing Mrs. Hume's Home Modification Needs Using a Rehabilitation Framework

In light of the previous description of the rehabilitation model, how would a therapist using this model address Mrs. Hume's home modification needs? The following questions will be used to guide this analysis:

+ What would be the therapist's primary focus?

+ How would a therapist using this model define Mrs. Hume's challenges?

+ What evaluation processes would be used with Mrs. Hume?

+ What interventions or services would be available to Mrs. Hume?

+ How would the therapist work with Mrs. Hume?

+ How would the environment be addressed in this model?

+ What outcomes would Mrs. Hume expect to achieve?

The extensive scientific and medical knowledge underlying the rehabilitation model would ensure that Mrs. Hume receives the very best medical care. This means that health professionals would actively manage her condition and that she could expect reduced inflammation, pain, and long-term damage to her joints. She would be under the care of a rheumatologist for the management of her arthritis and would be referred to other specialists as required. She is likely to be receiving the service of a physiotherapist to maximize her range of movement and muscle strength, and she is likely to be referred to an occupational therapist to maximize her function and independence in activities associated with daily living. She may also be referred to a hand therapist—or possibly a physiotherapist or occupational therapist—for splints to protect her joints. Within the rehabilitation model, Mrs. Hume would be identified primarily in terms of her health condition and would be provided services in line with protocols for that condition. Evaluation would commonly focus on defining her level of function, including measures of range of movement, grip strength, and independence. Mrs. Hume is also likely to receive ongoing evaluations of her physical and functional capacity as successive health professionals establish a baseline and periodically re-evaluate her condition to note improvements in her response to medications and remedial exercise and activities.

With a clear understanding of the health condition and its prognosis, the therapist would develop a treatment plan for Mrs. Hume and educate her about regaining function and maximizing independence. The goal of interventions would be to achieve maximum function, and Mrs. Hume is likely to be given exercises, taught compensatory joint protection strategies, and provided with splints and assistive devices to allow her to complete the activities of daily living (ADLs) considered "normal" for adults her age (e.g., all adults are expected to be independent in toileting). Assistive devices such as reachers and tap turners would commonly be recommended based on her diagnosis of rheumatoid arthritis (Mann & Lane, 1995) or in response to particular activity difficulties. Specific barriers to completing self-care activities in the home (e.g., low toilet and standard tap and door fittings) would result in recommended home modifications, such as installation of grab bars or lever taps and handles. The therapist might or might not make a home visit because potential environmental barriers could largely be determined from Mrs. Hume's known impairments, from identified functional capacities and performance difficulties in daily activities, and through discussion with Mrs. Hume about features in the home. Mrs. Hume would receive advice from the therapist about appropriate remedial strategies to continue with at home, as well as suitable assistive devices and modifications. Lack of compliance with recommended interventions would be attributed to Mrs. Hume's lack of motivation or understanding of her condition and the purpose of the interventions. In response, the occupational therapist would seek to educate Mrs. Hume about her condition and the benefits of adhering to recommendations. It would be anticipated that the recommended interventions would allow Mrs. Hume to function independently in self-care activities. Follow-up evaluations might be undertaken to confirm that she is completing tasks independently.

Implications of Using the Rehabilitation Model for Home Modifications

The rehabilitation model is not specific to occupational therapy, but it is a pervasive model in health, shaping the way health is understood and services are organized. However, the extensive knowledge of body structures and functions that underlies the rehabilitation model allows occupational therapists using this model to reduce the amount of residual impairment resulting from an injury or health condition and promote high levels of function and independence. Having grown out of a medical model, the rehabilitation model uses a "medical" or individual model of disability, which sees disablement as a personal problem resulting from disease, trauma, or other health condition and requiring care and individual treatment by medical professionals (WHO, 2001). Consequently, much of the evaluation process is focused on determining the degree of a person's impairment or specific deficits. Measures of function either rely on personal interpretations of normal function or refer to data that detail the maximum or average for any given age group. However, little is known about the strength or range-of-movement requirements for everyday tasks (Badley, 1995; Law & Baum, 2005), and assessment results might over- or underestimate the specific requirements of particular tasks for any given individual in his or her environment (Dunn, 2005). A deeper understanding of the specific difficulties someone experiences in daily activities would ensure that interventions are more appropriately tailored to the individual.

Often, many people are involved in providing specialized care and addressing specific deficits. This can leave the affected person feeling overwhelmed, fragmented, and disempowered. A focus on presenting physical problems can also mean that social and emotional needs are not acknowledged well within this model (Seidel, 1998). Evaluation and treatment protocols tend to focus on specific functions and often do not allow the occupational therapist to develop an understanding of the real person and their concerns and priorities. Rehabilitation goals of maximizing function and independence often take precedence over the client's unique concerns and goals. Whereas occupational therapists are concerned with ensuring that people can function without help, clients might be more worried about having control over their daily activities and making lifestyle decisions (Clough, Leamy, Miller, & Bright, 2004; Heywood, Oldman, & Means, 2002). Consequently, devices or modifications recommended by a rehabilitation therapist to promote independence in the shower, for example, might not be acceptable to the client because he or she might be more interested in conserving time and energy to engage in other chosen activities rather than being exhausted by routine self-care tasks. When clients do not embrace the interventions offered, it is often perceived that they lack motivation or understanding. However, because the professional largely determines goals and interventions with specific reference to the individual's performance deficits (Law, 1998), they might not be well suited to the person's requirements, preferences, or lifestyle.

It is often difficult for clients to shape and direct intervention in the rehabilitation model because therapists are usually the ones who have extensive knowledge of the injury or health condition, its pathology, and how it can be remediated. In addition, clients usually have little knowledge of the interventions available and are reliant on the expertise of the therapist for recommendations. Although it would be helpful to use this opportunity to educate the client about alternative options and their relative benefits, the focus instead is on increasing compliance (Law, 1998), assuming that once the person understands why the intervention is considered necessary, he or she will automatically accept it.

In the rehabilitation model, restoration of function is usually the primary focus of treatment, with remediation strategies, such as assistive devices and home modifications, receiving less attention. In the hierarchy of rehabilitation interventions, these strategies are frequently seen as part of discharge planning, and there is often insufficient time to effectively plan and implement the intervention before the person is discharged. With interventions focused primarily on a client's specific performance difficulties, little attention is given to how the environment can support and promote further engagement in activities. The restricted view of the environment as a physical entity means that its personal, cultural, and social aspects are often overlooked. Consequently, interventions might not be tailored as well as they could be to the home environment and could create challenges for the client and others instead.

The outcomes of rehabilitation are generally defined and evaluated by service providers (Law, 1998) and are traditionally focused on achieving a specific performance standard or complete independence. It is difficult to measure the success of modification outcomes, especially in terms of independence achieved, using the standardized tests currently in use because many measures of independence assign a penalty for using any assistance, including a device. For example, when using the Functional Independence Measure (Uniform Data System for Medical Rehabilitation, 1997), people can only achieve the highest score of 7 if they do not use a device or have any assistance to complete the task (Cook & Hussey, 2002). In addition, rehabilitation outcome measures such as the Functional Independence Measure do not assess the value of activities for the individual or the quality or acceptability of performance.

OCCUPATION-BASED MODEL

In an effort to differentiate itself from other health care professions and to articulate its unique scope of concern, occupational therapy developed its own models and frameworks for practice. These models aimed to unify the profession, which had been fractured by an explosion of new knowledge about the internal workings of the body and psyche and increasingly specialized practice structured around medical conditions. An overemphasis on techniques and the use of modalities prompted the profession to re-examine its direction and to reconnect with its original philosophy, beliefs, and focus on occupation (Schwartz, 2003). *Occupational performance*, a term first coined in the American Occupational Therapy Association (AOTA) grant report in 1973, became the unique and central concern of the profession because it focused on individuals' abilities to accomplish tasks related to their roles and developmental stage (AOTA, 1973; Reed, 2005). The Occupational Performance Model (OPM) was one of the earliest occupational therapy models to evolve from this shift in direction. It grew out of a series of AOTA task forces and committees in the 1970s and the writings of leaders in the profession about that time, such as Llorens, Mosey, and Reilly (Kielhofner, 2004; Llorens, 1989; Mosey, 1981; Pedretti, 1996). The OPM was primarily structured around the concepts of performance components (sensorimotor, cognitive/cognitive integration, psychosocial/psychological) and performance areas (ADLs, work/productive activities, and play/leisure). Figure 3-1 displays a graphical representation of the OPM as presented by Pedretti (1996). Failure or disruption in performance areas (ADLs and work/productive activities or play/ leisure) are assumed to result from deficits in performance components, task learning experience, and/ or an unsupportive life space or context. The temporal/environmental performance context (physical, cultural, and social) is acknowledged as important to successful occupational performance but is not developed as an integrated concept.

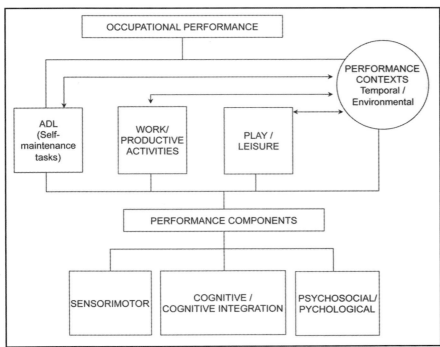

Figure 3-1. OPM. (Adapted with permission from *Occupational therapy: Practice skills for physical dysfunction*, Pedretti, L. W., Occupational performance: A model for practice in physical dysfunction, pp. 3-12. Copyright © Elsevier 1996.)

Although originally described as a frame of reference for practice and educational design (AOTA, 1973, 1974), the OPM detailed the profession's domains of concern, focus, and areas of expertise and has had a substantial and enduring influence on practice (Turpin & Iwama, 2011), especially in physical rehabilitation. The Model of Human Occupation, first published in 1985 (Kielhofner, 1985), was the first occupational therapy model to appear after the OPM, and although the OPM was particularly influenced by rehabilitation and focused on increasing a person's skills, the Model of Human Occupation initially addressed a conceptual gap that existed for practice areas in which clients had permanent impairments and disability and for which rehabilitation was not an appropriate model. Building on a growing awareness that a rehabilitation slant had overly influenced the profession's approach to occupational performance (thereby limiting the profession conceptually), a proliferation of occupational therapy models occurred in the 1990s, all centered on a more contextualized and broader notion of the concept of occupational performance.

One occupational therapy model that was developed at that time with occupational performance as its core concern was the CMOP (Canadian Association of Occupational Therapists, 1997). In its more recent iteration, published in *Enabling Occupation II: Advancing an Occupational Therapy Vision for Health, Well-Being and Justice* (Polatajko, Townsend, & Craik, 2007; Polatajko et al., 2013), the CMOP-E emphasizes the importance of engaging in occupation, regardless of whether an individual can perform it. For example, Townsend and Polatajko (2007) told the story of a father and his son with a severe disability who undertake marathons, triathlons, and iron man events together. The son engages in (rather than performing) the occupation as he is towed and pushed by the father.

Within the CMOP-E, the person is conceived of as an occupational being embedded in a broader context (Figure 3-2). People can influence their physical and mental health and their physical and social environment through participation in purposeful activity or occupation. They are "portrayed as having three performance components [the language of the OPM]—cognitive, affective, and physical—with spirituality at the core" (Polatajko et al., 2013, p. 23). Moving away from the individual focus of the OPM, the CMOP-E, a client-centered model, conceptualized the client in six ways: individuals, families, group, communities, organization, and populations.

From the perspective of the CMOP-E, the aim of occupational therapy is to enable any or all of the following through occupation: people's engagement in everyday life, people's occupational performance, and a just society in which all people are able to participate. Occupation is conceptualized as a bridge that links the person and environment. It is through their action that people connect with their environments. Occupation is important and has therapeutic value because it affects well-being, structures time and life more generally, and brings together individual and cultural aspects of the creation of meaning.

Figure 3-2. CMOP-E. (Reprinted with permission from Polatajko, H. J., Townsend, E. A., & Craik, J. [2007]. Canadian Model of Occupational Performance and Engagement. In E. A. Townsend & H. J. Polatajko [Eds.], *Enabling occupation II: Advancing an occupational therapy vision for health, well-being & justice through occupation* [2nd ed., pp. 13-36]. Ottawa, Canada: Canadian Association of Occupational Therapists.)

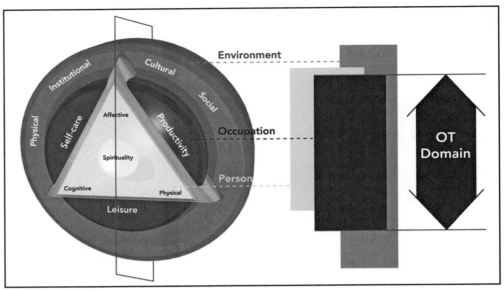

Although the model indicates that occupation can be categorized in a variety of ways (depending on its meaning and purpose for specific clients), it uses the three categories of self-care, productivity, and leisure (the OPM categories). It also emphasizes that occupational performance and engagement have a temporal dimension in that they are organized into patterns over days, weeks, years, and the whole of a person's life. The purpose of engaging in occupation is conceptualized as health, well-being, and justice. Using Trombly's (1995) distinction, occupation is understood as both ends and means. That is, being able to perform and engage in occupation is the end that occupational therapy aims to achieve, but occupation is also used as the means to achieve this aim.

Occupational performance and engagement are promoted by identifying challenges to them at both individual and societal levels and addressing these challenges. Assessment and intervention planning are closely linked in that assessment aims to identify challenges to the occupational performance and participation that is meaningful to the client and required in his or her roles, and intervention is targeted toward addressing those challenges. To come to understand valued occupational performance and engagement for a specific client, CMOP-E uses a "who, what, when, where, and why" framework (Polatajko et al., 2013). This framework guides occupational therapists to be client-centered in determining specifically who is doing what, when and where, and why it is important to them (because they want or need to). The Canadian Occupational Performance Measure (COPM; Law et al., 1998, 2014) can be used as an assessment tool to determine occupational goals. Intervention could be focused on the person, environment, and/or occupation.

The role of occupational therapists is to work collaboratively with clients, guided by the principles of enablement and client-centered (or person-centered) practice. The six enablement foundations outlined in this model (Townsend et al., 2013) are as follows:

1. Choice, risk, and responsibility, in which occupational therapists "enable safe engagement in just-right risk-taking"

2. Client participation

3. Visions of possibility, where both occupational therapists and their clients need to form visions of what might be possible

4. Change, emphasizing that occupational therapy goes beyond simply restoring function and preventing problems (the predominant focus of rehabilitation) but promotes change that facilitates the development or expansion of occupational patterns, balance, and transitions

5. Justice, where occupational performance and engagement are enabled by recognizing and addressing systematic injustices that affect people

6. Power sharing, emphasizing that occupational therapists work with clients in a collaborative and equal way

Intervention is underpinned by these six enablement foundations and uses the following 10 (alphabetically ordered) enablement skills: Adapt, Advocate, Coach, Collaborate, Consult, Coordinate, Design/Build, Educate, Engage, and Specialize. These enablement skills are outlined in the Canadian Model of Client-Centered Enablement. Townsend et al. (2013) also identified three categories of generic skills that underpin enablement. These are:

1. Process skills: analyze, assess, critique, empathize, evaluate, examine, implement, intervene, investigate, plan, reflect

2. Professional skills: comply with ethical and moral codes, comply with professional regulatory requirements, document practice

3. Scholarship skills: use evidence, evaluate programs and services, generate and disseminate knowledge, transfer knowledge

When describing the environment, Polatajko et al. (2013) stated, "The model depicts the person embedded within the environment to indicate that each individual lives within a unique environmental context—cultural, institutional, physical and social—which affords occupational possibilities" (p. 26). The environment is an important part of the "who, what, when, where, and why" framework in that it is not possible to separate the person/group and what is being done from where and when it is being done. Because the focus of the model is occupational performance and engagement, the environment is conceptualized as the context is what shapes this. It influences choice, organization, performance, and satisfaction but is not the focus of the model.

The outcomes of occupational therapy using this model are occupational performance and engagement. To evaluate the achievement of these, occupational therapists would compare the outcomes of intervention with the goals that were identified in the COPM, as well reflect on the question of whether occupational performance has been enabled (i.e., on the process as well as the end result).

Addressing Mrs. Hume's Home Modification Needs Using the CMOP-E

The focus of the therapist working with Mrs. Hume using the CMOP-E would be on enabling her performance of and engagement in meaningful daily activities and roles through occupation. Mrs. Hume would be viewed as someone who is actively engaging in occupations, and attention would be centered on occupations that are most meaningful to Mrs. Hume and relevant to her life stage and living situation. The therapist would interview Mrs. Hume and complete a COPM with her to identify her self-perception of performance in day-to-day activities and the importance of these to her. From this, the therapist would work with Mrs. Hume to identify goals and then negotiate with her to work on the goals related to the home environment. At the level of the person, the therapist would observe Mrs.

Hume undertaking meaningful and purposeful activities and roles in context and evaluate the impact of her condition (i.e., analyzing affective, cognitive, and physical performance components) on her occupational performance and engagement. At the level of the environment, the occupational therapist would undertake a home evaluation and examine the impact of physical, cultural, and social aspects of the home (and the influence of the institutional environment on the home) on Mrs. Hume's occupational performance and engagement. The attention given to various occupational categories such as self-care, productivity, and leisure would vary depending on reimbursement schedules and the priorities of the service organization and Mrs. Hume. For example, a home modification service would prioritize Mrs. Hume's self-care and productivity tasks related to her remaining safe and independent within the home and the immediate surroundings.

The therapist would work collaboratively with Mrs. Hume to tailor interventions in light of her unique situation and preferences. The home environment would be reviewed in terms of its ability to support occupational performance and engagement. Aspects of the physical environment, such as features of the building, furniture, fixtures, and fittings that can no longer be managed, would be identified and removed, replaced, or modified. Consideration would also be given to other people in the environment and to how roles may need to be reassigned or modified to assist Mrs. Hume in daily activities. Family members would be educated about Mrs. Hume's condition so that they can support her by undertaking more difficult activities. For example, her daughter might help Mrs. Hume and her sister prepare meals that could be frozen in smaller portions and then reheated in the microwave so that Mrs. Hume does not have to manage heavy saucepans. Cultural aspects of the home and community, such as customs and behavior standards, would be acknowledged when evaluating activities and roles and recommending changes. The occupational therapist may also encourage Mrs. Hume to write to the local council requesting that the sidewalk in front of her house en route to the local shop be repaired so that she and her neighbors of similar age can safely walk to get their daily supplies. At the completion of the intervention process, in which Mrs. Hume might also have been connected to community groups and other services, appropriate home modifications would have been collaboratively identified and undertaken that would promote her occupational performance and engagement. Occupational performance and engagement are then evaluated by returning to the COPM and ensuring that her initial concerns and goals have been addressed and further issues have not arisen. If the issues have not been adequately addressed, the occupational therapist may revisit the process and refine the intervention further.

Implications of Using the CMOP-E for Home Modifications

The CMOP-E offers occupational therapists a vehicle for defining their unique scope of practice. Much of the knowledge about body structures and functions gained by the profession during its alignment with the rehabilitation model provided the foundation for understanding and addressing function and skill development as it affects occupational performance. However, the CMOP-E moves away from a focus on body structures and functions and presents enablement through occupation as the core of occupational therapy. Conceptualizing occupation as the bridge linking person and environment means that promoting occupational performance and engagement drives any intervention targeting the person and/or environment. Occupational therapists consider people's physical, cognitive, and affective capacities, as well as their spiritual core, in the context of their everyday activities, tasks, and roles (grouped into the areas of self-care, productivity, and leisure) and in relation to their developmental stage, culture, and environment. As people are seen as embedded in an environmental context that "affords occupational possibilities" (Polatajko et al., 2013, p. 23), the environment is a powerful resource for promoting occupational performance and engagement.

The rich understanding of the environment as having cultural, institutional, physical, and social aspects means that, in home modification practice, consideration of the environment is not limited to the physical aspects of the home. Home modification would not be considered an end in itself but as a means to promote occupational performance and engagement. Concern for what people do drives consideration of how the environment could be modified to enable their occupational performance and engagement. Because occupation has unique meanings and purposes in different people's lives, home modification practice cannot simply be a procedural process of applying similar solutions. Instead, an occupational therapist would work with each client to understand his or her occupational patterns and priorities and negotiate and problem solve with the client to determine modifications that would facilitate these, making them easier, safer, and/or more likely.

At times, therapists experience difficulty attending to or prioritizing occupational performance issues because these issues may be perceived as being outside the scope of the service or not recognized within reimbursement schedules. In these situations, it is important that therapists remain mindful of the clients' priorities and target evaluation and interventions to address these, even if performance of and engagement in valued activities are not being addressed directly. If a therapist is primarily responsible for making modifications to the home for a client like Mrs. Hume, it is very important that these modifications be constructed with the client's occupational performance and roles in mind. For example, if gardening were an important occupation for Mrs. Hume, repairing the path to the garden would be important to her safety. It is also crucial that therapists see themselves as part of a continuum of care and refer clients to therapists in other services who have the focus and resources to address the client's specific concerns regarding occupational performance and engagement. For example, if Mrs. Hume would benefit from raised garden beds and this is outside the remit of the home modification service, referral to another agency would be required. When occupational performance and engagement are addressed in a holistic way, all of the factors affecting performance can be identified and the full range of suitable interventions determined. Even if the therapist is not in a position to provide the solutions, the client can be empowered to investigate assistance from elsewhere or purchase preferred solutions themselves, such as writing to the local council. If therapists are addressing only a defined part of occupational therapy's scope of concern, they need to ensure that clients understand what it is they can and cannot attend to. This is particularly important when client priorities are in conflict with or extend beyond the service focus. In such cases, clients should be redirected to services that are better aligned to their specific needs. It is also important that therapists work within the service to advocate for policy and service delivery changes that better reflect clients' occupational performance needs.

The main outcome measure used in the CMOP-E is the COPM. This measure is used to identify client goals and priorities. Because it takes a holistic approach to goal setting, it is likely to identify goals that would be beyond the scope of many home modification services, so it can be a very useful tool for determining other services that would be valuable in helping the client to achieve those goals. It would also be a valuable tool to use to evaluate the effectiveness of the home modifications undertaken in achieving the client's goals.

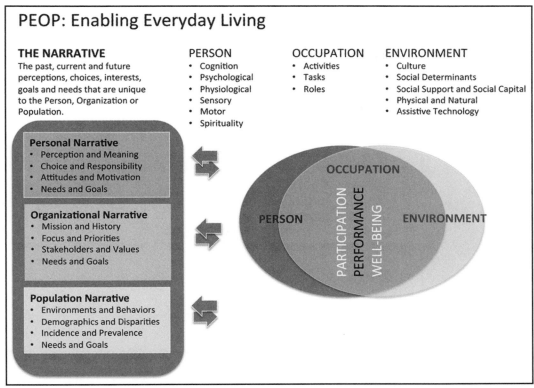

Figure 3-3. The Person-Environment-Occupation-Performance Model. (Reprinted with permission from Baum, C. M., Christiansen, C. H., & Bass, J. D. [2015]. The Person-Environment-Occupation-Performance [PEOP] Model. In C. H. Christiansen, C. M. Baum, & J. D. Bass [Eds.], *Occupational therapy: Performance, participation, and well-being* [4th ed., pp. 47-55]. Thorofare, NJ: SLACK Incorporated.)

The strength of the CMOP-E is its emphasis on client-centeredness and its broadening of the concept of occupational performance to include engagement. In contrast to the earlier OPM, it emphasizes that a person's occupational performance and engagement are contextualized within a cultural, institutional, physical, and social environment. However, central to the model is the notion of occupation as the bridge that connects person and environment. This differs from ecological models in which a transactive relationship exists among person, environment, and occupation.

ECOLOGICAL MODELS

In the 1990s, new occupational therapy models were developed that highlighted the importance of the context in which occupational performance occurs (Brown, 2014). Brown (2014) identified the following three ecological models: Ecology of Human Performance (EHP; Dunn, Brown, & McGuigan, 1994), Person-Environment-Occupation (PEO; Law et al., 1996), and Person-Environment-Occupation-Performance (PEOP; Baum & Christiansen, 2005; Baum, Christiansen, & Bass, 2015; Christiansen, 1991; Christiansen & Baum, 1997, with this model changing substantially in each version), although PEOP also conceptualizes occupation as a bridge (Figure 3-3). Referring to contemporary occupational therapy models at that time (largely influenced by the OPM), Dunn et al. (1994) stated, "In theory and in practice, context (as an area of concern for occupational therapists) has not received the same attention as performance components and performance areas" (p. 595). The term *ecological* refers to the interactions of organisms with each other and their environment ("Ecological," n.d.). The ecological models in occupational therapy particularly emphasized that occupational performance occurs in and is shaped by specific contexts. These models were "built on social science theory, earlier occupational therapy models, and the disability movement" (Brown, 2014, p. 495).

As with other occupational therapy models originally developed in the 1990s, ecological models consider occupational performance to be the primary interest of occupational therapists (with the latest

Figure 3-4. Person-Environment-Occupational Model. (Reprinted with permission from Law, M., Cooper, B., Strong, S., Stewart, D., Rigby, P., & Letts. L. [1996]. The person-environment-occupation model: A transactive approach to occupational performance. *Canadian Journal of Occupational Therapy, 63,* 9-23.)

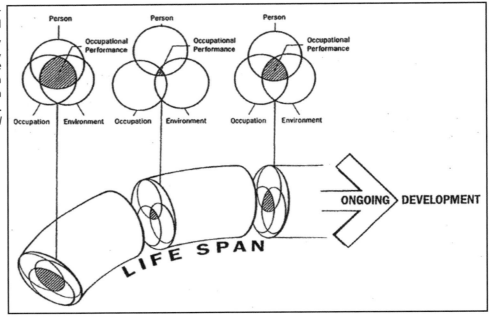

version of PEOP identifying participation, performance, and well-being as the central concern; Baum et al., 2015) and recognize the dynamic and reciprocal relationship among person, occupation, and environment. Ecological models, particularly the PEO, are founded on the notion of "goodness-of-fit" (Brown, 2014, p. 495), where occupational performance is optimized by a close match between the following elements: the person's skills and abilities and the affordances and demands of the occupation and environment (Figure 3-4). Because these elements are intertwined, they are not dealt with separately but as a whole. The various ecological models refer to the whole in different ways. For example, in PEO, an event is the unit of analysis (Law et al., 1996), in which the focus is on certain people doing particular things in specific places, at specific times. EHP uses the term *performance range* to refer to the tasks that are available to a specific person in a specific environment (Dunn et al., 1994). A change in any of the elements will cause alteration to their fit, resulting in changed occupational performance and participation (a change in the whole). Goodness-of-fit has a temporal dimension, and the elements of person, occupation, and environment will change over time (e.g., at different times in the life course and from moment to moment as people change what they are doing and move in and out of different environments; see Figure 3-4).

Ecological models build on the traditional occupational therapy concept of people as unique. Each person is viewed holistically and is acknowledged as bringing unique personal attributes, capacities,

and life experiences to the collaboration. However, using the example of the PEO, ecological models differ from occupation-based models such as the CMOP-E in that, rather than being client-/person-centered, the person is only one of three elements (person, environment, and occupation), the capacities, demands, and affordances of which must fit well together to promote occupational performance. From a transactional perspective, the person cannot be considered separately from their environment and, as Law et al. (1996) stated, "a person's contexts are continually shifting and as contexts change, the behaviors necessary to accomplish a goal also change" (p. 10).

Ecological models center on meeting goals for occupational performance and focus on the principle of goodness-of-fit when a person performs occupation in specific contexts. If any one or several of these elements change, then goodness-of-fit will alter. As people are constantly changing what they are doing and where, goodness-of-fit is not static but conceptualized as resulting from a dynamic process. All elements interact reciprocally and continuously across space and time to constrain or facilitate occupational performance (Brown, 2014).

Like all occupational therapy models, need is defined in terms of a person's specific concerns regarding occupation. Particular attention is paid to identifying the nature and extent of issues impeding the performance of occupations the person needs and wants to do (usually determined by his or her roles and preferred occupations; Law et al., 1996). Ecological models consider occupational performance breakdown as resulting from poor person-environment-occupation fit (PEO fit). Occupational therapists use both subjective and objective methods to evaluate performance, participation, and the PEO fit and to understand the value and acceptability of the performance to the person (Law et al., 1996). They examine PEO fit using skilled observation of the whole event (the person performing the occupation in the natural environment) and analyzing when, where, how, and why the performance is breaking down. The occupational performance difficulty might result from a change in the person's abilities, the way he or she undertakes the occupation or the demands of the environment, or some combination of these. Specific assessments may be undertaken to gain a more detailed understanding of any of the three elements: the person's capacity and how this might be contributing to performance breakdown; examination of specific aspects of the environment; and occupational and activity analysis, to determine the demands of preferred and necessary occupation. However, assessments in ecological models do not consider the elements separately, but together. Therefore, examples of ecological assessment would include observing people demonstrating how they perform an occupation in their own homes; identifying through interview that someone experiences a challenge when performing an occupation in one environment while having no difficulty in a different environment; hearing a client report that since acquiring an impairment, he or she is no longer able to perform an occupation in the same way as previously in a familiar environment.

The role of the occupational therapist in ecological models is to promote occupational performance by enhancing the PEO fit. These models encourage occupational therapists to use a broad range of intervention strategies aimed at making changes in the person, environment, and/or occupation (i.e., they are likely to be used in combination). When seeking to enhance the capacities of the person, they might use established rehabilitation principles, education, or tools to increase emotional well-being, such as motivational interviewing. If their intervention targets the environment, specific strategies might, for example, aim to change the various dimensions of the home. Interventions may be used to alter the demands of occupations such as grading and adapting and the provision of equipment. Dunn et al. (1994) outlined the following five principles of intervention: establish or restore an individual's skills and abilities, alter or change the environment in which occupational performance is being undertaken, adapt the contextual features or task demands, prevent

difficulties arising, and create "circumstances that promote more adaptable or complex performance in context" (Dunn et al., 1994, p. 604). However, Law et al. (1996) cautioned that changes in any one of these areas will have an impact on the others, but not in a way that can be predicted. Therefore, occupational therapists need to be alert to unanticipated consequences of their interventions.

In ecological models, the environment is one of three elements that lie in a transactive relationship. Drawing on theories of the environment from several disciplines, and also incorporating theories of environment-behavior (to provide a richer description of the relationship among people and their environments and occupations), ecological models conceptualize environmental contexts broadly as having cultural, temporal, social, socioeconomic, societal and institutional, and physical (natural and built environment) elements. Ecological models conceptualize the environmental context as shaping and being shaped by people (Turpin & Iwama, 2011). For example, the cultural environment shapes what people think and how they see the world, and this, in turn, shapes the cultural environment (often reinforcing shared culture; however, some strategies might specifically be employed to change attitudes). At an individual level, although EHP presents people as being surrounded by potential tasks, the environmental context will determine the specific performance range that is available to a person (often strongly influenced by that person's roles; Dunn et al., 1994).

The expected outcome of ecological models is that people will be able to perform the occupations that they need and want to do because the PEO fit has been enhanced. Evaluation measures that could be used include comparisons between assessments undertaken before and after intervention—goal-based assessments such as the COPM.

Addressing Mrs. Hume's Home Modification Needs Using an Ecological Framework

In using an ecological model in the case of Mrs. Hume, the occupational therapist first recognizes the uniqueness of her experience of her condition; the occupations and roles that are expected of and/or preferred by her; and the environments in which she lives, works, and recreates and considers how these combine to affect her occupational performance and participation. Mrs. Hume's occupational performance is likely to vary throughout the day, from one day to another, and into the future, depending on her capacities, the demands of her roles and occupations, and how the various environmental contexts constrain or enable performance and participation. The therapist will seek to optimize Mrs. Hume's occupational performance by enhancing the congruence among her capacities and motivations, her occupations and roles, and the environmental contexts in which they occur. Using discussion and observation, the therapist will identify the nature and extent of occupational performance concerns in collaboration with Mrs. Hume. He or she will obtain an occupational history and profile and observe and analyze performance using standardized performance, occupational, and environmental assessment tools. The occupational therapist will identify Mrs. Hume's occupational performance goals and, together with her, evaluate the quality of her performance to determine its acceptability and to ensure valued occupations are prioritized.

These models recognize Mrs. Hume's life experience, values, interests, personal attributes, and strengths and build on existing strategies and supports to develop interventions. With the notion of the goodness-of-fit in mind, the therapist will explore a range of alternative interventions with Mrs. Hume that could result in enhanced occupational performance and participation. These may include developing skills, exploring alternative ways of undertaking tasks, and making changes to the environment. Collaboration with Mrs. Hume is undertaken throughout so that a rich understanding of her life underpins the work of extending her involvement in occupations and roles and increasing her participation, where appropriate, in activities in the home and community. The therapist will work closely with Mrs. Hume to explore and evaluate various options to ensure that they fit with her requirements, preferences, personal style, and the way tasks are undertaken. In addition, the therapist will discuss the intervention options with Mrs. Hume to ensure that they will work within the cultural, socioeconomic, institutional, physical, and social aspects of her home environment and community. Therapists using these models are aware that any change to the person, occupation, or environment is likely to affect the other aspects in unanticipated ways. Hence, care is taken to examine these possibilities prior to recommending them and then to monitor unexpected outcomes following implementation. The occupational performance outcomes sought by Mrs. Hume form the foundation for evaluation, using tools that assess her satisfaction with her current performance as well as more objective measures of performance quality. In addition, measures of Mrs. Hume's participation in the household, neighborhood, and wider

community would be used. The therapist might encourage Mrs. Hume to write to her local council requesting improved accessibility to and additional seating in the shopping mall. Alternatively, the therapist might make representation to management of the local mall or local business community to advocate for better access or additional seating for older people and people with disabilities. The therapist might also join community or industry groups to advocate for more appropriate housing and better access to community facilities and services for older people and people with disabilities. People like Mrs. Hume would benefit if these were characteristic of their regular environmental contexts.

Implications of Using an Ecological Model for Home Modifications

Ecological models acknowledge the complexity and variability of occupational performance because of the dynamic transaction between the person, occupation, and environment. This closely reflects the reality of practice and enables occupational therapists to analyze and explain occupational performance in terms of the "goodness-of-fit" among person, occupation, and environment, rather than attributing problems to the individual. Ecological models also recognize the uniqueness of each person—their abilities, the way they perform tasks, and the personal nature of the home environment—and allow occupational therapists to understand and tailor interventions to specific situations. They shift the occupational therapists' focus from evaluating the detail of each of the elements separately to trying to understand how they interact in the whole situation.

Ecological models empower occupational therapists to take a holistic view of the person in context, attending carefully to what the person wants and needs to do and the specific features on the environments in which they need to perform these occupations. The models encourage therapists to gain a deeper understanding of each person's perceptions of performance issues in their specific environments and to work with people to identify priorities, as well as existing strengths and supports, that can be used to promote occupational performance and participation. Occupational therapists work collaboratively with people and acknowledge the experience and knowledge that each person brings to the partnership.

An understanding of the inevitable variability of occupational performance and participation (as outcomes) ensures that therapists develop solutions that are flexible enough to support performance across the day, the week, and into the future. By providing a range of alternative intervention options aimed at enhancing PEO fit by one or several of following—improving the person's capacity and skill, finding another way to perform the activity, or modifying the environment—therapists provide choices and assist individuals to build a repertoire of useful strategies to use in different situations. These models enable occupational therapists to work with individuals to deal with the complexity of the home environment and to determine how interventions might affect the cultural, socioeconomic, institutional, physical, and social aspects of the home environment and the community. They also require occupational therapists to look beyond just the home environment and to ensure that performance is supported in all of the environments in which the person operates. With an understanding of the complexity of the home environment and the uniqueness of each person, and knowledge that making a change in any of the three elements will alter the others, occupational therapists appreciate the need for follow-up to address any unexpected outcomes of interventions. The perceptions and experiences of the person are central to evaluating the success of the intervention, and the effectiveness of the solution is evaluated in terms of how well it reflects the goals and wishes of the individual and fits the unique PEO transaction. Finally, these models encourage therapists and the profession to look beyond the individual household and situation to examine how services, systems, and policies can be mobilized to further promote occupational engagement and performance, encouraging therapists to become involved in communities and systems to ensure all members of the community can fully participate in society (Brown, 2014).

The image of the difference between maps and schedules when travelling is useful for considering the potential difficulties of using ecological models. Using this analogy, ecological models are more like maps than schedules. They are particularly valuable for taking an expanded, contextual view of occupational performance, but they might need to be combined with detailed assessment and intervention methods when putting them into practice.

CULTURALLY SENSITIVE MODEL

In response to the general lack of cultural relevance of existing occupational therapy models to the Japanese context, a group of Japanese occupational therapists led by Michael Iwama developed the Kawa model (Iwama, 2006). They found that existing occupational therapy models, all of which

had been developed in Western countries, were based on a very different worldview from that of Japanese culture. In particular, the focus on the individual and the notion of a centralized self had little resonance with the collectivist culture of Japan. In essence, the Kawa model is also an ecological model but adds extra symbolism, which can be useful to describe concepts of occupational therapy practice. The concepts of *occupation* and *occupational engagement* can be difficult to describe, particularly in other cultures where these terms are often confused with *activity* and *function*; although similar concepts, they do not reflect the full scope of occupational therapy practice. The model was initially developed to address the cultural relevance of occupational therapy models for Japanese society; however, it has found resonance in and been used with other collectivist cultures (e.g., Australian Aboriginal and Torres Strait Islander peoples) and with those from individualist cultures as well.

The Kawa model uses the image of a river as a symbolic representation of life (Figure 3-5A). Just as a river flows from the mountains to the sea, a person's life energy "flows" from birth to death. Water is used to represent this life energy, and the flow of water represents life flow. In a river, the flow of water is both shaped by the contours of the landscape through which the river flows and shapes that terrain. Thus, the river metaphor presents an individual's life as deeply contextualized, shaped by and shaping the surroundings.

In this model, the view of the person is informed by a collectivist rather than individualist viewpoint. In a collectivist culture, belonging is the most important aspect of life, and being and doing flow from this. This is in stark contrast to many occupational therapy models that prioritize doing, conceptualizing humans as occupational beings. The Kawa model emphasizes the interconnectedness of people and how their occupations are affected by this. As Iwama (2006) explained, "one's own or one's group's occupations are interwoven and connected to the occupation of others."

The main focus of the model is promoting *sukima*, a Japanese word referring to the spaces between obstructions. Iwama (2006) refers to this as "where life energy still flows: the promise of occupational therapy" (p. 151). The strengths-based nature of the Kawa model is evident in its central concern. By focusing on the spaces, occupational therapists can build upon what is working for people in their particular contexts and work toward enhancing life flow for that person in that particular context. Turpin (2017) outlined the six steps followed when using this model:

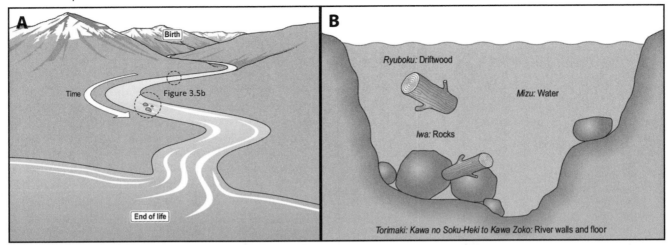

Figure 3-5. Kawa Model. (Reprinted with permission from Iwama, M. [2006]. *The KAWA Model: Culturally relevant occupational therapy.* Philadelphia, PA: Elsevier Health Sciences.)

1. Determine the relevance of the model and, if relevant, who should draw the river diagram

2. Clarify the context through discussion with the person(s) who draws the river

3. Prioritize issues according to the person's perspective

4. Assess the focal points for intervention

5. Undertake intervention

6. Evaluate using person-centered goals

Identifying current challenges facing the client is undertaken through drawing or conceptualizing the river. Although this will involve drawing the length of the river (to that point in the person's life), a transection of that person's "river" enables the occupational therapist to explore the current challenges the client experiences (Figure 3-5B). In the transection, the river elements and their relationships are presented through the various objects in and characteristics of the river. The Kawa model originally identified four elements of the river: water, river walls and floor, rocks, and driftwood (Iwama, 2006). To facilitate a strengths-based approach, two additional elements were later added: Orange Tang fish and sparkles. The river walls and floor shape the course and flow of the river, and objects in the river may obstruct or aid water flow. Each element is described as follows:

+ Water (Miso): Emphasizing the interconnectedness of people and their surroundings, life flow is represented by water, a liquid. In a collectivist society such as Japan, the group rather than the individual is often the primary focus. However, regardless of whether the social context is collectivist or individual, the liquid nature of water emphasizes that all people live within a context that shapes their lives (a liquid conforms to the shape of the container). Iwama (2006) explained that, in Japan, some of the meanings and functions of water are "fluid, pure, spirit, filling, [and] cleansing and renewing," and he emphasized that the culturally specific understandings of the elements are important to elicit because they "will have significant bearing on the utility of this model in one's practice" (p. 144).

+ The river walls and bottom (Kawa no sky-high and Kawa no Zoko, respectively): These elements, plus water, together form the central concern of the Kawa model. The river walls and floor represent the environment. In a collectivist culture, the social environment is emphasized, with particular attention paid to the social group to which a person belongs. In all cultures, the environments in which people live shape their lives (their life flow). Using the river metaphor, the sides and floor could be wide and deep, allowing water to flow easily, or they could be narrow and shallow, restricting its flow.

+ Rocks (Iwa—Japanese for large rocks and crags): In the model, these refer to life circumstances that impede life flow and are perceived by the person as "problematic and difficult to remove" (Iwama, 2006, p. 147). These could include conditions that have been present from birth (e.g., congenital conditions) or that have developed during a person's life (e.g., acquired conditions). As Iwama stated, "Some of these rocks remain unremarkable until they butt up against certain aspects of the social and physical environment" (p. 147) (e.g., a condition might not be problematic in some environments, but a person might be quite "disabled" in other environments).

✦ Driftwood (Ryuboku): This represents personal attributes and resources. Examples include a person's character, personality, values, and skills, as well as material (e.g.. wealth, equipment) and immaterial (e.g.. friends and family) assets. Driftwood can positively and negatively affect circumstances and life flow in that, using the river metaphor, they could enhance water flow when they knock obstructions out of the way or impede the flow of water when caught on the river walls or other obstructions.

✦ Orange Tang and sparkles: These elements have been added since the original book on the Kawa model. The images of thriving fish and sparkling, clean water are associated with healthy environments. In the Kawa model, these elements represent those aspects of a person's life that are going well. Their purpose is to emphasize the strengths basis of this model, rather than simply taking a deficit view.

When using the Kawa model, the role of the occupational therapist is to promote life flow. This could be done in a wide variety of ways. Taking a strengths approach, occupational therapists would aim to build on aspects of the person's life where life flow is occurring (sukima). From this starting point, they might explore with the person ways that obstacles (rocks) could be removed or altered to increase life flow and how personal attributes and resources (driftwood) could be strengthened or used to address obstacles (e.g., driftwood can be used to lever rocks). Occupational therapists might work with the collective or the individual, as most appropriate, and the first task is to determine who should draw the river (as this may not be confined to the person receiving services).

In the Kawa model, once a good understanding of sukima and the river and its elements is obtained, a broad range of intervention strategies could be used. Intervention could be aimed at the context (river walls and floor) so that it better supports occupation. As context is understood very broadly and often includes a collectivist culture, intervention addressing the context is likely to include physical components, interpersonal elements (especially family), and the expectations associated with the social roles a person plays in society. Interventions could also aim to remove or alter obstacles to occupation and strengthen personal attributes and resources. Examples might include taking on new social roles that will provide further opportunities for occupation or relinquishing others that obstruct occupation, teaching skills that will enhance personal attributes, and facilitating the acquisition of resources such as programs and equipment.

Evaluation of intervention is important. As with the ecological models, because the Kawa model takes a holistic perspective, intervention targeting one aspect of the "river" will inevitably alter other aspects of it. As Iwama stated, "When change is introduced in any point in the context, all other parts of the whole are affected and also subject to change" (2006, p. 171). Therefore, occupational therapists need to be alert to unanticipated outcomes.

Addressing Mrs. Hume's Home Modification Needs Using a Culturally Sensitive Framework

In the Kawa model, the central concern is promoting the person's flow of life energy, which is conceptualized as shaped by and shaping the context in which he or she lives. Consequently, the occupational therapist would seek to understand how well Mrs. Hume feels her life energy is flowing within her broader life context, which will particularly include those with whom she shares her life. The focus would be on life within and around the home and community, with particular interest taken in Mrs. Hume's roles and related occupations and how these are interwoven and connected to the roles and occupation of others. This contextual understanding, in which both strengths and challenges are identified, would be developed using the river drawing. The whole household might be involved in drawing a cross-section of the river at the current time, identifying obstacles, resources, and supports to life within the home. Mrs. Hume and her sister, who live in the house, and her daughter who visits regularly, could all contribute to the river drawing by sitting down together and talking about the various elements of the river. This process allows them to think about life in the home (the water—life flow) and what aspects of the house facilitate or restrict their lives (river walls and floor). The river metaphor facilitates discussion on the life they want and the areas of the home that support it (where the river is wide) or restrict it (narrowing of the river). The conversation can explore life within and around the home and how roles, occupations, and dimensions of the environment contribute. Mrs. Hume and her family might identify areas of the home where they are well supported to enjoy their valued roles and occupations, such as the lounge room where they read, watch television, and take an interest in the activities in the neighborhood. The bathroom and toilet might be identified as challenging because Mrs. Hume and her sister struggle with the existing layout and floor surfaces, which create uncertainty or restrict their enjoyment because they are worried about slipping and being injured, which would then prevent Mrs. Hume from continuing in her volunteer roles in the community. Mrs. Hume's daughter might also highlight her growing anxiety about the safety and well-being of her mother and aunt when managing their medications and in day-to-day activities such as house maintenance. This discussion of the river drawing aims to generate a detailed understanding of each person's viewpoint so that it provides an accurate representation of the household as a whole.

In the cross-section of the river, the challenging and supportive elements of the home are identified and represented using rocks and driftwood. Using this strengths-based approach, evaluation and intervention are very closely intertwined because the evaluation focuses on identifying what is working well and what is not working (narrowing of the river), and interventions aim to enhance what is working well, thus expanding sukima (spaces where the water flows) while addressing identified challenges. During this process, the occupational therapist listens carefully to discussions in order to understand life within the home and to understand the family and their priorities, resources, and openness to alternatives. By encouraging people to discuss issues, the therapist develops a clear understanding of each person's perspective and works with them as a group to ensure the drawing adequately represents their experiences.

In developing the drawing, Mrs. Hume's concerns about using the bathroom are raised by the group. Her reduced balance and agility are represented as rocks and the wet, slippery tiles are shown as narrowed river walls. The interaction between Mrs. Hume's balance and mobility and the bathroom environment creates a high-risk situation, which may be addressed by changing the environment to reduce the risk and increase her ability to safely and confidently take a shower. This increases life flow by enhancing the spaces (sukima) between the rocks and river walls. Mrs. Hume currently manages her showering routine by being careful (driftwood) as she uses existing structures such as the shower screen and taps for support and always ensures her sister is at home when she is in the shower. Mrs. Hume's late husband was a builder and, although she is open to suggested modifications, she is sensitive to making changes to the house he built (driftwood). The daughter who lives nearby is very supportive and has the capacity to house Mrs. Hume and her sister (driftwood) while the modifications are being made to the bathroom. Mrs. Hume and her sister are both resourceful people (driftwood) and willing to actively explore alternative strategies, the use of equipment, or other resources in the environment with the occupational therapist. Mrs. Hume has savings that she is happy to invest in making the modification suit her preferences. Her family is able to contribute financially.

In addition to the drawing and associated discussion, the occupational therapist uses observation and evaluation tools to examine occupational performance in various areas of the home to quantify the magnitude of issues and ascertain their quality and nature. For example, the therapist might ask Mrs. Hume to demonstrate her showering routine to identify tasks within the activity where her safety is at risk to then discuss where further supports could address these risks and enhance her showering experience. The therapist then presents a range of recommendations that address observed problems while building on strengths. Because Mrs. Hume already uses structures in the bathroom to keep herself safe while showering, the therapist can capitalize on this and introduce safer structures into the bathroom, such as well-placed grab bars, where she is currently seeking support. However, because the shower screen cannot support a grab bar, the therapist would suggest reversing the direction of the shower door opening so that a grab bar can be attached to the wall to provide support as Mrs. Hume or her sister step over the hob. The occupational therapist would discuss the implications of this potential change for both Mrs. Hume and her sister to ensure that any changes would increase the sukima for everyone in the household.

The drawing and subsequent discussions would be undertaken in the home, around a table, with all relevant people present. The conversation would acknowledge the social aspects of the environment and the roles each person plays in the household, family, and community. The interpersonal relationships are privileged in the discussion, allowing everyone to contribute to the creation of solutions. The physical environment is modified to reduce barriers and promote occupation according to the solutions that were chosen. The outcomes of a home modification would be examined in terms of how it contributes to the life flow for Mrs. Hume and her sister. A new river drawing following the modification could be compared with the initial drawing to discuss the extent to which changes increased life flow and enhance roles and occupation and whether any changes have occurred that may have narrowed the river unexpectedly. These would be addressed by revisiting the collaborative process previously outlined.

Implications of Using a Culturally Sensitive Approach to Home Modifications

The Kawa model is essentially an ecological model that is culturally sensitive, seeing people within their context. Although it was originally designed to work with people from a collectivist culture, it also provides a transformative framework for working with households undertaking home modifications in individualist cultures. It recognizes the pervasive impacts of any changes to home on the whole household. The home is a collective of people who are intertwined financially, socially, physically, and through the rhythms of daily occupations, as well as past experiences and future aspirations.

The relevance of drawing a river to home modification practice may not immediately be clear to some occupational therapists and clients because the expectations would be for the therapist to provide solutions rather than engage in a collaborative process. However, drawing the river provides an opportunity for all members of the household to contribute to the conversation about life within the home. It shifts the focus from identifying problems for an identified individual and implementing specific interventions to considering how the household works as a whole and how best to support a rich and healthy home life. Although this process might appear to be more time consuming, it allows the occupational therapist to develop a richer and more comprehensive understanding of the home life, which may save time negotiating options that are unacceptable to the people in the household because the context of the home was not well enough understood. It also increases the likelihood that all people in the household have a vested interest in the solutions that are developed.

This visual tool allows the client to engage in a collaborative, creative process and to own and control the process and discussion because he or she is doing the drawing rather than being the recipient of a litany of targeted questions from the occupational therapist. The metaphor of the river allows the household to identify issues to address without being constrained by a professional lens. This is particularly useful when working with families who have children with a disability. For example, a family might want their daughter with a disability to have the experience of being involved in preparing the family dinner. This issue might not have been raised if the therapist's protocol was driving the encounter. Working with families using the Kawa model ensures interventions are appropriate to the rich ecosystem of the household and the lives people want, rather than being focused on the needs of a particular individual. Being a strengths-based model, it recognizes and builds on what is working well and what people want to achieve rather than defining and addressing problems.

The potential difficulty in using the Kawa model is that it is based on a very different worldview than most other occupational therapy models and is thus less familiar for Western occupational therapists. Although it can be used as "simply another person-environment-occupation model," when occupational therapists take on this different worldview, the true transformative nature of this model can be realized. However, the task of seeing the world from a different vantage point is a difficult one that requires deep reflection on one's own culture and way of seeing the world.

CONCLUSION

Occupational therapists use models, either implicitly or explicitly, to define their scope of concern and role, identify and understand issues or problems, determine appropriate evaluation and intervention strategies, and evaluate outcomes. Conceptual models provide overview concepts and describe the relationships between the identified elements, and procedural models specify a procedure for attending to issues and elements. Therapists need both conceptual and procedural models to operate effectively because practice requires therapists to have an understanding of all of the elements of concern and their interactions, as well as a plan of action. However, therapists need to be aware of the models they draw on in practice and ensure that their actions echo their stated focus and goals. Each model presented in this chapter conceptualizes the person, occupational performance, environment, and interaction between these in different ways, all of which have an impact on how occupational therapists engage with issues and implement environmental interventions.

The rehabilitation model provides therapists with knowledge of body structures and functions and allows them to reduce the amount of residual impairment resulting from an injury or health condition and to promote function and independence. However, without a deeper understanding of the particular difficulties an individual is experiencing in daily activities, interventions are not tailored to the specific needs of the individual and may result in changes that are ineffective or unacceptable in the home environment.

In shifting the focus of therapy to occupational performance and engagement, the CMOP-E guides occupational therapists in a client-/person-centered approach to enabling occupation. The goal of an occupational therapist using this model is to enable people's engagement in everyday life, their occupational performance, and a just society in which all people are able to participate. People's occupational performance and engagement are conceptualized as embedded within a cultural, institutional, physical, and social environment.

The ecological models, with their understanding of the dynamic transaction among person, occupation, and environment, provide a holistic framework for addressing the complexities that individuals encounter when undertaking everyday activities in the home and community. They recognize the continual change that occurs because people continuously change their occupations and the environments in which they are performed. Recognition of the environment as a means of limiting and creating occupational performance opportunities also enables therapists to actively use the environment to promote participation within the home and community. Both ecological models and the CMOP-E encourage therapists to move beyond working with individuals to becoming agents of change within the community, thus ensuring equitable participation for all.

The Kawa model is an ecological model that differs from most occupational therapy models in its symbolism and worldview. Based on a collectivist worldview, it encourages occupational therapists to consider the interconnectedness of their clients' occupations with those of others in their lives.

Models provide a framework for thinking and clinical decision making and a structure that ensures systematic and comprehensive practice. When therapists are aware of the concepts shaping their practice, they are well placed to reflect on their practice and articulate their unique contribution to stakeholders. Selection of evaluation and intervention strategies is also thoughtful and well informed, and the goal and outcomes of interventions are clearly defined. Occupational therapy has a rich history of describing and refining the models that shape practice. It is important that these continue to be thoughtfully applied to achieve good home medication outcomes for clients.

REFERENCES

American Occupational Therapy Association. (1973). *Project to delineate the roles and functions of occupational therapy personnel*. Rockville, MD: Author.

American Occupational Therapy Association. (1974). *A curriculum guide for occupational therapy educators*. Rockville, MD: Author.

Auriemma, D., Faust, S., Sibrian, K., & Jimenez, J. (1999). Home modifications for the elderly: Implications for the occupational therapist. *Physical and Occupational Therapy in Geriatrics, 16*(2-4), 135-144.

Badley, E. M. (1995). The genesis of handicap: Definition, models of disablement and the role of external factors. *Disability and Rehabilitation, 17*, 53-62.

Baum, C. M., & Christiansen, C. H. (2005). Person-environment-occupational performance: An occupation-based framework for practice. In C. H. Christiansen, C. M. Baum, & J. Bass-Haugen (Eds.), *Occupational therapy: Performance, participation and well-being* (3rd ed., pp. 243-266). Thorofare, NJ: SLACK Incorporated.

Baum, C. M., Christiansen, C. H., & Bass, J. D. (2015). The person-environment-occupational performance (PEOP) model. In C. H. Christiansen, C. M. Baum, & J. D. Bass (Eds.), *Occupational therapy: Performance, participation and well-being* (4th ed., pp. 47-55). Thorofare, NJ: SLACK Incorporated.

Brown, C. E. (2014). Ecological models in occupational therapy. In B.A.B. Schell, G. Gillen, & M. E. Scaffa (Eds.), *Willard and Spackman's occupational therapy* (12th ed., pp. 494-504). Philadelphia, PA: Wolters Kluwer Lippincott Williams & Wilkins.

Canadian Association of Occupational Therapists. (1997). *Enabling occupation: An occupational therapy perspective*. Ottawa, ON: CAOT Publications ACE.

Christiansen, C. (1991). Occupational therapy: Intervention for life performance. In C. Christiansen & C. Baum (Eds.), *Occupational therapy: Overcoming human performance deficits* (pp. 3-43). Thorofare, NJ: SLACK Incorporated.

Christiansen, C. H., & Baum, C. M. (1997). Person-environment occupational performance: A conceptual model for practice. In C. H. Christiansen & C. M. Baum (Eds.), *Occupational therapy: Enabling function and well-being* (2nd ed., pp. 46-71). Thorofare, NJ: SLACK Incorporated.

Clough, R., Leamy, M., Miller, V., & Bright, L. (2004). *Housing decisions in later life*. New York: Palgrave Macmillan.

Cook, A., & Hussey, S. (2002). *Assistive technologies: Principles and practice* (2nd ed.). St. Louis, MO: Mosby.

Dewsbury, G., Clarke, K., Randall, D., Rouncefield, M., & Sommerville, I. (2004). The anti-social model of disability. *Disability and Society, 19*(2), 145-158.

Duncan, E. A. S. (2011). *Foundations for practice in occupational therapy* (5th ed.). London: Churchill Livingstone Elsevier.

Dunn, W. (2005). Measurement issues and practices. In M. Law, C. Baum, & W. Dunn (Eds.), *Measuring occupational performance: Supporting best practice in occupational therapy* (pp. 21-32). Thorofare, NJ: SLACK Incorporated.

Dunn, W., Brown, C., & McGuigan, A. (1994). The ecology of human performance: A framework for considering the impact of context. *American Journal of Occupational Therapy, 48*, 595-607.

Ecological. (n.d.). In *Oxford Dictionary online*. Retrieved from https://en.oxforddictionaries.com/definition/ecological

Heywood, F., Oldman, C., & Means, R. (2002). *Housing and home in later life*. Buckingham, UK: Open University Press.

Iwama, M. (2006). *The KAWA Model: Culturally relevant occupational therapy*. Philadelphia, PA: Elsevier Health Sciences.

Kielhofner, G. (1985). *A model of human occupation: Theory and application*. Baltimore, MD: Williams & Wilkins.

Kielhofner, G. (2004). The development of occupational therapy knowledge. In G. Kielhofner (Ed.), *Conceptual foundations of occupational therapy* (3rd ed., pp. 27-63). Philadelphia, PA: F. A. Davis.

Law, M. (1998). *Client-centered occupational therapy*. Thorofare, NJ: SLACK Incorporated.

Law, M., Baptiste, S., Carswell, A., McColl, M., Polatajko, H., & Pollock, N. (1998). *Canadian occupational performance measure* (3rd ed.). Toronto, ON: CAOT Publications ACE.

Law, M., Baptiste, S., Carswell, A., McColl, M., Polatajko, H., & Pollock, N. (2014). *Canadian occupational performance measure* (5th ed.). Ottawa, ON: CAOT Publications ACE.

Law, M., & Baum, C. M. (2005). Measurement in occupational therapy. In M. Law, C. Baum, & W. Dunn (Eds.), *Measuring occupational performance: Supporting best practice in occupational therapy* (pp. 3-20). Thorofare, NJ: SLACK Incorporated.

Law, M., Cooper, B., Strong, S., Stewart, D., Rigby, P., & Letts. L. (1996). The person-environment-occupation model: A transactive approach to occupational performance. *Canadian Journal of Occupational Therapy, 63*, 9-23.

Llorens, L. A. (1989). Health care system models and occupational therapy. *Occupational Therapy in Health Care, 5*(4), 25-37.

Mann, W. C., & Lane, J. P. (1995). *Assistive technology for persons with disabilities* (2nd ed.). Bethesda, MD: American Occupational Therapy Association.

Mosey, A. C. (1981). *Occupational therapy: Configuration of a profession*. New York: Raven Press.

Owen, A., Adams, F., & Franszen, D. (2014). Factors influencing model use in occupational therapy. *South African Journal of Occupational Therapy, 44*(1), 41-47.

Pedretti, L. W. (1996). Occupational performance: A model for practice in physical dysfunction. In L. W. Pedretti (Ed.), *Occupational therapy: Practice skills for physical dysfunction* (pp. 3-12). St. Louis, MO: Mosby.

Polatajko, H. J., Townsend, E. A., & Craik, J. (2007). Canadian model of occupational performance and engagement (CMOP-E). In E. A. Townsend & H. J. Polatajko (Eds.), *Enabling occupation II: Advancing an occupational therapy vision of health, well-being & justice through occupation* (p. 23). Ottawa, ON: Canadian Association of Occupational Therapists.

Polatajko, H. J., Davis, J., Stewart, D., Cantin, N., Amoroso, B., Purdie, L., & Zimmerman, D. (2013). Specifying the domain of concern: Occupation as core. In E. A. Townsend & H. J. Polatajko (Eds.), *Enabling occupation II: Advancing an occupational therapy vision for health, well-being & justice through occupation* (2nd ed., pp. 13-36). Ottawa, ON: Canadian Association of Occupational Therapists.

Pynoos, J., Tabbarah, M., Angelelli, J., & Demiere, M. (1998). Improving the delivery of home modifications. *Technology and Disability, 8*, 3-14.

Reed, K. (1998). Theory and frame of reference. In M. E. Neistadt & E. B. Crepeau (Eds.), *Willard and Spackman's occupational therapy* (9th ed., pp. 521-524). New York: Lippincott-Raven.

Reed, K. (2005). An annotated history of the concepts used in occupational therapy. In C. H. Christiansen, C. M. Baum, & J. Bass-Haugen (Eds.), *Occupational therapy: Performance, participation, and well-being* (3rd ed., pp. 567-626). Thorofare, NJ: SLACK Incorporated.

Schwartz, C. B. (2003). The history of occupational therapy. In E. B. Crepeau, E. S. Cohn, & B. A. Boyt Schell (Eds.), *Willard and Spackman's occupational therapy* (10th ed., pp. 5-14). Philadelphia, PA: Lippincott Williams & Wilkins.

Seidel, A. C. (1998). Theories derived from rehabilitation perspectives. In M. E. Neistadt & E. B. Crepeau (Eds.), *Willard and Spackman's occupational therapy* (9th ed., pp. 536-542). New York, NY: Lippincott-Raven.

Tabbarah, M., Silverstein, M., & Seeman, T. (2000). A health and demographic profile of non-institutionalized older Americans residing in environments with home modifications. *Journal of Aging and Health, 12*(2), 204-228.

Tamaru, A., McColl, M. A., & Yamasaki, S. (2007). Understanding "independence": Perspectives of occupational therapists. *Disability and Rehabilitation, 29*(13), 1021-1033.

Townsend, E. A., Beagan, B., Kumas-Tan, Z., Versnel, J., Iwama, M., Landry, J., . . . Brown, J. (2013). Enabling: Occupational therapy's core competency. In E. A. Townsend & H. J. Polatajko (Eds.), *Enabling occupation II: Advancing an occupational therapy vision for health, well-being & justice through occupation* (2nd ed., pp. 87-134). Ottawa, ON: Canadian Association of Occupational Therapists.

Townsend, E. A., & Polatajko, H. J. (Eds.). (2007). *Enabling occupation II: Advancing an occupational therapy vision for health, well-being & justice through occupation*. Ottawa, ON: Canadian Association of Occupational Therapists.

Trombly, C. A. (1995). Occupation: Purposefulness and meaningfulness as therapeutic mechanisms. *American Journal of Occupational Therapy, 49*(10), 960-972.

Turpin, M. (2017). Occupational therapy practice models. In M. Curtin, M. Egan, & J. Adams (Eds.), *Occupational therapy for people experiencing illness, injury or impairment: Promoting occupation and participation* (7th ed., pp. 115-133). New York: Elsevier.

Turpin, M & Iwama, M. (2011). *Using occupational therapy models in practice: A fieldguide*. Edinburg, UK: Churchill Livingstone, Elsevier.

Uniform Data System for Medical Rehabilitation. (1997). *Functional independence measure* (Version 5.1). Buffalo, NY: Buffalo General Hospital, State University of New York.

World Health Organization. (1980). *The international classification of impairments, disabilities and handicaps (ICIDH)*. Geneva, Switzerland: Author.

World Health Organization. (2001). *International classification of function, disability and health*. Geneva, Switzerland: Author.

Legislation, Regulations, Codes, and Standards Influencing Home Modification Practice

4

Elizabeth Ainsworth, MOccThy, Grad Cert Health Sci;
Desleigh de Jonge, MPhil (OccThy), Grad Cert Soc Sci; and Jon Sanford, MArch, BS

This chapter provides an overview of the worldwide range of legislation and guidelines relevant to promoting the rights of people with a disability through access to the built environment. Human rights conventions and disability discrimination legislation have shaped community values, design and construction practice, and service delivery to ensure that older people and people with a disability are afforded equitable access to goods, services, and the built environment within the community. In particular, building regulations, building codes, and access standards that incorporate access and mobility requirements have sought to address discrimination that might occur because of barriers in public facilities and spaces. Although legislation and guidelines have focused primarily on public facilities, they are not without impact on housing. Legislation and guidelines relating to the design of accessible housing continue to emerge in a range of countries through the efforts of people concerned about the lack of inclusive environments. With an enhanced understanding of the relevance and application of individual rights and building legislation, occupational therapists will be better equipped to promote the inclusion of older people and people with a disability into everyday home and community life and to empower them to claim their rightful place in society.

CHAPTER OBJECTIVES

By the end of this chapter, the reader will be able to:

✦ Describe the development of international human rights conventions and the implications for older people and people with a disability

✦ Discuss disability discrimination and building legislation and their impact on the design of public and private built environments

✦ Understand the relevance and application of rights-based legislation and building legislation to the design and modification of the home environment

✦ Understand the application of the complaints and remedial processes that are used in relation to rights-based legislation and building legislation

Ainsworth, E., & de Jonge, D. *An Occupational Therapist's Guide to Home Modification Practice, Second Edition (pp. 63–81).*
© 2019 SLACK Incorporated.

INTERNATIONAL FRAMEWORK FOR THE CREATION OF INCLUSIVE ENVIRONMENTS

Integrating people with a disability into the community and enabling them to live in homes they can call their own requires an understanding of the international convention on the rights of people with a disability and the emergence of rights-based legislation over time. Though people with a disability were once seen as being dependent on welfare, social assistance, or charity, they are now regarded primarily as citizens with equal rights and obligations. The following discussion briefly describes recent changes in the definition and models of disability, how these have influenced the development of legislation, and service delivery to people with a disability.

Definition of Disability

The definition of disability has changed significantly in recent decades. Prior to the end of the 20th century, disability was defined using the medical model that attributed disability to health conditions. Disability was seen as a problem within the person—a result of an individual's physical or mental limitations. A traditional definition of disability, widely promulgated by the World Health Organization (WHO), described disability as "any restriction or inability resulting from a disturbance or loss of bodily or mental function associated with disease, disorder, injury, or trauma, or other health-related state" (WHO, 1980, p. 143).

In the last decade of the 20th century, a number of new models of disability began to emerge based on Nagi's work (1965, 1976) that defined disability as the outcome of an interaction between impairment and environmental factors (Institute of Medicine, 1991, 1997; National Center for Medical Rehabilitation Research, 1993). Social models of disability emerged that differed slightly from the medical model regarding the relationship among medical conditions, impairments, functional limitations, and the effects of the interaction of the person with the environment. Generally, these models agreed that disability was a function of the interaction of the person with the environment (Brandt & Pope, 1997). Social models of disability continued to develop and evolve as people with a disability, their advocates, and organizations supporting them sought to use these to stimulate change in society (Office of the United Nations High Commissioner for Human Rights, 2006; Swain, 2004).

As a result, the WHO (2001) has adopted a social definition of disability. The new *International Classification of Functioning, Disability and Health* not only defines disability as the interaction of body function and structure with contextual (i.e., environmental and personal) factors, but it has extended it to include the activity and participation outcomes that result from this interaction. The environment is viewed as either a barrier or facilitator to activities and participation in social roles (WHO, 2001). Simply put, for an individual with an impairment (e.g., cannot ambulate), the typical home environment (e.g., stairs) can pose barriers to everyday activity (e.g., getting in and out of the house) and participation in social roles (e.g., neighbor interaction), whereas home modifications (e.g., ramp) can facilitate these outcomes.

Importance of Social Models of Disability

Social models of disability have encouraged a shift in focus from flaws or deficits in the individual (as described in the medical model or individual model of disability) to activity restrictions or barriers created by a society that excludes people from participating in everyday life in the community (Harrison & Davis, 2001; Oliver, 1990, 1996). These models describe disability as a complex phenomenon created, in part, by features of the physical, economic, and political environment and not simply a manifestation of a person's impairment (Australian Institute of Health and Welfare, 2003; Dickson, 2007; Harrison & Davis, 2001; Samaha, 2007). The environment is seen to facilitate participation that enables the fulfillment of roles appropriate to age, gender, and social and cultural identity. Alternatively, it can contribute to isolation, limiting achievement of daily activities and restricting participation in social, cultural, and community activities (WHO, 2001).

The social models of disability provide frameworks for the formulation of appropriate recommendations to create reasonable and necessary environments that provide appropriate access for people with a disability (Kornblau, Shamberg, & Kein, 2000). It challenges occupational therapists to reconsider their individualistic and medical approaches to occupational performance problems and encourages them to identify and eliminate social and environmental barriers to performance and participation (Whalley Hammell, 2001).

Though social models of disability have facilitated a shift from focusing on individual deficits to examining disabling environments and practices, they are under increasing scrutiny. Like the medical model and other theorizations of disability, these models by no means provide a comprehensive description of the experience of disability and are considered reductionist in nature (Imrie, 1996). In particular, social models have a tendency to ignore how impairment, in and of itself, has the potential to debilitate, regardless of the environmental and social conditions (Imrie & Hall, 2001a; Shakespeare & Watson, 2001).

Although it is undeniable that environments and social practices can alienate and disable people, addressing these issues alone might not eliminate the difficulties people with impairments experience (Shakespeare & Watson, 2001). Further, environmental design and social manipulations cannot always prevent the personal experience of physical and intellectual restrictions (Imrie & Hall, 2001a). It is therefore important to take appropriate action to address impairment in conjunction with removing environmental barriers and disabling practices (Shakespeare & Watson, 2001). Whatever model of disability is used, it is critical that all of the dimensions of the person's experiences are considered, including those of a physical, psychological, cultural, social, and political nature, rather than simplifying disability and operating within a medical or social model (Shakespeare & Erickson, 2000).

DISABILITY LEGISLATION

The social models of disability, with their recognition of the environment's influence on the experience of disability, has influenced the development of specific legislation and guidelines aimed at protecting the rights of people with a disability in a range of countries. The creation of a variety of international declarations, rules, or conventions and national legislative acts protects the human and civil rights of people with a disability throughout the world (Hurst, 2004).

Human Rights Protections

Human rights are those rights that are inherent in an individual's humanity. They sit above human-made laws and exist whether there are national laws to uphold them or not (Hurst, 2004). The universal establishment of human rights is regarded as the single most important political development influencing social change.

The rights of people with a disability have been the subject of much attention in the United Nations (U.N.; Office of the United Nations High Commissioner for Human Rights, 2006). Through the creation of various declarations, rules, and conventions, people with a disability are now recognized as legitimate citizens in society. The first indicators of international concern regarding the rights of people with a disability were described in the *U.N. Declaration on the Rights of Mentally Retarded Persons* (1971) and in the *U.N. Declaration on the Rights of Disabled Persons* (1975). Although these declarations did not detail the monitoring mechanisms or the reporting obligations of the international community, they served as the framework for human rights protections for people with a disability worldwide. As a result, they are regarded as the most important milestones in the development of equal rights for people with a disability (Imrie & Hall, 2001a).

The 1975 *U.N. Declaration on the Rights of Disabled Persons* clearly called for national and international action to protect the rights of individuals with a disability. It specifically stated that

> Disabled persons have the right to live with their families or with their foster parents and to participate in social, creative or recreation activities. No disabled person shall be subjected, as far as his or her residence is concerned, to differential treatment other than that required by his or her condition or by the improvement which he or she may derive therefrom. If the stay of a disabled person in a specialized establishment is indispensable, the environment and living conditions therein shall be as close as possible to those of the normal life of a person of his or her age. (U.N., 1975)

In the following decades, the U.N., through various activities, continued to promote human rights for people with a disability. The U.N. General Assembly proclaimed 1981 the International Year of the Disabled. In 1982, the General Assembly adopted the World Program of Action Concerning Disabled Persons, which established a world strategy to promote equality and full participation by people with a disability in social life and development. In 1983, the U.N. declared the ensuing 10 years to be the U.N. Decade of Disabled Persons (1983–1992).

Because of the experience gained during the Decade of Disabled Persons, the U.N. adopted a resolution entitled *Standard Rules on the Equalization of Opportunities for People With Disabilities* in 1993. The purpose of the resolution was to ensure that people with a disability could exercise the same rights and have the same obligations as others (Degener &

Quinn, 2000; Mooney Cotter, 2007). It established broad principles to guide nation states in developing domestic antidiscrimination and equal opportunities legislation (Imrie & Hall, 2001a).

Although the *Standard Rules on the Equalization of Opportunities for People With Disabilities* are considered to be the key moral imperative for change on a worldwide basis (Degener & Quinn, 2000), they were, nonetheless, nonbinding. As a result, disability rights activists and scholars have pressed for the adoption of a new worldwide convention on the elimination of discrimination against people with a disability (Degener & Quinn, 2000). In response, the U.N. Convention on the Rights of Persons With Disabilities and its Optional Protocol were adopted on December 13, 2006, at the U.N. headquarters in New York and were opened for signature and ratification on March 30, 2007. The convention is considered the first comprehensive human rights treaty of the 21st century (U.N., 2008).

The convention marks a "paradigm shift" in attitudes and approaches to people with a disability, moving them from being viewed as "objects" of charity requiring medical treatment and social protection to "subjects" with rights, who are capable of claiming those rights (U.N., 2008). Further, the convention emphasizes that people with a disability can make decisions about their lives based on their free and informed consent, as well as being full and active members of society (U.N., 2008). Unlike the *Declaration on the Rights of Mentally Retarded Persons* (U.N., 1971) and the *Declaration on the Rights of Disabled Persons* (U.N., 1975), the convention boldly sets out a plan of action for countries to enact laws and take other measures to improve disability rights and to eliminate legislation, customs, and practices that discriminate against people with a disability.

The U.N. declarations have also highlighted the rights of people with a disability to have access to the physical environment. The move to incorporate accessibility requirements into the various declarations, rules, and conventions is considered one mechanism by which people's citizenship can become a tangible outcome. The most recent U.N. *Convention on the Rights of People With Disabilities* (2008) details specific requirements with respect to accessibility to the built environment. However, it does not describe what accessibility should look like or how it should be created, leaving it up to the various nations that sign and ratify the convention to detail specifications and develop mechanisms for implementation and monitoring compliance. As a result, there continues to be a great deal of political diversity and complexity in providing appropriate access, conditioned by country-specific social,

institutional, and political attitudes and values (Imrie & Hall, 2001a). Some countries have legislation in place to ensure there is appropriate access to public buildings; however, the convention does not stipulate how nations should meet their responsibilities in terms of access to adequate housing. Further work is needed at an international level to ensure that well-designed housing is available for people with a disability (Imrie & Hall, 2001b). Nations might use a range of strategies to facilitate the creation of appropriate housing, including the following:

+ Building publicly funded housing and accommodation programs
+ Ensuring building regulation and certification through national, state, or local government programs
+ Enforcing antidiscrimination laws
+ Introducing industry incentives
+ Providing education and awareness training (Ozdowski, 2005)

Disability Discrimination Legislation and Civil Rights

Although changes to the built environment go some way to providing people with a disability access to facilities and services in the community, they cannot fully eradicate misconceptions and disablist attitudes in society. Such values and structures are better influenced through the pursuit of civil rights for people (Imrie, 1996). One of the basic human rights is freedom from discrimination, and antidiscrimination legislation ensures that this right, through civil rights laws or others, such as social welfare, constitutional, or criminal laws, can be enforced (Hurst, 2004).

Historically, people with a disability have been excluded from or marginalized in the community through discrimination. Disability discrimination means treating a person with a disability less favorably for a reason related to that person's disability, without justification (Hendricks, 1995; Williams & Levy, 2006). To ameliorate disability discrimination, many countries have enacted legislation to mandate that people with a disability be afforded the right to fully participate in all aspects of society. Although many countries have some form of disability discrimination legislation, the enforcement method, strength, and effectiveness of this legislation vary considerably (Gleeson, 2001). In an analysis of international disability discrimination legislation, Degener and Quinn (2000) identified that the scope of the terminology and definitions differs substantially between countries. They identified that some of the most comprehensive disability discrimination laws exist in Australia, Canada, Hong Kong, the Philippines, the United Kingdom, and the United States. Their analysis included employment, provision of goods and services, and transport. Additional areas specified included housing (Canada and Australia), education (United States and Australia), land possession (Australia), access to premises (Canada, United Kingdom, and Australia), and telecommunications (United States and Australia).

The strength of disability rights legislation can be attributed to different forces in different countries. In the United States, the empowerment and influence of disability advocacy groups, such as Vietnam veterans returning from war championing the need for change (Barnes, Mercer, & Shakespeare, 1999), was instrumental in moving welfare reform toward civil rights law (Degener & Quinn, 2000; Waddington & Diller, 2007). In the United Kingdom, civil rights laws focused less on individual rights and more on the achievement of social-policy gains (Gleeson, 2001). Because there is no written constitution in Britain, the rights-based advocacy model, Gleeson points out, has not been adopted. Whereas the widespread politicization of people with a disability and an advocacy group approach has been used successfully in the United States to bring about legislative change, other countries, such as the United Kingdom where various disability groups have not been as unified and effective in influencing change (Imrie, 1996), have relied on charities to drive the process (Gleeson, 2001). In contrast, Australia and New Zealand have secured improved civil rights and social structural change, largely through initiatives in state-government policy regimes (Gleeson, 2001).

The United States was one of the first countries to adopt antidiscrimination legislation and civil rights laws, starting with scattered equality provisions in various laws (Degener & Quinn, 2000). Legislation within the United States began with general civil rights legislation in 1964. This seminal piece of legislation did not specifically target people with a disability, but instead served as the basis for a series of disability-specific laws that covered both the U.S. federal government and the country as a whole (Fletcher, 2004; Peterson, 1998). The push for civil rights legislation in the United States continued with the development of more comprehensive laws, such as the Americans With Disabilities Act (ADA) in the 1990s. Table 4-1 outlines the history of the development of U.S. legislation, regulations, and standards.

The ADA (1990) represents not only the centerpiece of U.S. civil rights legislation related to people with a disability, it is also a landmark piece of legislation throughout the world. The intent of this legislation is to ensure that people with a disability experience equal opportunity, full participation, independent living, and economic self-sufficiency, and it is considerably more extensive in its coverage than other U.S. legislation (Department of Employment, Education, Training, and Youth Affairs, 1997). Not only does it give people with a disability the same protection as other groups, it also seeks to integrate people with a disability into the social mainstream and to break down barriers created by prejudice (Waddington & Diller, 2007). The ADA requires planners to consider access as being more than a technical or design issue and to understand its role in social injustice (Imrie, 1996). As rights-based legislation, it has heightened society's awareness of the built environment and the part it has played, and continues to play, in isolating and alienating people with a disability (Imrie, 1996). Further, it has increased the visibility of people with a disability in society, provided them with legal and often moral means of influence, and transformed some aspects of service provision for people with a disability (Imrie & Hall, 2001a).

TRANSLATING LEGISLATION INTO REGULATIONS

In the United States, when Congress passes a piece of legislation, it becomes a law. Laws dictating social policy alone, such as the ADA (1990), are generally insufficient to achieve accessibility. Consequently, building laws and state legislation that allow states to enforce building codes (including accessibility provisions) have also been promulgated to protect the rights of individuals with a disability. There are also design guidelines to assist developers to fulfill the requirements of these laws. These guidelines then serve as the basis for nominating the standards that detail the technical information. Figure 4-1 illustrates the relationship between laws, guidelines, and standards.

The ADA is a comprehensive but complex law and is considered to have a "patchwork quilt" of regulations associated with it (Ostroff, 2001). For example, the Architectural Barriers Act (ABA) of 1968 was initially developed to ensure access to facilities designed, built, altered, or leased with federal funds. This law was one of the first efforts to ensure access to the built environment; however, unlike the ADA, it did not have its basis in equal rights.

Under the ABA and ADA, the Access Board develops and maintains accessibility guidelines. These guidelines specify minimum or baseline

Table 4-1. Developments in U.S. Legislation, Standards, and Design Documentation

LEGISLATION	STANDARDS AND DESIGN DOCUMENTATION
1964 Civil Rights Act **1966** 30 states pass the accessibility legislation to use A117.1 **1968** National Commission on Architectural Barriers to Rehabilitation of the Handicapped (NCABRH) report, Design for All Americans, establishes groundwork for future accessibility legislation **1968 ABA** (Public Law 90-480)—Those buildings and facilities designed, constructed, altered, or leased with federal funds required to be fully accessible	**1961 ANSI A117.1 Making Buildings Accessible For and Usable by the Physically Handicapped** (American National Standards Institute [ANSI], 2003)—Voluntary access standards unless adopted by state or local governments **1965** Formation of the NCABRH (1967)
1973 49 states pass accessibility legislation to use ANSI A117.1 **1973 Rehabilitation Act** **1978** Rehabilitation Act amended—Authorizes the Access Board to establish minimum accessibility guidelines under the ABA and to ensure compliance with requirements	**1973** Access Board created under Section 504 of the Rehabilitation Act 1973
1988 Fair Housing Amendments Act (FHAA)—Expands the coverage of the Civil Rights Act 1968 to cover families with children and people with disabilities; access required for multifamily dwellings consisting of four or more units, both public and private	**1980 ANSI A117.1** revision **1982 Minimum Guidelines and Requirements for Accessible Design (MGRAD)**—Access Board issues minimum guidelines under the ABA that form the basis for enforceable standards **1984 Uniform Federal Accessibility Standards (UFAS)**—Four federal agencies jointly adopt standards to enforce the ABA, based on MGRAD, and cover newly constructed or renovated buildings built with federal funding, including public housing **1986 ANSI A117.1** revision
1990 ADA (Public Law 101-336)—Extends civil rights protection to people with disabilities; prohibits discrimination in the full and equal enjoyment of goods, services, facilities, privileges, advantages, or accommodations of any place of public accommodation (Title III) and state or local government (Title II). New building construction and alterations to be accessible, publicly and privately funded. Access requirements applicable to common areas for multiunit accommodation.	**1991 ADA Accessibility Guidelines (ADAAG)**—Covers access in new construction and alterations to places of public accommodation and commercial facilities covered by the ADA; also applicable to state and local government facilities. Guideline serves as the baseline of standards used to enforce the ADA; the Access Board issued supplements to ADAAG covering state and local government facilities (1998), children's environments (1998), play areas (2000), and recreation facilities (2002). **1991 Fair Housing Accessibility Guidelines (FHAG)** (Housing and Urban Development)—Guides design requirements for multifamily housing **1992 Council of American Building Officials (CABO)/ANSI A117.1** revision **1998 CABO/ANSI A117.1** revision **2003 International Code Council/ANSI A117.1** revision **2004 ADA-ABA Guidelines**—The Access Board jointly updates its guidelines under the ADA and ABA to make them more consistent. Enforcing agencies under the ADA and ABA adopt new standards based on these updated guidelines.

design criteria for regulations and standards to fulfill the requirements of these laws, but they are not enforceable unless a recognized agency adopts them as regulations. Prior to 2004, the ADA and ABA had separate guidelines. For example, the MGRAD (Architectural and Transportation Barriers Compliance Board, 1981) was first issued in 1982 as the accessibility guidelines for the ABA. Similarly, the ADAAG (1991) was developed by the Access Board to support civil rights legislation (ADA) by addressing accessibility to all public facilities, regardless of whether they receive federal funding (Nishita, Liebig, Pynoos, Perelman, & Spegal, 2007). These were periodically revised and, in 2004, were combined to form a uniform set of guidelines—the *ADA-ABA Accessibility Guidelines*—to cover both acts and to be more compatible with ANSI A117.1 (2003), the model accessibility code that is referenced in most U.S. building codes. By 2009, all federal agencies, with the exception of the U.S. Department of Housing and Urban Development (HUD), had adopted the ADA-ABA Accessibility Guidelines as mandatory to ensure building accessibility in the public and private sectors.

Guidelines developed to reinforce the ADA and ABA serve as a baseline for the development of standards. Standards provide the technical information required to make spaces or elements accessible. This includes detailing specifications, such as dimensions, materials, and slope or gradient requirements (Bowen, 2009). In 1984, the UFAS (1988) was developed to enforce the ABA and Section 504 of the Rehabilitation Act (1973) for buildings constructed with federal funding, including public housing. UFAS was the result of combining accessibility standards developed by four separate federal agencies to comply with the Architectural and Transportation Barriers Compliance Board's MGRAD (1981). Similarly, in 1994, the ADA standards were developed by the Department of Justice to enforce the ADA legislation and to ensure equal access in and out of commercial buildings and places of accommodation. The ADA standards have their basis in the ADAAG developed by the Access Board.

Over time, the Access Board has combined both the ADA and ABA Guidelines into one unified set of guidelines (ADA-ABA Accessibility Guidelines, 2004). By 2009, some of the federal agencies vested with enforcing the ABA adopted the new ADA-ABA guidelines. However, by 2009, neither enforcing authority for the ADA had adopted the new version of the ADAAG as *ADA Accessibility Standards*. As a result, the new guidelines are not mandatory unless adopted by these authorities. Because federal laws (ADA) and regulations take precedence over state

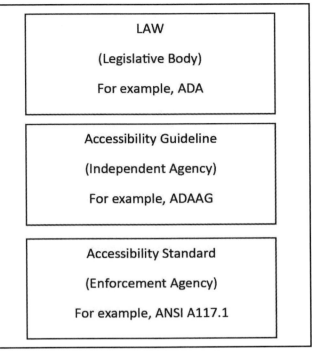

Figure 4-1. Hierarchy of enforceable regulations to support legislation.

and local laws and regulations, state/local laws/ regulations have to meet the minimum requirements of the federal laws, although they can specify higher standards (Rogerson, 2005).

There is a complex array of legislation covering various building types in the United States. For example, building works addressed by various pieces of legislation include the following:

+ Construction or alteration of state and local government and commercial facilities (ADA)

+ Access to buildings constructed, leased, or funded by the federal government (ABA)

+ Access to public spaces in multifamily housing (ADA)

+ Construction or renovation of public housing (Rehabilitation Act)

+ Construction or modifications to federally funded, designed, leased, or altered accommodation (ADA)

+ Construction and modifications to multifamily housing through specific housing legislation (FHAA)

+ Construction and modification of federally assisted single-family housing and townhouses, (Eleanor Smith Inclusive Home Design Act— revised 2013)

Table 4-2. Types of Facilities Addressed by Various Laws, Guidelines, and Standards

LAW	GUIDELINES	STANDARD	TYPE OF FACILITIES
ADA (civil law)	1991: ADAAG 2004: ADA-ABA Guidelines	1992, 1998, 2003: ANSI A117.1	Construction or alteration of facilities in both public (state and local government facilities) and private (places of public accommodation and commercial facilities) sectors, including places of public accommodation and commercial, state, and local government buildings and public spaces within multifamily housing
ABA (building law)	1982: MGRAD	1988: UFAS	All buildings constructed by or on behalf of the United States leased by the federal government or financed by federal dollars
504 Rehabilitation Act (civil law)		UFAS	New construction or renovation to a building using assistance from the federal government, including public housing
Fair Housing Act (FHA) 1968 (building law)	FHAG (1991)	ANSI A117.1	Sale, rental, and financing of private and public housing as well as the physical design of multifamily housing—four units of more or as few as two attached units that are not owner occupied
FHAA 1988 (building law)	FHAAG (1991)	ANSI A117.1	Residential structures of four or more units. Newly constructed multifamily dwelling units.
Visitability (selected states)			Private, single-family residences

Each of these laws has associated guidelines and standards that address design requirements of the specific facilities covered by the legislation (Table 4-2).

IMPLEMENTING AND MONITORING ACCESS REQUIREMENTS

There are various mechanisms for implementing and monitoring compliance with legislation and building regulations. As discussed in the previous section, the design of guidelines and standards is fundamental to ensuring buildings and facilities allow equitable access. These standards and guidelines assist designers, developers, and builders in the design and building of accessible facilities. Building on the requirement of Section 504 of the 1973 Rehabilitation Act, the ADA requires that government entities receiving federal funds ensure access to all new facilities and develop plans to correct deficiencies in existing facilities. To promote accessibility, there is training in ADA requirements, design guidelines and standards, and technical assistance via toll-free hotlines and publications (Ostroff, 2001). To check compliance, builders can undertake activities, including engaging experts to review plans, changing contract documents with design and construction firms to ensure proper responsibility, and completing construction site inspections and post-construction inspections.

In most countries, the two main ways authorities can monitor compliance are through pre-construction approval and a post-construction complaints-based process. Pre-construction approval requires that plans be submitted to an authority for endorsement (the issuance of a building permit that allows construction to take place) before building can commence (Richard Duncan, personal communication, July 23, 2009). This ensures that the design complies with local or state building codes (not necessarily civil rights laws) prior to construction. A post-construction complaints-based process, which generally follows compliance with the provisions of the civil rights laws and their guidelines, allows complaints about a facility's inaccessibility to be filed with a suitable authority once the problems have been identified. Enforcing disability discrimination law is often the task of public administrative agencies and the courts (Degener & Quinn, 2000), though complaints and lawsuits can be brought by private individuals, groups, and other private entities. Some countries, such as Australia, have a national construction code that requires all new public facilities and major renovations to comply with referenced access standards. This code mandates that plans be endorsed as complying with accessibility requirements prior to construction. Such a process ensures that all public buildings meet essential accessibility requirements and that the design and building industry is clear about their responsibility to provide accessibility. This requirement also reduces the likelihood of a post-construction complaint process occurring relating to discrimination; however, it does not preclude it. The disability discrimination legislation is used to deal with post-construction–based complaints.

Disability discrimination legislation takes precedence over, and provides a broader mandate than, building codes and regulations. Further, lawsuits involving accessibility issues are usually based on human or civil rights legislation (Ringaert, 2003). A building might be built according to a building code and/or standard, but if it excludes a targeted user or protected class of people, certain entities could sue because human or civil rights legislation would indicate that a person could not be discriminated against in the built environment on the basis of that person having a disability (Ringaert, 2003).

In the United States, there are no pre-construction approval processes for ADA compliance; rather, the ADA is enforced after construction when a complaint is filed. Individuals who believe they have been discriminated against may file a complaint with the relevant federal agency or federal court (Disability Rights Education & Defense Fund, 2008). Enforcement agencies encourage informal mediation and voluntary compliance (Disability Rights Education & Defense Fund, 2008). Yee and Golden (2007) describe enforcement of the law as playing a large role in the ADA's success in raising public awareness of the rights of people with disabilities. The Disability Rights Section of the Civil Rights Division of the U.S. Department of Justice is given the lead federal role in enforcing the legislation, and they investigate complaints lodged by the public, undertake periodic compliance reviews, and bring civil enforcement action (Mooney Cotter, 2007; Yee & Golden, 2007). However, the Department of Justice is authorized to bring a lawsuit where there is a pattern or practice of discrimination in violation of the legislation (Mooney Cotter, 2007). In enacting the ADA, Congress encouraged the use of alternative means of dispute resolution, including mediation, to resolve disputes. If mediation is unsuccessful, the various parties can pursue all legal remedies provided under the legislation, including private lawsuits (Mooney Cotter, 2007).

Under the provisions of the ADA, existing structures that have been built prior to the ADA's enactment also need to have accessibility improvements when possible. In the United States, barriers have to be removed only when it is readily achievable or structurally practicable. Readily achievable means that the changes are easily accomplished and can be carried out with little difficulty or expense. Examples include the simple ramping of a few steps or the installation of grab bars where only routine reinforcement of the wall is required. In determining whether an action to make a public accommodation accessible would be readily achievable, the overall size and cost of the proposed changes to the development are considered. Full compliance is considered structurally impracticable only in those circumstances where the incorporation of accessibility features is not easily accomplished and able to be carried out without much difficulty or expense.

In the United Kingdom, the Equality Act, a civil law, came into force on October 1, 2010 (except in Ireland, where the Disability Discrimination Act [DDA, 1995] is still in place and enforcement monitored by the Equality Commission for Northern Ireland). The Equality Act has two main purposes: to harmonize discrimination law and to strengthen the law to support progress on equality. The DDA 1995 has been combined with over 100 other pieces of legislation into this one act that provides a legal framework to protect the rights of individuals and advance equality of opportunity for all people. Technical guidance, rather than a strict compliance document, is provided. This guidance is considered to be a nonstatutory version of a code that provides comprehensive legal interpretation of sections of the act and the requirements of the legislation. As a result, it allows the requirements of the legislation to alter in line with changes in national best practice guidelines with regard to disability.

The U.K. Equality and Human Rights Commission (1995) has a role to eliminate discrimination against people with a disability and to promote equality of opportunity (Sawyer & Bright, 2007). Under the legislation, Disability Committees have been established in England, Scotland, and Wales because of the highly distinctive nature of disability equality law. The Disability Committees have decision-making powers in relation to those matters that solely concern disability, and the commission must seek the advice of the committee on all matters that relate to disability in a significant way. An Equality Advisory and Support Service provides online advice about discrimination and rights to people who have experienced discrimination, including handling of complaints. If complaints have not been resolved, individuals may take the issue to the Government Equalities Office for review. It has replaced the helpline service previously provided by the Equality and Human Rights Commission.

Prior to the introduction of the Equality Act (2010) in England, Scotland, and Wales, the DDA in the United Kingdom was considered by some to be more progressive in some areas than the ADA; it introduced a wide range of regulations to ensure accessibility and that reasonable adjustments are made (Imrie & Hall, 2001b). New design and planning benchmarks are emerging (Gooding, 1996; Imrie & Hall, 2001b). Access auditing of public premises has also increased over time, and businesses are questioning the implications of the DDA for their service (Gooding, 1996; Imrie & Hall, 2001b).

In Australia, access to the built environment is monitored through the DDA (1992) through a post-construction complaints-based process overseen by the Australian Human Rights Commission. The DDA requires that action plans be developed by the operators or owners of the public premises and lodged with the Australian Human Rights Commission to ensure that complaints are not submitted post-construction. The Australian DDA recognizes that equitable access for people with disabilities could cause unjustifiable hardship for the owner or operator of the premises. The DDA does not require that access be provided in the built environment if it would impose unjustifiable hardship on the person who would have to provide the equitable access. The Federal Court or Federal Magistrates Service determines what constitutes unjustifiable hardship. Issues considered in the claims of unjustifiable hardship can include cost to the proprietor; technical limits; topographical restrictions; the positive and negative effect on other people; safety, design, and construction issues; and the benefit for people with a disability. The Disability (Access to Premises—Buildings) Standards 2010 (the Premises Standards) have been created by the Australian Human Rights Commission to ensure that dignified, equitable, cost-effective, and reasonably achievable access to public buildings and the facilities and services within buildings is provided for people with a disability, and to give certainty to building certifiers, developers, and managers that, if the standards are complied with, they cannot be subject to a successful complaint under the DDA in relation to those matters covered by the Premises Standards (Australian Human Rights Commission, 2015). The Australian Human Rights Commission handles complaints about discrimination and uses a process of conciliation. If issues are unresolved, they may be taken to the Federal Magistrates Court or the Federal Court of Australia.

The Canadian Charter of Rights and Freedoms, with the federal and provincial human rights legislation, is a different approach to the complaints-based human rights approach followed in Australia and the United States (Department of Employment, Education, Training, and Youth Affairs, 1997). The Canadian Human Rights Act (1985) emphasizes the need to accommodate people with a disability unless doing so causes undue hardship (Mallory Hill & Everton, 2001). Case law has shown that upholding this accommodation is a right and not a privilege (Mallory Hill & Everton, 2001). Undue hardship is measured against health, safety, and cost (Mallory Hill & Everton, 2001). The Canadian Human Rights Commission is responsible for human rights issues and their application at the federal level. Separate provincial and territorial human rights commissions are responsible for enacting the provisions of the Human Rights Code within each province and municipality (Mallory Hill & Everton, 2001).

Private Housing Legislation

Similar legislative and regulatory mechanisms exist in the residential sector, although there are few accessibility regulations that cover residential facilities and even fewer that comprehensively regulate the design and modification of private housing, specifically for people who are older or who have a disability (Hyde, Talbert, & Grayson, 1997). Nonetheless, there is a growing movement in some countries to extend accessibility regulations to private housing. A number of countries have adopted disability discrimination legislation, which has proven useful in situations where complaints have been made by people with a disability who have not been able to access the common areas of multifamily complexes. Countries such as Canada, which has specifically omitted residential design and construction from national legislation, have left residential accessibility up to local jurisdictions (Clarke Scott, Nowlan, & Gutman, 2001; Mallory Hill & Everton, 2001; Rogerson, 2005). The United States is one of the few countries in the world with civil rights legislation that covers private (multifamily) housing (Starr, 2005). Further, the ABA and the Rehabilitation Act (1973) require a small percentage (5%) of housing constructed with public funds to have accessible dwelling units, and these are generally made available only to people who are eligible for publicly funded housing (Maisel, Smith, & Steinfeld, 2008).

Specifically, in the United States, the FHA, originally passed as Title VIII of the Civil Rights Act of 1964, prohibits discrimination in the sale, rental, and financing of private and public housing, as well as the physical design of newly constructed multifamily housing, based on race, color, religion, gender, or national origin (FHA, 1968). Title VIII was amended in 1988 by the FHAA, which expanded coverage of the act to prohibit discrimination based on disability or family status. The FHAA significantly expanded the scope of the original legislation and strengthened its enforcement mechanisms to cover public and private multifamily housing (accommodation with more than four units; FHAA, 1988). Consequently, under this legislation, property owners are required to allow a tenant with a disability to undertake modifications within certain guidelines to accommodate his or her individual need (Newman & Mezrich, 1997). However, tenants would be required to pay for the alterations, comply with the building codes, and, if requested, return the property to its original condition when they leave (Lawlor & Thomas, 2008).

To reinforce the FHAA (1998), the U.S. Department of HUD released technical requirements for multifamily housing in 1991. The FHAG are designed to help builders comply with accessibility requirements as required by the government (International Code Council, 2007). It refers regularly to ANSI A117.1 (2003) and guides developments that may or may not have elevators.

The FHAG cover newly constructed multifamily homes constructed by builders, private property owners, and publicly assisted landlords (Imrie, 2006). Exempt properties include newly constructed townhouses or fewer than four housing unit complexes and properties constructed in locations with unusual terrain or other site characteristics that limit accessibility (Mooney Cotter, 2007; Newman & Mezrich, 1997; Nishita et al., 2007).

Builders constructing four or more owner-occupied dwelling units in buildings with one elevator or more have to make all units accessible or have to ensure accessibility to ground-floor units only if there is no elevator (Imrie, 2006; Newman & Mezrich, 1997). Accessible design required in newly constructed housing (rather than in existing housing) includes accessible common-use areas (e.g., via at least one accessible entrance, doors that are wide enough for wheelchairs to pass through, and kitchens and bathrooms that allow a person using a wheelchair to maneuver). It also includes other adaptable features within the housing (e.g., an accessible route to and through the dwelling, light switches, thermostats, and other controls in accessible locations) and reinforcement in bathroom walls for future installation of grab rails (U.S. Department of Justice, 2005). The owner of newly constructed buildings must be an active participant in making the building accessible and usable by people with a disability compared with the more passive role played by owners of existing properties (Newman & Mezrich, 1997).

Under the FHAG, access to public spaces in multifamily housing (e.g., exterior spaces, elevators, corridors, and interior common spaces) is mandated by the technical requirements for public spaces in the *ADA-ABA Accessibility Guidelines*. If a facility does not comply with these requirements, residents with disabilities can request reasonable modifications to common interior or exterior areas at the property owner's expense (Newman & Mezrich, 1997).

One goal of the FHAA (1988) is to facilitate home modifications in rental housing (Steinfeld, Levine, & Shea, 1998) by providing people with disabilities the right to reasonable accommodation. This means that a landlord cannot prevent a tenant from adding home modifications to a housing unit to increase its accessibility (National Association of Home Builders Research Center, 2007), though these changes must be negotiated. There is a requirement that tenants pay for these modifications themselves and that they use a licensed contractor to complete the work. At the end of their tenancy, they must return the area to its original condition, again at the cost of the tenant who installed the original modifications (National Association of Home Builders Research Center; Steinfeld et al., 1998). However, modifications might be made to the interior of the home that do not have to be removed if they do not affect the next tenant's use of the apartment (Steinfeld et al., 1998). The section of the bill that deals with retrofitting existing multiunit dwellings calls for "reasonable accommodation" for people with disabilities, but it is vague on the responsibility of the owner to pay for changes, even in the common areas (Pynoos & Nishita, 2006, p. 284).

As previously indicated, federal U.S. law requires access for people with mobility and other impairments to all new multifamily residences and to a small percentage of single-family homes constructed with public funds (Maisel et al., 2008). Consequently, current housing policy in the United States does not address the vast majority of single-family homes (as well as duplexes, townhomes, and triplexes) in which most people live (Maisel et al., 2008). As a result, "visitability" legislation has been developed and implemented in the United States over the past two decades, most of it occurring at state and local levels (Spegal & Liebig, 2003). The visitability movement seeks to increase the supply of housing that people with disabilities can visit or live in for a short term. Design features include the incorporation of a zero-step entrance, wide doorways, and at least one bathroom on the main floor of the home (Maisel et al., 2008).

Visitability programs have also begun to spread throughout the United States, using mandates, incentives, and voluntary-based codes to encourage visitable design to be adopted in new housing. To date, visitability legislation has been created in at least 27 U.S. cities (Maisel et al., 2008). Little is known about the outcomes of these programs because of the following:

+ Not all locations use the term *visitability* in their enactments

+ There is no pattern of organizations accountable for the oversight of the ordinances

+ Agencies responsible for the implementation of the approach are not specified

+ There is no one method of keeping track of how many homes have been built (Spegal & Liebig, 2003)

The extent to which visitability is adopted depends on local municipalities "buying" into the idea and ensuring it is included in local ordinances or building codes. Much of the approach is being adopted unevenly, depending on the political stance of the various states. Visitability is continuing to face opposition because of concerns about cost and consumer perception (Kochera, 2002).

Because of the fragmented adoption of visitability on the state and local level, the visitability movement has inspired the creation of the Inclusive Home Design Act that was first introduced into the U.S. Congress as a bill in 2003, 2005, 2007, and then as the Eleanor Smith Inclusive Home Design Act in 2015 (now known as *HR 4202*). Although Congress has not yet passed the bill, it has the potential to ensure that single-family homes receiving assistance from the federal government incorporate visitable features (Maisel et al., 2008).

The U.S. Supreme Court Olmstead decision (1999) has also affected accessible housing because it requires states to administer services, programs, and activities for people with disabilities in "integrated" settings (Maisel et al., 2008). The decision has led to more homes being made accessible, with some states using funding from federal grant programs for home modifications for people moving from institutions into the community (Maisel et al., 2008).

Implementing and Monitoring Access Requirements

The FHAA (1988) established administrative enforcement mechanisms to enable the HUD attorneys to bring actions before administrative law judges on behalf of people experiencing housing discrimination. Complaints filed with HUD are investigated by the Office of Fair Housing and Equal Opportunity (Mooney Cotter, 2007). The Department of Justice can take over the role of the department in seeking resolution on behalf of aggrieved people if it proceeds as a civil action (Mooney Cotter, 2007). A United States administrative law judge may preside over the case unless any party to the charge elects to have the case heard in federal district court (U.S. Department of HUD, 2015).

Similar to disputes in the public sector, disability discrimination legislation also takes precedence over building codes and regulations in residential settings (Ringaert, 2003). Consequently, a building constructed according to a building code and/or standard may still result in a complaint or lawsuit if a person is discriminated against in the built environment based on that person having a disability (Ringaert, 2003).

EVALUATION OF CURRENT LEGISLATION AND STANDARDS

The rights-based approach to access policy used in the United States has also been identified as having limitations (Gooding, 1994; Higgins, 1992; Imrie, 1996; Young, 1990). First, this type of approach reinforces the individual conceptualization of disability, emphasizing the problem as belonging to the individual rather than a problem being the norms embedded in society (Higgins, 1992; Imrie, 1996). Second, it presumes that the current situation that works for the majority is the ideal; therefore, it should be available and acceptable to all (Higgins, 1992; Imrie, 1996). Third, it is underpinned by a form of legal individualism that ignores or denies the structural inequalities that perpetuate discrimination against people's disabilities (Imrie, 1996). The onus remains with the "victim" to establish harm has been done in each situation (Imrie, 1996; Young, 1990). Rights legislation also attempts to provide equal protection to distinctly unequal groups and does not recognize the potential value of positive discrimination in addressing structural disadvantages (Gooding, 1994; Imrie, 1996). Although legislation can contain overt discrimination, it cannot eradicate it fully (Doyle, 1995; Imrie & Hall, 2001a). Consequently, the political and economic power of people with disabilities needs to be restored to enable them to influence government and corporate attitudes and practice (Imrie & Hall, 2001b).

There is a great deal of diversity and complexity in the way discrimination and civil rights legislation and building legislation regulations, codes, and standards have been developed, operationalized, and monitored across the world. Consequently, international legislative frameworks have also had varying meaningful impacts on design practice and people with a disability. For example, the civil status of people with a disability is markedly different between the United States and the United Kingdom. Despite this difference, there continues to be a struggle for this group in both countries to gain strong and binding antidiscrimination legislation that influences service delivery and the design of the built environment (Imrie, 1996). Access issues in the United States are regarded as matters of social justice, a problem relating to a person's civil liberties (Imrie, 1996). In the United Kingdom, the government sees access as a technical or compensatory matter that can be dealt with through redistributive measures (Imrie, 1996), and U.K. developers have noted that people with a disability have limited financial impact on their services and are reticent to build in features that meet their needs (Harrison & Davis, 2001).

Almost all of the countries and territories have not yet made the access requirements of people with a disability and older people an integral part of development plans relating to different features of the built environment (U.N., 1995). There are separate approaches to formulating access legislation distinct from existing relevant laws, bylaws, codes, rules, and regulations in countries and territories such as China, the Islamic Republic of Iran, Hong Kong, Japan, the Republic of Korea, and Vietnam (U.N., 1995). In contrast, Australia, Malaysia, and Singapore adopted an integrated approach in formulating their respective access legislation by incorporating access standards for people with a disability into relevant existing building regulations (U.N., 1995).

Another issue is that various pieces of legislation do not address the issues of creating livable and usable living spaces (Imrie & Hall, 2001b) that provide inclusive communities. There is evidence of failure to incorporate access considerations in urban and rural development projects and a focus on access to buildings rather than the overall development (Imrie, 2006). Although access legislation of Malaysia and Singapore applies to all types of buildings, including domestic buildings, legal instruments of other countries and territories tend to apply to public buildings only (U.N., 1995).

The use and enforcement of access law worldwide is inconsistent and uneven within and between regulatory authorities (Centre for Housing Research, 2007; Mazumdar & Geis, 2001; Newman & Mezrich, 1997; Switzer, 2001). There is a perception that there have been inadequate staffing and budgetary resources at various government levels to implement and enforce the legislation (Hinton, 2003; Mazumdar & Geis, 2001). Further, there is evidence that there is a high level of ignorance about how and when to use the regulations, particularly among those people who are in roles of enforcement (Barnes, 2007; Centre for Housing Research, 2007; Steinfeld et al., 1998). For example, confusion exists in relation to how building

regulations interface with disability discrimination legislation, resulting in design responses that are often limited or confused (Imrie & Hall, 2001a). Builders and owners are required to have an understanding of how their buildings meet the broad civil rights requirements of the law, and yet many have never studied law or civil rights interpretations (Salmen, 2001). There is a view that even when owners understand the law, they might not understand their responsibilities (Steinfeld et al., 1998).

Ambiguities, exemptions, and get-out clauses characterize access statutes, thus diminishing their coverage and effectiveness (Barnes, 2007; Imrie & Hall, 2001a; Milner & Madigan, 2001; Newman & Mezrich, 1997). For example, the ADA has get-out clauses such as "undue hardship," "readily achievable," and "unreasonable financial costs," which can be used to justify not making built environments accessible (Imrie, 1996). This and other legislation have stipulations on reasonable provision of access for people with disabilities that are vague and open to interpretation (i.e., there appears to be multiple interpretations of the word *reasonable*, which is used frequently in legislation in this area; Imrie & Hall, 2001a).

The complaint process relies on people with a disability contacting the relevant authorities. However, they often do not understand the intent and application of the legislation, regulations, and standards and experience a great deal of difficulty in navigating the complaints system. The complaints process can often be protracted and poorly articulated or promoted. At times, people with a disability do not have the emotional energy to cope with the process and can fear negative or inadequate responses to their requests, making them feel even more disempowered (Frank, 2005; Newman & Mezrich, 1997). Further, some legal systems, such as those in the United States, are adversarial in nature, influencing people's perceptions of or reactions to the complaint process (Mazumdar & Geis, 2001).

Finally, agencies and groups participating in formulating access legislation have varied greatly between countries (Nielsen & Ambrose, 1998; U.N., 1995). Consequently, legislation has tended to form without a comprehensive understanding of the needs of all people with a disability (Milner & Madigan, 2001; U.N., 1995). There is an emphasis on adults in wheelchairs and a focus on the medical conception of disability that is abstract and generalized (Imrie & Hall, 2001a). There is also a generalization of access requirements across groups of people (Imrie & Hall, 2001a). Building regulations also fail to take account of the diverse and changing needs of people with disabilities (Imrie & Hall, 2001a). Attitudes toward people with disabilities are still being framed by the concept of the "undeserving poor," or buildings are being designed to provide minimum standards of access (Imrie, 2003). Architects have been described as making accessibility a legal rather than moral imperative (Mazumdar & Geis, 2001). Consequently, attitudinal and architectural barriers continue to exist that limit the participation of people with disabilities in society (Switzer, 2001).

Private Homes

To support disability rights, civil rights legislation has included provisions for the removal of physical barriers to activity and participation, as well as the designation of authorities to enforce those accessibility requirements. As pointed out at the beginning of this chapter, the jurisdiction for these regulations is primarily public buildings and facilities. There are few regulations that cover residential facilities and even fewer that comprehensively regulate the design and modification of private housing, specifically for older people and people with a disability (Hyde et al., 1997). Nonetheless, there is a growing movement in some countries to extend accessibility regulations to private housing. In some countries, in the absence of specific legislation, the design guidelines and standards produced for public buildings are often used as a guide when modifying private homes. As explained in the chapter on access standards (Chapter 11), this can be problematic if property developers, design and construction professionals, and occupational therapists are not familiar with the limitations associated with the use of these standards. This can include, for example, the potential mismatch between the functional ability of the person and the responsiveness of the accessible design to that person's needs (Sanford & Megrew, 1999).

Worldwide, approaches to ensuring housing accessibility are continuing to develop. For example, in Europe, housing accessibility has been secured by three main strategies:

1. Mainstreaming, where all new dwellings must meet accessibility standards (e.g., Denmark, Sweden, Norway, the Netherlands)

2. Exclusive legislation, which is applied to only certain categories of users such as wheelchair users (e.g., United Kingdom, Austria, Germany, Portugal, Luxembourg)

3. A progressive approach in which increasing degrees of accessibility and adaptability are stipulated for different building types and users (e.g., Italy; Nielsen & Ambrose, 1998)

Although many countries have adopted various requirements for new housing, such as the United States, these requirements are typically intended for new multifamily housing (Kochera, 2002). Countries with multifamily accessibility policies include Italy, the Netherlands, France, Spain, Greece, and Sweden (Kochera, 2002). As an exception to this, since 2004, London, England, has had a policy that requires all new homes (including houses and flats of varying sizes in both the public and private sectors) be built to the Lifetime Homes Standard, with 10% built to wheelchair accessible standard. In Wales and Northern Ireland, the Welsh Assembly and the Northern Ireland Housing Executive require the Lifetime Homes Standard in their funded developments. The Lifetime Homes Standard is generally higher than that required by Part M of the Building Regulations (which deals with accessibility), although some elements of Part M are equal to the Lifetime Homes requirements or need relatively minor changes to comply (Lifetime Homes, 2015).

Although it is easy to provide incentives and regulations for new stock, most older people and people with long-term disabilities live in established housing and cannot readily afford to purchase new dwellings. The following are examples of countries that have building regulations requiring accessibility in private homes (Imrie, 2006):

+ Norway: Building regulations require an accessible entry and external approach to the common entrance of a building that has more than four dwellings and toilets in all new dwellings, regardless of whether they are single-family homes or multiunit developments.

+ Sweden: Building regulations state that there must be wheelchair access to all units in a residential building of three stories or more, including an accessible path of travel from the pavement to the building entrance, accessible thresholds, and the provision of a lift (there is no requirement for this in single-family homes).

+ Denmark: Building regulations stipulate that single-family homes that are self-built have to be constructed to minimum levels of accessibility, including having a no-step entrance.

+ Australia, Willoughby Council, New South Wales: New developments with more than nine dwellings are to incorporate adaptable housing design (AS4299); this is similar for multiunit developments for Waverley and Ryde Councils in New South Wales.

+ Japan: All new housing, both public and private, are to be built to universal design standards.

The U.S. approach to accessible housing is poor and underdeveloped. No single U.S. law or program regulates comprehensively for the design and adaptation of housing specifically for older people and people with a disability, although a patchwork of federal programs and mechanisms supports the implementation of home modifications (Hyde et al., 1997; Milner & Madigan, 2001). Regulations and design standards typically focus on the needs of wheelchair users with little consideration for the diverse needs of the population of older people and people with a disability. Little research exists on the changes in wheelchair size and shape and the impact of the introduction of new technology to improve the mobility of the equipment and comfort of the user, let alone the needs of the broader population of people with a disability whose access needs might differ significantly from the wheelchair user. Inevitably, future adaptations to homes designed specifically for wheelchair users are necessary to ensure better accessibility within the home and to cater to the needs of a broader range of people with a disability (Imrie, 2006).

A progressive approach, with use of increasing degrees of universal, accessible, and adaptable design for different building types and older people and people with a disability, can ensure housing accessibility. For example, Italy has various laws and ministerial decrees rather than a building code or building regulations. It stipulates three levels of accessibility: accessible (access to a building, including common areas, through the entry and use spaces within the building safely and independently); visitable (access to the principle spaces within buildings and to where there is at least one accessible toilet); and adaptable design (modification to the built environment at little cost; Christophersen, 2001; D'Innocenzo & Morini, 2001). This progressive approach has developed from the movement to integrate people with a disability into the community. Details and technical prescriptions have been added gradually to existing regulations over the years, resulting in professionals needing to keep in mind the design requirements of people with a disability while developing solutions (D'Innocenzo & Morini, 2001). Initially, public buildings were introduced to access regulations; that has now been extended to include public residential buildings and neighborhoods (D'Innocenzo & Morini, 2001). Different design approaches for different building types were selected based on the needs and priorities of the neighborhood. People's varying differences have been driving a "policy of differences" for design practice rather than designing to suit the "average man" (D'Innocenzo & Morini, 2001, p. 15.20). Though there are gaps in the practice of this progressive design approach in Italy, a strong societal belief that every person has the right to access his or her own house and external built environments has emerged (D'Innocenzo & Morini, 2001).

Regulations, incentives, and information have been the three mechanisms used to promote adaptable housing for people of all ages and abilities in Europe (Nielsen & Ambrose, 1998). However, statutes in relation to providing accessible housing vary in form and content and are stronger in social-housing schemes or where the government has significant influence over the construction process (Imrie, 2006). The legal basis for ensuring access to housing is generally ineffectual, with limited means of enforcement (Imrie, 2006). Consequently, some view nonlegislative means as the fastest way to improve building practice (Nielsen & Ambrose, 1998). There is a perception that regulations increase cost, stifle design creativity and innovation, and decrease responsiveness to the market (Imrie, 2006). However, although there is a clear demand for accessible housing, there has been a poor market response. Some believe nonlegislative approaches such as voluntary guidelines, branding of universal designs, and information campaigns to be the least successful strategies for encouraging the development of more accessible housing in communities (Centre for Housing Research, 2007). The countries that have been most successful in producing a market response, such as the United States, Japan, and Norway, have systematically combined regulatory, incentive, and collaborative capacity building strategies (Centre for Housing Research, 2007). Countries where populations have been growing older faster have had regulations for new housing in place for a considerable length of time (Centre for Housing Research, 2007).

IMPLICATIONS FOR OCCUPATIONAL THERAPISTS

Occupational therapy services will continue to be in demand to provide home modification advice as older people and people with a disability struggle with built environments that require design improvements. Occupational therapists understand that older people and people with a disability constitute a diverse population that does not suit a "one-size-fits-all" design approach. They have an awareness of the limitations of the access standards that are used as the basis for public building and private home design, and they have an important role in informing builders and developers about the individual design needs of clients in relation to the person's home environment.

An understanding of human rights and building legislation will equip occupational therapists with knowledge and information that can be shared with older people and people with disabilities who may need to negotiate with builders and government authorities about appropriate design solutions in the public and private sectors. Therapists can encourage and empower older people and people with a disability to advocate for their own needs and provide their perspective on improvements needed during design and planning processes. Occupational therapists are also well suited to influencing the values and perspectives of design and construction professionals and advocating for better-designed environments within the community by educating these professionals about the diverse needs of older people and people with a disability, discussing the implications of designs, and challenging builders and designers to build more creatively and to universal design goals and principles. Therapists are also well placed to contribute to the evaluation of the effectiveness of various built environments and the impact of the environment on occupational performance, health, safety, independence, quality of life, and home and community participation outcomes. They also hold a professional responsibility to monitor and respond to proposed legislative changes and to support calls for improvements to legislation, guidelines, and standards.

CONCLUSION

This chapter has provided an overview of the worldwide range of legislation and guidelines relevant to promoting the rights of older people and people with a disability through access to the built environment. Information has been given on the move from the medical model to social models of disability, their advantages, and their limitations.

This chapter has described how human rights and disability discrimination legislation has attempted to shape community values, design and building practice, and service delivery to ensure people with a disability are afforded equitable access within the community. Information has been provided on the ADA as a landmark piece of legislation in the civil rights struggle for people with a disability in the United States. In some countries, such as the United Kingdom, building regulations and standards that incorporate access and mobility requirements have sought to address discrimination that might occur from barriers in public facilities and spaces. Very few countries have required their legislation to include mandatory accessible design of private homes.

This chapter has highlighted that the emergence of home environments that do not further disable people is far from being realized. Although disability discrimination, civil rights, and building legislation in various countries have influenced the design of public buildings, they have not made private accessible housing available to everyone requiring it, nor have they eliminated attitudinal barriers (Switzer, 2001). Current legislation around the world is not likely to make a dramatic change to the housing circumstances of older people and people with a disability. Rather, significant action is required to transform attitudes and value systems to positively influence housing quality and design for diverse populations (Imrie, 2006). Occupational therapists are well qualified and experienced to make a valuable contribution to transforming these attitudes and values. They can influence the values and perspective of design and construction professionals as they work in collaboration to design a more comprehensive use of dwelling spaces by people with diverse needs. In addition, they have a valuable role to advocate for older people and people with a disability and to empower them to influence design and construction practice in the community.

REFERENCES

American National Standards Institute. (2003). *ICC/ANSI A117.1-2003: Accessible and usable buildings and facilities*. New York: Author.

Americans With Disabilities Act. (1990). ADA home page. Retrieved from http://www.usdoj.gov/crt/ada/adahom1.htm

Americans With Disabilities Act Accessibility Guidelines. (1991). ADA accessibility guidelines for buildings and facilities (ADAAG). Retrieved from http://www.access-board.gov/adaag/html/adaag.htm

Americans With Disabilities Act and Architectural Barriers Act Accessibility Guidelines. (2004). ADA and ABA accessibility guidelines for buildings and facilities. Retrieved from http://www.access-board.gov/ada-aba/final.cfm

Architectural Barriers Act. (1968). The Architectural Barriers Act (ABA) of 1968. Retrieved from http://www.access-board.gov/about/laws/aba.htm

Architectural and Transportation Barriers Compliance Board. (1981). Minimum guidelines and requirements for accessible design. *Federal Register, 46*(11), 4270-4304.

Australia Disability Discrimination Act. (1992). Disability Discrimination Act 1992. Retrieved from http://www.dredf.org/international/Ausdda.html

Australian Human Rights Commission. (2015). Guidelines on application of the Premises Standards. Retrieved from https://www.humanrights.gov.au/guidelines-application-premises-standards

Australian Institute of Health and Welfare. (2003). *Disability: The use of aids and the role of the environment*. Canberra, Australia: Author.

Barnes, C. (2007). Education, citizenship and social justice. Retrieved from http://esj.sagepub.com/cgi/reprint/2/3/203

Barnes, C., Mercer, G., & Shakespeare, T. (1999). *Exploring disability: A sociological introduction*. Cambridge, UK: Polity Press.

Bowen, I. (2009). Access basics: The laws, the regulations, the standards (and where they come from): The Americans With Disabilities Act and Section 504. Retrieved from http://ada-one.com/pdf/AccessBasics.pdf

Brandt, E., & Pope, A. M. (Eds.). (1997). *Enabling America: Assessing the role of rehabilitation science and engineering*. Washington, DC: National Academy Press.

Canadian Human Rights Act. (1985). Canadian Human Rights Act (R.S., 1985, c. H-6). Retrieved from http://laws.justice.gc.ca/en/h-6/index.html

Centre for Housing Research. (2007). Housing and disability: Future proofing New Zealand's housing stock for an inclusive society. Prepared by CRESA/Public Policy & Research/Auckland Disability Resource Centre for Centre for Housing Research, Aotearoa, New Zealand, and the Office of Disability Issues.

Christophersen, J. (2001). Accessible housing in five European countries: Standards and built results. In W.F.E. Preiser & E. Ostroff (Eds.), *Universal design handbook* (pp. 13.1-13.14). New York: McGraw-Hill.

Civil Rights Act. (1964). Teaching with documents: The Civil Rights Act of 1964 and the Equal Employment Opportunity Commission. Retrieved from http://www.archives.gov/education/lessons/civil-rights-act

Clarke Scott, M. A., Nowlan, S., & Gutman, G. (2001). Progressive housing design and home technologies in Canada. In W.F.E. Preiser & E. Ostroff (Eds.), *Universal design handbook* (pp. 36.1-36.15). New York: McGraw-Hill.

Degener, T., & Quinn, G. (2000). A survey of international, comparative and regional disability law reform. Retrieved from http://www.dredf.org/international/degener_quinn.html

Department of Employment, Education, Training, and Youth Affairs. (1997). *Comparison of international provisions on disability discrimination in education*. Canberra, Australia: Author.

Department of Housing and Urban Development. (1991). Fair housing accessibility guidelines. *Federal Register, 56*(44), 9472-9515.

Dickson, E. (2007). Equality of opportunity for all? An assessment of the effectiveness of the Anti-Discrimination Act 1991 (Queensland) as a tool for the delivery of equality of opportunity in education for people with impairments (Unpublished thesis). T. C. Beirne School of Law, University of Queensland.

D'Innocenzo, A., & Morini, A. (2001). Accessible design in Italy. In W. F. E. Preiser & E. Ostroff (Eds.), *Universal design handbook* (pp. 15.1-15.23). New York: McGraw-Hill.

Disability Rights Education & Defense Fund. (2008). A comparison of ADA, IDEA, and Section 504. Retrieved from http://www.dredf.org/advocacy/comparison.html

Doyle, B. (1995). *Disability, discrimination and equal opportunities: A comparative study of the employment rights of disabled persons*. London: Mansell.

Equality and Human Rights Commission. (1995). The law about disability discrimination. Retrieved from http://www.equalityhumanrights.com/your-rights/disability/the-law-about-disability-discrimination

Fair Housing Act. (1968). United Stated Department of Justice Civil Rights Division: Fair Housing Act. Retrieved from http://www.usdoj.gov/crt/housing/title8.php

Fair Housing Amendments Act. (1988). FHEO programs. Retrieved from http://www.hud.gov/offices/fheo/progdesc/title8.cfm

Fletcher, V. (2004). American access. *Green Places*, February 24-25.

Frank, J. J. (2005). Barriers to the accommodation request process of the Americans with Disabilities Act. *Journal of Rehabilitation, 71*(2), 28-39.

Gleeson, B. (2001). Disability and the open city. *Urban Studies, 38*(2), 251-265.

Gooding, C. (1994). *Disabling laws, enabling acts*. London: Pluto Press.

Gooding, C. (1996). *Blackstone's guide to the Disability Discrimination Act 1995*. London: Blackstone Press.

Harrison, M., & Davis, C. (2001). *Housing, social policy and difference: Disability, ethnicity, gender and housing*. Bristol, UK: The Policy Press.

Hendricks, A. (1995). The significance of equality and non-discrimination for the protection of the rights and dignity of disabled persons. In T. Degener & Y. Koster-Dreese (Eds.), *Human rights and disabled persons: Essays and relevant human rights instruments* (pp. 40-62). Leiden, the Netherlands: Martinus Nijhoff Publishers.

Higgins, P. C. (1992). *Making disability: Exploring the social transformation of human variation*. Springfield, IL: Thomas.

Hinton, C. A. (2003). The perceptions of people with disabilities as to the effectiveness of the Americans With Disabilities Act. *Journal of Disability Policy Studies, 13*(4), 210-220.

Hurst, R. (2004). Legislation and human rights. In J. Swain, S. French, C. Barnes, & C. Thomas (Eds.), *Disabling barriers—Enabling environments* (pp. 297-230). London: Sage Publications.

Hyde, J., Talbert, R., & Grayson, P. J. (1997). Fostering adaptive housing: An overview of funding sources, laws and policies. In S. Lanspery & J. Hyde (Eds.), *Staying put: Adapting the places instead of the people* (pp. 223-236). Amityville, NY: Baywood Publishing Company, Inc.

Imrie, R. (1996). *Disability and the city: International perspectives*. New York: St. Martin's Press.

Imrie, R. (2003). Architects' conceptions of the human body. *Environment and Planning D: Society and Space, 21*, 47-65.

Imrie, R. (2006). *Accessible housing: Quality, disability and design*. London: Routledge Taylor & Francis Group.

Imrie, R., & Hall, P. (2001a). An exploration of disability and the development process. *Urban Studies, 38*(2), 333-350.

Imrie, R., & Hall, P. (2001b). *Inclusive design: Designing and developing accessible environments*. London: Spon Press.

Institute of Medicine. (1991). *Disability in America: A national agenda for prevention* (A. M. Pope & A. R. Tarlov, Eds.). Washington, DC: National Academy Press.

Institute of Medicine. (1997). *Enabling America: Assessing the role of rehabilitation science and engineering* (E. N. Brandt & A. M. Pope, Eds.). Washington, DC: National Academy Press.

International Code Council. (2007). Improving the accessibility of buildings for people with disabilities. Retrieved from http://www.iccsafe.org/safety/Pages/accessibility-1.aspx

Kochera, A. (2002). Accessibility and visitability features in single family homes: A review of state and local activity. Retrieved from http://assets.aarp.org/rgcenter/il/2002_03_homes.pdf

Kornblau, B., Shamberg, S., & Kein, R. (2000). Occupational therapy and the Americans With Disabilities Act (ADA). *American Journal of Occupational Therapy, 54*(6), 622-625.

Lawlor, D., & Thomas, M. (2008). *Residential design for ageing in place*. Hoboken, NJ: John Wiley.

Lifetime Homes. (2015). Policy and regulation. Retrieved from http://www.lifetimehomes.org.uk/pages/policy-and-regulation.html

Maisel, J. R., Smith, E., & Steinfeld, E. (2008). Increasing home access: Designing for visitability. Retrieved from http://assets.aarp.org/rgcenter/il/2008_14_access.pdf

Mallory Hill, S., & Everton, B. (2001). Accessibility standards and universal design developments in Canada. In W.F.E. Preiser & E. Ostroff (Eds.), *Universal design handbook* (pp. 16.1-16.17). New York: McGraw-Hill.

Mazumdar, S., & Geis, G. (2001). Interpreting accessibility standards: Experiences in the US courts. In W.F.E. Preiser & E. Ostroff (Eds.), *Universal design handbook* (pp. 12.1-12.8). New York: McGraw-Hill.

Milner, J., & Madigan, R. (2001). The politics of accessible housing in the UK. In S. M. Peace & C. Holland (Eds.), *Inclusive housing in an ageing society: Innovative approaches* (pp. 77-100). Bristol, UK: The Policy Press.

Mooney Cotter, A. (2007). *This ability*. Hampshire, UK: Ashgate Publishing Ltd.

Nagi, S. Z. (1965). Some conceptual issues in disability and rehabilitation. In M. B. Sussman (Ed.), *Sociology and rehabilitation* (pp. 100-113). Washington, DC: American Sociological Association.

Nagi, S. Z. (1976). An epidemiology of disability among adults in the United States. *Milbank Memorial Fund Quarterly, 54*, 439-468.

National Association of Home Builders Research Center. (2007). *Safety first: A technical approach to home modifications: Rebuilding together training workshop student guide*. Upper Marlboro, MD: Author.

National Center for Medical Rehabilitation Research. (1993). *Research plan for the National Center for Medical Rehabilitation Research*. Washington, DC: National Institutes of Health.

National Commission on Architectural Barriers to Rehabilitation of the Handicapped. (1967). Design for all Americans: A report of the National Commission on Architectural Barriers to Rehabilitation of the Handicapped. Retrieved from http://www.eric.ed.gov/ERICWebPortal/search/detailmini.jsp?_nfpb=true&_&ERICExtSearch_SearchValue_0=ED026786&ERICExtSearch_SearchType_0=no&accno=ED026786

Newman, S. J., & Mezrich, M. N. (1997). Implications of the 1988 Fair Housing Act for the Frail Elderly. In S. Lanspery & J. Hyde (Eds.), *Staying put: Adapting the places instead of the people* (pp. 237-252). Amityville, NY: Baywood Publishing Company, Inc.

Nielsen, C. W., & Ambrose, I. (1998). Lifetime adaptable housing in Europe. Retrieved from https://iospress.metapress.com/content/clcxwwxappgwdhpg/resource-secured/?target=fulltext.pdf

Nishita, C. M., Liebig, P. S., Pynoos, J., Perelman, L., & Spegal, K. (2007). Promoting basic accessibility in the home: Analyzing patterns in the diffusion of visitability legislation. *Journal of Disability Policy Studies, 18*(1), 2-13.

Office of the United Nations High Commissioner for Human Rights. (2006). Standard rules on the equalization of opportunities for persons with disabilities. Retrieved from http://www2.ohchr.org/english/law/opportunities.htm

Oliver, M. (1990). The individual and social models of disability. Paper presented at Joint Workshop of the Living Options Group and the Research Unit of the Royal College of Physicians. Retrieved from http://www.leeds.ac.uk/disability-studies/archiveuk/Oliver/in%20soc%20dis.pdf

Oliver, M. (1996). *Understanding disability, from theory to practice*. London: Macmillan.

Ostroff, E. (2001). Universal design practice in the United States. In W. F. E. Preiser & E. Ostroff (Eds.), *Universal design handbook* (pp. 12.1-12.8). New York: McGraw-Hill.

Ozdowski, S. (2005). Submission to the VBC/ABCB consultation on accessible housing. Retrieved from http://www.human-rights.gov.au/disability_rights/accommodation/housesub.htm

Peterson, W. (1998). Public policy affecting universal design. *Assistive Technology, 10*, 13-20.

Pynoos, J., & Nishita, C. M. (2006). Home modifications. In R. Schulz, L. S. Noelker, K. Rockwood, & R. Sprott (Eds.), *The encyclopedia of aging* (4th ed., pp. 528-530). New York: Springer.

Rehabilitation Act. (1973). The Rehabilitation Act Amendments of 1973, as amended. Retrieved from http://www.access-board.gov/enforcement/Rehab-Act-text/intro.htm

Ringaert, L. (2003). Universal design of the built environment to enable occupational performance. In L. Letts, P. Rigby, & D. Stewart (Eds.), *Using environments to enable occupational performance* (pp. 97-116). Thorofare, NJ: SLACK Incorporated.

Rogerson, F. (2005). *A review of the effectiveness of Part M of the building regulations*. Dublin, Ireland: National Disability Authority.

Salmen, J.P.S. (2001). US accessibility codes and standards: Challenges for universal design. In W.F.E. Preiser & E. Ostroff (Eds.), *Universal design handbook* (pp. 12.1-12.8). New York: McGraw-Hill.

Samaha, A. D. (2007). What good is the social model of disability? Retrieved from http://lawreview.uchicago.edu/issues/archive/v74/74_4/Samaha.pdf

Sanford, J. A., & Megrew, M. B. (1999). Using environmental simulation to measure accessibility for older people. In E. Steinfeld & S. Danford (Eds.), *Measuring enabling environments* (pp. 183-206). New York: Plenum Press.

Sawyer, A., & Bright, K. (2007). *Access manual: Auditing and managing inclusive built environments*. London: Blackwell Publishing Ltd.

Shakespeare, T., & Erickson, M. (2000). Different strokes: Beyond biological determinism and social constructionism. In H. Rose & S. Rose (Eds.), *Alas poor Darwin* (pp. 229-247). New York: Harmony Books.

Shakespeare, T., & Watson, N. (2001). The social model of disability: An outdated ideology? In S. N. Barnartt & B. M. Altman (Eds.), *Research in social science and disability, Vol. 2. Exploring theories and expanding methodologies* (pp. 9-21). New York: Elsevier Science Ltd.

Spegal, K., & Liebig, P. (2003). *Visitability: Trends, approaches and outcomes*. Los Angeles; University of Southern California: The National Resource Centre on Supportive Housing and Home Modification.

Starr, A. (2005). *Churchill fellowship report*. Canberra, Australia: The Winston Churchill Memorial Trust of Australia.

Steinfeld, E., Levine, D. R., & Shea, S. M. (1998). Home modifications and the fair housing law. *Technology and Disability, 8*, 15-35.

Swain, J. (2004). International perspectives on disability. In J. Swain, S. French, C. Barnes, & C. Thomas (Eds.), *Disabling barriers—Enabling environments* (pp. 54-60). London: Sage Publications.

Switzer, J. V. (2001). The Americans With Disabilities Act: Ten years later. *Policy Studies Journal, 29*(4), 629-632.

Uniform Federal Accessibility Standards. (1988). Uniform federal accessibility standards (UFAS). Retrieved from http://www.access-board.gov/ufas/ufas-html/ufas.htm

United Kingdom Disability Discrimination Act. (1995). Disability Discrimination Act 1995. Retrieved from http://www.opsi.gov.uk/acts/acts1995/1995050.htm

United Nations. (1971). Declaration on the rights of mentally retarded persons. Retrieved from http://www2.ohchr.org/english/law/res2856.htm

United Nations. (1975). United Nations declaration on the rights of disabled persons. Retrieved from http://www2.ohchr.org/english/law/res3447.htm

United Nations. (1993). The standard rules on the equalization of opportunities for persons with disabilities. Retrieved from http://www.un.org/esa/socdev/enable/dissre00.htm

United Nations. (1995). The promotion of non-handicapping environments for disabled and elderly persons in the Asia and Pacific Region—Chapter 1. Retrieved from http://www.unescap.org/esid/psis/disability/decade/publications/z15008cs/z1500802.htm

United Nations. (2008). Convention on the rights of persons with disabilities. Retrieved from http://www.un.org/disabilities/default.asp?navid=12&pid=150

United States Department of Housing and Urban Development. (2015). HUD charges South Dakota property owners with discriminating against resident with disabilities. Retrieved from http://portal.hud.gov/hudportal/HUD?src=/press/press_releases_media_advisories/2015/HUDNo_15-091

United States Department of Justice. (2005). A guide to disability rights laws. Retrieved from http://www.ada.gov/cguide.htm

United States Supreme Court. (1999). Olmstead V.L.C. (98-536) 527 U.S. 581 (1999) 138 F.3d 893.

Waddington, L., & Diller, M. (2007). Tensions and coherence in disability policy: The uneasy relationship between social welfare and civil rights models of disability in American, European and international employment law. Retrieved from http://www.dredf.org/international/waddington.html

Whalley Hammell, K. (2001). Changing institutional environments to enable occupation among people with severe physical impairments. In L. Letts, P. Rigby, & D. Stewart (Eds.), *Using environments to enable occupational performance* (pp. 35-54). Thorofare, NJ: SLACK Incorporated.

Williams, P. J. G., & Levy, D. (2006). New DDA duties of property owners and managers. Access by Design. *Centre for Accessible Environments, 106*, 6-9.

World Health Organization. (1980). *The international classification of impairments, disabilities and handicaps (ICIDH)*. Geneva, Switzerland: Author.

World Health Organization. (2001). *The international classification of function, disability and health: ICF*. Geneva, Switzerland: Author.

Yee, S., & Golden, M. (2007). Achieving accessibility: How the Americans with Disabilities Act is changing the face and mind of a nation. Retrieved from http://www.dredf.org/international/paper_y-g.html

Young, I. M. (1990). *Justice and the politics of difference*. Princeton, NJ: Princeton University Press.

The Home Modification Process

5

Elizabeth Ainsworth, MOccThy, Grad Cert Health Sci
and Desleigh de Jonge, MPhil (OccThy), Grad Cert Soc Sci

This chapter describes the home modification process as undertaken by occupational therapists. Overall, the process involves screening and prioritizing referrals, evaluating occupational performance in the home environment, planning and negotiating interventions, and monitoring and evaluating outcomes. More specifically, occupational therapists arrange appointments, visit clients, listen to clients' stories of their experiences in the home, gather information, evaluate occupational performance, research interventions, negotiate and recommend intervention options, seek technical advice, and evaluate the effectiveness of the interventions in relation to client outcomes. At each stage of the process, occupational therapists adopt a dynamic occupation-based and client-centered approach, which is influenced by specific models of practice and guided by professional reasoning. Such practice ensures that the health and level of participation of each client is maintained or enhanced through engagement in occupation or valued daily activities.

CHAPTER OBJECTIVES

By the end of this chapter, the reader will be able to:

+ Describe the process occupational therapists use when undertaking a home modification

+ Explain the contribution of the occupational therapist, the client, and other stakeholders to the home modification process

+ Explain the complexity associated with the minor modification process and the important role of the occupational therapist in this area of practice

INTRODUCTION

The home environment provides the context for many roles and activities and is an important setting for occupational therapists to examine when seeking to promote a person's occupational performance (Siebert, Smallfield, & Stark, 2014; Stark, 2003). With careful planning, people can remain in their own homes and continue to participate in community life (Law & Baum, 2005). Occupational therapists work with older people and people with disabilities to promote their health, well-being, and participation through engagement in everyday life activities (occupations) for the purposes of enhancing or enabling participation in roles, habits, and routines in the home and community (American Occupational Therapy Association [AOTA], 2014). In this work, therapists develop an understanding of the interaction between the following:

Ainsworth, E., & de Jonge, D. *An Occupational Therapist's
Guide to Home Modification Practice, Second Edition (pp. 83-110).*
© 2019 SLACK Incorporated.

✦ The clients' physical, sensory, cognitive, neu-
robehavioral, and psychological capacities

✦ Their physical, social, cultural, societal, personal, and temporal contexts

✦ The occupations, activities, tasks, and roles
that clients identify as important (AOTA, 2014;
Law & Baum, 2005)

Occupational therapists take a specific approach
to home modification practice that is guided by a
range of various models, the client-centered and
collaborative approach, and professional reasoning.
Of significance to the occupational therapy process
is the importance and meaning that clients assign
to their homes and the value associated with completing the home modification assessment in this
environment.

Recently, ecological or transactional models in
occupational therapy have recognized the dynamic
relationship between the person, their environment, and their occupations and regard occupational performance (the ability of a person to carry out
activities of daily life) as a result of the transaction
between the client, the activity, and the environment or context (AOTA, 2014; Brown, 2009). The
focus of home modifications intervention, using
these models, is to optimize occupational performance. Occupational therapists establish a picture
of a person's occupational performance by creating
an occupational profile that is a summary of a client's occupational history and experience, patterns
of daily living, interests, values, and needs (AOTA,
2014). Then, by observing how the client performs
activities relevant to desired occupations, the therapist evaluates occupational performance, taking
note of the effectiveness of performance and performance patterns (AOTA, 2014). The various ecological
transactional models that guide this process provide
the theoretical basis, or underlying concepts, that
guide evaluation and the selection of environmental
interventions for use to optimize occupational performance (Stark, 2003).

Occupational therapists use a client-centered and
collaborative approach to ensure that they develop a
deep appreciation of the client's experience and how
each is managing the occupations of everyday life
in the home and community. A client-centered and
collaborative approach allows therapists to work in
partnership with clients throughout all stages of the
home modification process, including evaluation,
planning, and negotiating interventions, and monitoring and measuring the outcomes (Law, Baptiste, &
Mills, 1995). This approach honors the contributions

of both the client and the occupational therapist
(AOTA, 2014; Law, 1998). Clients bring their stories to
the process, identifying and sharing their concerns
and priorities, while therapists contribute their
knowledge of occupational performance and the
person-environment-occupation transaction (AOTA,
2014; Law, 1998).

Professional reasoning skills are used by therapists as they listen to clients and observe them
interacting with their environment to plan, direct,
perform, and reflect on the care of clients (Schell
& Schell, 2008). A framework of scientific, narrative, pragmatic, ethical, and interactive reasoning is
used during the home modification process to frame
issues and guide problem solving and decision making (Schell, 2014). This framework also guides therapists in selecting and negotiating interventions in
collaboration with the client (Crabtree, 1998; Schell,
2014).

Throughout the home modification process, therapists remain mindful that the home is a private
living space and that clients attach meaning to the
home, the spaces, and the objects within it (Aplin, de
Jonge, & Gustafsson, 2013). Interventions can have a
significant impact on the home environment, which
can influence clients' acceptance and adjustment to
changes in the home (Aplin, de Jonge, & Gustafsson,
2015). Consulting with the client's family, friends,
caregivers, or other relevant stakeholders can also
optimize collaboration, agreement with recommendations, and satisfaction and improve overall client
outcomes (Law, 1998). Consulting with these stakeholders is required when a client is not able to make
informed choices and decisions about their home
modifications.

To ensure that home modifications are tailored to
the specific needs of each client, the occupational
therapy evaluation is undertaken in the home where
the activities are customarily performed (Corcoran,
2005; Law, King, & Russell, 2005; Siebert, 2005;
Siebert et al., 2014). Interviewing and observing people in their home environment provide occupational
therapists with an opportunity to observe activities and interactions as they occur in that setting
rather than relying on reports about the situation
(Corcoran, 2005) or on evaluations undertaken in an
unfamiliar environment. Interviewing the client in
his or her own home also enhances the occupational
therapist's understanding of the environmental context in which the client operates (Aplin et al., 2013;
Corcoran, 2005).

INFLUENCES ON OCCUPATIONAL THERAPY PRACTICE

Home modification practice varies across the world in terms of the extent and types of services provided. Differing funding and service priorities mean that some communities have well-developed home modification services, whereas others rely on a patchwork of local resources to attend to people's specific needs. The legislative context and building regulations in different jurisdictions can also affect which services are provided and how they are delivered. In some regions, home modifications are provided within health and home care services; in other locations, these services are provided within the housing and building sector.

Within services, the types and levels of occupational therapy services provided for people requiring home modifications depend on the following:

✦ The service delivery requirements of the programs

✦ The source and level of funding available

✦ The range of intervention options supported by the service

Furthermore, occupational therapists working in a private practice might provide a specific range of home modification services, depending on reimbursement schedules or the level of funding available for their time. Occupational therapists' competence in home modification practice varies greatly because of different types and levels of experience and the availability and quality of home modification training and education and building advice.

Although occupational therapists might not be involved in the whole home modification process, they could still be required to provide the client with assistance and advice at any stage. For example, occupational therapists may be contacted to undertake the whole home modification process; they may be required to work with the client up to the point of identifying interventions; they may need to check modifications proposed by alternative parties to provide advice on their suitability or whether changes are required; or they may need to visit the client to train him or her in the use of the home modification after it has been installed. At times, the therapist might be required to visit a person's home to examine a modification that is not achieving the desired outcome to suggest alternative interventions. The timing and extent of occupational therapists' involvement during the home modification process depend on whether the referrer and other stakeholders understand the role or contribution of occupational therapists in the home modification process and whether occupational therapists have sufficient knowledge and expertise in the area. With a good understanding of the role of occupational therapists, other parties concerned, such as clients, health and community care professionals, program administrators, insurance companies, lawyers, and design and construction professionals, can involve therapists constructively throughout the process. Occupational therapists with appropriate knowledge and experience can demonstrate the benefits of their involvement at various stages and can be called on repeatedly to contribute their expertise.

ROLE AND VALUE OF THE OCCUPATIONAL THERAPIST IN RECOMMENDING MINOR MODIFICATIONS

Minor Modifications: It's Not as Simple as "Do It Yourself"

A minor modification is sometimes considered a simple solution that can be implemented through a "do-it-yourself" approach, but many situations are more complex than is immediately apparent. Minor and major home modifications have not been clearly or comprehensively defined in much of the international legislation informing policy and service development. This has resulted in a divergence of opinion about how home modification services should be defined and delivered and who needs to be involved in recommending and installing these alterations. There is a limited understanding outside the profession of the value of minor home modifications. Further, there is ongoing debate both outside and within the profession about the role of occupational therapists in working with consumers to make minor home modifications. Naive understandings of the home modification practice result in the perception that minor modifications are simple and able to be undertaken by anyone. This approach can be problematic, especially considering the complexity associated with the process of determining the most appropriate solution. When the complexity of the process is not acknowledged and addressed and an occupational therapist is not considered or included in this process, poor home modification outcomes may result.

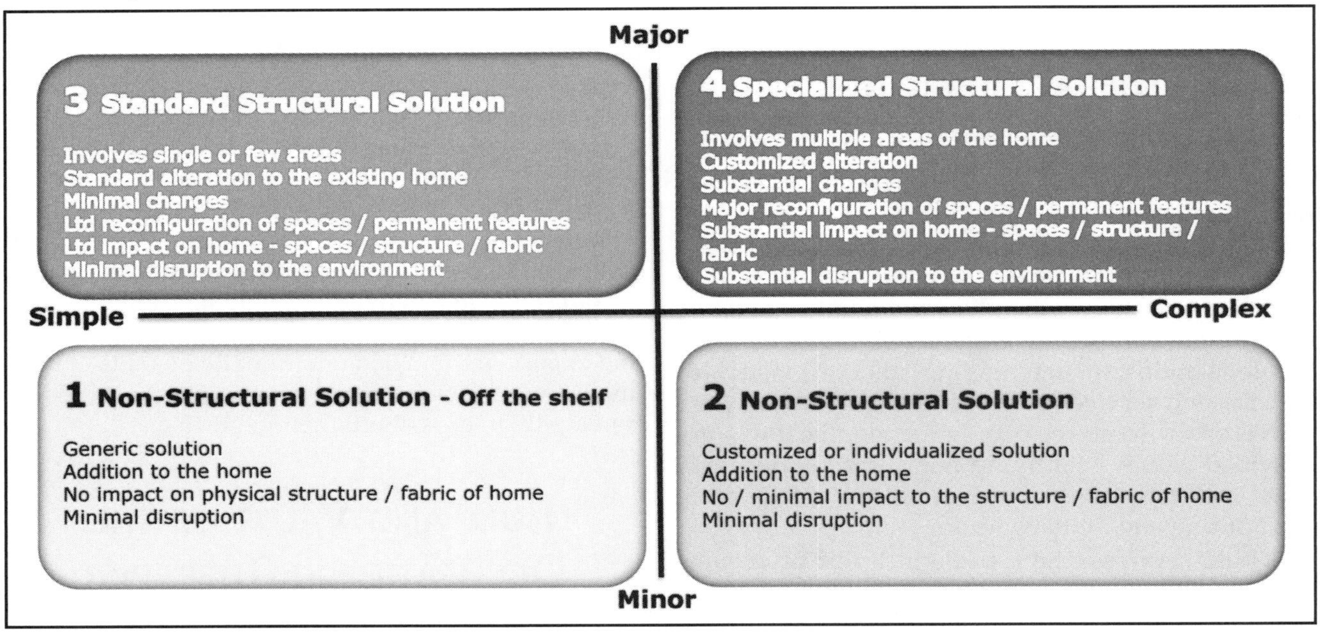

Figure 5-1. Framework of complexity associated with minor modification recommendations.

The Complexity in Home Modification Decision Making

The simplicity of a home modification does not always reflect the simplicity of the situation it is addressing. Figure 5-1 presents a framework for differentiating between the simplicity and complexity of the solution versus the simplicity and complexity of the situation. A minor modification may be considered a simple solution, but the process used to determine this minor modification may be complex. Complexity may arise from factors associated with the person, their occupation, and/or how the environment presents. The complexity of the situation (i.e., the person's circumstances, the way in which they undertake activities in the home, and the immediate and broader socioeconomic/legislative environment) affect home modification decisions and outcomes. Achieving good outcomes requires a well-considered home modification approach that includes a clear understanding of products and design solutions so they can be matched to the needs of the consumer and the household. Occupational therapists possess the knowledge and skills necessary to assist people in identifying the best home modification solution. Further information about this issue and this complexity is detailed in Appendix A.

STAGES OF THE HOME MODIFICATION PROCESS

There are a number of stages in the home modification process, from the initial referral to the final evaluation of the home modification and the education and training of the person in its use after installation. The specific stages of the home modification process include the following:

+ Receiving and analyzing the referral information
+ Prioritizing referrals
+ Arranging the home visit with the client
+ Preparing for the home visit
+ Traveling to the home and meeting the client
+ Entering the property
+ Interviewing and observing the client
+ Inspecting the home
+ Measuring the client and his or her equipment and/or caregiver
+ Photographing, measuring, and drawing the built environment
+ Planning, selecting, and negotiating a range of interventions
+ Concluding the home visit
+ Seeking technical advice

+ Writing the report and completing concept drawings

+ Submitting the report to the referrer

+ Educating and training clients in the use of home modifications

+ Evaluating home modifications and client outcomes after installation

Occupational therapists can enter and exit at various points of the home modification service delivery process, depending on the type and level of service required by the referrer, their knowledge and level of expertise, and the expertise of other stakeholders involved in the process.

Receiving and Analyzing the Referral Information

The home modification process begins with the occupational therapist receiving and analyzing the referral information (Figure 5-2). There is a range of reasons for seeking home modification advice from occupational therapists. Clients might have a newly diagnosed health condition, or they might have experienced a recent injury that requires changes to their existing home environment before they can be discharged from care. Individuals might be aging and experiencing increasing difficulty coping in their current home situation. Home modifications might be sought when people move to a new environment that does not adequately support their occupational performance. Alternatively, there might be changes to someone's social context or roles that affect the fit between their performance skills and patterns, activity demands, and the environment (Siebert, 2005).

Requests for a home modification evaluation are generally received from health practitioners and community and home care service providers; however, increasingly, informed clients and caregivers are contacting occupational therapists for home modification services. At times the need for home modifications may be identified as part of discharge planning from an inpatient or rehabilitation facility (Siebert et al., 2014). Referrals can arrive by phone, e-mail, fax, or letter and can contain variable amounts of information. Most contain a general request for a home evaluation because of an individual's health condition, injury, or increasing frailty. Some referrals seek a specific environmental intervention (e.g., grab bars beside the toilet) or are requested as a prevention strategy (e.g., to reduce the risks of falls; Siebert et al., 2014).

The referral stage signals the start of information gathering. As therapists review referrals, they note

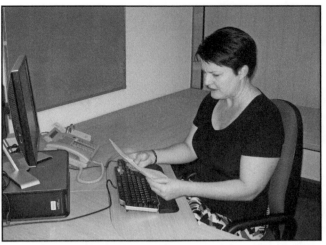

Figure 5-2. Receiving and analyzing the referral information.

essential information, such as the client's name, address, and age. This background information and other details, such as the person's disability, health condition, or age-related changes, might be entered into a service database to assist with recording and tracking service requests and events. Existing records, if available, are to be reviewed to determine whether clients have been seen previously and the nature of services they have accessed. Prior to the visit, therapists might need to carry out research on specific disabilities or health conditions, their presentation, and functional implications to understand them more fully in order to develop hypotheses about their likely impact on occupational performance and potential environmental barriers. Such information can help therapists think through the range of suitable interventions in advance of the home visit. Further, an understanding of prognoses alerts therapists to future equipment and support requirements and/or alternative ways of undertaking tasks that might need to be considered when planning interventions.

Other referral information of interest is whether the person is currently using equipment or receiving assistance in the home. If occupational therapists are not familiar with the equipment information provided, they might have to undertake background research to ensure that they are well informed about the specifications of the equipment and how such devices can be used. Caregiver or family support information provides a prompt for the occupational therapist to ensure that these people are present at the time of the home visit and to engage them in the home-visit process (Klein, Rosage, & Shaw, 1999). It is also important to note who lives at home with the client and whether there are any regular visitors or guests. People who use the home environment regularly will also need to be consulted when devising environmental interventions, especially if substantial changes are to be made to the home that may affect how they interact with and use the environment.

Information about the treating doctor, therapist, nurse, or other service providers is also required to ensure that relevant providers can be contacted for further information, such as details about medical treatment, rehabilitation, or equipment that might be prescribed, or to discuss the suitability of proposed interventions. It should be noted, however, that informed consent must be obtained from the client before making contact with these providers.

The referral might include information about the style of home and any environmental barriers being experienced. The details about the style of home can provide an indication of any other environmental barriers in addition to those already documented. For example, knowing that a person with mobility impairment is living in an older, two-story house alerts the therapist to examine the condition of the stairs, stair usage, and range of activities undertaken on the upper level.

Some specialist home modification providers and private therapists have developed a dedicated home modification referral information form to gather referral information and document other background information essential to providing timely and appropriate service. The quality of referral information varies greatly in detail and quality. Referrers generally provide information on client demographics, background information on the person's disability and/or health condition, and a general statement of need. However, in order to prepare effectively for the visit, therapists require additional detail, including the following:

+ The referrer and accompanying documentation
+ The current use of equipment and health and community services
+ The style of the home and existing environmental barriers
+ The type of modification/service requested
+ The ownership of the home
+ The need for an interpreter or formal or informal decision maker
+ The presence of other household members

In addition, to assist therapists in establishing timelines for service provision, they:

+ Require critical time frames (e.g., the client's expected discharge date)
+ Need to know the level of safety and risk to the client in his or her current situation (e.g., the

prevalence or likelihood of accident or injury, restricted activity, or unwanted dependence)

Figure 5-3 is a sample home modification referral information form. When therapists make their initial phone calls to clients to set up a time for their home visit, this is a good opportunity to discuss occupational performance issues experienced in the home and to explain the role of the occupational therapist. Clients' expectations can be clarified in relation to the home modification and the timing, duration, and process of the home visit. Information gathered during these calls might also highlight additional issues (e.g., that the client is not eligible for a particular service and might require a referral to an alternative service).

Prioritizing Referrals

Occupational therapists often have to prioritize their work and allocate their time judiciously, especially if their services are in demand. Referrals are generally prioritized in light of the urgency of each individual client's need, as well as the relative importance with respect to other referrals (Bradford, 1998). Factors to consider when prioritizing referrals are listed in Table 5-1.

When considering the urgency of referrals, therapists consider whether clients are at risk of being involved in an adverse event resulting in reduced activity, injury, institutionalization, or premature death if they are not visited immediately. Those who are at a high risk are prioritized as being urgent. For example, an urgent home visit may be required if a referral indicates that the client has had falls in the home, has been hospitalized, and is not able to return home without adequate services and modifications. Alternatively, a visit may be considered nonurgent if the client has activity limitations that can be improved in the short term with the use of equipment that can be purchased or borrowed or if they have care support in the home. Once the urgency of each client is determined, clients are then prioritized based on the degree of risk in relation to other people on the waiting list.

When determining the level of urgency, therapists need to determine and record the likelihood of an adverse event occurring and the consequences of an event. For example, in the urgent case described earlier, the therapist would record that the client was highly likely to receive an injury resulting in further hospitalization should he or she return home without appropriate interventions. The nonurgent case would be recorded as being unlikely to result in an adverse event in the form of an injury and that any activity restrictions could be mitigated by the use of equipment while awaiting a home modification assessment (Table 5-2).

Occupational Therapy Home Modification Referral Information Form

Demographic Information

Client name:

Address:

Phone number:

Date of birth:

Gender:

ID number:

Referral Information

Date of referral:

Referral source (including contact details):

Client's advocate or spokesperson (including contact details):

Does the client require an interpreter?

Does the client wish to have a particular person at the interview? If so, please provide the person's name and contact details.

Type of Referral

Home modification:

Postmodification evaluation:

Other:

List of Documentation Received

Confidential medical report from a doctor or other medical personnel:

Authority to request or disclose client information:

Other:

Health Condition or Disability Information

List client's health condition or disability or details about any age-related changes:

Is the client's condition permanent, improving, deteriorating, temporary, or stable?

Has the client experienced a recent significant change in function or mobility? Describe.

Has there been a recent significant change in function or mobility?

What medication is the client taking for their conditions?

How many times has the client been hospitalized in the last 12 months?

What were the reasons for the client's hospitalization?

Is the client receiving family or informal caregiver assistance or community services to assist with self-care or household tasks, or access within the community?

What community services or informal support services are being received by the client (include information on the treating doctor, therapist, nurse, or other service providers)?

Does the client live alone, with a caregiver who is well, or with a caregiver who is aging or has a health or medical condition?

Figure 5-3. Sample occupational therapy home modification referral information form. *(continued)*

Description of the Client's Equipment

List the items of equipment that the client is currently using in the home and community to assist with mobility and day-to-day activities:

Description of the Home Environment

Describe the style of the client's home:

Is home owned or rented? If rented, state length of lease.

Description of the Environmental Barriers

Describe the environmental barriers being encountered by the client:

Describe the impact these barriers have on client or caregiver functioning:

Description of the Client's Home Modification Request:

Urgency of Home Visit

Provide an opinion on home modifications requirements:

Describe urgency of need for home modifications:

Occupational Therapist's Comments:

Signature Block

Staff Person Receiving Referral

   Name:

   Position Title:

   Signature:

   Date:

   Facility or Agency:

   Program:

Occupational Therapist Receiving or Reviewing Referral

   Name:

   Signature:

   Date:

   Facility or Agency:

   Program:

Figure 5-3 (continued). Sample occupational therapy home modification referral information form.

Table 5-1. Considerations When Prioritizing Referrals

PRIORITY	High	Moderate	Moderate to low	Low
RESPONSE	See within the week	See within few weeks	See within 2 months	See within 6 months
CONSEQUENCE	Event likely to result in death or hospitalization	Event likely to result in compromised health or performance	Event likely to compromise independence	Event likely to affect quality of life and participation
LIKELIHOOD	High likelihood of adverse event	Moderate likelihood of adverse event	Low likelihood of adverse event	Adverse event unlikely
TYPE OF LIMITATION	Transfers, mobility, and hygiene activities such as toileting and bathing	Other self-care activities such as eating and dressing	Cleaning, shopping, cooking, laundry	Leisure and community participation
ABILITY TO FUNCTION	Unable to perform essential elements of the activity	Difficulty performing essential elements of the activity	Difficulty performing some essential elements of the activity	Little difficulty performing essential elements of the activity
ALTERNATIVES	No viable alternative possible	Alternative method or equipment option possible, but does not address issue fully	Alternative method or equipment option can temporarily address issue	Alternative method or equipment option possible
AVAILABLE SUPPORT	No alternative support available	No alternative support available onsite, but can be purchased	No alternative support available onsite, but can be accessed at no cost	Alternative support available onsite
TIMING	Palliative condition	Chronic/lifelong condition	Fluctuating condition	Acute, short-term condition
SOLUTION TYPE	Minor and/or major modifications	Minor and/or major modifications, equipment	Minor modifications and equipment	Equipment only

Table 5-2. Client Examples Illustrating Prioritization Information and Resulting Level of Urgency for a Visit

NAME	SUSPECTED ENVIRONMENTAL HAZARD/BARRIER	CONSEQUENCE	LIKELIHOOD	URGENCY OF HOME VISIT
Mrs. Jones	Slippery bathroom floor	High—injury because of a fall	Likely—already been hospitalized	High
Mrs. Smith	Low toilet	Minor—reduced activity performance	Low—can be managed with additional equipment or caregiver support in interim	Low

Where cases are not easily assessed as being high or low risk, various resources and tools are available to assist with decision making. For example, as illustrated in Figure 5-4, any event that is considered likely or almost certain with a major or critical consequence would be considered extreme and therefore classified as extremely urgent. Any event that results in a moderate, major, or critical level of consequence and could be unlikely, possible, likely, or almost certain to occur is also considered to be high risk and therefore urgent. When events are likely to be rare to almost certain to occur and have a range of consequence from insignificant to major, they are considered a lower risk and priority to those listed

Figure 5-4. Risk assessment chart. (Adapted from Australian Standard for Risk Management [AS/NZS ISO 31000:2009].)

Likelihood	Consequence				
	Insignificant	Minor	Moderate	Major	Critical
Almost Certain	Medium	Medium	High	Extreme	Extreme
Likely	Low	Medium	High	High	Extreme
Possible	Low	Medium	High	High	High
Unlikely	Low	Low	Medium	Medium	High
Rare	Low	Low	Low	Low	Medium

Consequence	Description of Consequence
1. Insignificant	No treatment required
2. Minor	Minor injury requiring First Aid treatment (e.g. minor cuts, bruises, bumps)
3. Moderate	Injury requiring medical treatment or lost time
4. Major	Serious injury (injuries) requiring specialist medical treatment or hospitalisation
5. Critical	Loss of life, permanent disability or multiple serious injuries

Likelihood	Description of Likelihood
1. Rare	Will only occur in exceptional circumstances
2. Unlikely	Not likely to occur within the foreseeable future, or within the project lifecycle
3. Possible	May occur within the foreseeable future, or within the project lifecycle
4. Likely	Likely to occur within the foreseeable future, or within the project lifecycle
5. Almost Certain	Almost certain to occur within the foreseeable future or within the project lifecycle

earlier. Events that have insignificant to major consequence but are rarely likely or are likely to occur are low risk and priority.

Unfortunately, services may not have prioritization tools to assist clients and occupational therapy practice. The presence of these tools depends on the concern of organizations in relation to client wait lists, and their policies and procedures in relation to delivery of client services. Prioritization tools are required to ensure that services direct their resources to meet client need without disadvantaging people and being challenged about their service delivery processes. Prioritization tools are important for occupational therapists to use when justifying services and bidding for resources. They provide clear guidance to funding bodies as to why some clients are seen before others.

Considerations affecting the prioritization of clients include:

✦ The service context (e.g., hospital, community, or private practice) and the overall priorities of the service (e.g., the care requirements of clients in relation to the safety of caregivers)

✦ Other available services that the client might be referred to while awaiting an occupational therapy visit

✦ Whether a phone call to a client with discussion about interim options can assist in the initial stages of the referral, particularly if there is a wait list for services

Arranging the Home Visit With the Client

Once the priority of the referral has been determined, the occupational therapist contacts the client by phone, e-mail, text message, or letter within the recommended time frame that may be established by the therapist or the organization to arrange the home visit (Figure 5-5). Alternatively, the client may be advised that he or she has been placed on a waiting list and will be contacted in the future to arrange an appointment, assuming personal needs do not change. If clients are on a waiting list, they should be advised to contact the home modification program and the occupational therapist should their situation change. Clients might need to be reprioritized if their need for a visit becomes urgent or if their risk of accident, injury, or institutionalization increases.

An informal or formal decision maker, service provider, guardian, or family member might need to be contacted if the client requires assistance to communicate their requirements. In such cases, documented informed consent should be sought from these representatives before information is gathered about the client.

The Timing and Duration of the Home Visit

The timing of the home visit is generally determined by the urgency of the client's situation and the availability of the client and other members of the household to meet. Clients at high risk of injury will need to be seen urgently, whereas others can be scheduled routinely. The timing of the home visit might also need to be planned around the expected date of discharge from the hospital. If the client requires urgent home modifications to ensure his or her safety, the occupational therapist might undertake a home visit before or immediately after discharge. If it is not possible to complete all the required work in time, the therapist might recommend basic modifications and plan a second visit to discuss other interventions after the client has returned home. In some instances, when the person has recently acquired a disabling condition, the occupational therapist might delay the visit until after the person has been living in the home for a short period and has had time to settle into his or her new routine and identify the environmental barriers. This can help the client make well-informed decisions about the issues and interventions required. When arranging home visits around the availability of the client, it is important to be aware that clients are often reliant on others for help with their self-care and home management routine and medical appointments. Therefore, occupational therapists may need to arrange the visit around other scheduled activities.

The duration of home visits varies and should be negotiated with the client when making the appointment. Generally, occupational therapists can anticipate the time required for the visit based on the referral or the initial conversation. Alternatively, the service or reimbursement system may allocate a specific amount of time for home visits as defined by the client's health condition or the identified need. However, sometimes the complexity of the situation might only become evident during the visit.

A range of issues can affect the timing and duration of the home visit. These include the following:

+ The energy levels of the client: The client might have limited physical, cognitive, or psychological capacity, which means that he or she can only manage short visits or visits conducted at times during the day or week.

+ The number of people in attendance to contribute to the decision-making process: The occupational therapist might need to negotiate an appointment time to suit several people and spend considerable time listening to the views of the client and others when gathering information and negotiating a range of intervention options.

+ The amount of equipment used: The occupational therapist might need time to undertake extensive measurement of the client, his or her equipment, and the home environment to determine the person's body dimensions, reach range, circulation, and storage space and

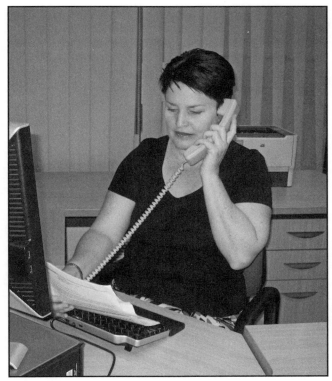

Figure 5-5. Contacting the client to arrange a home visit.

dimensions and location of fittings and fixtures in the environment.

+ The number and nature of occupational performance difficulties being experienced: If the person is having trouble with several activities, the occupational therapist will need to allocate a reasonable time frame to ensure that performance in each activity is adequately evaluated.

+ The number and type of barriers in the home environment: Some houses present numerous barriers to performance; others present challenges to being modified. The occupational therapist might need to take numerous photos and approximate measurements and seek technical advice from design or building professionals before proposing interventions. The greater the number and extent of environmental and construction barriers, the more time required to problem solve and plan the interventions.

If considerable time is required to evaluate the person, his or her occupational performance, and the home environment, the visit time may need to be extended or additional visits booked (Silverstein & Hyde, 1997). If the occupational therapist has been allocated only a limited time for the home visit, he or she will need to negotiate with the client and formulate a mutually agreeable structure for the interview, allocating a specific time for each stage of the visit, including the interview, observation, measurement, walk-through of the home, and discussion of intervention options.

Clients should be advised to have all concerned parties present at the visit. Involving the various stakeholders in the home modification process ensures that all relevant issues are discussed and carefully considered and that intervention options developed are acceptable and useful to everyone affected by them (Klein et al., 1999). Further, involving stakeholders at the time of the visit is likely to reduce the number of discussions and meetings, phone calls, and/or subsequent visits required to consult with various parties.

If clients rely on equipment to undertake different activities in the home, they need to be advised to have devices available at the time of the home visit. This allows the occupational therapist to measure the items and observe their use in the home. Further home visits might be required if the client does not have his or her equipment available at the time of the initial home visit, particularly if the equipment dimensions and space requirements (with or without a caregiver using the equipment) are likely to affect the design of the home modification.

Preparing for the Home Visit

Being well prepared ensures that the home visit is productive and efficient. Occupational therapists prepare for home visits by doing the following:

+ Filling in interview forms with relevant referral information in advance of the visit

+ Gathering required home visiting resources

+ Compiling appropriate forms and evaluation tools for information gathering

+ Collecting evaluation and environmental measurement tools

+ Collating information on various intervention options

Prior to the visit, therapists should read the referral information and any other background information on record and transfer relevant information onto forms to be used during the visit. It is also useful to take the referral documentation on the visit to confirm and clarify information with the client.

Therapists should ensure that they gather a range of resources that can be used during a home visit, including the following:

+ Personal identification information, such as an identification badge

+ A clipboard and pens or computer technology, such as a laptop or tablet

+ Occupational therapy evaluation tools, including interview guides, checklists, and report forms (if they are not on a computer or tablet)

+ Paper and pencils for drawing diagrams

+ A cell/mobile phone

+ A street directory or satellite navigation system for directions to the property

+ Water

+ Written information on whom to contact in the event of an emergency, such as a car breakdown

+ A first-aid kit in the vehicle

The forms that need to be taken on home visits can include an interview form with prompts, a home visit checklist with specific features in different areas of the home, and privacy and consent forms for use when information needs to be sought from other service providers, such as the doctor, hospital therapists, or home and community care nurses. Occupational therapists may need to take photos of the person and/or areas of the home, which might require the client's written permission.

Evaluation tools such as the Canadian Occupational Performance Measure (Law et al., 1998), Performance Assessment of Self-Care Skills (Rogers & Holm, 2007), Safer-Home (Chiu & Oliver, 2006), Housing Enabler (Iwarsson & Slaugh, 2001), In Home Occupational Performance Evaluation (Stark, Somerville & Morris, 2010), and other standardized tools can be used to establish a picture of the person-environment-occupation transaction and provide a base measure of performance for comparison with outcomes measures (Law & Baum, 2005).

The choice of environmental measurement tools depends on the environmental barriers highlighted in the referral information. It is useful to have a kit that holds the following tools, with appropriate instruction sheets and forms in hard copy or electronic format, on all home visits:

+ 18-ft (5-m) tape measure to measure dimensions

+ Electronic distance meter to measure long distances

+ Camera (and spare batteries) for photos of the environmental barriers and the client's equipment to keep as a record from the visit and to incorporate into the home modification report

+ Light meter to measure lighting levels

+ Force measure to measure the amount of force required to open doors and drawers

+ Electronic clinometer to measure the horizontal gradients of landings, paths, ramps, floors

✦ Pegs, string line, and spirit level for setting out the proposed configuration of an outdoor ramp

Prior to the visit, therapists also need to research and collate resource information to take with them to assist with intervention planning. The resource information might include the following:

✦ Concept drawings (site and floor plans or elevations) or photos of modified environments to show the client examples of completed work

✦ Access standards or guidelines and/or local building codes relevant to the type of home being visited (to discuss specific design requirements with the client)

✦ Photos and product information (e.g., brochures or information from the internet) to show the client illustrations of home modification designs and products and equipment solutions

✦ Products such as taps and grab rails to enable the client to see and feel items

✦ Equipment such as an over-toilet frame or a bath board that can serve as a less-costly alternative to a home modification. These items may be taken on the home visit to try and evaluate their suitability for the client and the environment.

Safety Considerations

Prior to the visit, it is important that occupational therapists evaluate potential risks to themselves and the client during the home visit and ensure that safety measures are put in place.

Communicating the Home Visit Schedule

As a safety precaution, occupational therapists should advise their fellow workers of their schedule, including the addresses and phone numbers of the clients they will be visiting, the time and expected duration of these visits, and their cell/mobile phone number. Staff working in private practice might need to identify a suitable contact and advise this person of the time of their visits and their exact whereabouts, especially if they work on their own, outside of business hours, or in isolated locations.

Identification and Clothing

Occupational therapists should have personal identification on them at all times. They should also ensure that their appearance and clothing are appropriate and reflect community standards, in particular those that meet the expectations of the older generation. For example, when visiting older people, it is advisable for female occupational therapists to wear trousers rather than skirts to enable them to maintain their modesty while moving into various positions during measuring. It is also preferable that occupational therapists not wear shirts with plunging necklines or shorts or jeans that are low cut or ripped. Therapists should also wear enclosed shoes with low heels because they are likely to be walking on a variety of surfaces, both within and outside of the home. Shoes that can be slipped on and off easily allow occupational therapists to remove shoes before entering the house. When visiting construction sites, clothing and shoes should comply with work health and safety requirements. In such situations, occupational therapists may need to wear hard hats for head protection and steel-tip boots for foot protection.

Personal Safety, Training, and Support

Therapists need to be conscious of the environments they are entering and the background of the people they are visiting. They need to gather information about the home environment such as the location and available phone reception, whether there are animals present and if they will pose a threat to safety, and the person's current health status prior to their visit to ensure the therapist is safe at the visit.

It is always advisable for occupational therapists to carry a mobile phone at the time of the home visit. On arrival, they need to ensure that their vehicle is in a safe, well-lit, easy-to-access location near the premises. The car should be parked on the street or in a designated parking area in the direction of exit from the street and should not block residents or caregivers needing access to and from the home.

A visual check of the property on entry can also provide information about whether there are pets that might pose a safety risk to visitors. Discussion might be needed about restraining pets if the therapist is concerned about the animal or feels that it might disrupt the home visit.

Inside the premises, therapists should ensure that they position themselves between the client and the exit to ensure obstacle-free egress in the event of an adverse event. If the client or other householders exhibit any suspicious or unusual behavior, it may be prudent to conclude the visit and exit the premises. It is advisable to record this information on file or report it to a supervisor on returning to the office. Similarly, if an adverse incident occurs at the time of the home visit, the therapist must advise a supervisor as soon as the home visit is completed and make a record of the incident on file.

Where therapists are dealing with remote, complex, or challenging clients, it is advisable for them to undergo personal safety training. At times, it might

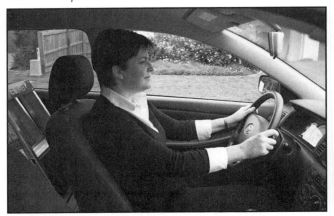

Figure 5-6. Driving to the client's home.

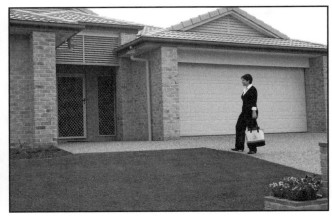

Figure 5-7. Entering the property.

be necessary to take another person along on a visit. For example, if a client lives in a remote region that requires hours of driving, a second person might be required to share the driving and ensure safety in a remote location. When clients are frail, unwell, or live alone, the occupational therapist might require assistance to assess the person's safety in performing a range of activities in their environment. If an occupational therapist is visiting a client who has just left a mental health facility or prison or has a history of becoming aggressive toward others, he or she might need another staff member for support.

Traveling to the Home and Meeting the Client

The home visit process begins well before the therapist reaches the front door of the client's home (Figure 5-6). Occupational therapists survey the community and gather information en route to the person's home (Klein et al., 1999). They observe the location of local facilities in relation to the client's premises; type and location of public transport; general topography of the district; presence and condition of footpaths, curbs, and roads in the surrounding area; and style and condition of housing in the neighborhood. By observing the client's surroundings, therapists can gain an understanding of why people may choose not to relocate, particularly if they are located close to community facilities or support services. Reviewing the surroundings also provides detail of the potential environmental barriers to participation in the community. It enables therapists to ensure that modifications to the exterior of the home will fit with the look of the rest of the street and neighborhood.

Entering the Property

Prior to the visit, occupational therapists should ensure that they have the client's permission to enter the property (Figure 5-7). On walking to the front door, the therapist may notice aspects of the external layout of the home that might affect the client's occupational performance. For example, the therapist might note the slope of the land just outside of the boundary for street access to the site, height and style of fencing for privacy, slope of the land within the boundary, and presence of any paths and steps. It can also be noted whether paths are free of hazards and obstacles, the number of risers on the stairs, the condition of the steps and handrails, the presence of light fittings, and the age and style of the home. These are potential barriers to occupational performance that may require further discussion and consideration (Figure 5-8). The wider dimensions of home also should be considered when entering the property, taking note of the appearance and style of the exterior of the home, for example.

If the client is not at home or does not answer the door, the therapist might call the client's phone number provided. If there is no answer, the therapist might leave a business card with a note indicating the time of the visit. If there is evidence that the client may be at home and there may be concerns about this person's personal safety, the therapist might call the contact person listed in their documentation or the police to seek assistance.

When meeting the client at the front entry, the therapist should introduce him- or herself, show identification, and confirm that the client is available to begin the home visit and is comfortable with the therapist entering the home. As a courtesy, it is suggested to ask whether shoes need to be removed before entering the home.

On entry, the therapist should observe the environment to ascertain his or her level of personal safety. If there is any feeling of unease for any reason during the home visit, the therapist needs to discontinue the visit and exit the premises. If there are no perceived threats, the visit can proceed and the therapist can establish a presence in the home. The occupational therapist should ask the client and other householders where they would be most comfortably seated and ensure that this location is well suited to conducting an interview and viewing resource materials. The occupational therapist then takes the seat suggested by the client. The therapist may politely request that seating be rearranged, the radio or television be turned off, or lights be turned on to create a more conducive interview environment.

If the client offers a drink, the therapist can accept it and use this time to establish a rapport. It is also an opportunity to begin to understand the client's experience of home, commenting on, for example, the view; the décor; or the prints, objects, or photos on display. Using this approach, clients come to understand that the occupational therapist is interested in their story and that he or she values their experiences and meaning of home. This is an important first step in creating a collaborative relationship with clients, where they feel valued as experts in their own lives and homes. A useful opening question to gather a wealth of information about the client's connection to home is, "How long have you lived here?" This often allows people to share their history of home, whether it is home with many memories and a place they wish to remain, or a place that is new to them that they are not familiar with or perhaps a place that they do not enjoy living in. The therapist might also use this opportunity to observe the client as he or she prepares the refreshments, noting any concerns about mobility and ability to structure and complete the task, as well as concentration and communication during the activity. The therapist should be aware that performance during this activity may not be representative of the person's usual performance and that hypotheses formulated at this time need to be confirmed through further evaluation. The therapist might note the layout and condition of the home, existing obstacles, and color and lighting of the rooms and discuss issues of concern with the client as they become relevant during the interview.

When the client is finally seated, the therapist makes a full introduction, providing information about the home modification program, his or her role, and the purpose of the visit. The therapist should introduce him- or herself to everyone present and develop an understanding of each person's relationship with the client and his or her place in the home and its routines. The therapist may also need

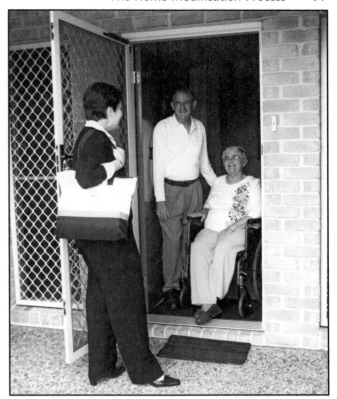

Figure 5-8. Observing the property features and the client.

to clarify each person's role in any decision making to do with modification of the home environment. For example, the client's husband might have been involved in building and maintaining the home and would therefore need to be consulted about changes; a community care nurse might provide assistance during bathing and would therefore need to be consulted about modifications to the bathroom; the client's daughter might be concerned about disruptions to the household that would necessitate her accommodating her parents if major modifications are undertaken.

In different situations, the occupational therapist might have to vary the way the visit is conducted. For example, the therapist might sit and complete the interview first before asking the client to show how he or she currently undertakes activities in various areas of the home. Alternatively, the client may be anxious to discuss his or her concerns and show the problem areas in the home first to ensure that the occupational therapist is clear about the issues. The therapist might also decide that viewing the home is important before the interview because it could provide important information on the layout of the home and specific fixtures and fittings. Regardless of the order of events, it is essential that the therapist gains all of the information required before discussing interventions.

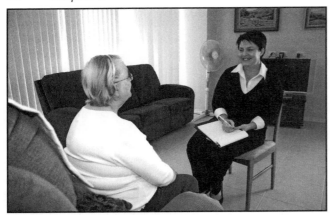

Figure 5-9. Interviewing the client.

Interviewing the Client

At the start of the interview process, the occupational therapist discusses his or her role in ensuring the privacy and confidentiality of the information gathered and asks the client to sign the consent forms. The therapist confirms the referral information and the background details with the client to ensure these are accurate (Figure 5-9). During the interview, the therapist listens to the person's story to understand the following:

+ The person's health condition and concerns

+ Activities, routines, and roles within the home and community

+ Use of the various areas of the home

+ The personal meaning of the home, including objects, spaces, and features within the home

+ The history of the home

+ The person's future hopes and dreams in relation to his or her home (Siebert, 2005)

The occupational therapist can use a series of open and closed questions to develop a deeper understanding of the person, his or her occupations, and occupational performance concerns and barriers in the home environment. This questioning process involves identifying and defining issues of importance to the client and understanding the history and routines within the household and how these may influence the nature, feasibility, and appropriateness of interventions (Siebert, 2005). The client's wants, needs, occupational risks, and problems are evaluated, and information is gathered, synthesized, and framed from an occupational perspective (AOTA, 2014). This information is then considered as the occupational therapist observes the client undertaking various activities in the home at a later stage in the visit.

Information gathered at the time of the interview is documented to ensure a record of the detail is retained (Stark, 2003). Occupational therapists may use one or more of the following to document information:

+ A notebook for handwritten interview notes or drawings

+ Paper forms with key headings or checklists to guide the interview process

+ Personal computers (handheld or laptop or tablet) that contain documents with key headings or checklists. This technology may be used to type in responses directly or convert handwriting to text and upload photos so that changes can be drawn on the photo directly.

+ Digital pens and dedicated documents with key headings or checklists. The digital pens can record handwriting and concept drawings or convert these to text and electronic diagrams.

The type of technology used depends on a range of factors, including the therapist's experience with and confidence in using technology; the cost, availability, and reliability of the technology; the organization's position on its use for home visiting; and access to technical support.

Inspecting the Home

During the visit, the therapist examines the environment carefully to develop a full understanding of its layout, structure, fixtures and fittings, and the barriers to occupational performance (Figures 5-10 through 5-16). Of interest will be:

+ External access around the home: Access to the mailbox, trash cans, clothesline, pool, greenhouse, front, and back yards, and the front gate; the quality and type of paths, stairs, ramps, and driveway areas

+ Internal access within the home: The layout of the home (open plan or with corridors); location and number of internal stairs; number of bedrooms and route of access to the various areas of the home; changes in floor levels and the types of floor finishes

+ Kitchen, bathroom, laundry, and bedrooms: Layout and the types of fittings and fixtures

+ Car parking facilities: Space, lighting, and access

+ Access to the vehicle or public transport: Access from the car parking facility to the home, the distance to public transport facilities

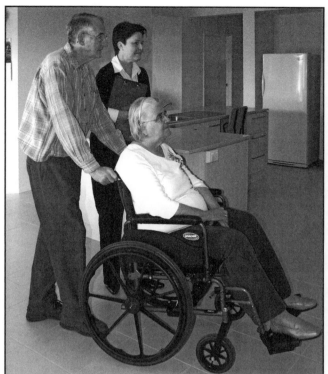

Figure 5-10. Inspecting the home with the client.

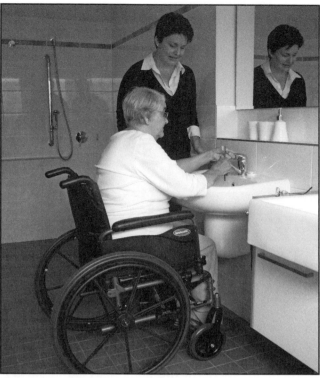

Figure 5-11. Observing the client.

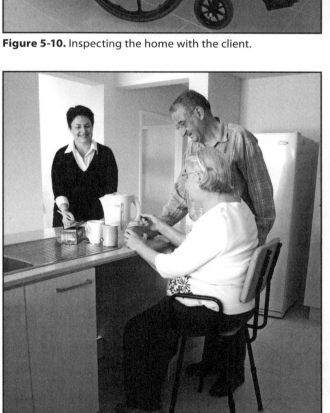

Figure 5-12. Observing the client.

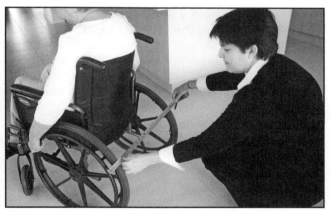

Figure 5-13. Measuring the client's equipment.

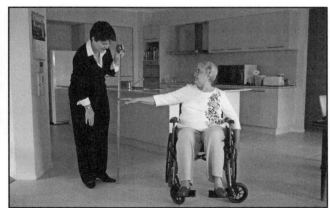

Figure 5-14. Measuring the client's reach range.

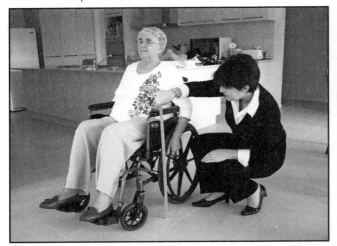

Figure 5-15. Measuring the client's equipment.

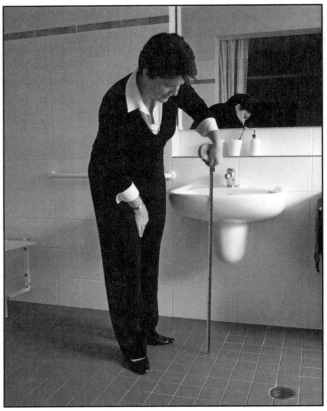

Figure 5-16. Measuring the environment.

A walk-through also offers an opportunity to gather information about the dimensions of the home to understand what might be important about the home for the client and their family and how this may affect decision making. For example, the aesthetic and style of the home may be important to consider when thinking about the appearance of grab rails or a ramp. A walk-through of the different areas with the client will enable the occupational therapist to analyze the physical environment and its potential to enhance or constrain occupational performance (Siebert, 2005). It will also afford the client an opportunity to show where occupational performance difficulties occur. The occupational therapist then uses skilled observation and occupational analysis to analyze the client's occupational performance as he or she demonstrates activities of concern or simulates elements of activities, such as transfers, bending, lifting, and reaching (Klein et al., 1999). The therapist listens to the client's concerns and then observes his or her performance, analyzing the sequence of activities and discussing how, when, where, and why the difficulties occur with the client (Ohta & Ohta, 1997). This ensures that the hypotheses formulated by the therapist about the person's capacity at the time of referral and interview are fully explored and validated or refuted as appropriate. Examining occupational performance in different areas of the home with the client ensures that he or she understands how the current design and layout of the home, or the existing fittings and fixtures, might hamper occupational performance and allows the therapist to discuss potential interventions.

Measuring the Client, Equipment, and Caregiver

The occupational therapist might need to measure the client, his or her equipment, and the caregiver to determine the required size of openings and circulation spaces and the location of fittings and fixtures (see Figures 5-14 through 5-16).

When the client's dimensions are required, the therapist measures the following:

+ Height, width, and length of various body parts
+ Reach range in seated and/or standing positions
+ Eye height and examines his or her visual fields

In addition, the therapist measures the height, length, width, and circulation space of the equipment and caregivers. The therapist also checks the positioning and movement of the client with the equipment and caregivers in relation to managing the spaces, fittings, and fixtures. This information ensures that spaces can be designed to optimize the ease of approach and use and that fixtures and fittings are within reach.

If there are going to be multiple users of a specific area, the anthropometrics of all users will need to be

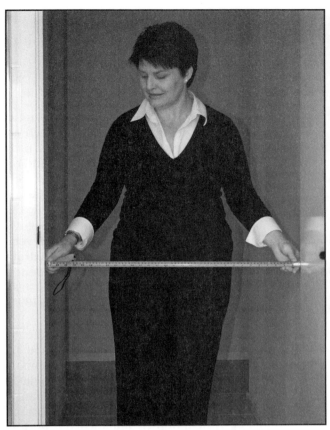

Figure 5-17. Measuring the environment.

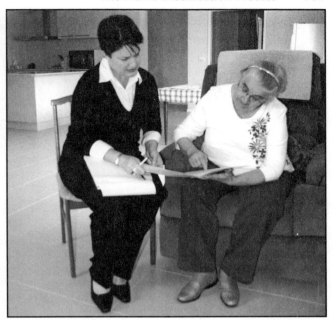

Figure 5-18. Planning, selecting, and negotiating interventions.

considered in the redesign of space and placement of fittings and fixtures, with adjustable options being integrated into the design if necessary.

Photographing, Measuring, and Drawing the Environment

Concept drawings and photographs can become a valuable record of the home visit and can be used to complement the written detail in the report. Therapists are reminded to seek permission from clients to photograph, measure, and draw areas of the home.

Photographs

Therapists may take photos of key areas and features in the home from various angles to ensure that comprehensive information is collected. Photographs can be useful in reports because they add visual detail about the home and environmental barriers. Digital photographs can be easily inserted into word processing or presentation software/apps and can be annotated by hand or electronically to highlight barriers and illustrate where the modifications are to be installed.

A digital photo might also be useful for the therapist to discuss the environmental barriers and range of solutions with the client if he or she is not able to access an area of the home. Printouts can be drawn on to illustrate the location of the proposed modifications or shown on the screen of a portable device. Photos can also serve as a record of the environment before, during, and after the home modification and can be a visual aid for informing other clients, their families, and caregivers about alternative environmental interventions.

Measurements

The occupational therapist needs to collect a comprehensive set of measurements of the problem areas in the home environment (Figures 5-17 and 5-18). Measurements of features that are working well for the client should also be taken so that these dimensions can be incorporated in any redesign.

The type of measurements taken will depend on the environmental barriers or enablers identified. Measurements can include lengths, widths, depths, and heights of fittings, fixtures, and the circulation spaces in problem areas of the home. It might also be necessary to measure the spaces adjacent to or along a path of travel to these areas, as these areas might need to be incorporated in the final redesign. It is advisable to collect any additional measurements that might be useful if alternative solutions need to be explored at a later stage.

All relevant measurement information, including concept drawings of the layout of specific areas in

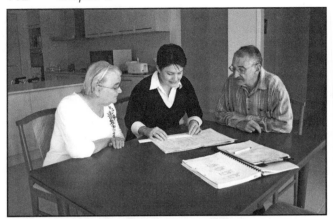

Figure 5-19. Reviewing the professional drawings.

floor plan and elevation views, is recorded at the time of the visit and is incorporated in the design of the modification.

Chapter 7 provides further information about measuring the person and the environment.

Concept Drawings

Measurements of the environment are recorded on a concept drawing, which can be used when communicating design requirements to various stakeholders.

Therapists employ various drawing methods, depending on their expertise and the type of work they do. They may choose to take only approximate measurements and create concept sketches to send on to a skilled contractor or building design professional to refine and develop into scale architectural drawings. Alternatively, therapists may develop simple concept drawings, drawn to scale, to ensure that there is adequate space for circulation and fixtures and fittings in the proposed design before passing it on to building and design professionals for detailed drawings. Therapists should check the level of service they are required to provide with their licensing boards to ensure that they do not work outside of their scope of practice with respect to the creation and provision of drawings.

Once a draftsperson or builder has developed a scale drawing, the therapist needs to review the drawing and evaluate the usefulness of the design for the client and other people involved in the household. Consequently, a plan review may be undertaken with the client and others. A scale ruler is used during a plan review to confirm that required clearances and circulation spaces have been included in the design and that the plan supports the movement of the person, their equipment, and carer during activities.

Chapter 8 provides information on drawing the built environment.

Planning, Selecting, and Negotiating Interventions

An individual's occupational performance can be enhanced through a range of interventions, such as seeking alternative ways to undertake activities, providing assistive devices and social supports, and/or modifying the home environment (Figure 5-19). Once therapists have a clear understanding of the client's occupational profile and his or her key occupational performance issues, they can select, review, negotiate, plan, and implement a range of suitable interventions. When designing interventions, therapists draw on theory, practice models, and research evidence and use professional reasoning to choose the best solution for each situation (AOTA, 2014; Fisher, 1998; Schell, 2014).

Occupational therapists collaborate with clients to establish short- and long-term goals related to occupational performance in the home and community (Grayson, 1997). Short-term goals might include addressing problems associated with performance components or environmental issues; long-term goals might be to maintain or enhance the performance of daily occupations related to performing different roles in the home and community (Law & Baum, 2005). Once the client's goals are identified and prioritized, the therapist works with him or her to identify the interventions to address these goals (AOTA, 2014).

When an extensive number of changes is required, staff may need to discuss the list of recommendations with clients and, if relevant, caregivers, so that items can be prioritized (Connell & Sanford, 1997; Silverstein & Hyde, 1997). Prioritizing home modifications is especially important if there are issues relating to costs, funding, and timing of the work.

Factors Influencing Intervention Options

The process of planning and discussing intervention options with the client can be a complex undertaking influenced by a range of factors: client related, therapist related, and environment related.

Client-Related Factors

Occupational therapists should consider various areas of the home as they talk through the range of intervention options. Clients may be unable to change when and how specific activities are undertaken and therefore may be reluctant to consider some intervention options. However, they can also grow accustomed to reduced levels of performance and underestimate the barriers in the home environment (Pynoos, Sanford, & Rosenfelt, 2002; Wylde, 1998). Interventions can also have an impact on the physical, social, cultural, personal, spiritual, and temporal elements of the home environment, which should be considered carefully when selecting and negotiating modifications (Aplin et al., 2015; Hawkins & Stewart, 2002).

Other factors that can affect the selection, negotiation, and acceptance of home modifications include the following:

+ The cost of the modification: Clients might not have the funds to make changes to their home, especially if most of the home modifications are to be self-funded, as they generally are (American Association of Retired Persons [AARP], 2000). In addition, some modifications require additional structural or maintenance work to be undertaken before the modification is completed, which is often at a cost clients can ill afford (Jones, de Jonge, & Phillips, 2008).

+ The person's knowledge of the range of possible intervention options: Without a clear understanding of what is possible, clients are often not able to envision how their situation can be improved (Jones et al., 2008).

+ The person's perception of the need, usefulness, and acceptability of the intervention: Clients are more likely to accept an intervention if they believe it supports their sense of personal identity. Conversely, interventions that undermine their sense of identity are unlikely to be welcomed (McCreadie & Tinker, 2005).

+ The availability of information about arranging the work: Clients are better able to undertake a modification if they understand the building process: how to choose and engage a contractor, how the work would be done, how to manage in the home while the work is underway, and how to cope with any mess caused by contractors (AARP, 2000; Duncan, 1998; Pynoos & Nishita, 2003).

+ The amount of disruption the intervention is likely to cause: Clients are sometimes reluctant to undertake extensive work in areas such as the bathroom if it will be out of commission for a period.

Therapist-Related Factors

Interventions recommended by occupational therapists are likely to be influenced by their own level of knowledge, skill, and experience in the home modification field, as well as their model of practice. For example, occupational therapists with a wide-ranging knowledge of domestic products, design standards or guidelines, and resources and who undertake postmodification evaluation of previous work are likely to have a wealth of valuable information and experience that they can draw on. Therapists who use an ecological or transactive model of practice are also more likely to address occupational performance difficulties using environmental interventions than therapists who use models focused on remediating performance components.

Environment-Related Factors

When considering modifications for the home, the team and the client need to consider a range of factors relating to the suitability of the dwelling for alteration, including the following:

+ The cost-effectiveness of any changes, given the size, value, age, and structural suitability of the home (Connell & Sanford, 1997; Silverstein & Hyde, 1997)

+ Building rules and regulations relevant to the redesign of the area to ensure compliance with the law

+ The fit of any modification with the style and design of the dwelling and existing streetscape, if the work is located outside of the home

+ The long-term viability of the design and suitability to current and future householders. Current design trends, such as universal design, aim to ensure that products and designs are "useable by all" (Center for Universal Design, 1997) and reduce the likelihood that the modification needs to be altered or removed later as the needs change (Ringaert, 2003).

+ The dimensions of the home (outlined in Chapter 1) provide a comprehensive list of environmental factors that have been found to influence home modification decision making.

Other Factors

In most services, there are policies and procedures relating to home modification recommendations and a specific range of resources available to assist in the planning of interventions. Legislation, industry standards, and design guidelines might also guide the design and implementation of environmental interventions (Ringaert, 2003).

Chapter 4 provides information on legislation influencing home modification practice, and Chapter 11 provides details about access standards and their role in guiding interventions.

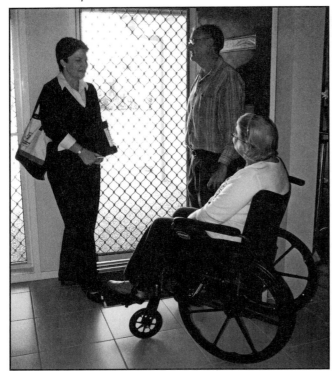

Figure 5-20. Concluding the home visit.

Educating Clients About Proposed Interventions and the Modification Process

Throughout the process of selecting and negotiating interventions, the therapist has a responsibility to inform the client about the extent of change to an area required, the range of people to be involved in the process and their respective responsibilities, and the expected time frame for the modification work. In addition, the therapist should discuss the expected impact of the home modification on the way activities would be undertaken and the expected appearance of the final modification. The therapist might show the client photos and diagrams of the layout of a room to help him or her better understand how it will look and how he or she might be able to move through or use the area.

Some occupational therapists find it useful to take clients to facilities that have already been modified to allow them to move around in the space and try the fittings and fixtures. This may include visiting:

+ A demonstration home or display center to view and try accessible design features

+ A hydrotherapy center to try an accessible toilet, vanity unit, and shower recess

+ A shopping center to try the gradients of accessible ramps

+ Another client's home to see the home modifications

Information gleaned from these trials can be used to confirm or guide the redesign of proposed home modifications.

Chapter 9 provides information on developing suitable interventions, and Chapter 10 provides detail about sourcing and evaluating products and designs.

Concluding the Home Visit

At the conclusion of the home visit, the therapist should provide the client with a brief verbal summary of the outcomes from the visit and confirm the full range of issues and options to be included in the home modification report (Figure 5-20). It is also beneficial to leave a brief written summary of the proposed interventions and an action plan stating who is responsible for each step of the plan. At this time, it is important to ensure that the client agrees with the recommendations. If the client does not agree, the therapist should extend the visit or make another time for further discussion and negotiation with the client and other stakeholders. If technical advice is required on the proposed modification, the therapist might also arrange to visit with a designer or builder before the interventions are finalized and the home modification report is written and submitted to the relevant body for approval.

Seeking Technical Advice

Technical building advice is sometimes required, particularly where home modification work is expected to be extensive or if the client and occupational therapist are not clear about whether the home can structurally accommodate the modification. Because occupational therapists do not receive training in construction and renovation of buildings, they consult with experts, such as design or building professionals, who provide expertise on design and building matters. For example, a therapist might need to know whether:

+ A wall can support a grab bar

+ A wall can be removed to allow more circulation space without compromising the integrity of the roof

+ Light fittings and power points can be of a particular type and positioned in specific locations in a bathroom under national plumbing and electrical code requirements

+ A garage can be converted into an extra bedroom under local building regulations

+ A ramp can be designed with an appropriate gradient to suit an area with limited space or if the yard has a slope

+ A proposed extension of a home is possible under local building regulations

+ A stair lift can be installed on stairs leading to several units under the building regulations

Design or building professionals generally contribute to the design and construction of modifications by:

+ Noting environmental barriers and constraints, including property boundaries, immovable structures, or items that will affect the design (e.g., protected trees and fire-rated or load-bearing walls)

+ Systematically measuring relevant areas and noting the position of services and other permanent fittings and fixtures, such as windows and doors

+ Deciding on the structural work required, such as modifying the levels or finishes of the floor and removing, moving, or installing new walls, doorways, or windows

+ Deciding on the changes required to services, such as the location of electrical points, water pipes, or drains

+ Planning the location of fittings and fixtures

+ Drawing the redesigned area to scale

+ Finalizing product finishes, such as flooring and surfaces, lighting, and color options

+ Providing an estimated cost of the works

Issues discussed among the occupational therapist, design or building professional, and client might include the following:

+ The feasibility of the proposed environmental modification, such as whether the home modification is reasonable given the age and type of construction of the home or whether the changes can be easily and stylishly included in the existing layout of the home

+ The existing dimensions and space for the home modifications, such as adequate floor area to incorporate the home modification

+ The required dimensions of the modifications, such as length, height, width, or depth of spaces, fixtures, and fittings

+ The range of products and features to be incorporated into the alterations, with consideration

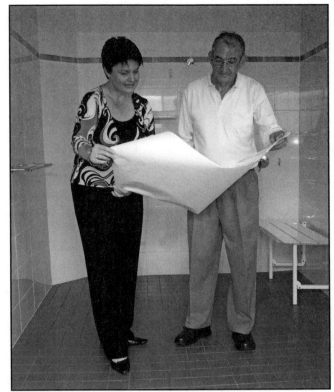

Figure 5-21. Checking the built environment against the plans.

given to the specific needs of the client as well as other people in the household

+ The cost and design of the proposed work in relation to the household budget and the degree of design elegance associated with the cost of the proposed modification

The information gathered from discussions with the design and building professional might be included in the therapist's report, or the design and building professional might provide a written technical specification report with accompanying drawings and photos. If the technical specification report and drawings have more technical detail than the therapist's home modification report, these should be used by the contractor for quoting and completing the work.

Reviewing Professional Drawings

To ensure that the developed drawings are consistent with those agreed to by the therapist in collaboration with the client, the therapist compares them with those created by the design or building professional (Figure 5-21). The therapist ensures that all relevant information is included and that there are no discrepancies, omissions, or inadequate adherence to recommendations or design guidelines or standards. Once the plans are reviewed, the therapist provides a report on how the proposed design will or will not meet the client's needs and either endorses the drawings or provides a report about the discrepancies noted on the plans. This report provides feedback to the design or building professional and ensures the drawings are revised to suit the client's specific requirements. It may be necessary to undertake a plan review process with the client to double-check the layout and measurements, particularly if equipment was being scripted at the time when drawings were being developed, or if the client's physical and functional changes require alteration of features and fittings, new equipment, or a greater level of carer support (i.e., one rather than two carers).

Role Differences

It is important to note that design or building professionals are not trained to have an understanding of a client's health conditions and disabilities and the associated impact on occupational performance; hence, they have no expertise in evaluating the specific needs of clients. They are not trained to analyze the person-environment-occupation transaction, to identify a specific cause of performance difficulties, or to determine how occupational performance can be further enabled using a range of interventions. Further, they are not skilled in measuring a person with or without equipment and do not have expertise in determining future equipment and carer requirements in relation to the person's health condition or disability. The information that is gleaned from measuring the person, the equipment, and carer and anticipating future need can affect the current and proposed layout of areas within and outside the home.

Building and design professionals do possess important technical expertise on the design and construction of buildings and surrounding environments, which can assist in the planning of environmental interventions. They are also experts at providing drawings, specifications for other building and design professionals, and costings for works completion. Consequently, it is imperative that a team approach is used in home modification practice so that various professionals can contribute their unique expertise to the process and the design of environmental interventions (Pynoos et al., 2002).

Writing the Report and Completing the Drawings

Occupational therapists should document the findings and recommendations as soon as possible after the home visit. This will ensure that the details of the visit are captured accurately in the report. Notes and photos taken at the time of the visit can also assist with recall.

The occupational therapy report should summarize information gathered at the time of the home visit. It is also important that the therapist contacts the client, family, or people assisting the client to make decisions, or other service providers after the visit to seek further information about the client's health condition or disability and their functional capacity. As stated earlier, permission should be sought from the client prior to contacting relevant stakeholders. Some services require that client permission be recorded in writing and placed on file for future reference.

It is important that therapists are clear about the documentation requirements of the original referrer (the program or individual who will receive the report) because each might have their own reporting expectations. The report should be in politically correct language and worded simply so that it can be clearly understood by the intended reader. Details about whether information has been reported by the client, family, caregivers, or others or observed by the occupational therapist should be included. More essentially, the report should provide a record of the professional and clinical reasoning and decision-making process and not just the outcomes of the home visit. If required, photos and drawings should be incorporated into the report to provide a detailed picture of the client's circumstances and the areas of the home environment requiring alteration. Finally, the report should provide the client with a record of the visit, including the issues and solutions discussed and the final recommendations.

The Structure of a Home Modification Report

Not all occupational therapists or home modification services stipulate a structure for home modification reports; however, it is recommended that they establish a structure for these documents. For example, some services might choose to document the occupational therapy report in two sections as follows.

The first section of the report should provide background information about the client; their disability or medical condition; and any personal or environmental impacts on their occupational performance, valued roles, occupations, and day-to-day activities. Other background information can include details of the equipment being used by the client in the home and, where appropriate, the dimensions of these items with and without the client. Information on the client's current living situation and use of support services should also be included in this first section.

The report should detail the issues identified and discussed during the interview as well as the options explored. Justification for the final option should also be provided, explaining why this is the best option for the client and his or her situation. This section should detail the specific needs of the client and the physical, social, cultural, personal, and temporal aspects of the home that affect decision making. A statement might need to be made against each recommendation, detailing the consequence of not proceeding with the home modification, to ensure the reader is clear about the proposal.

The second section of the report is a guide for the building professional when undertaking the home modification work. This section should incorporate a general list of the modifications required, including the location and dimensions of features, circulation spaces and clearances, and performance requirements of products and finishes (Bradford, 1998). The building professional does not need to read the confidential information about the client contained in the first section; he or she requires only the technical information to undertake the home modification work. It is therefore necessary that this second section provides sufficient detail for the modification work to be undertaken successfully and, where appropriate, include the detailed specification and plans provided by the builder or architect. This section of the report should be able to stand alone in its own right and have sufficient detail to guide a builder, particularly if the building professional's drawings and specifications become detached from the occupational therapy report. It is not satisfactory for the therapist to refer the reader to the builder's or architect's report and not include a detailed summary of the home modification requirements in that report. If the builder's report is lost or goes missing, there would then be no detail in the therapist's report to guide the same or another builder. Further, this section of the therapist's report may be used by several builders for quoting. It is not industry standard for builders to quote off another builder's documentation, but it is acceptable to use the therapist's documentation.

When making recommendations, it is preferable that therapists indicate only the performance requirements of products rather than specify brands to ensure no one company has a competitive advantage over others and to prevent the therapist from being sued if there is product failure. This practice also ensures that the builder can select from a range of products. There might be specific occasions when the client requires a particular product to suit his or her needs. In such situations, occupational therapists might have to provide product information in their report to ensure that the client's needs are met (Bradford, 1998).

It is important that therapists develop an intimate knowledge of the wide range of products suitable for use in home modifications. They should be familiar with industry standards on how the product should be manufactured, tested for safety, and labeled for correct use.

Therapists can provide each client with a copy of the report and its recommendations to ensure he or she has a record to refer to while the work is being undertaken. The therapist should be mindful that the report, and any other associated documentation relating to the client on file, is a legal document and might one day be used in court. It is therefore important to consider the extent and type of information to be kept on file and included in reports. Organizations have a specific policy in relation to the release of reports that therapists need to consider before providing documentation.

Submitting the Report

In the next step of the home modification process, therapists submit the report for approval and action. Some services require information only for the builder and do not need the client's background information. In this instance, therapists can keep notes on file for future reference and to comply with the legislative requirements for storage of client records.

If therapists have provided sufficient justification for the recommendations and details of the modification in the report, the work can be approved and started. On occasion, the person or program providing the funding for the home modification might not approve the modification; the alterations might be considered too costly, too invasive, an inappropriate intervention given the client's requirements, or outside the scope of the provision of the program. There might be requested changes to the recommendations, which would require another home visit to renegotiate the interventions with the client. It is important that therapists be clear about the parameters of the program before making recommendations because this will inevitably save time. However, they should always ensure that their recommendations are in the best interests of their clients and provide them with sufficient information to make informed choices. Clients might decide to fund their preferred option themselves. Alternatively, therapists might refer clients to another service should their needs fall outside the scope of the existing service or funding.

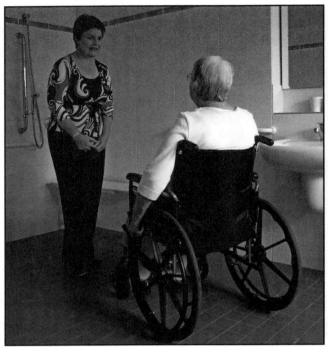

Figure 5-22. Reviewing the impact of the home modifications on the client's occupational performance.

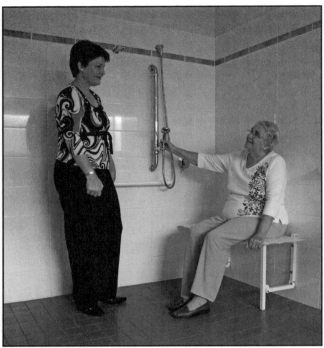

Figure 5-23. Observing the client using the home modifications.

If therapists are in doubt about what might be approved, they could propose a range of options in the home modification report, from the least costly and least invasive option through to the ideal solution that may be more expensive. It is important that therapists clearly document their clinical reasoning in relation to the proposed interventions, the level of importance or priority assigned to these interventions, and the consequence of each for the client. Documentation is also to include details about the consequence of not proceeding with the recommendations. This information will provide helpful detail for the decision maker as he or she reads the report.

Further information about ethical, legal, and reporting issues can be found in Chapter 12.

Educating and Training Clients in the Use of Home Modifications

Occupational therapists have a role in educating and training clients in the use of modifications once they have been installed. This training is particularly relevant in situations where:

+ The modifications have been extensive

+ The person's impairments are newly acquired

+ The person's occupational performance has declined over time

+ A range of equipment has been considered in the planning of the modification

+ Caregivers need to use the modification when assisting the client (Siebert, 2005)

Further education and training in the use of modifications may be required if the client has demonstrated difficulty managing alternative interventions. This training may need to be delivered over several sessions depending on how the clients manage with the initial instruction for use.

Therapists might also provide contact information for repair or maintenance (Bradford, 1998) so that the client can contact the supplier or builder for assistance if problems arise during the warranty period.

Evaluating Home Modifications and Client Outcomes After Installation

The home modification process concludes with the occupational therapist inspecting the modification and other interventions to determine whether the home modifications have been installed properly and that they have achieved the desired outcomes for the client, are effective, and have not presented any unexpected impacts or difficulties (Figures 5-22 and 5-23). The therapist also confirms that the modifications and interventions have met client expectations and fit in with the look and feel of the home and household routines. In addition, they discuss whether the client's occupational performance has been supported or enhanced through the new interventions. Further changes might have to be made if the modification has not helped the person's occupational performance or if it has created further environmental barriers.

The postmodification inspection can involve therapists taking a walk-through of the property with clients to examine the effectiveness of the modifications and/or comprise a formal evaluation of the outcomes of the modification using a standardized evaluation tool. In the first instance, occupational therapists might complete a detailed review of the products and finishes installed and check the specific measurements to ensure that the home modification has been completed per the therapist's documented recommendations and drawings or per the design or building professional's specification and drawings.

Therapists should inform clients (or advocates) if they identify problems resulting from poor workmanship, incorrect installation of fittings and fixtures, or delays with work completion by tradesmen. To act in this capacity, they will need to understand the relevant legislation, such as building or antidiscrimination legislation, to help resolve issues. They will also need some knowledge of advocacy and building service organizations that can assist in the resolution of disputes.

Improved occupational performance is the expected outcome of occupational therapy interventions (Backman, 2005). Performance outcomes discussed during the initial evaluation process (at the time of interviewing and observing the client) can be revisited after the modification to note any change in that performance. By using standardized tools to identify goals and evaluate performance, therapists can assess the extent of change following the modification. This information is invaluable in informing practice and demonstrating the effectiveness of home modification practice.

Further information about evaluating client outcomes can be found in Chapter 13.

At the conclusion of this process, the occupational therapist discusses the discontinuation of services with the client to ensure they are clear about the process. Services from the therapist should cease if the occupational performance goals have been achieved or if the goals have not been met but the person has progressed as far as he or she can toward these goals, if he or she has received the maximum benefit of occupational therapy services, if unforeseen circumstances arise (such as the client

relocating or dying), and if no further home modifications are required (Siebert et al., 2014).

Conclusion

This chapter described how occupational therapists receive and analyze referral information with a view to prioritizing their visit in relation to other referrals. After contacting clients to arrange a suitable time and preparing and collating required resources in advance of the visit, therapists travel to the clients' homes, where they complete interviews; inspect the homes; measure the clients and their equipment and/or caregivers; and photograph, measure, and draw the built environment. They sit with the clients to plan, select, and negotiate a range of interventions before concluding the first visit.

This chapter has also discussed how technical advice may be required from professionals with design or construction expertise before the report and drawings are finalized and submitted to the individual or organization providing funding approval. Information has been provided on the valuable role of occupational therapists in educating and training the client in the use of the home modification and evaluating its effectiveness after installation and use by the client.

References

American Association of Retired Persons. (2000). *Fixing to stay: A national survey on housing and home modification issues.* Washington, DC: Author.

American Occupational Therapy Association. (2014). Occupational therapy practice framework: Domain and process (3rd ed.). *American Journal of Occupational Therapy, 68,* S1-S48. doi:10.5014/ajot.2014.682006

Aplin, T., de Jonge, D., & Gustafsson, L. (2013). Understanding the dimensions of home that impact on home modification decision making. *Australian Occupational Therapy Journal, 60*(2), 101-109.

Aplin, T., de Jonge, D., & Gustafsson, L. (2015). Understanding home modifications impact on clients and their family's experience of home: A qualitative study. *Australian Occupational Therapy Journal, 62*(2), 121-131.

Backman, C. L. (2005). Outcomes and outcome measures: Measuring what matters is in the eye of the beholder. *Canadian Journal of Occupational Therapy, 72*(5), 259-261.

Bradford, I. (1998). The adaptation process. In R. Bull (Ed.), *Housing options for disabled people* (pp. 78-113). Cambridge, MA: Athenaeum Press.

Brown, C. E. (2009). Ecological models in occupational therapy. In E. B. Crepeau, E. S. Cohn, & B. A. Boyt Schell (Eds.), *Willard and Spackman's occupational therapy* (11th ed., pp. 435-445). Philadelphia, PA: Wolters Kluwer Lippincott, Williams & Wilkins.

Center for Universal Design. (1997). *The principles of universal design, version 2.0.* Raleigh, NC: North Carolina State University. Retrieved from http://www.design.ncsu.edu/cud/about_ud/udprinciplestext.htm

Chiu, T., & Oliver, R. (2006). Factor analysis and construct validity of the SAFER-HOME. *Occupational Therapy Journal of Research: Occupation, Participation and Health, 26*(4), 132-142.

Connell, B. R., & Sanford, J. A. (1997). Individualizing home modification recommendations to facilitate performance of routine activities. In S. Lanspery & J. Hyde (Eds.), *Staying put: Adapting the places instead of the people* (pp. 113-148). Amityville, NY: Baywood Publishing Company Incorporated.

Corcoran, M. (2005). Using qualitative measurement methods to understand occupational performance. In M. Law, C. Baum, & W. Dunn (Eds.), *Measuring occupational performance: Supporting best practice in occupational therapy* (pp. 65-78). Thorofare, NJ: SLACK Incorporated.

Crabtree, M. (1998). Images of reasoning: A literature review. *Australian Occupational Therapy Journal, 45*, 113-123.

Duncan, R. (1998). Funding, financing and other resources for home modifications. *Technology and Disability, 8*, 37-50.

Fisher, A. G. (1998). Uniting practice and theory in an occupational framework. *American Journal of Occupational Therapy, 52*(7), 509-520.

Grayson, P. J. (1997). Technology and home adaptations. In S. Lanspery & J. Hyde (Eds.), *Staying put: Adapting the places instead of the people* (pp. 55-74). Amityville, NY: Baywood Publishing Company Incorporated.

Hawkins, R., & Stewart, S. (2002). Changing rooms: The impact of adaptations on the meaning of home for a disabled person and the role of the occupational therapist in the process. *British Journal of Occupational Therapy, 65*(2), 81-87.

Iwarsson, S., & Slaugh, B. (2001). *The housing enabler: An instrument for assessing and analyzing accessibility problems in housing.* Navlinge och Staffanstorp, Sweden: Veten & Stapen HB & Slaug Data Management.

Jones, A., de Jonge, D., & Phillips, R. (2008). *The impact of home maintenance and modification services on health, community care and housing outcomes in later life.* Melbourne, Australia: Australian Housing and Urban Research Institute.

Klein, S. K., Rosage, L., & Shaw, G. (1999). The role of occupational therapists in home modification programs at an area agency on aging. In E. D. Taira & J. L. Carlson (Eds.), *Aging in place: Designing, adapting, and enhancing the home environment* (pp. 19-38). Binghamton, NY: The Haworth Press.

Law, M. (1998). *Client-centered occupational therapy.* Thorofare, NJ: SLACK Incorporated.

Law, M., Baptiste, S., Carswell, A., McColl, M., Polatajko, H., & Pollock, N. (1998). *Canadian occupational performance measure* (3rd ed.). Toronto, ON: Canadian Association of Occupational Therapists.

Law, M., Baptiste, S., & Mills, J. (1995). Client-centered practice: What does it mean and does it make a difference. *Canadian Journal of Occupational Therapy, 62*, 250-257.

Law, M., & Baum, C. (2005). Measurement in occupational therapy. In M. Law, C. Baum, & W. Dunn (Eds.), *Measuring occupational performance: Supporting best practice in occupational therapy* (pp. 3-20). Thorofare, NJ: SLACK Incorporated.

Law, M., King, G., & Russell, D. (2005). Guiding therapist decisions about measuring outcomes in occupational therapy. In M. Law, C. Baum, & W. Dunn (Eds.), *Measuring occupational performance: Supporting best practice in occupational therapy* (pp. 33-44). Thorofare, NJ: SLACK Incorporated.

McCreadie, C., & Tinker, A. (2005). The acceptability of assistance technology to older people. *Ageing and Society, 25*(1), 91-110.

Ohta, R. J., & Ohta, B. M. (1997). The elderly consumer's decision to accept or reject home adaptations: Issues and perspectives. In S. Lanspery & J. Hyde (Eds.), *Staying put: Adapting the places instead of the people* (pp. 79-89). Amityville, NY: Baywood Publishing Company Incorporated.

Pynoos, J., & Nishita, C. J. (2003). The cost and financing of home modifications in the United States. *Journal of Disability Policy Studies, 14*(2), 68-73.

Pynoos, J., Sanford, J., & Rosenfelt, T. (2002). A team approach to home modifications. *OT Practice, 7*(7), 15-19.

Ringaert, L. (2003). Universal design of the built environment to enable occupational performance. In L. Letts, P. Rigby, & D. Stewart (Eds.), *Using environments to enable occupational performance* (pp. 97-115). Thorofare, NJ: SLACK Incorporated.

Rogers, J. C., & Holm, M. B. (2007). The performance assessment of self-care skills (PASS). In I. E. Asher (Ed.), *An annotated index of occupational therapy evaluation tools* (3rd ed., pp. 102-110). Bethesda, MD: American Occupational Therapy Association.

Schell, B.A.B. (2014). Professional reasoning in practice. In B.A.B. Schell, G. Gillen, M. E. Scaffa, & E. S. Cohn (Eds.), *Willard & Spackman's occupational therapy* (12th ed., pp. 384-397). Philadelphia, PA: Wolters Kluwer/Lippincott Williams & Wilkins.

Schell, B.A.B., & Schell, J. W. (2008). Professional reasoning as the basis for practice. In B. A. Boyt Schell & J. W. Schell (Eds.), *Clinical and professional reasoning in occupational therapy* (pp. 3-12). Philadelphia, PA: Lippincott, Williams & Wilkins.

Siebert, C. (2005). *Occupational therapy practice guidelines for home modifications.* Bethesda, MD: American Occupational Therapy Association.

Siebert, C., Smallfield, S., & Stark, S. (2014). *Occupational therapy practice guidelines for home modifications.* Bethesda, MD: The American Occupational Therapy Association Press.

Silverstein, N. M., & Hyde, J. (1997). The importance of a consumer perspective in home adaptation of Alzheimer's households. In S. Lanspery & J. Hyde (Eds.), *Staying put: Adapting the places instead of the people* (pp. 91-111). Amityville, NY: Baywood Publishing Company.

Stark, S. (2003). Home modifications that enable occupational performance. In L. Letts, R. Rigby, & P. Stewart (Eds.), *Using environments to enable occupational performance* (pp. 219-234). Thorofare, NJ: SLACK Incorporated.

Stark, S., Sommerville, E. K., & Morris, J.C. (2010). In-Home Occupational Performance Evaluation (I-HOPE). *American Journal of Occupational Therapy, 64*, 580-589.

Wylde, M. A. (1998). Consumer knowledge of home modifications. *Technology and Disability, 8*, 51-68.

6

Evaluating Clients' Home Modification Needs and Priorities

Desleigh de Jonge, MPhil (OccThy), Grad Cert Soc Sci and
Melanie Hoyle, BSc (Psych), MOccThySt, Grad Dip Health Sci, Post Grad Dip Psych

In occupational therapy, evaluation is viewed as a collaborative process that aims to understand people as occupational beings and how they create meaning in their lives through occupation (Cohn, Schell, & Neistadt, 2003). A home evaluation seeks to understand and analyze the dynamic transaction between people, their occupational patterns, and the home environment. Using a top-down approach and an occupation-based framework, occupational therapists analyze occupational performance by first seeking to understand the roles and occupations of importance to the person and the impact of the injury, impairment, or health condition on the person's life. The therapist then observes and examines the person's performance, the home environment, and occupational elements (activities, tasks, and sequences) to identify barriers and facilitators to performance. Clients are considered central to the evaluation process, actively contributing to the therapist's understanding of their experience and capacities, the value of the activities they engage in, and the intricacies of the home environment.

Given the unique and complex nature of occupational performance in the home, therapists rely heavily on professional reasoning to deal with the diversity of information they gather during the evaluation process. This chapter describes the range of reasoning styles therapists use and how they are used throughout the process to develop and test hypotheses, understand the client's perspective, and determine what is achievable to ensure the best possible outcomes. The chapter also details the variety of evaluation strategies therapists use to understand and interpret occupational performance in the home, including informal and structured interviews, skilled observation, and standardized assessment tools, and discusses what each strategy contributes to the home modification process. Criteria are also provided to guide therapists when they are selecting and evaluating standardized assessment tools.

CHAPTER OBJECTIVES

By the end of this chapter, the reader will be able to:

+ Describe the purpose of a home evaluation
+ Explain the framework therapists use for evaluating occupational performance in the home
+ Describe how professional reasoning is used throughout a home evaluation
+ Identify the types of evaluation strategies occupational therapists use during a home visit and what each contributes to the evaluation process
+ Identify important considerations in choosing standardized assessment tools for home modifications

Ainsworth, E., & de Jonge, D. *An Occupational Therapist's Guide to Home Modification Practice, Second Edition (pp. 111-144).*
© 2019 SLACK Incorporated.

PURPOSE OF EVALUATION

When providing a home modification service, the purpose of an occupational therapy evaluation is to gain an understanding of the clients' skills and abilities and the barriers that prevent them from successfully completing the necessary and valued activities in their home. The home is a natural environment in which the therapist and client can develop a shared understanding of occupational performance issues. It is here that therapists can observe their clients undertaking everyday activities and see what is completed and how and where they are usually done. By using a range of evaluation strategies, the therapist identifies "misfits" involving the person, occupations, and the environment. Throughout the visit, the therapist monitors the environment and talks with people who live in the home to understand the dimensions of the home environment that influence occupational performance and are likely to affect decision making.

Therapists undertake evaluations in the home to:

+ Ensure that clients being discharged from a hospital or institution are safe and able to undertake basic self-care activities independently

+ Identify fall risks, especially in the homes of older people and people with a history of falling

+ Ensure that people with congenital and acquired impairments (e.g., cerebral palsy, stroke, spinal or head injury, Parkinsonism) are able to mobilize safely and function effectively in their home environments

+ Ensure that older people, including those with and without an identified health condition, are able to remain living in their homes for as long as possible

+ Assist families to care for children, teenagers, or adults with impairments

Home is where many and varied occupations are undertaken (Rigby, Trentham, & Letts, 2014). It is where people commonly eat; rest; look after themselves and others; and manage their finances, goods, and resources. It is where they develop and maintain relationships or refresh and replenish their energies through a range of restful and active leisure pursuits. It is the base from which they engage in the community and explore the world. Some activities happen routinely on a daily or weekly basis, whereas others happen seasonally or periodically. Home evaluations generally involve an assessment of the person's ability to perform valued and important occupations in the home. Depending on the person's roles, goals, and priorities, an evaluation would generally include an assessment of self-care and household activities, as well as those to do with leisure and community participation. Some evaluations focus primarily on the accessibility or safety of the home and community.

Evaluations generally take a number of forms. First, they are used as a means of screening (i.e., determining whether a person requires occupational therapy services and how urgently). Evaluations also assist therapists to analyze and identify the nature and, in some cases, the extent of the occupational performance issue. Finally, evaluation allows therapists to determine whether there has been a change in occupational performance as a result of occupational therapy intervention. This is commonly referred to as *outcome measurement*. Each of these evaluation approaches uses different strategies, although some traverse a number of purposes.

Screening

Screening involves a cursory evaluation of the person's occupational performance to determine whether a more thorough evaluation is required (Shotwell, 2014). This can take the form of a brief, informal interview with the person (or the referrer) to determine whether he or she has any specific occupational performance concerns or is at risk of developing associated problems. Therapists commonly use structured questioning to understand the nature of the person's impairment or health condition and its current and future impact on occupational performance. Therapists also briefly explore the demands of various roles and activities and the nature of the home environment and potential impacts on occupational performance (Law & Baum, 2017). Alternatively, they use standardized tools to evaluate the person's capacity to perform a range of activities or identify environmental hazards that may place the person at risk of occupational performance difficulties in the home. Both informal and structured questioning rely on the therapist's experience and professional judgment to decide whether the client requires a service and how urgently it should be delivered. The information gathered using standardized assessments provides a mechanism for determining the extent of a performance problem, which can be used to justify and prioritize service provision. In addition, information gained from screening all referrals can assist in determining the extent of need generally in the community.

Analyzing and Diagnosing Occupational Performance

Therapists are primarily familiar with using evaluations to analyze and diagnose occupational performance difficulties. These evaluations require a thorough approach to information gathering and analysis and are essential to designing effective interventions. Therapists generally use a range of evaluation strategies to understand the precise nature of the occupational performance difficulties being experienced and to identify aspects of the person-environment-occupation transaction that are contributing factors.

Therapists use a range of evaluation strategies to identify and analyze occupational performance issues. Informal and structured interviews provide background information on clients and their living environment and help therapists develop an understanding of client concerns and their perspective on the nature and impact of occupational performance problems. Therapists also use skilled observation to closely examine occupational performance, identify where performance is ineffective or hazardous, and investigate factors contributing to inadequate performance. These observations are often undertaken in a semistructured way with performance described qualitatively, which relies heavily on the professional experience and judgment of the therapist. Therapists also use standardized assessment tools to measure the extent of the performance problem and diagnose the cause of the presenting problem.

Evaluation of Outcomes

Outcome evaluation assists therapists to determine the effectiveness of home modification interventions. These evaluations are undertaken to confirm that the changes have produced the desired improvements in occupational performance and to ensure there are no adverse consequences resulting from the introduced changes. The consistent use of outcome measures is also fundamental to evidence-based practice (Law & Baum, 2017). These evaluations inform therapists about the most effective interventions in a range of situations and build a body of evidence of their value and effectiveness. This information is being used increasingly by policy makers and management to make decisions about policy directions and the future funding of various service programs (Law & Baum, 2017). Outcomes can be evaluated qualitatively and quantitatively. Qualitative evaluation provides an opportunity to record the client's and therapist's perception of the impact of the intervention. Quantitative evaluation can demonstrate the extent of impact and establish whether there have been any measurable changes as a result of the intervention, especially if standardized measures are used before and after the event.

FRAMEWORK FOR EVALUATION

In home modification practice, it is important that the evaluation strategies chosen reflect client-centered practice so that clients are empowered by the process and have a sense of ownership of the modifications undertaken in their home. Evaluation methods should allow clients to identify their specific concerns about valued occupations, record their unique occupational performance requirements, and document the impact of interventions on their lives (Law, Baum, & Dunn, 2017). This requires that evaluation strategies do the following:

+ Allow occupational performance issues or problems to be identified by the client and household members and not solely by the therapist and team
+ Permit the unique nature of each person's participation in occupations to be recognized
+ Provide opportunities for both the subjective experience and the observable qualities of occupational performance to be recorded
+ Afford the client (and relevant others) to have a say in evaluating the outcomes of the interventions
+ Recognize the unique qualities of the home environment
+ Assist clients and household members to develop a mutual understanding of therapists' safety, prevention, or health maintenance concerns (Law & Baum, 2017)

Client-centered evaluation requires that evaluation strategies extend beyond the measurement of performance components. Evaluation strategies need to be able to measure the extent of occupational engagement, giving due recognition to the uniqueness of each person's valued roles and occupations. They should also allow the client and therapist to jointly plan interventions (Law & Baum, 2017) and to determine the effectiveness and value of these to the client in the short and long term.

Evaluation should also accurately reflect the scope and focus of the profession and its practice frameworks. When using the occupational therapy practice framework, evaluation focuses on understanding the person's occupational history and experiences and his or her patterns of daily living, interests, values, and needs, as well as his or her priorities and concerns about occupational performance (American Occupational Therapy Association [AOTA], 2014). Occupational performance is observed in context in order to determine supports/facilitators or barriers to performance, giving due consideration to body structures and function, performance skills and patterns, and activity demands as well as the environment. The therapist, in collaboration with the client, then determines concerns and risks and identifies problems and the probable causes.

When using an ecological approach, evaluation should focus on the quantity and quality of occupational performance using both objective and subjective methods. It examines the "fit" of the person, environment, and occupations, acknowledging that these are constantly changing and evolving. These models recognize the unique personal attributes, capacities, and life experiences each individual brings to the collaboration. Evaluations need to examine the physical, sociocultural, personal, and temporal elements of the environment and the potential impact of these on occupational performance. It would also consider these environmental domains from an individual, household, neighborhood, and community perspective.

Professional Reasoning

As a result of the individual and complex nature of home modification practice, therapists rely heavily on professional reasoning throughout the evaluation and intervention process. Whereas medical settings refer to clinical reasoning, the term *professional reasoning* has evolved to acknowledge the range of practice settings occupational therapists work in. This section focuses on the use of professional reasoning during evaluation. The role of professional reasoning in designing acceptable, effective, and workable home modification interventions will be discussed further in Chapter 9; however, good reasoning in the evaluation process is critical to developing a thorough understanding of the issues, which then contributes to developing effective interventions and achieving good client outcomes.

Therapists use a "whole body" process (Schell, 2014) to understand occupational performance in the home, identify factors that constrain performance, and create a home environment that enables occupational engagement. Using a combination of theoretical knowledge and personal and professional experience, therapists analyze copious amounts of diverse information to fully understand each person and his or her occupational performance

issues. They can then recommend interventions that will fit well with each unique person-environment-occupation transaction.

Therapists use a combination of thinking approaches to understand occupational performance issues in the home environment: scientific, narrative, pragmatic, ethical, and interactive reasoning (Schell, 2014). For example, from the moment therapists receive a referral, they begin to gather information and use scientific reasoning to anticipate occupational performance difficulties or generate hypotheses from their bank of theoretical knowledge of impairments and health conditions and the role the environment plays in creating disability. Therapists continue to use scientific reasoning throughout the evaluation process when choosing appropriate evaluation methods and analyzing and interpreting behavior. When talking with their clients and listening to their stories, therapists use narrative reasoning to develop a deeper understanding of people's lifestyles, aspirations, concerns, and valued occupations. They then work with their clients throughout the visit to develop a rich understanding of their experiences and environments and to explore and create a new future. Pragmatic reasoning assists therapists to use their personal resources to their best advantage, understand the service delivery context, and work sensibly and effectively within the policy framework and available resources. Ethical reasoning ensures that the therapist maintains respect for the values and rights of all clients and provides the best possible service in every situation. Finally, interactive reasoning promotes the development of a strong therapeutic relationship between the therapist and the client, which builds a collaborative alliance and enhances the potential for success of therapeutic interventions. Professional reasoning has been described as "a dynamic process simultaneously influenced by the client and therapist's characteristics, experience, and background" (Radomski, 2008, p. 45). The dynamic nature of professional reasoning is particularly evident when therapists use a client-centered approach, where they need to be flexible and responsive to the uniqueness of each person and his or her home environment.

Scientific Reasoning

What Is Scientific Reasoning?

Scientific reasoning is described as "a logical process that parallels scientific inquiry" (Schell, 2014, p. 388). Two forms of scientific reasoning are described in the literature: diagnostic reasoning and procedural reasoning (Schell, 2014). Diagnostic reasoning is concerned with sensing and defining professional problems (Schell, 2014), and procedural reasoning is the thinking that comes from choosing suitable evaluation and intervention approaches (Fleming, 1991, 1994). In combination, these processes assist therapists to progress from defining to resolving occupational performance problems (Chapparo & Ranka, 2000). Drawing on relevant bodies of knowledge, the therapist seeks and interprets cues and then generates and tests hypotheses (Rogers & Holm, 1991) about the person's occupational performance difficulties and contributing factors.

How Is It Used?

The process begins with the therapist gleaning cues from the written referral, case file, preliminary conversation with the client, presentation of the neighborhood, appearance and design of the home, and initial encounter with the client. For example, Glenda, an older woman with osteoporosis, is referred for a home assessment following a fall. The therapist would initially determine her age, living situation, general health, and whether she sustained any injuries from the fall by reading the referral or file. He or she would ask Glenda about her health (including her vision, physical condition, memory, cognition, medication use, etc.) and the circumstances of the fall to identify potential precipitating and contributing factors. During the visit, the therapist would note the age, design, and state of repair of the house, and he or she would scan the environment for known hazards. He or she would also observe the client as she walks outside and within the house and note her agility and ability to negotiate obstacles and changes in lighting levels and flooring. These are the cues that provide therapists with initial information about clients and their physical and functional status, their occupations, and their home environments, which assist them to generate hypotheses about the person's occupational performance.

How Does It Influence the Evaluation Process?

The cues sought and noted by therapists are shaped by their knowledge, experiences, and models of practice. For example, a therapist's knowledge of factors that contribute to falls would direct him or her to collect information about a client's fall history, number of medications, and so forth. Knowing about the consequences of a fall for someone with osteoporosis also alerts the therapist to investigate this and other comorbidities. Therapists with experience working with people with a history of falls would be alert to features in the environment that could be injurious during a fall. The various models to which therapists ascribe also define what they attend to and what they understand to have contributed to the observed problem. A rehabilitation therapist might focus primarily on measuring the extent of the person's functional impairment; therapists using an occupational performance model would focus on understanding how the person undertakes activities, whereas those using an ecological model would examine the environment and how well it supports activity engagement. Within clinical practice, therapists often draw on a number of models to develop a comprehensive understanding of the person and his or her situation.

When using diagnostic reasoning, therapists draw on existing knowledge to acquire and interpret cues and generate and test hypotheses. From a given diagnosis, therapists can anticipate functional difficulties and hypothesize about how these are likely to affect occupational performance and progress in the long term. In addition, therapists analyze and interpret behavior in an effort to understand what is contributing to it. If Glenda were to trip when walking to the bathroom during the home visit, the therapist might attribute this to wearing poor footwear, being distracted, a developing dementia or neurological impairment, vision loss, reduced sensation, or uneven carpet. These hypotheses would then be tested or adjusted as further cues are sought and interpreted. For example, the therapist might ask Glenda to demonstrate how she gets in and out of the shower recess. By asking her to remove her shoes and talking about how her legs and feet feel on the floor and shower recess surface, the therapist can test whether the problem persists without footwear. Allowing her to concentrate on the task allows the therapist to observe her performance without distractions. Observing her capacity to notice and lift her feet over obstacles or level changes on the floor enables the therapist to test her concerns about Glenda's physical and cognitive function. Her ability to negotiate changes in floor level and uneven carpet allows the therapist to examine the impact of environmental barriers on Glenda's performance.

Procedural reasoning is used to choose appropriate evaluation strategies, including valid and reliable assessment tools (Radomski, 2008). Therapists select strategies and tools that allow them to gather information about the person, his or her occupations and the environment, and the transaction between them. A combination of observation, assessment, and discussion allows various hypotheses to be modified and tested until the therapist develops a clear understanding of occupational performance and the person-environment-occupation transaction.

What Does It Offer the Therapist and Client?

Scientific reasoning allows therapists to draw on their knowledge and experience to gather, analyze, and interpret vast amounts of information. When therapists are well informed and able to use this information to generate a number of hypotheses, they are well placed to observe and interpret the person-environment-occupation transaction and understand how and why occupational performance difficulties occur. This complex process is often easier for experienced therapists who have integrated their model(s) of practice, have acquired a broad knowledge base through experience and reading, and have developed the capacity to attend to and simultaneously process a diverse range of information. Less experienced therapists often struggle to use their model(s) of practice and limited knowledge effectively, to attend to a number of cues at the same time, and to generate multiple hypotheses. This can result in a tendency for them to jump to conclusions quickly if time is not taken to critically reflect on assumptions (Chapparo & Ranka, 2000). Experienced therapists are also at risk of "contracting" to routine practices if they over-rely on experience, do not keep their knowledge current, or actively reflect on their reasoning processes (Chapparo & Ranka, 2000).

Although scientific reasoning might appear to be the realm of the therapist, clients also benefit from this form of reasoning. When therapists are able to share their knowledge and articulate their reasoning, they can engage clients in a meaningful and informative discussion about risks and potentially contributing factors. This allows the client to be an active part of the issue identification and decision-making process rather than feeling uninformed, disempowered, and pressured by "expert" opinion.

Narrative and Conditional Reasoning

What Is Narrative Reasoning?

Occupational therapy has been described as both an art and a science (Peloquin, 1994; Townsend & Polatajko, 2013). Narrative reasoning, which addresses the art of the profession, contrasts with and compliments scientific reasoning. Narrative reasoning is used to understand and describe a person's unique experience of his or her situation and to work with that person to create an impelling future. It assists therapists to make sense of each person's situation and imagine the impact of the illness, injury or health condition, aging, or disability on their lives (Schell, 2014).

How Is It Used?

Throughout the home visit, therapists engage in natural conversations with the householder, making comments about spaces in the house and asking questions such as, "Did you decorate this room yourself?" and "Are these photos of your family?" This generally elicits storytelling that assists in developing rapport and gaining a richer understanding of the home and the people living in it. Therapists also use semistructured interviews to gather information. These interviews can include open-ended questions that allow clients to describe their experience in the home. This allows therapists to draw information from these stories to enrich their understanding of the impact of the health condition or impairment on a client's engagement in activities in the home and gain information about his or her occupational history. It also provides the client with an opportunity to introduce new or unexpected elements to the story that might not have been uncovered through direct or closed questioning. Active and empathetic listening is also important in building rapport and encouraging clients to openly share their experiences and aspirations. Creating a safe space for disclosure might be as simple as agreeing to have a cup of tea and listening without interjecting, instead allowing the client to discuss things that are important to him or her.

By taking the time to talk with and listen to Glenda, the older woman described previously in this chapter, the therapist develops a rich understanding of the impact of her condition on her day-to-day roles, routines and activities, and the significance of her home environment. He or she would learn that Glenda was experiencing an increasing number of falls and that this was making her feel unsafe in her home and reluctant to go out without someone accompanying her. Consequently, she finds herself doing less and feeling even more uncertain. The therapist also learns that Glenda had lived in the house for 45 years of her married life and had raised five children in this home. Of significance is that she now lives alone in the home that her recently deceased husband built. Glenda is reluctant to make changes because the home provides her with a strong connection to him and their family. She also looks after two of her young grandchildren after school, bathing and feeding them before her daughter collects them after work.

Narrative reasoning is not only useful for developing a deeper understanding of each person and his or her personal preferences and priorities, it is also valuable in assisting clients to explore and create a new future for themselves. When discussing issues, the therapist has an opportunity to share stories with a client and create new possibilities and a future for him or her. For example, therapists can sometimes assist clients to articulate and analyze their concerns by sharing stories about other people's experiences. Stories also help clients envision possibilities and create goals that may have been long abandoned. For example, when discussing a recent experience with a client with similar reservations about going out into the community, the therapist shared a story about how a simple modification to the front entry of the house had provided the client with greater confidence and a sense of security when entering and exiting the house. This story allowed Glenda to contemplate developing goals she might not otherwise have considered.

How Does It Influence the Evaluation Process?

Spending time developing a deeper understanding of each client and his or her home environments allows therapists to contextualize and make sense of information gathered during the evaluation. For example, understanding the value a client places on furniture and other objects in the home assists the therapist to acknowledge that they are more than environmental hazards. It allows them to remain open and respectful and to anticipate issues where their evaluation of risk might differ from that of their client.

Narrative reasoning can often be an automatic and unconscious process for both novice and expert therapists. For example, informally observing people in their homes can reveal a great deal about their life stories. A well-tended garden informs the therapist that the householder appreciates plants and that they spend a great deal of time either tending to the garden themselves or paying someone else to do it. Photographs on the wall reveal personal connections. Shelves and floor space cluttered with valued objects and trinkets alert the therapist to the attachment that the person has to his or her belongings. These observations are different from the cues sought in scientific reasoning, where therapists seek cues to generate and test hypotheses and then filter information through their scientific knowledge to analyze or diagnose issues. In narrative reasoning, the therapist absorbs information from people's stories and from the environment to build an understanding of their life experience and the personal and social culture of the home environment.

What Does It Offer the Client and Therapist?

Narrative reasoning allows clients to examine their issues and air their concerns in a safe environment. It also enables therapists to develop a deep understanding of each client's unique experience of his or her situation. The trust and rapport developed in this process makes it easier for the client to disclose personal information and to have faith in the therapist's evaluation of the issues because it is founded on a deep understanding of the situation. This type of reasoning also allows therapists to explore the symbolic meaning of home with the client and to ensure that modifications are life enhancing, as well as rational and pragmatic. It shifts the focus from simply addressing issues of safety, function, and independence to developing a rich and deep understanding of the person, his or her valued occupations, and the home environment. It also affords clients the opportunity to be the authors of their own life story.

Pragmatic Reasoning

What Is Pragmatic Reasoning?

Pragmatic reasoning is the consideration given to the practical realities encountered in practice. It assists therapists to work sensibly and effectively within their own personal resources as well as within the resources available in the practice context (Schell, 2014). Therapists bring personal experiences, professional competencies, and a level of commitment to professional practice that affect their capacity to deliver a service. The demands on therapists' time within the service and outside work will also influence their availability. In addition, the practicalities and logistics of delivering services within a particular setting (in this case, the home) and the processes and resources within the service organization (Schell & Cervero, 1993) influence the type and level of service that can be delivered.

How Is It Used?

In daily practice, therapists use pragmatic reasoning to make the best use of their personal resources such as knowledge, skills, abilities, time, and level of commitment, as well as service resources such as evaluation resources, structures and processes, reimbursement schedules, and policy directives. For example, a therapist might have limited experience in dealing with people like Glenda who have an increased falls risk, so he or she would dedicate time prior to the visit to reading about, training in, and becoming familiar with known falls risks. This would ensure the most effective use of visit time. If a specific time was allocated for the visit by the service or reimbursement schedule, the therapist would try to structure it to ensure that all issues were addressed and prioritized efficiently. If the service did not have resources dedicated to assessing falls risk, the therapist might borrow them from another center to use in this instance, with plans to order them for the service should more clients with falls risks require assistance. The constraints placed on the evaluation by the client and the environment would also need to be considered in order to maximize the effectiveness of the visit (e.g., advising Glenda of the length of time required for the visit and negotiating a mutually convenient time where both the therapist and Glenda have the necessary time available). If the environment has many hazards, the therapist might need to spend more time at Glenda's house and postpone the next client visit scheduled for that day or book a second visit to discuss issues of concern.

How Does It Influence the Evaluation Process?

During the evaluation process, therapists use their knowledge of and experience with various evaluation strategies to identify and define occupational performance issues. The diversity of experience and competency among therapists leads to variability in the nature and quality of evaluation, especially in a continually developing area of practice such as home modification. It is therefore important that, as a profession, therapists develop and share practice knowledge and evaluation tools and protocols to ensure that professional practice and service delivery are consistent and of a high quality. Therapists with limited experience should consult with more experienced colleagues to ensure that they have been effective in identifying all of the relevant issues in the complex practice environment.

Therapists need to be flexible and responsive to the specific needs and circumstances of each client and therefore use pragmatic reasoning to choose the most appropriate strategies for any given situation. The home setting presents particular challenges to traditional evaluation methods and assessment tools. Being a private space, the client or homeowner might have sensitivities or preferences that affect which, and how, things can be evaluated. This requires therapists to search for new evaluation strategies that accommodate the diversity of issues and circumstances they encounter in this complex environment.

The time available for a home visit can also influence the nature of evaluation undertaken. Time-limited or one-off home visits can make it difficult for therapists to develop a deep understanding of the person-environment-occupation transaction and to be entrusted sufficiently to recommend changes to personal routines and spaces. Consequently, therapists use pragmatic reasoning to assist clients to prioritize issues to ensure that the most important matters are attended to in the time available for the visit.

Service organizations often have a particular focus and assessment protocols that might or might not align well with professional practice. In these situations, therapists fulfill their employment responsibilities by clarifying what they are able to offer the client within this service and referring him or her to other services that can address additional needs. Therapists can then work with the organization to refine and develop procedures and protocols within the service so that they are more in line with current professional knowledge or best practice.

What Does It Offer the Therapist and Client?

Therapists are faced with a considerable number of pragmatic considerations when undertaking home modification evaluations. They are acutely aware of the many factors in the practice context that impinge on home modification practice and use pragmatic reasoning to manage the many competing demands on their time and resources. When managed well, therapists can optimize the use of their time and resources to address occupational performance issues in the home. However, sometimes pragmatic issues can significantly constrain practice. A focus on budget, cost-effectiveness, and efficient use of resources, including therapists' time, can sometimes result in an emphasis on throughput and short-term outcomes. The home is a very personal and private environment and, as such, sufficient time is required to allow the therapist to get to know the client and to allow him or her to focus and direct the evaluation process. The challenge for therapists is to achieve a balance between working within available resources and working long term to maximize the resources available, which includes building the capacity of therapists and services to respond to people's diverse home modification needs. Therefore, pragmatic reasoning necessarily requires therapists to provide ongoing input to facilitate the development of service policies, procedures, and resources to ensure that home modification services are as effective as they are efficient.

Ethical Reasoning

What Is Ethical Reasoning?

Ethical reasoning, often the culmination of the reasoning process, identifies "what should be done" from possibilities generated from other reasoning forms (Schell, 2014). When the art and science of occupational therapy meet reality, therapists call on their personal and professional values to ensure that quality services are delivered to all clients. Ethical reasoning is the thinking that therapists undertake to synthesize knowledge and evidence, client values and goals, an appraisal of his or her competencies, and practical aspects of service delivery to provide the best possible care (Radomski, 2008). When dealing with the many competing forces that affect their thinking and decision making, therapists filter decisions through the core values and attitudes of the profession and its code of ethics. The profession holds a number of enduring values, one of which is that all humans are unique. This value challenges therapists to appreciate each individual's experiences, values, and goals over theoretical understandings and routine procedures and implores them to make time and use evaluation strategies that recognize and understand each person's distinctive nature.

How Is It Used?

When considering scientific, narrative, and pragmatic aspects of practice, therapists are often confronted with conflicting information and demands. Ethical reasoning requires therapists to critically reflect on competing perspectives to ensure that their actions manifest ethical practice. The *Occupational Therapy Code of Ethics* of the AOTA identifies six Principles and Standards of Conduct, which require therapists to:

1. Demonstrate a concern for the well-being and safety of the recipients of their services (beneficence)

2. Refrain from actions that cause harm (nonmaleficence)

3. Respect the right of the individual to self-determination, privacy, confidentiality, and consent (autonomy)

4. Promote fairness and objectivity in the provision of occupational therapy services (justice)

5. Provide comprehensive, accurate, and objective information when representing the profession (veracity)

6. Treat clients, colleagues, and other professionals with respect, fairness, discretion, and integrity (fidelity; AOTA, 2015, pp. 2-8).

When visiting clients' homes, therapists are privy to a great deal of information about their clients. For example, on entering Glenda's home, the therapist becomes aware of a number of hazards that put her at a high risk of falling. Ethical reasoning alerts the therapist to his or her responsibility to address each of these before leaving the home. The therapist is also aware that he or she should not introduce any additional risks by placing equipment in Glenda's path or asking her to perform an activity that would unnecessarily place her at risk. At the same time, the therapist has to respect Glenda's right to privacy and control in her own home and can therefore not enter rooms without permission or impose solutions that are not welcomed. Additionally, the therapist must not disclose information to others about Glenda and her living situation without her permission. Ethical reasoning also impels the therapist to provide a high quality of service to all clients, regardless of race, social circumstances, or attitude, and ensures that clients are well informed about what can and cannot be provided by the particular service. The therapist would also ensure that Glenda is referred to more appropriate services should her needs fall outside of his or her responsibilities.

How Does It Influence the Evaluation Process?

It is not uncommon that the values of therapists or service organizations sometimes differ from those of clients. These conflicts are inevitable and require the therapist to use sound reasoning to resolve differences of opinion. Respectful and open discussion with the client ensures that the therapist understands his or her perspective and collaborates to achieve a mutually satisfying outcome. Therapists also need to critically reflect on their personal and professional values in order to "confront, understand and work toward resolving the contradictions within his/her practice between what is desirable and actual practice" (Johns, 2000, p. 34). An evaluation with sound ethical reasoning ensures that the therapist evaluates the right things using the best possible approach for the particular situation, regardless of the challenges presented. Further information on frameworks for ethical decision making is provided in Chapter 12.

What Does It Offer the Therapist and Client?

Ethical reasoning provides the therapist with a systematic way of addressing conflicts between what should be done and what can be done (Doherty, 2009). It also ensures that all clients are treated respectfully and receive high-quality service, regardless of the situation. Within the evaluation process, ethical reasoning allows the therapist to fully explore the client's perspective and work collaboratively with them to define and prioritize issues.

Interactive Reasoning

What Is Interactive Reasoning?

The therapeutic relationship, defined as "a trusting connection and rapport established between therapist and client through collaboration, communication, therapist empathy and mutual understanding and respect" (Cole & McLean, 2003, p. 33-34), is an essential element of occupational therapy practice. The importance of this relationship between therapist and client has been well established as influential for the outcomes of therapy, such that without the relationship, interventions may be compromised (Bonsaksen, Vøllestad, & Taylor, 2013). To this end it is critical to success that the therapeutic relationship or alliance is established and maintained until goals are achieved (Tickle-Degnen, 2002). Interactive reasoning is "thinking directed toward building positive interpersonal relationships, permitting collaborative problem identification and problem solving" (Schell, 2014, p. 389). Schell states that it largely involves automatic acts that influence and form the interpersonal behaviors and communication skills used by the therapist in the creation and maintenance of a therapeutic relationship in which occupational therapy can take place with a client. It might be conscious when the therapist thinks specifically about the relationship, such as supporting a client when he or she is thinking through the challenges to day-to-day function in the home.

How Is It Used?

In order to build trust, a foundational basis of the therapeutic relationship, the therapist must enter the client's life world (Crepeau, 1991) and employ strategies that are designed to engage and encourage the client (Schell, 2014). To successfully achieve this, the therapist must use interactive reasoning to choose, enact, understand, and account for the range of automatic and conscious interpersonal and communicative skills employed to establish and foster a connection with the client. This enables the therapist to make best use of communication strategies that the client responds to positively (Schell, 2014). Further, this reasoning is necessary in order to preserve the therapeutic relationship and enable the client and therapist to work in collaboration toward the resolution of performance problems and achievement of occupational goals (Schell, 2014).

Due to the importance of the therapeutic relationship to the success of occupational therapy outcomes, interactive reasoning is vital, and therapists need to ensure that they consider and attend to communicative and behavioral choices that they implement when working with a client. For example, when conducting the initial evaluation with Glenda, the therapist may choose to use an open body position, active listening skills, paraphrasing, inclusion of clarifying questions, etc. that demonstrate that he or she is eager to hear about the Glenda's needs, priorities, and concerns and to understand the situation from her perspective. These choices are made to convey to Glenda that the therapist is open to working together and will assist in establishing rapport and the base of trust on which an effective therapeutic relationship can be built.

Although some of the outcomes of interactive reasoning, such as the communication skill choices mentioned, are conscious and easily identified, some are a result of more automatic acts (Schell, 2014). Therapists need to work at becoming aware of their more unconscious tendencies, as these, too, can affect the therapeutic relationship. An example might be if a therapist automatically touches Glenda on the arm to convey sympathy when she mentions that her husband is deceased, which, depending on Glenda's preferences, she might find comforting or intrusive. Due to the presence of both more conscious and automatic influences, it can at times be easiest to see the significance of interactive reasoning when an error in reasoning occurs and negatively affects the therapeutic relationship (Schell, 2014). Despite this, it is an essential aspect of professional reasoning requiring attention, as it underpins the therapeutic relationship, which enables the collaboration and sharing of information between client and therapist that are necessary for the other reasoning types.

How Does It Influence the Evaluation Process?

Interactive reasoning, as previously mentioned, enables the development and continuation of the therapeutic relationship, which is central to the occupational therapy process and vital to the successful outcomes of interventions. If a strong and allied relationship that is focused on working with the client is not established or maintained, it can jeopardize all aspects of the occupational therapy process, including the gathering of information, therapist understanding of client needs and priorities, establishing goals, professional reasoning, etc., as well as associated interventions and outcomes. In order to obtain and understand the information on which the other reasonings are based, interactive reasoning is necessary to ensure a relationship between the therapist and client that enables collaboration and two-way communication. In addition, if there are problems within or a breakdown of the therapeutic relationship, interactive reasoning can be utilized to examine communication skills or interpersonal behaviors, identify potential difficulties/issues, and enable the therapist to improve upon or rebuild the therapy relationship or, if necessary, refer the client on to another therapist or service.

What Does It Offer the Therapist and Client?

Interactive reasoning draws the therapist's attention to the importance of the therapeutic relationship to ensure successful outcomes in occupational therapy practice. It provides a means to review the communication skills and interpersonal behaviors that are used to establish and maintain a trust-based relationship that enables collaboration and facilitates ongoing therapy with a client. It also provides the therapist with a course of inquiry and action if there are difficulties within the therapeutic relationship that are hindering the occupational therapy process. It ensures that the client is afforded the opportunity to be a valued partner in the therapeutic relationship. This enables them to be understood as a person; their needs, preferences, priorities, and concerns to be heard; and therapy to be carried out in an environment where they are respected and approached with empathy. The successful use of interactive reasoning contributes to the establishment of a solid alliance between therapist and client, which enhances the potential for the best possible outcome(s) from therapy and can be beneficial to both client and therapist alike. A good relationship builds client trust, whereby they feel listened to, thus enabling them to have confidence that the recommendations will address their needs and improve their circumstances.

Types of Evaluation Strategies

Therapists use a range of evaluation strategies, such as informal and structured interviews, skilled observation, and standardized assessments, to gather information about the client and his or her home and to test hypotheses.

Informal Interview

Home modification evaluations generally begin with the therapist engaging in an informal discussion with the client about the home, the reason for referral, or concerns the client has about his or her occupational performance. Interviewing is an essential step in the evaluation process and generally serves a dual purpose. First, interviews allow therapists to gather information; hear clients' stories; and understand their experiences, concerns, goals, and aspirations (Henry & Kramer, 2009). Second, interviews afford therapists an opportunity to build collaborative relationships with their clients and gain their trust (Henry & Kramer, 2009). Interviewing is used by therapists to create a shared understanding of each client's situation so that the home modification process can address his or her individual concerns and priorities.

Informal interviews are useful in gathering qualitative information about the client and the home, which is essential in providing a client-focused service. These interviews can be unstructured and/or semistructured but generally take the form of a conversation, where questions are asked and information is provided without adhering to a predetermined format. This two-way communication is commonly guided by broad goals or, at most, a set of prompts that direct therapists through a range of topics. However, to explore issues further, therapists often develop additional questions in response to the client's comments or responses. This style of questioning is used at the start of the visit to explore clients' priorities and aspirations and then throughout the visit as they move through the home and demonstrate performance in specific areas to gather further insights into clients' concerns and experiences.

Although individual therapists are likely to have their own personal style of communication, a range of strategies can be used to increase the effectiveness of informal interviews. At the outset, it is essential to create a safe and accepting interpersonal climate for the interview. Finding a quiet, comfortable place in the house where the client and therapist can sit close to each other (3- to 4-ft apart and at right angles) is an important first step. It is equally important, however, that the therapist allows the initial conversation to flow freely while both parties are settling into the interview and becoming comfortable with each other. It can be valuable to let the client raise the topic of conversation, because the therapist can learn more about the client and what he or she feels is important. This also provides the therapist with an opportunity to demonstrate genuine interest in the client's concerns and value his or her perspective.

Once the interview climate has been established, the therapist uses a range of questioning techniques, such as open and closed questions and probing, to encourage discussion and to explore occupational performance issues in greater depth. Regardless of the quality of the interview questions, therapists need to constantly monitor the effectiveness of each interview and the quality of the information acquired. Informal interviews are difficult to conduct without a lot of experience; however, they are likely to be most effective when the interviewer:

+ Is knowledgeable about the content of the interview
+ Structures a purposeful and well-rounded interview
+ Is open and responsive to topics introduced by the interviewee
+ Uses clear communication that can be understood by everyone involved in the interview
+ Employs a gentle approach that allows the interviewees sufficient time to consider their responses and reply

+ Is empathetic and listens attentively to what is being said, how it is said, and what is not said

+ Has sensitive responses to the interviewees' expressed opinions and concerns

+ Is able to take positive control of the direction of the interview or steer the interview, based on agreed goals for the interaction

+ Is able to critique or challenge what is said if inconsistencies occur or issues require closer examination

+ Remembers what has been said previously and relates back to information obtained at different parts of the interview

+ Clarifies information gained and explores the client's perceptions of events without imposing meaning or overinterpreting information (Kvale, 1996)

Informal interviews allow clients to provide therapists with a wealth of information at their own pace; however, this information can be easily overlooked or lost if it is not adequately managed or recorded. However, when utilized effectively, these types of interviews enable therapists to explore, probe, and analyze the nature of difficulties clients are experiencing. It takes time and experience to learn to use informal interviewing well because it can be difficult to obtain the right information and integrate the information provided, especially when clients are eager to talk about a broad range of topics. Equally, it can take a great deal of skill to coax reserved clients to disclose personal information, which is often required in home modification practice. Experienced therapists who have developed an internalized framework and procedure for interviewing are comfortably placed to use informal interviewing well. However, without a systematic approach and regular review, informal interviewing can result in some issues being explored haphazardly or being neglected altogether.

Informal interviewing generally allows therapists to learn a great deal about clients' particular concerns and requirements and the impact of occupational performance difficulties. Although this information is invaluable in shaping decision making and negotiations with clients, it is often not recorded formally. This lack of documentation results in "underground practice" (Mattingly & Fleming, 1994; Pierre, 2001), where discrepancies occur between what therapists do and what they record. Consequently, the complexity of issues considered when making home modification decisions is often not acknowledged and documented by therapists or recognized

within services. Even if this qualitative information was effectively recorded, it is not in a form that readily allows the outcomes of home modification interventions to be measured. With the growing focus on evidence-based practice, therapists need to ensure that the client's perspective, which occupational therapy claims to be vital, is recorded. It is crucial that this perspective is not lost in the search for standardized evaluation tools in determining the nature and extent of need and quantifying the effectiveness of interventions.

Structured Interviews and Checklists

Many occupational therapy services develop structured forms and checklists that are targeted at identifying occupational performance issues in the home for a particular client group. In clinical practice, these are frequently used to screen for the presence/absence of occupational performance issues and to establish the extent and urgency of the concerns. These forms provide therapists with a structure for collecting demographic information, health and/or disability history, roles and routines, and self-reported ability and support required to undertake personal and instrumental activities of daily living (ADLs). In organizations that offer home modification services, information is also gathered on the age, materials, structure, design, layout and features of the house, and the surrounding environment. A number of environmental checklists can assist therapists to identify environmental features that are potential hazards or barriers to people with specific impairments or health conditions. These tools are a useful guide for therapists who are new to the service or area of practice because they help them collect all information relevant to the particular service. With the many distractions that can occur in a home environment, these tools can ensure that therapists address everything on the form during the interview or environmental inspection. The structure of these tools ensures some consistency in the information gathered and makes it easier when clients are transferred to other therapists within the service or revisit the service at a later date. Although these tools are not standardized and do not often provide the quantitative information required for evaluating the effectiveness of an intervention, they do provide information on the preintervention situation. When clients or other staff view the information collected using these tools, the domain of concern of occupational therapy becomes immediately apparent.

Although structured forms and checklists are useful, they do have a number of limitations. It has been said that "what occupational therapists do looks simple, what they know is quite complex" (Mattingly & Fleming, 1994, p. 24). The use of set forms to ensure consistent information gathering often oversimplifies what occupational therapists really do. Two-dimensional information about the person, activity performance, or the environment belies the complexity of the person-environment-occupation transaction. Often, these forms and checklists do not reflect the breadth and depth of information that therapists gain when interviewing clients, which misrepresents the nature of information therapists operate from. Second, once a form has been developed, it is often assumed that anyone could collect the information, which leads to services sometimes questioning why other staff could not be trained to do a home assessment. Third, in the interest of comprehensiveness, these forms frequently require therapists to collect additional nonspecified information to address the specific concerns of the client at the time of the interview. This may result in an unnecessary invasion of the person's privacy, especially when information about irrelevant medical conditions is collected or spaces in the house are inspected unnecessarily. Finally, these tools are often not reviewed regularly enough in light of new evidence, theoretical knowledge, or changes in service practice, which results in traditional practices often persisting well beyond their use-by date.

Skilled Observations and Occupational Analysis

Observing clients in their homes, where they perform their usual daily activities, provides a wealth of valuable information more comprehensive and detailed than can be gained from interviewing alone. During the course of the home visit, occupational therapists observe clients as they move and perform various activities around the home (e.g., answering the door, moving through the home, completing transfers, and making refreshments). These general observations, often automatic to experienced therapists, provide a basis for discussing the impact of the health condition or impairment on life within the home. However, therapists also ask clients to perform specific occupations, in particular, those identified as problematic, during the initial interview. By skillfully observing occupational performance, therapists can observe behavior in its natural environment and identify factors that are either contributing to or interfering with performance (Dunn, 2000).

Occupational therapists have specialized knowledge and skills that allow them to analyze and evaluate occupational performance (Dunn, 2000), and they use different theoretical lenses to understand occupational performance and factors that contribute to performance difficulties (Crepeau, Schell, Gillen, & Scaffa, 2014). For example, when using an ecological model such as person-environment-occupation or person-environment-occupation-performance, therapists focus on analyzing the fit between the person, the occupation, and the environment. Occupational therapists also use their skills in occupational and activity analysis to identify the important elements of various occupations in the home and where and how breakdowns in performance occur.

Occupational Analysis

Occupational analysis is core to occupational therapy practice. It allows therapists to analyze occupations of value and concern to clients in the actual context in which they are performed and to gain an understanding of their possible meaning, component tasks, specific performance requirements, and potential facilitators and barriers to performance (Crepeau et al., 2014). This qualitative information allows therapists to identify the particular aspects of the task that result in difficulties or compromise. Using whole-body reasoning, therapists then examine aspects of the individual's performance, occupational, and/or environmental demands that are impinging on successful completion. This type of analysis acknowledges the unique meaning and purpose of the activity for the individual and recognizes the distinctive way tasks are performed, depending on the purpose of the task, the experience and preferences of the person, and the demands and structure of the occupation and environment.

Activity analysis, on the other hand, analyzes activities in a more abstract sense so as to assist therapists in anticipating potential difficulties in performance (Crepeau et al., 2014). When undertaking an activity analysis, therapists tend to identify common components of the task and capacities and environmental elements required for successful completion. This alerts therapists to the specific aspects of the task where breakdowns in performance are likely and helps them to understand possible contributions to difficulties and errors. For example, a simple activity such as going to the toilet incorporates a number of tasks, and there can be a breakdown at any stage of this activity if there is a poor person-environment-occupation fit. Table 6-1 details the procedural component tasks of going to the toilet.

Task breakdown can occur if the person has specific impairments that make it difficult to anticipate

Table 6-1. Activity Analysis of Going to the Toilet

Register need to go to the toilet
Locate and find way to toilet
Open the door
Enter the room
Turn on the light
Close the door
Travel, turn, and position at front of pedestal
Undress
Sit down onto toilet
Reach for toilet paper/release sheet
Transfer weight for wiping
Attend to personal hygiene
Move from sitting to standing
Don and adjust clothing
Turn and flush toilet
Clean toilet bowl
Open door
Negotiate doorway
Find way to sink to wash hands
Turn on faucets
Wash hands
Dry hands
Turn lights on and off at night
Note potential for collapse or assistance need

a toileting need, mobilize to the toilet, locate the toilet, see various fixtures and fittings, and use the toilet. In addition, there may be aspects of the environment that make it difficult for the person to carry out the activity (e.g., too great a distance, convoluted or obstructed path of travel, unfamiliar toileting environment, high positioning of door handles and locks, unfamiliar or inaccessible positioning of light fittings, low toilet pan, inoperable flush button, hard-to-reach or difficult-to-tear toilet paper, or lack of space between the entry door and toilet bowl). Therapists commonly observe people performing various aspects of activities and analyze performance difficulties as they occur. This is not a formalized process but rather one where each therapist uses an individual approach to analyzing tasks and interpreting problems.

Some standardized tools, such as the Performance Assessment of Self-Care Skills (PASS; Rogers & Holm, 1994; Rogers, Holm, & Chisholm, 2016) and Comprehensive Assessment and Solution Process for Aging Residents (CASPAR; Sanford, Pynoos, Tejral, & Browne, 2002), provide a framework for analyzing and evaluating various household activities. These tools present essential task elements and a structure for examining and recording difficulties experienced and assistance required for successful completion. Although this type of analysis provides a foundation for identifying potential performance breakdowns and contributing factors, these and other activity analysis frameworks tend to focus on the physical and immediately observable aspects of activities. Less attention is paid to the sensory, cognitive, and emotional demands of activities: preparing for, initiating, and terminating activities and the routines and habits required when undertaking daily tasks in the home. There needs to be further evaluation to determine when, where, and how people undertake tasks, their experience of the performance, and the specific qualities of performance that are important to them.

Therapists generally use a combination of activity and occupational analysis when observing occupational performance in the home (Crepeau et al., 2014). Using a blended approach to analysis allows therapists to understand the particular importance and issues for specific clients, as well as the factors contributing to performance difficulties and how these can be addressed (Crepeau et al., 2014). Because skilled observation is generally undertaken qualitatively, it can be difficult to measure changes in performance objectively. The nature and quality of analysis are also dependent on the therapist's clinical experience. Furthermore, it is important to be aware that an individual's performance is likely to vary throughout the day as his or her capacities and environmental conditions change, and therapists need to account for this variability when evaluating an individual's performance in various household activities.

Rogers and Holm (2009) have identified a number of parameters that therapists examine when analyzing occupational performance: value, independence, adequacy, and safety.

Value

Value is the importance or significance of the occupation to the individual. When resources are limited, people generally establish priorities and reserve their energies for highly valued occupations (Rogers & Holm, 2009). The relative value of tasks is often addressed in the interview or other assessment processes and assists in identifying client goals and priorities. However, the therapist may review and revise these priorities in collaboration with the client if further performance concerns become evident while activities are being performed.

Independence

Independence generally refers to a person's ability to complete activities without assistance. A person's level of dependence is measured in terms of the type of assistance he or she requires to complete an activity. Assistance is commonly assessed as progressing from low levels of support, in the form of using assistive devices and the need for supervision or task setup, to high levels of support, such as another person providing verbal or physical prompting or physical assistance. People's confidence in their ability to perform activities in the home is another facet of independence (Rogers & Holm, 2009). If they believe they cannot perform a task, it is likely that their performance will be compromised. Though independence is the primary goal of many services and therapists, it may not be important to the client. Some people with a disability prefer to receive assistance with routine daily living tasks to allow time and energy for activities they prefer, such as working or spending quality time with loved ones (Baum, Bass, & Christiansen, 2005). Sacrificing independence in one activity can result in more autonomy in overall lifestyle and a greater quality of life.

Adequacy

Adequacy refers to the efficiency and acceptability of the process and outcome of the activity (Rogers & Holm, 2009). Efficiency refers to minimizing the amount of effort required to achieve a given outcome. Rogers and Holm (2009) evaluate efficiency by examining the degree of difficulty, pain, fatigue, and dyspnea exhibited or experienced during the task as well as the amount of time taken. Acceptability of the outcome is evaluated in terms of social standards, personal satisfaction, and presence of aberrant behaviors (Rogers & Holm, 2009).

The ease and comfort with which an individual undertakes activities are important considerations when analyzing occupational performance because they affect his or her personal experience of daily life within the home, which can subsequently influence overall quality of life. Therapists generally gather information about the experience of the performance from clients, informally asking whether they experience any difficulty, pain, fatigue, and dyspnea during performance. Therapists can also obtain information on the level of difficulty or discomfort experienced by using standardized tools such as the following:

+ The Usability Rating Scale (Pitrella & Kappler, 1988; Steinfeld & Danford, 1997): A 7-point bipolar measure of difficulty ranging from -3 (very difficult) to +3 (very easy), with 0 providing a neutral point at the center of the scale

+ The Brief Pain Inventory (Cleeland & Ryan, 1994): A measure of the intensity and interference of pain

+ The Faces Pain Scale/The Faces Pain Scale—Revised (Bieri, Reeve, Champion, Addicoat, & Ziegler, 1990; Hicks, von Baeyer, Spafford, Van Korlaar, & Goodenough, 2001): A picture scale of pain intensity

Alternatively, therapists can use customized scales in the form of Likert scales and semantic differentials or picture scales. Although customized scales might not be standardized, they provide therapists with a mechanism for identifying and discussing clients' experiences of performance and perceptions of difficulty or discomfort.

A typical 5-level Likert scale is set out as follows: How difficult is your current showering routine?

1. Very difficult

2. Difficult

3. Neither easy nor difficult

4. Easy

5. Very easy

Semantic differential scales usually feature descriptive adjectives with opposite meanings at either end of a scale. For example:

No pain |___|____|____|___| Worst pain imaginable

No difficulty |___|____|____|___| Severe difficulty

Therapists also monitor clients for clinical signs of exertion (e.g., increased effort, pallor, sweating, or labored breathing). Tools such as wearable devices and monitors can also be useful in gauging increased effort. The duration of activities can be measured using a stopwatch; however, the ideal time required for various household tasks is yet to be calculated and is likely to vary from one person to another (Rogers & Holm, 2009). It is likely that clients and their significant others will report whether the time taken for the activity is acceptable or manageable.

The acceptability of the outcome is determined by establishing the person's level of satisfaction with the end product and comparing the result with social expectations (Rogers & Holm, 2009). Overall satisfaction can be evaluated using qualitative comments, customized scales, or a standardized measure such as the Canadian Occupational Performance Measure (COPM; Law et al., 1998, 2014), or the In-Home Occupational Performance Evaluation (I-HOPE; Stark, Somerville, & Morris, 2010), which measure the client's perception of performance and satisfaction with performance. It is difficult to clearly define socially acceptable performance. Therapists generally rely on the client's level of satisfaction but would be concerned when outcomes vary significantly from social standards and place an individual at risk of social alienation from his or her family, friends, and peer group. The therapist would then discuss with the person his or her perception of performance to confirm whether the outcome required improvement. Therapists also use skilled observation to note behaviors that interfere with the process or outcome and vary greatly from the way tasks are typically performed, such as confusion in the order of the procedure, repetitive checking, inappropriate use of fixtures and fittings, and impulsive or disruptive behavior. These are then discussed with the client and significant others.

Safety

In home modification practice, therapists are routinely required to assess the safety of individuals in their homes. Safety is defined as the level of risk that individuals are exposed to when they are performing specific tasks and is a product of the interaction between the capacity of the individual at any given moment, the nature of the task he or she is performing, and the challenges presented by the environment (Rogers & Holm, 2009). Although safety is a complex parameter to measure and control for, it is also critical to the success of the home modification process. If it is not addressed adequately, there could be potentially catastrophic consequences for the client.

A risk management framework is a useful structure for evaluating and managing risks in the home in a logical and systematic manner. Risk management involves developing processes, structures, and a culture to manage adverse events and optimize opportunities for safety (Standards Association of Australia, 2009). It is a recognized process within a range of settings and is used by a variety of organizations. Risk management is a consultative process that involves all stakeholders and, in particular, the person exposed to the risk. This ensures that all views are considered in identifying and evaluating risk and that everyone involved has ownership of the measure to be undertaken to manage the risk. Risk management in the home is likely to include consultation with the client and, in many cases, to extend to the people he or she lives with, family, health providers, personal assistance providers, and advocates.

When undertaking a risk management process, it is important to define the context and determine the purpose of the risk management activity. The context refers to the internal and external environment and, in home modification practice, involves understanding the goals and priorities of clients, their capacities, their social resources, and the physical environments in which they live. The purpose of the risk management activity in this setting is to minimize risk of injury and maximize opportunities for meaningful activity in the home—two purposes that sometimes conflict. Negotiations may need to be undertaken to achieve a balanced plan that meets the needs and wants of the client. For example, a client may wish to soak in a bath regularly to relieve joint pain but may be exposed to a number of risks getting in and out of the bath. The occupational therapist or the organization for which he or she works might also be concerned about their duty of care and potential litigation in relation to the recommendations made. This may lead to risk minimization at the expense of the client's quality of life. Therapists can use a systematic and inclusive approach to risk management to meet their duty of care while still allowing clients to take responsibility for the levels of risk they wish to include in their daily lives. This process involves identifying, analyzing, evaluating, managing, monitoring, and reviewing risks.

Identifying Risks

Identifying risks involves establishing which events are likely to have adverse or uncertain outcomes. When identifying risk in the home environment, it is necessary to observe the person performing the relevant tasks in his or her home. Self-report is not an adequate method of determining risk because people might not always be aware of potential risks in their home. Neither is a simple audit of the physical environment sufficient because, although an audit might identify hazards (i.e., events or situations that are the source of danger with the potential to cause harm or injury) it does not determine the degree of risk involved with the hazard. Risk is the likelihood of harm resulting from exposure to a hazard. Simply auditing the physical environment for hazards does not take into account the likelihood of exposure to the hazard and the capacities, vulnerabilities, and experience of the person and how these interact with the environment.

Analyzing Risks

Once the potential hazards have been identified, it is necessary to develop an understanding of the level of risk. Analyzing each risk involves all of the stakeholders making a judgment about the likelihood of an adverse event occurring and the consequences of such an event. When determining the level of risk, the therapist, client, and other relevant stakeholders need to consider the following:

+ Frequency: How often the person is exposed to the hazard

+ Probability: The probability of an adverse event occurring

+ Consequences: The likely consequences of an adverse event
+ History: Previous experience of an adverse event (Pybus, 1996)

In a home evaluation, a qualitative analysis of risk is undertaken in consultation with the client and other household members. For example, if we were to analyze the risk of falling or tripping on the front stairs, the client and the therapist would need to determine how often the stairs are used, the chances of the person tripping or falling, the consequences of an incident, and whether an incident has occurred in the past and how often. Levels of risk vary from one situation to another. For example, the risk would be low where a fit and agile older person lived in a dwelling in good repair, rarely used the front stairs, and had no history of tripping on the stairs. In another situation, where an older person with osteoporosis lived in a house in poor repair, used the stairs frequently, and had tripped on the stairs previously, the risk would be high. Even if this person used the stairs only intermittently (e.g., to collect the mail) the potential consequences of a fall would warrant management of the risk. The process of identifying and discussing the frequency of exposure, probability of an event, likely consequences, and history of incidents provides a useful structure for therapists to discuss their concerns and understand the client's perception of the risk. By affording clients an opportunity to discuss the frequency of exposure and history of adverse events, therapists can gain a deeper understanding of the potential risk.

Evaluating Risks

Once a judgment has been made about the level of each identified risk, it is then possible to decide which risks need to be addressed and their order of priority. In home modifications, the decisions will need to take into account the level of risk, the personal priorities of the client, the role of the organization providing the service, and the resources available for managing the risk.

Managing Risks

In selecting the most appropriate risk management option, therapists generate a range of options and collaborate with clients and other stakeholders to agree on the most effective and acceptable solutions. Several risk management strategies are employed:

+ Avoiding the risk: In the home, one option for managing a risk is to avoid that area of the home or the activity completely. For example, a person might choose to use another entry to the house exclusively and avoid the flight of stairs in need of repair.

+ Reducing the likelihood of the risk: Possibly the most common is to reduce the likelihood of an accident by providing modifications, assistive equipment, alternative ways of performing tasks, or any combination of these strategies. However, an additional evaluation will then be required to ensure that additional or different risks are not being introduced.

+ Changing the consequences: Changing the consequences to reduce the extent of injury is another approach. For example, the person might take medication, wear protective equipment to reduce the risk of fracture, or wear a personal alarm to call for help.

+ Sharing the risk: The risk could be shared, for example, by getting someone else to collect the mail or enlisting some help in using the stairs.

+ Retaining the risk: This is a valid choice where the activity is highly valued by the individual and other risk management strategies are neither feasible nor acceptable to the client. For example, people may choose to continue to use the stairs to collect mail, regardless of falls risks, because they have done so all their lives and would not entertain having someone else do it for them (Standards Association of Australia, 2009).

Therapists, and the organizations they work for, might be averse to this last option because of concerns about meeting their duty of care and possible litigation. However, imposing unacceptable risk-management strategies on the client is counterproductive because they are likely to cause distress and/or not be used. In these situations, it is imperative that the therapist works with the client to ensure he or she fully understands the probability of an event occurring and the consequences involved. It is also important that the client is fully informed on how to manage the risk and knows where to seek further assistance if required.

Monitoring and Reviewing Risks

It is essential that therapists maintain an ongoing review of risk management strategies to ensure that the management plan is sustainable and remains effective. Factors that affect the probability and consequences of an outcome will inevitably change over time and affect the suitability of a strategy. Therefore, it is important to follow up once a management strategy has been put in place and then again at regular intervals to ensure it continues to manage the risk. Alternatively, clients should be encouraged to contact the service should they feel that the probability or consequences of a risk have changed. Outcome measures can be used to monitor and review the effectiveness of risk management strategies. For further information on risk management in home modification practice, please refer to Chapter 5.

Skilled observation allows therapists to analyze the person-environment-occupation fit and to identify where and how breakdowns are occurring, which then provides the foundation for developing successful interventions. This form of evaluation requires highly developed skills in observation, occupational analysis, and risk management and is often difficult for students and inexperienced therapists to use effectively. Because of the complexity of the information gathered and the qualitative nature of it, it is difficult to assess the quality of evaluations undertaken by various therapists and quantify the effectiveness of interventions. Once again, without clear documentation of the evaluation undertaken, the profession is not able to articulate its unique approach and contribution to service delivery.

Standardized Assessment

The Nature of Standardized Assessment

Standardized assessments, whether qualitative or quantitative in nature, are developed and tested to ensure that the information collected is comprehensive, trustworthy or valid, and consistent or reliable. *Trustworthiness* is a term used to refer to ensuring the credibility and quality of qualitative data. For quantitative measures, validity ensures that the tool measures what it is intended to and that there is agreement about what it is measuring; reliability ensures that the measures are consistent (Magasi, Gohil, Burghart, & Wallisch, 2017). Standardized assessments ensure effective, systematic, and consistent information gathering (Law & Baum, 2005). They provide therapists with a mechanism for appraising or calculating the magnitude, quantity, or quality of a particular characteristic or attribute (Law & Baum, 2017). These tools provide a uniform procedure for administering the assessment by specifying the conditions, tools, instructions, and questions. Some standardized assessments are norm referenced, whereas others are criterion referenced (Dunn, 2017). Norm-referenced tools compare individual test scores with those of a comparison sample or an ideal (Dunn, 2017). These tools are useful for diagnosis or screening because they assist the therapist in determining the extent of impairment or difficulty and whether performance warrants further investigation. Criterion-referenced assessments are especially useful for occupational therapists because they measure performance against an identified standard rather than an "ideal" (Dunn, 2017). These

tools can be used to identify and specify the goals and needs of individuals and allow therapists to evaluate the effectiveness of an intervention. When using standardized tools, it is imperative that therapists understand the focus and purpose of the tool and select "the most appropriate measure with the best psychometric properties" (Cooper, Letts, Rigby, Stewart, & Strong, 2005, p. 316). In home modification practice, assessment tools need to be sensitive to changes in occupational performance and ensure that the environment is adequately acknowledged.

Traditional Assessment Tools

The use of standardized assessments can result in therapists measuring "variables that can be measured rather than what should be measured" (Corcoran, 2005, p. 65). Traditionally, occupational therapists have used a range of standardized tools to assess clients' functional capacities, independence in ADLs, or accessibility or safety of the environment (Table 6-2). Assessing the functional capacities of an individual, such as motor (sensorimotor), process or cognitive, communication, and interaction or social capacities in a standardized environment assists therapists in anticipating performance issues or understanding aspects of the person that are likely to constrain occupational performance. Establishing the person's level of dependence in a range of ADLs also alerts the therapist to potential occupational performance concerns in the home environment. Therapists can develop an awareness of challenges to occupational performance in the home by using standardized tools to identify barriers and hazards in the home environment. Table 6-2 provides an overview of a range of standardized assessments available to therapists.

Historically, the person, occupation, and environment have been viewed as discrete elements that could be assessed independently (Cooper et al., 2005). However, the interdependent relationship between these elements is increasingly being acknowledged. Occupational performance is considered to be the result of all three elements working together and affecting each other. These traditional assessments tell us little about the person-environment-occupation transaction in the home and how this affects occupational performance, something that is considered critical in assessing occupational performance in this natural environment (Law & Baum, 2005). They often have a specific purpose and focus, which make it difficult to address the unique needs of individual clients, the person's occupational experience and interests, the specific demands of the activity, the fit between the person and the environment, or the capacity of the environment to support specific occupations (Law & Baum, 2005).

Table 6-2. Standardized Measures of Functional Capacity, Independence, Occupational Performance, and the Environment

FUNCTIONAL CAPACITIES	REFERENCE
Audition Screening Tool	Popelka, G. R. (1997). *High and low pitch sounds: A screening tool.* Unpublished manuscript.
Caregiver Strain Index	Robinson, B. C. (1983). Validation of a caregiver strain index. *Journal of Gerontology, 38*(3), 344-348.
Modified Caregiver Strain Index	Thorton, M., Travis, S.S. (2003). Analysis of the reliability of the Modified Caregiver Strain Index. *The Journal of Gerontology, Series B, Psychological Sciences and Social Sciences, 58*(2), S129.
Functional Reach Test	Duncan, P. W., Weiner, D. K., Chandler, J., & Studenski, S. (1990). Functional reach: A new clinical measure of balance. *Journal of Gerontology: Medical Sciences, 45*(6), M192-M195.
Geriatric Depression Scale	Yesavage, J. A., Brink, T. L., Rose, T. L., Lum, O., Adey, M., Leirer V.O. (1983). Development and validation of a geriatric depression screening scale: A preliminary report. *Journal of Psychiatric Research, 17*(1), 37-49.
Geriatric Depression Scale: Short Form	Sheikh, J. I, & Yesavage, J.A. (1986). Geriatric Depression Scale (GDS). Recent evidence and development of a shorter version. In T.L. Brink (Ed.). *Clinical gerontology: A guide to assessment and intervention* (pp., 165-173). New York: The Haworth Press, Inc.
Lighthouse Near Acuity Card	Ferris, F. L., Kassoff, A., Bresnick, G. H., & Bailey, I. (1982). New visual acuity charts for clinical research. *American Journal of Ophthalmology, 94,* 91-96.
Lighthouse International Functional Vision Screening Questionnaire	Horowitz, A., Teresi, J., & Cassels, L. A. (1991). Development of a vision screening questionnaire for older people. *Journal of Gerontological Social Work, 17*(3/4), 37-56.
	Lighthouse International, 111 East 59th Street, New York, NY, 10022. Tel: (212) 821-9525, Fax: (212) 821-9706
Mini-Mental State Examination	Folstein, M. F., Folstein, S. E., & McHugh, P. R. (1975). "Mini-Mental State": A practical method for grading cognitive state if patients for the clinician. *Journal of Psychiatric Research, 12,* 189-198.
Montreal Cognitive Assessment www.mocatest.org	Nasreddine, Z. S., Phillips, N. A., Bédirian, V., Charbonneau, S., Whitehead, V., Collin, I., . . . Chertkow, H. (2005). The Montreal Cognitive Assessment, MoCA: A brief screening tool for mild cognitive impairment. *Journal of the American Geriatrics Society, 53*(4), 695-699.
Patient Health Questionnaire—9	Kroenke, K., Spitzer, R. L., & Williams, J. B. W. (2001). The PhQ-9: Validity of a brief depression severity measure. *Journal of General Internal Medicine, 16*(9), 606-613.
Short Blessed Test	Katzman, R., Brown, T., Fuld, P., Peck, A., Schechter, R., & Schimmell, H. (1983). Validation of a short orientation-memory-concentration test of cognitive impairment. *American Journal of Psychiatry, 140*(5), 734-739.
Timed Up-and-Go Test	Podsiadlo, D., & Richardson, S. (1991). The timed "up-and-go": A test of basic mobility for frail elderly persons. *Journal of the American Geriatrics Society, 39,* 142-148.
Zarit Burden Interview	Zarit, S. H., Reever, K. E., & Bach-Peterson, J. (1980). Relatives of the impaired elderly, correlates of feeling of burden. *Gerontologist, 20*(6), 649-655.
Zarit Burden Interview—Revised	Zarit, S. H., Orr, N. K., & Zarit, J. M. (1985). *The hidden victims of Alzheimer's disease: Families under stress.* New York: New York University Press.

(continued)

Table 6-2. Standardized Measures of Functional Capacity, Independence, Occupational Performance, and the Environment (continued)

LEVEL OF INDEPENDENCE	REFERENCE
ADL Staircase	Sonn, U., & Hulter-Åsberg, K., (1991). Assessment of activities of daily living in the elderly. *Scandinavian Journal of Rehabilitation Medicine, 23*, 193-202.
ADL Staircase—Revised	Iwarsson, S., & Isacsson, Å., (1997). On scaling methodology and environmental influences in disability assessments: The cumulative structure of personal and instrumental ADL among older adults in a Swedish rural district. *Canadian Journal of Occupational Therapy, 64*, 240-251.
Modified Barthel Index	Shah, S., Vanclay, F., & Cooper, B. (1989). Improving the sensitivity of the Barthel Index for stroke rehabilitation. *Journal of Clinical Epidemiology, 42*, 703-709.
Functional Independence Measure (FIM)	Uniform Data System for Medical Rehabilitation. (2009). *The FIM system clinical guide—Version 5.2.* Buffalo, NY: UDSMR, State University of New York at Buffalo.
Katz Index of Activities of Daily Living	Katz, S., Ford, A. B., Moskowitz, R. W., Jackson, B. A., & Jaffe, M. W. (1963). Studies of illness in the aged: The index of ADL: A standardized measure of biological and psychosocial function. *Journal of the American Medical Association, 185*(12), 914-919.
Functional Independence Measure for Children (WeeFIM)	Msall, M. E., DiGaudio, K., Rogers, B. T., LaForest, S., Catanzaro, N. L., Campbell, J., . . . Duffy, L. C. (1994). The Functional Independence Measure for Children (WeeFIM): Conceptual basis and pilot use in children with developmental disabilities. *Clinical Pediatrics, 33*(7), 421-430.
OCCUPATIONAL PERFORMANCE	REFERENCE
COPM	Law, M., Baptiste, S., Carswell, A., McColl, M., Polatajko, H., & Pollock, N. (2014). *Canadian occupational performance measure* (5th ed.). Ottawa, ON: CAOT Publications ACE.
Occupational Circumstances Assessment—Interview and Rating Scale	Forsyth, K., Deshpande, S., Kielhofner, G., Henriksson, C., Haglund, L., Olson, L., . . . Kulkarni, S. (2005). *The Occupational Circumstances Assessment Interview and Rating Scale (OCAIRS)—Version 4.0.* Chicago, IL: Model of Human Occupation Clearing House, University of Illinois at Chicago.
Occupational Performance History Interview II (OPHI II)	Kielhofner, G., Mallinson, T., Crawford, D., Nowak, M., Rigby, M., Henry, A., & Walens, D. (2004). *The Occupational Performance History Interview-II—Version 2.1.* Chicago, IL: Model of Human Occupation Clearinghouse, University of Illinois at Chicago.
Occupational Self-Assessment (OSA)	Baron, K., Kielhofner, G., Ienger, A., Goldhammer, V., & Wolenski, J. (2006). *Occupational Self-Assessment—Version 2.2.* Chicago, IL: Model of Human Occupation Clearinghouse, University of Illinois at Chicago.
QUALITY OF PERFORMANCE	REFERENCE
Assessment of Motor and Process Skills (AMPS)	Fisher, A. G., & Jones, K. B. (2011). *Assessment of Motor and Process Skills: Development, standardization, and administration manual* (7th ed. Rev.). Fort Collins, CO: Three Star Press.
Client-Clinician Assessment Protocol (C-CAP)	Lilja, M. (2002). *Riktlinjer för användning av Client-Clinician Assessment Protocol (C-CAP). [Guidelines for Using the Client-Clinician Assessment Protocol (C-CAP)].* Stockholm, Sweden: Karolinska Institutet.
PASS Clinic and PASS Home	Rogers, J. C., Holm, M. B., & Chisholm, D. (2016). *The Performance Assessment of Self-Care Skills (PASS)—Version 4.1.* Pittsburgh, PA: University of Pittsburgh.

(continued)

Table 6-2. Standardized Measures of Functional Capacity, Independence, Occupational Performance, and the Environment (continued)

ACCESSIBILITY, USABILITY, AND SAFETY OF THE ENVIRONMENT	REFERENCE
CASPAR	Sanford, J. A., Pynoos, J., Tejral, A., & Browne, A. (2002). Development of a comprehensive assessment for delivery of home modifications. *Physical & Occupational Therapy in Geriatrics, 20*(2), 43-55.
Dimensions of Home Measure (DOHM)	Aplin, T., Chien, C. W., & Gustafsson, L. (2016). Initial validation of the dimensions of home measure. *Australian Occupational Therapy Journal, 63*(1), 47-56.
Home and Community Environment	Kaysor, J., Jette, A., & Haley, S. (2005). Development of the Home and Community Environment (HACE) instrument. *Journal of Rehabilitation Medicine, 37*(1), 37-44.
Home Environmental Assessment Protocol	Gitlin, L. N., Schinfeld, S., Winter, L., Corcoran, M., Boyce, A., & Hauck, W. (2002). Evaluating home environments of persons with dementia: inter-rater reliability and validity of the home environmental assessment protocol (HEAP). *Disability and Rehabilitation, 24*(1), 59-71.
Home Occupational Environment Assessment	Baum, C. M., & Edwards, D. F. (1998). *Guide for the Home Occupational-Environmental Assessment.* St. Louis, MO: Washington University Program of Occupational Therapy.
Home Falls and Accidents Screening Tool	Mackenzie, L., Byles, J., & Higginbotham, N. (2000). Designing the Home Falls and Accidents Screening Tool (HOME FAST): Selecting the items. *British Journal of Occupational Therapy, 63*(6), 260-269.
Housing Enabler (HE)	Iwarsson, S., & Slaug, B. (2001). *The Housing Enabler: An instrument for assessing and analyzing accessibility problems in housing.* Navlinge och Staffanstorp, Sweden: Veten & Stapen HB & Slaug Data Management.
I-HOPE	Stark, S. L., Somerville, E. K., & Morris, J. C. (2010). In-Home Occupational Performance Evaluation (I-HOPE). *American Journal of Occupational Therapy, 64*(4), 580-589.
Safety Assessment of Function and the Environment for Rehabilitation	Oliver, R., Blathwayt, J., Brackley, C., & Tamaki, T. (1993). Development of the Safety Assessment of Function and the Environment for Rehabilitation (SAFER) tool. *Canadian Journal of Occupational Therapy, 60*(2), 78-82.
Safety Assessment of Function and the Environment for Rehabilitation—Health Outcome Measurement and Evaluation	Chiu, T., Oliver, R., Ascott, P., Choo, L., Davis, T., Gaya, A., . . . Letts, L. (2006). *Safety assessment of function and the environment for rehabilitation: Health outcome measurement and evaluation (SAFER-HOME) version 3 manual.* Toronto, ON: COTA Health.
Usability in My Home	Fänge, A., & Iwarsson, S. (1999). Physical housing environment: Development of a self-assessment instrument. *Canadian Journal of Occupational Therapy, 66*, 250-260. Fänge, A. (2002). *Usability in My Home manual.* Lund, Sweden: Lund University, Division of Occupational Therapy.
Westmead Home Safety Assessment	Clemson, L. (1997). *Home fall hazards. A guide to identifying fall hazards in the homes of elderly people and an accompaniment to the assessment tool the Westmead Home Safety Assessment.* Victoria, Australia: Co-ordinates Publications.

Measures of Occupational Performance

There are few standardized assessment tools that quickly and accurately assess many of the parameters of interest for occupational therapists and their clients (Corcoran, 2005), in particular, occupational performance and the person-environment-occupation transaction. When measuring occupational performance, occupational therapists need to capture both the subjective experience and the objective performance (McColl & Pollock, 2017). They require tools that allow them to understand the specific needs of the individual and assist them to explain behavior. A number of structured and semistructured interview schedules have been developed that guide therapists to systematically examine the individual's experience of occupation (e.g., the COPM [Law et al., 1998, 2014], OSA [Baron, Kielhofner, Ienger, Goldhammer, & Wolenski, 2002, 2006], and the OPHI-II [Kielhofner et al., 1998, 2004]). Whereas the OPHI-II and the OSA both examine the impact of the environment on occupational performance, the COPM focuses primarily on defining occupational performance issues and relies on the client and therapist exploring the impact of the environment on performance through informal discussion and observation. A detailed description and review of these tools is available in McColl and Pollock (2017). These standardized tools allow therapists to develop an understanding of clients' past and present experiences and perceptions of their occupational performance and assist in the development of occupation-focused goals (Fasoli, 2008). The client-centered nature of these tools engages the client in identifying occupational performance issues, thus increasing his or her involvement in the evaluation process and the therapist's understanding from the client's perspective. These tools also allow individualized intervention plans to be developed and the impact of these to be evaluated.

Occupational therapists frequently use standardized assessments to assess occupational performance in relation to personal and instrumental ADLs and community participation. Assessments of ADLs usually focus on determining the level of independence across a range of tasks for the purposes of screening or measuring outcomes (e.g., the Modified Barthel Index [Shah, Vanclay, & Cooper, 1989], FIM [Uniform Data System for Medical Rehabilitation (UDSMR), 1997, 2009], WeeFIM [Msall et al., 1994], Katz Index of Activities of Daily Living [Katz, Ford, Moskowitz, Jackson, & Jaffe, 1963], ADL Staircase [Sonn & Hulter-Åsberg, 1991], and the ADL Staircase—Revised [Iwarsson & Isacsson, 1997]). Generally, these global measures of independence do not provide information on the quality of performance or problematic aspects of the tasks (Gitlin, 2005). Though they may be useful as screening tools, they are not designed to analyze or diagnose occupational performance issues or evaluate home modification outcomes.

Recently, a number of performance-based assessments have been designed to assist therapists to objectively analyze the quality of performance and identify barriers to valued occupations. A detailed description of assessments of personal and instrumental ADLs and community participation is available in Law et al. (2017). Some of these tools rely on self or proxy report. However, tools that use performance observation are of particular interest to home modification therapists because they allow them to evaluate the quality of occupational performance in daily activities and the factors that contribute to this. Tools of particular interest are the AMPS (Fisher, 1995; Fisher & Jones, 2011a, 2011b) and PASS (Chisholm, Toto, Raina, Holm, & Rogers, 2014; Rogers & Holm, 1994). Therapists using these tools can select tasks relevant to the client in his or her own environment and diagnose the precise moment and nature of performance breakdown. They examine the quality of performance rather than focusing solely on the outcome of performance. The AMPS is used by therapists who undergo extensive training to examine an individual's ability to perform specific motor and process skills within meaningful personal and instrumental ADLs selected from a bank of more than 120 standardized ADL tasks (Fisher & Griswold, 2014). This tool allows therapists to diagnose specific performance difficulties that clients experience when undertaking activities but does not measure the impact of the environment or environmental interventions on performance.

The PASS is one of the few tools that examines safety and adequacy of performance in addition to level of independence on a 4-point scale (Gitlin, 2005). The PASS is available in a clinic and home version, and both include 26 core tasks related to functional mobility (5), personal self-care (3), instrumental ADLs with cognitive emphasis (14), and instrumental ADLs with physical emphasis (4) (Furphy, & Stav, 2014; Holms, & Rogers, 2017). Each task is criterion referenced, detailing the subtasks required for successful completion (Figure 6-1). Therapists can select specific tasks depending on the client's priorities or lifestyle or use the task development template to develop a new task. The tool allows therapists to identify the precise point of task breakdown and to provide verbal support, nondirective or directive verbal support, gestures, task and environmental modification, demonstration, physical guidance, physical support, or total assistance to support task completion.

Task # H3: FM: Toilet Mobility and Management

HOME CONDITIONS: Bathroom area and
1. Toilet, "as is"
2. Elastic-waist shorts (extra-large size) available if needed
3. Client positioned facing the toilet

HOME INSTRUCTIONS:

"Now let's go into the bathroom to assess morning care activities." [Wait for Client to locate bathroom]

[As Client enters the bathroom] "For this task you do not need to remove your clothing, however, if you do not wish to lower your pants/slacks here is a pair of shorts you can put over your pants/slacks before you begin. Do you know what you are to do?" [Wait for response]

"First I'd like you to show me how you manage clothing as you prepare to sit down on the toilet." [Wait for response]

"Now show me how you sit down on the toilet and how you reach for and gather toilet paper. Put the toilet paper into the toilet as you normally would. Do you know what you are to do?" [Wait for response]

"Now show me how you get up from the toilet and pull up your clothing." [Wait for response]

SCORE	INDEPENDENCE	SAFETY	ADEQUACY	
			PROCESS	QUALITY
3	No assists given for task initiation, continuation, or completion	Safe practices were observed	Subtasks performed with precision & economy of effort & action	Optimal (performance matches the quality standards listed in each subtask)
2	No Level 7-9 assists given, but occasional Level 1-6 assists given	Minor risks were evident but no assistance provided	Subtasks generally performed w/ precision & economy of effort & action; occasional lack of efficiency, redundant or extraneous action; no missing steps	Acceptable (Performance, for the most part, matches or nearly matches the quality standards listed in each subtask)
1	No Level 9 assists given; or occasional Level 7 or 8 assists given; or continuous Level 1-6 assists given	Risks to safety were observed and assistance given to prevent potential harm	Subtasks generally performed w/ lack of precision and/or economy of effort & action; consistent extraneous or redundant actions; steps may be missing	Marginal (Performance, for the most part, does not match the quality standards listed in each subtask)
0	Level 9 assists given; or continuous Level 7 or 8 assists given; or unable to initiate, continue, or complete subtask or task	Risks to safety of such severity were observed that task was stopped or taken over by assessor to prevent harm	Subtasks are consistently performed w/ lack of precision and/or economy of effort & action so that task progress is unattainable	Unacceptable (Performance does not match the quality standards listed in each subtask, perhaps with few exceptions)

Task # H3: FM: Toilet Mobility and Management		INDEPENDENCE DATA											SAFETY DATA	ADEQUACY DATA		SUMMARY SCORES
Assistive Technology Devices (ATDs) used during task: 1. 2. 3. Total # of ATDs used:____	No Assistance	Verbal Supportive (Encouragement)	Verbal Non-Directive	Verbal Directive	Gestures	Task or Environment Rearrangement	Demonstration	Physical Guidance	Physical Support	Total Assist	INDEPENDENCE subtask scores	Unsafe Observations	PROCESS: Imprecision, lack of economy, missing steps	QUALITY: Standards not met / improvement needed		
Assist level →	0	1	2	3	4	5	6	7	8	9						
Subtasks	Subtask Criteria															
1	Locates bathroom efficiently (goes directly to bathroom)															
2	Turns to position self in front of toilet & maintains balance (does not grab sink for support; does not grab towel rack for support)															
3	Manages clothing sufficiently (so it does not get soiled), and maintains balance appropriately (does not lose balance/fall forward/drop to toilet seat)															
4	Lowers self onto toilet in a controlled manner (does not "plop" down; buttocks are centered on & touching seat)															
5	Reaches for & gathers (grasps and folds) toilet paper, & maintains balance (does not fall forward or sideways)															
6	Places toilet paper into toilet & maintains balance (does not fall forward or sideways)															
7	Raises self from toilet in a controlled manner (does not "rock" to gain momentum; no loss of balance) & achieves & maintains standing balance (does not sway or "catch" self on sink or other object)															
8	Manages clothing sufficiently (fits as it should at waist), and maintains balance appropriately (does not lose balance/fall forward/drop to toilet seat)															

Summary Scores: INDEPENDENCE MEAN SCORE ↑, SAFETY SCORE ↑, ADEQUACY SCORE ↑

Figure 6-1. Extract from PASS—functional mobility: toilet transfers. (Reprinted with permission from J. C. Rogers and M. B. Holm, University of Pittsburgh, Pittsburgh, PA.)

The C-CAP (Lilja, 2002; Petersson, Fisher, Hemmingsson, & Lilja, 2007) uses both self-report and observation to evaluate an individual's performance in terms of independence, difficulty, and safety of activities, including mobility (14) and personal (10) and instrumental (12) ADLs (Thomas Jefferson University, n.d.). It has four parts: Part I provides questions to build rapport and explore routines and support systems. Part II is a client self-report of perceived ability to perform daily life tasks and records assistive devices currently in use (see extract in Figure 6-2). Part III examines the client's readiness to change, and Part IV consists of occupational therapist observations and rating of the client's ability to perform daily life tasks (Petersson et al., 2007). The tool provides therapists with a structure for exploring the client's current experience, perceptions of performance, and readiness to change and setting goals for home modification interventions.

Environmental Assessments

With the growing recognition of the role of the environment in disablement, a number of assessments have been developed to examine the environment in relation to the person and his or her ability to operate effectively in that environment. For a comprehensive review of quality environmental measures, refer to Cooper et al. (2005). Cooper et al. note it is difficult for any one tool to assess this multifaceted and complex entity comprehensively. Consequently, it is important to be clear about the purpose and focus of the tools available and what each can contribute to an understanding of the impact of the environment on occupational performance. There are tools designed specifically to analyze the home environment: the HE (Iwarsson & Slaug, 2010), *Maintaining Seniors' Independence: A Guide to Home Adaptations* (Canada Mortgage and Housing Corporation [CMHC], 2012), the CASPAR (Sanford et al., 2002), the I-HOPE (Stark et al., 2010), and the DOHM (Aplin et al., 2013).

The HE is based on the Enabler developed by Steinfeld in the 1980s (Fänge, Risser, & Iwarsson, 2007) and is particularly useful for examining the congruence between the person's functional capacities and his or her physical environment. There is a particular focus on assessing the accessibility of the home environment for people with a range of functional and mobility impairments, such as difficulty interpreting information, severe loss of sight, complete loss of sight, severe loss of hearing, prevalence of poor balance, incoordination, limitations of stamina, difficulty in moving head, difficulty in reaching with arms, difficulty in handling and fingering, loss of upper extremity skills, difficulty bending or kneeling, reliance on walking aids, reliance on wheelchair, and extremes of size and weight (Figure 6-3). This tool (demonstration version available at www.enabler.nu) allows therapists to identify potential accessibility barriers in the home, which can then be examined further through additional performance testing (Cooper et al., 2005).

The HE is administered in three steps:

1. Using a combination of interview and observation, the functional limitations (13 items) and dependence in mobility (2 items) are identified.

2. The physical barriers in the home and immediate outdoor environment (188 items) are noted.

3. The accessibility score is calculated using a complex matrix and specialized software to examine the profile of functional limitations and mobility dependence against the accessibility barriers in the environment, where a predefined severity score has been provided for each barrier. The severity of accessibility barrier is rated 1 through 4, with higher points awarded to items that are likely to present more severe problems to people with that limitation (Figure 6-4). The final score indicates the magnitude of accessibility problems in the environment. Scores higher than zero indicated the presence of accessibility problems (Iwarsson & Slaug, 2010).

Currently, this tool is used to evaluate the suitability of accommodation for people with a range of functional and mobility impairments to assist in municipal planning (Fänge et al., 2007) and in research to identify the number and magnitude of accessibility problems in housing for older people and its relationship to healthy aging outcomes (Fänge & Iwarsson, 2005; Iwarsson, 2005; Iwarsson, Horstmann, & Slaug, 2007). Although the accessibility measures in this tool are based on the Scandinavian accessibility standards, this tool directs therapists to environmental features that are potential accessibility barriers to people with a range of mobility and functional impairments.

Maintaining Seniors' Independence: A Guide to Home Adaptations (CMHC, 2012) was designed for occupational therapists to identify:

+ Self-care and household activities that people have difficulty completing independently

+ Obstacles in the home that can impede activities from being undertaken

+ Home improvements and minor adaptations that are inexpensive and easy to complete

PART II: SELF-REPORT

Client Perceived Level of Functioning- For each task ask client:
1. *"How difficult is it for you to perform the activity?"*
2. *"How important is it to you to learn <u>new strategies</u> to (bathe) to make this easier for you?"*

1. FUNCTIONAL MOBILITY

ASK: *How difficult is it for you to:*			**ASK:** *"How important is it for you to learn a way to make this easier for you?"*	
TASK	**Difficulty** 1=no diff., 2=a little diff., 3=mod. diff., 4=a lot of diff., 5=unable to do	**Do You:** 1 = Use a device 2 = Use personal assistance 3 = Use both a device and personal assistance 4= NO DEVICE/NO ASSISTANCE N/A=not applicable	**Important to Learn New Strategies** 1=not at all, 2=a little, 3=moderate, 4=very much	**OT Comments**
Walk indoors/getting around the house				
Walk a block				
Maintaining balance while showering				
Stoop, crouch or kneel to retrieve item				
Bending over from standing position to pick up clothing off of floor				
Reaching for items above shoulder level				
Climb 1 flight of stairs				
Move in and out of a chair				
Move in and out of a bed				
Move in and out of bath/shower				
Get on and off of toilet				

Figure 6-2. Extract from the C-CAP (Gitlin et al., 2006; Lilja, 2002; Petersson, Fisher, Hemmingsson, & Lilja, 2007). (Reprinted with permission from Laura Gitlin.)

FUNCTIONAL LIMITATIONS AND DEPENDENCE ON MOBILITY DEVICES

Yes No

□	□	A.	Difficulty interpreting information
□	□	B1.	Visual impairment
□	□	B2.	Blindness
□	□	C.	Loss of hearing
□	□	D.	Poor balance
□	□	E.	Incoordination
□	□	F.	Limitations of stamina
□	□	G.	Difficulty in moving head
□	□	H.	Reduced upper extremity function
□	□	I.	Reduced fine motor skill
□	□	J.	Loss of upper extremity function
□	□	K.	Reduced spine and/or lower extremity function

                                                        A B C*
□ □ L. Dependence on walking aid(s)   □ □ □
□ □ M. Dependence on wheelchair   □ □ □

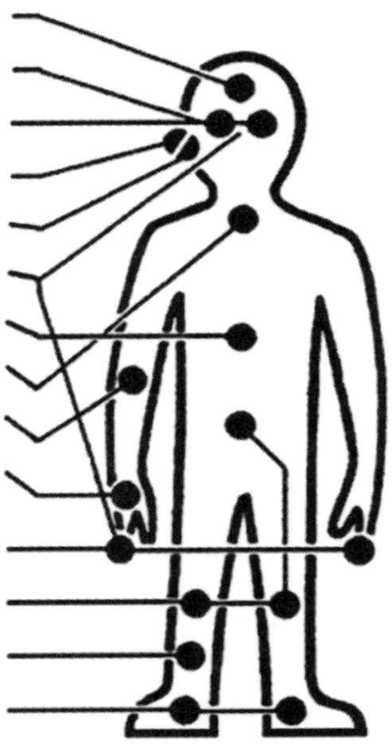

*Section in the environmental component: A. Exterior surroundings. B. Entrance. C. Indoor environment

Figure 6-3. HE—functional limitations form. (Reprinted with permission from Iwarsson, S., & Slaug, B. [2010]. *The Housing Enabler: A method for rating/screening and analysing accessibility problems in housing* [2nd ed.]. Lund and Staffanstorp, Sweden: Veten & Skapen HB and Slaug Enabling Development.)

Personal component / functional profile	Yes / No / Bygg ikapp, page ref.	A	B1	B2	C	D	E	F	G	H	I	J	K	L	M	RATING
A. Exterior surroundings																
General **A1.** Paths narrower than 1.5 m. *A width of 1.0 m is acceptable provided there are 1.5 m turning zones at least every 10 m.*	p. 304					3	3							3	3	□ Yes □ No □ Not rated
A2. Irregular/uneven surface. (irregular surfacing, joins, sloping sections cracks, holes; 5 mm or more).	p. 305		2	3		1	1		3				1	3	3	□ Yes □ No □ Not rated
A3. Unstable surface (loose gravel, sand, clay, etc). *Mark if it causes difficulties e.g. when using a wheelchair or rollator.*			2	3		3	3	2					1	3	4	□ Yes □ No □ Not rated

Figure 6-4. HE—environmental assessment form. (Reprinted with permission from Iwarsson, S., & Slaug, B. [2010]. *The Housing Enabler: A method for rating/screening and analysing accessibility problems in housing* [2nd ed.]. Lund and Staffanstorp, Sweden: Veten & Skapen HB and Slaug Enabling Development.)

BATHING AND PERSONAL HYGIENE

Do you perform the following activities alone and without difficulty:

16. Turn faucets "on"/"off"?

☐ No ☐ Yes ☐ N.A.

Functional Limitations	Home Check-List	Recommendations	
	Check:	**Housing**	**Other**
☐ Poor grip/dexterity	■ Access to wash-basin, faucets	☐ Lever type faucet handles	
☐ Limited range (upper limbs)	■ Type of faucets	☐ Single action faucets	
☐ Muscle weakness		☐ Technical aids: — extended faucet handle — "faucet turner"	
☐ Wheelchair dependent		☐ Clear space underneath sink/insulate plumbing	
		☐ Move faucets to side or closer to front	

Comments: _____

17. Regulate the water temperature?

☐ No ☐ Yes ☐ N.A.

Functional Limitations	Home Check-List	Recommendations	
	Check:	**Housing**	**Other**
☐ Poor grip/dexterity	■ Hot water temperature	☐ Set hot water temperature to 46°C	
☐ Poor coordination (upper limbs)	■ Hot/cold water control or adjustment	☐ Single action faucet	
☐ Sensory loss		☐ Extended faucet handle	

Comments: _____

Figure 6-5. Extract from *Maintaining Seniors' Independence: A Guide to Home Adaptations*. (Reprinted with permission from Canada Mortgage and Housing Corporation. [2012]. *Maintaining seniors' independence: A guide to home adaptations*. Ottawa, ON: Author.)

The guide uses semistructured interview and observations of the client undertaking various activities within the home and can take 1 to 2 hours. It includes 73 items grouped under topics such as general accessibility; getting up, dressing, and tidying the bedroom; bathing and personal hygiene at the basin; taking a shower; taking a bath; using the toilet; preparing meals; doing the laundry; cleaning the house; using the telephone; enjoying leisure/doing business; and taking medication. Figure 6-5 shows an extract of items from bathing and personal hygiene at the basin.

The assessment tool is aimed at working with older people who are experiencing changes in their physical autonomy (i.e., the ability to independently undertake the various ADLs due to motor, organic,

sensory, or speech difficulties). It has not been designed to meet the particular needs of persons with mental or major psychological deficiencies (confusion, perceptual problems). The tool is mostly intended for people living in apartments and single-family homes. The suggested minor adaptations require the clinical judgment of an occupational therapist to determine suitability and tailoring to the specific requirements of the individual, and more elaborate adaptations require engagement with consultants in architectural design and residential construction (CMHC, 2012).

The CASPAR (Sanford et al., 2002) is a client-directed assessment that enables an older adult, family, or nonspecialist therapist to identify problems in undertaking tasks in the home. This tool examines

3.4 Using the Bathroom				
Tasks	**Problem**	**Help**	**Device**	**Comments**
Toileting				
Getting close enough to any toilet.	☐	☐		
Getting on/off any toilet.	☐	☐		
Reaching the toilet paper at any toilet.	☐	☐		
Flushing any toilet.	☐	☐		
Other (specify):	☐	☐		
	☐	☐		
	☐	☐		
Bathing/Showering				
Getting close enough to any bathtub/shower.	☐	☐		
Getting in/out of any bathtub/shower.	☐	☐		
Lowering down to/rising up from the bottom of any bathtub.	☐	☐		
Standing while showering in any shower.	☐	☐		
Reaching the faucet and turning the water on/off in any bathtub/shower.	☐ ☐	☐ ☐		
Reaching the water, soap, shampoo, etc. in any bathtub/shower.	☐	☐		
Other (specify):	☐	☐		
	☐	☐		

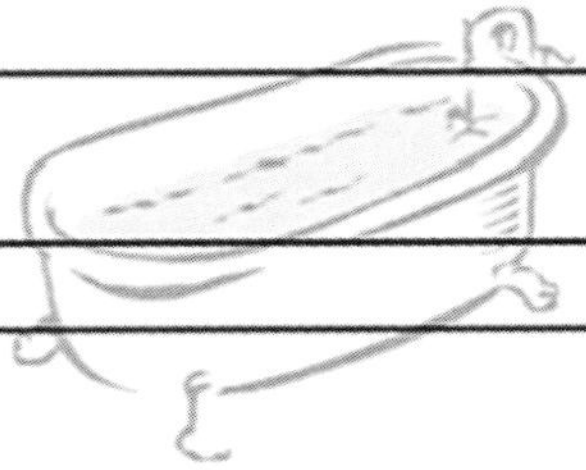

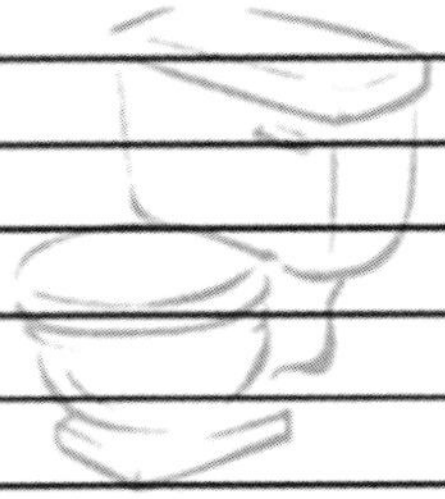

Figure 6-6. Example of CASPAR item. (Reprinted with permission from Extended Home Living Services, Wheeling, IL.)

the person's interaction with the specific elements in the built environment when accessing the house; mobilizing throughout the house; managing controls such as lighting and temperature controls; getting in and out of bed; and undertaking daily living tasks such as toileting, bathing, grooming, cooking, and washing. Figure 6-6 provides an extract from the CASPAR, which examines the use of the bathroom.

The CASPAR allows therapists to record instances where the client experiences a problem with specific task elements, receives help, or uses a device for assistance. This tool provides a useful structure for documenting problems and prioritizing person-environment issues but does not allow therapists to document or record changes in the quality of performance. It does, however, provide detailed diagrams to guide therapists in measuring specific aspects of the built environment related to common problems and modifications.

The I-HOPE is a performance-based measure that focuses on home-based activities that are essential for aging in place (Stark et al., 2010). It was developed in response to the author's identification that there was an absence of assessments that reviewed function in relation to the environment. To address this, this measure was designed to examine the fit between the person and environment in the home, encouraging the identification and review of the effects of "person-environment misfits" (Stark et al., 2010). While acknowledging the influence of the environment on performance, this measure also considers the client's perspective on and satisfaction with their performance in their activity participation and enables the observation of changes in the person-environment fit before and after home modification.

This measure enables a trained therapist to establish current activity patterns, ascertain activities that are difficult but important to the person, and identify environmental barriers that affect specific

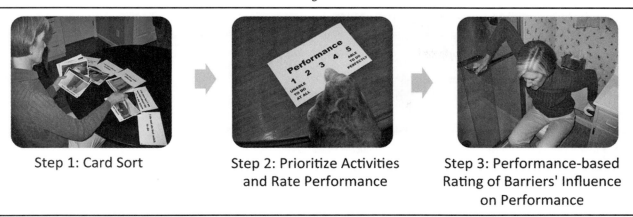

Step 1: Card Sort → Step 2: Prioritize Activities and Rate Performance → Step 3: Performance-based Rating of Barriers' Influence on Performance

Figure 6-7. The I-HOPE process.

activities. It achieves this by using a three-step process, including (Figure 6-7):

1. An activity card sort in which 44 activities are sorted into five categories: (1) I do not do/do not want to do; (2) I do now with no problem; (3) I do now with difficulty; (4) I do not do but wish to do; and (5) I am worried about doing in the future

2. Client ranking of problematic activities to measure subjective performance and associated satisfaction with performance on a 5-point scale

3. Therapist observation of client performing activities in the relevant environmental context to enable identification of environmental barriers. Therapists then rate the impact of the barriers on performance on a 6-point scale, with 0 = independent with or without a device, 1 = standby assistance/independent with difficulty/unsafe, 2 = minimal assistance, 3 = moderate assistance, 4 = maximum assistance, and 5 = no activity.

From the completion of this assessment process, four subscales are derived, including an activity participation score, client's rating of performance score, client's satisfaction with performance score, and severity of environmental barriers score (Stark et al., 2010).

The I-HOPE demonstrates sound psychometric properties and enables therapists to reliably determine a client's participation in daily activities, ability to perform activities, satisfaction with their performance, and the influence of environmental barriers on activity performance (Stark et al., 2010). This tool was designed for older adults (60 years and older) and may not be generalizable because the designated activities may not be applicable to other populations. Furthermore, it is limited to evaluating clients in their current environment, as the client must be present at the time of assessment. Despite this, the I-HOPE appears to be clinically useful and encourages the follow-up and review of outcomes postmodification as it has the potential for measuring change in performance, satisfaction, and environmental barrier scores between preintervention and postintervention.

As home modification practice becomes more person-centered, occupational therapists want to understand the dimensions of home that influence decision making and ensure that modifications are not negatively affecting the experience of home. The DOHM, based on a literature review and an extensive qualitative study (Aplin, de Jonge, & Gustafsson, 2013, 2015), was developed to examine the six dimensions of home that are important considerations in the home modification process and that can be affected by changes to the home environment. The DOHM is a self-report tool that consists of 36 items (Table 6-3) measuring various dimensions of home: personal (11 items), social (4 items), occupational (5 items), temporal (3 items), physical (12 items), and societal (a single item measuring clients' comfort with the cost of the modifications; Aplin, Chien, & Gustafsson, 2016). Each statement is related to aspects of each dimension (see Table 6-3) and is rated on a progressive 5-point Likert scale, with response descriptors being 1 = strongly disagree, 2 = disagree, 3 = unsure, 4 = agree, and 5 = strongly agree (Aplin et al., 2016).

Although still early in its development, the DOHM has established content validity following a review by six expert occupational therapists and academics, who rated the tool as being comprehensive in its overall measurement of the dimensions of home with inter-rater agreement of 0.83 (Aplin et al., 2013). The unidimensionality of the DOHM's subscales has been

Table 6-3. Dimensions of Home Measure (DOHM) Items

PERSONAL DIMENSION: PRIVACY, SAFETY, AND FREEDOM

- I have the privacy I want from others in my home.
- I have enough privacy from neighbors and other people in the street.
- I feel safe living in this home.
- I feel safe while moving around and doing activities in and around my home.
- I feel independent that I am able to do the things I want to myself.
- My home allows me to get out as much as I want.
- I can be myself at home.

PERSONAL DIMENSION: IDENTITY AND CONNECTEDNESS

- I am happy with the appearance of my home.
- My home reflects who I am.
- I feel connected to my home.
- My home contains special memories for me.

SOCIAL DIMENSION: FAMILY AND FRIENDS

- I can easily have friends and family visit if I want.
- I have good relationships with those I live with or who visit often.
- The modifications will/do suit others who use my home.
- It is easy for me to do activities with my friends and family at my home.

OCCUPATIONAL DIMENSION: HOME AS A PLACE OF ACTIVITIES

- My home is easy to clean.
- I can easily move around in my home.
- I can easily do the activities I need to in my home (e.g., shower, toilet).
- I can easily do the activities I enjoy at home (e.g., leisure activities).
- It is easy for my carers to help me with the activities for which I need help.

TEMPORAL DIMENSION: HOME NOW AND IN THE FUTURE

- I am happy with my daily/weekly routine at home.
- I know where everything is and how it works in my home.
- With how things are at the moment, I am well set up for the future in my home.

PHYSICAL DIMENSION: STRUCTURE, SERVICES, AND FACILITIES

- The wiring in my home is in a good condition.
- The ventilation in my home is in good working order.
- The plumbing in my home is in good working order (e.g., drainage in the bathroom).
- I am happy with the layout of my home.
- My home has no structural problems.
- The materials and finishes in my home are in good condition (e.g., the flooring, taps, sink, and tiles).

PHYSICAL DIMENSION: AMBIENCE AND SPACE

- I enjoy the ambience of my home (e.g., a view, breeze, or sunshine).
- I can easily keep warm/cool enough in my home.
- I have enough space in my home for my needs.
- I have enough storage space in my home.
- I have good light in my home.
- When coming and going from my home, I am protected from the weather.

SOCIETAL DIMENSION: COST

- I am comfortable with the cost of the modifications (e.g., initial installation costs, maintenance).

supported by Rasch-based principal component analysis and item-fit analysis. Hierarchical results of item difficulties, however, revealed that more items would be needed to capture the full range of a participant's experiences of home (Aplin et al., 2016).

Selecting and Evaluating Standardized Assessment Tools

When choosing an assessment tool, it is critical to understand the purpose and focus of the tool and to ensure that these align with the intended application (Cooper et al., 2005). Unfortunately, there are few tools that address the issues of concern of occupational therapists and their clients and assess them in the way they need to be assessed. Once a suitable standardized tool has been identified, therapists investigate the psychometric properties of the tool to ensure that it has adequate validity, reliability, sensitivity for its purpose and clinical utility for use in home modification practice. Using valid and reliable measures allows therapists to determine the extent of the problem and evaluate the effectiveness of interventions in addressing them. Standardized evaluation tools ensure consistency and assist those therapists with limited experience to identify and address issues thoroughly and systematically. However, standardized tools may have limited flexibility when used to address clients' specific concerns; the complex interaction between the person, environment, and occupations; and the unique situations encountered in home environments. It is often challenging to use standardized tools effectively in the home because time is often limited, and it is difficult to follow instructions rigidly in an unfamiliar and unstructured environment (Gitlin, 2005). Some tools require specialist training and have specific setup requirements. Many standardized measures are not sensitive to the changes that can result from interventions, such as decrease in time taken and making the client feel safer, and can penalize the use of standard interventions, such as the use of an assistive device. These limit their usefulness in evaluating outcomes. For example, the FIM (UDSMR, 1997, 2009) is considered a gold standard in terms of its psychometric properties. While it may be a useful tool for screening level of independence, it does not provide therapists with useful information about the adequacy and safety of performance or the person-environment-occupation transaction, and it is not responsive to changes resulting from typical occupational therapy interventions, such as assistive devices (Johansson, Lilja, Petersson, & Borell, 2007). Regardless of its psychometric properties, the FIM is useful only in specific circumstances (e.g., screening and measuring the outcomes of remediation interventions) and is potentially detrimental in demonstrating the efficacy of adaptive interventions. When standardized tools are not available or not appropriate, therapists should use qualitative evaluation strategies, such as interviews and skilled observations that are trustworthy and consistent (Law & Baum, 2005) and ensure that information gathered using these invaluable strategies is adequately documented.

CONCLUSION

Evaluation serves a number of purposes. Primarily, therapists use evaluation to identify and examine misfits between the person, occupations, and environment. However, it is also valuable in screening referrals to identify people with potential occupational performance issues and to measure the magnitude of change in occupational performance resulting from home modification interventions. Professional reasoning is used throughout the evaluation process. Drawing on relevant practice frameworks and existing bodies of knowledge, therapists seek and interpret cues and generate and test hypotheses about the person's occupational performance difficulties and contributing factors. They use narrative reasoning to understand and describe each client's unique experience of his or her situation and to work with him or her to create an impelling future. Pragmatic reasoning assists therapists to work sensibly and effectively within their personal resources, as well as the resources available in the practice context, and ethical reasoning requires therapists to reflect on their personal and professional values when dealing with the many competing forces that affect thinking and decision making. Finally, interactive reasoning supports the development of a strong therapeutic relationship between the therapist and the client, enabling a collaborative alliance between the two parties that enhances the potential for success of therapeutic interventions.

Therapists use a range of evaluation strategies to gather information about the client, his or her occupational performance, and his or her home. Informal interviewing is used to develop two-way communication between the therapist and the client, allowing therapists to build collaborative partnerships; earn clients' trust and confidence; gather information; hear stories; and understand clients' experiences, concerns, goals, and aspirations. Structured interviews provide therapists with a framework for collecting demographic information, medical history, and self-reported ability to undertake ADLs, as well as information on the age, design, and features of the house. Dedicated checklists prompt therapists to identify potential hazards or barriers for older people and people with specific impairments, health conditions, or disabilities.

Skilled observation allows therapists to observe occupational performance in the client's natural environment and identify factors that are contributing to, or interfering with, performance. General observations provide a basis for discussing the impact of aging and/or their health condition, impairment, or disability on life within the home, and analysis of specific occupations (in particular, those identified as problematic during the initial interview) allows therapists to examine the value, independence, adequacy, and safety of performance. A growing number of standardized assessments are available to therapists to ensure that the information collected is comprehensive, trustworthy or valid, and consistent or reliable. Using valid and reliable measures allows therapists to determine the extent of the problem and evaluate the effectiveness of interventions in addressing the identified problem or concern.

REFERENCES

American Occupational Therapy Association. (2014). Occupational therapy practice framework: Domain and process (3rd ed.). *American Journal of Occupational Therapy, 68*(Suppl. 1), S1-S48.

American Occupational Therapy Association. (2015). Occupational therapy code of ethics. *American Journal of Occupational Therapy, 69*(Suppl. 3), S1-S8.

Aplin, T., Chien, C.-W., & Gustafsson, L. (2016). Initial validation of the dimensions of home measure. *Australian Occupational Therapy Journal, 63*(1), 47-56.

Aplin, T., de Jonge, D., & Gustafsson, L. (2013). Understanding the dimensions of home that impact on home modification decision making. *Australian Occupational Therapy Journal, 60*(2), 101-109.

Aplin, T., de Jonge, D., & Gustafsson, L. (2015). Understanding home modifications impact on clients and their family's experience of home: A qualitative study. *Australian Occupational Therapy Journal, 62*(2), 123-131.

Baron, K., Kielhofner, G., Ienger, A., Goldhammer, V., & Wolenski, J. (2002). *Occupational Self-Assessment—Version 2.1*. Chicago, IL: Model of Human Occupation Clearinghouse, University of Illinois at Chicago.

Baron, K., Kielhofner, G., Ienger, A., Goldhammer, V., & Wolenski, J. (2006). *Occupational Self-Assessment—Version 2.2*. Chicago, IL: Model of Human Occupation Clearinghouse, University of Illinois at Chicago.

Baum, C. M., Bass J. H., & Christiansen, C. H. (2005). Person-environment-occupational-performance: A model for planning interventions for individuals and organizations. In C. H. Christiansen, C. M. Baum, & J. H. Bass (Eds.), *Occupational therapy: Performance, participation and well-being* (3rd ed., pp. 373-392). Thorofare, NJ: SLACK Incorporated.

Bieri, D., Reeve, R. A., Champion, G. D., Addicoat, L., & Ziegler, J. B. (1990). The Faces Pain Scale for the self-assessment of the severity of pain experienced by children: Development, initial validation, and preliminary investigation for ratio scale properties. *Pain, 41*, 139-150.

Bonsaksen, T., Vøllestad, K., & Taylor, R. R. (2013). The Intentional Relationship Model—Use of the therapeutic relationship in occupational therapy practice. *Ergoterapeuten, 56*(5), 26-31.

Canada Mortgage and Housing Corporation. (2012). *Maintaining seniors' independence: A guide to home adaptations*. Ottawa, ON: Author. Retrieved from https://www.cmhc-schl.gc.ca/odpub/pdf/61042.pdf?fr=1499654340236

Chapparo, C., & Ranka, J. (2000). Clinical reasoning in occupational therapy. In J. Higgs & M. Jones (Eds.), *Clinical reasoning in the health professions* (pp. 128-137). Oxford, UK: Butterworth-Heinemann.

Chisholm, D., Toto, P., Raina, K., Holm, M., & Rogers, J. (2014). Evaluating capacity to live independently and safely in the community: Performance Assessment of Self-care Skills. *British Journal of Occupational Therapy, 77*(2), 59-63.

Cleeland, C. S., & Ryan, K. M. (1994). Pain assessment: Global use of the Brief Pain Inventory. *Annuals of the Academy of Medicine Singapore, 23*(2), 129-138.

Cohn, E. S., Schell, B. A., & Neistadt, M. E. (2003). Introduction to evaluation and interviewing. In E. B. Crepeau, E. S. Cohn, & B. A. Boyt Schell (Eds.), *Willard & Spackman's occupational therapy* (10th ed., pp. 279-285). Philadelphia, PA: Lippincott, Williams & Wilkins.

Cole, M. B., & McLean, V. (2003). Therapeutic relationships redefined. *Occupational Therapy in Mental Health, 19*(2), 33-56.

Cooper, B., Letts, L., Rigby, P., Stewart, D., & Strong, S. (2005). Measuring environmental factors. In M. Law, C. Baum, & W. Dunn (Eds.), *Measuring occupational performance: Supporting best practice in occupational therapy* (2nd ed., pp. 315-344). Thorofare, NJ: SLACK Incorporated.

Corcoran, M. (2005). Using qualitative measurement methods to understand occupational performance. In M. Law, C. Baum, & W. Dunn (Eds.), *Measuring occupational performance: Supporting best practice in occupational therapy* (2nd ed., pp. 65-80). Thorofare, NJ: SLACK Incorporated.

Crepeau, E. B. (1991). Achieving intersubjective understanding: Examples from an occupational therapy treatment session. *American Journal of Occupational Therapy, 45*(11), 1016-1024.

Crepeau, E. B., Schell, B. A. B., Gillen, G., & Scaffa, M. E. (2014). Analyzing occupations and activity. In B. A. B. Schell, G. Gillen, M. E. Scaffa, & E. S. Cohn (Eds.), *Willard & Spackman's occupational therapy* (12th ed., pp. 234-248). Philadelphia, PA: Wolters Kluwer/Lippincott Williams & Wilkins.

Doherty, R. F. (2009). Ethical decision making in occupational therapy practice. In E. B. Crepeau, E. S. Cohn, & B. A. Boyt Schell (Eds.), *Willard & Spackman's occupational therapy* (11th ed., pp. 274-285). Philadelphia, PA: Wolters Kluwer/Lippincott Williams & Wilkins.

Dunn, W. (2000). Best practice occupational therapy assessment. In W. Dunn (Ed.), *Best practice occupational therapy: In community services with children and families* (pp. 79-108). Thorofare, NJ: SLACK Incorporated.

Dunn, W. (2017). Measurement concepts and practices. In M. Law, C. Baum, & W. Dunn (Eds.), *Measuring occupational performance: Supporting best practice in occupational therapy* (3rd ed., pp. 38-49). Thorofare, NJ: SLACK Incorporated.

Fänge, A., & Iwarsson, S. (2005). Changes in ADL dependence and aspects of usability following housing adaptation: A longitudinal perspective. *American Journal of Occupational Therapy, 59*, 296-304.

Fänge, A., Risser, R., & Iwarsson, S. (2007). Challenges in implementation of research methodology in community-based occupational therapy: The Housing Enabler example. *Scandinavian Journal of Occupational Therapy, 14*, 54-62.

Fasoli, S. E. (2008). Assessing roles and competence. In M. V. Radomski & C. A. Trombly Latham (Eds.), *Occupational therapy for physical dysfunction* (6th ed., pp. 65-90). Philadelphia, PA: Wolters Kluwer/Lippincott, Williams & Wilkins.

Fisher, A. (1995). *Assessment of motor and process skills*. Fort Collins, CO: Three Star Press.

Fisher, A. G., & Griswold, L. A. (2014). Performance skills: Implementing performance analyses to evaluate quality of occupational performance. In B. A. B. Schell, G. Gillen, M. E. Scaffa, & E. S. Cohn (Eds.), *Willard & Spackman's occupational therapy* (12th ed., pp. 249-264). Philadelphia, PA: Wolters Kluwer/Lippincott Williams & Wilkins.

Fisher, A. G., & Jones, K. B. (2011a). *Assessment of Motor and Process Skills: Development, standardization, and administration manual* (7th ed. Rev.). Fort Collins, CO: Three Star Press.

Fisher, A. G., & Jones, K. B. (2011b). *Assessment of Motor and Process Skills: User manual* (7th ed. Rev.). Fort Collins, CO: Three Star Press.

Fleming, M. H. (1991). The therapists with a three track mind. *American Journal of Occupational Therapy, 45*(11), 1007-1014.

Fleming, M. H. (1994). Procedural reasoning: Addressing functional limitations. In C. Mattingly & M. H. Fleming (Eds.), *Clinical reasoning: Forms of inquiry in a therapeutic practice* (pp. 137-177). Philadelphia, PA: Davis.

Furphy, K. A., & Stav, W. B. (2014). Occupational performance assessments. In I. E. Asher (Ed.), *Asher's occupational therapy assessment tools: an annotated index* (4th ed., pp. 29-64). Bethesda, MD: American Occupational Therapy Association.

Gitlin, L. (2005). Measuring performance in instrumental activities of daily living. In M. Law, C. Baum, & W. Dunn (Eds.), *Measuring occupational performance: Supporting best practice in occupational therapy* (2nd ed., pp. 227-248). Thorofare, NJ: SLACK Incorporated.

Gitlin, L. N., Winter, L., Dennis, M. P., Corcoran, M., Schinfeld, S., & Hauck, W. W. (2006). A randomized trial of a multi-component home intervention to reduce functional difficulties in older adults. *Journal of the American Geriatrics Society, 54*(5), 809-816.

Henry, A. D., & Kramer, J. M. (2009). The interview process in occupational therapy. In E. B. Crepeau, E. S. Cohn, & B. A. Boyt Schell (Eds.), *Willard & Spackman's occupational therapy* (11th ed., pp. 342-358). Philadelphia, PA: Wolters Kluwer/Lippincott Williams & Wilkins.

Hicks, C. L., von Baeyer, C. L., Spafford, P., van Korlaar, I., & Goodenough, B. (2001). The Faces Pain Scale—Revised: Toward a common metric in pediatric pain measurement. *Pain, 93*, 173-183.

Holms, M. B., & Rogers, J. C. (2017). Measuring performance in instrumental activities of daily living. In M. Law, C. Baum, & W. Dunn (Eds.), *Measuring occupational performance: Supporting best practice in occupational therapy* (3rd ed., pp. 305-332). Thorofare, NJ: SLACK Incorporated.

Iwarsson, S. (2005). A long-term perspective on person-environment fit and ADL dependence among older Swedish adults. *Gerontologist, 45*, 327-336.

Iwarsson, S., Horstmann, V., & Slaug, B. (2007). Housing matters in very old age—Yet differently due to ADL dependence level differences. *Scandinavian Journal of Occupational Therapy, 14*, 3-15.

Iwarsson, S., & Isacsson, Å., (1997). On scaling methodology and environmental influences in disability assessments: The cumulative structure of personal and instrumental ADL among older adults in a Swedish rural district. *Canadian Journal of Occupational Therapy, 64*, 240-251.

Iwarsson, S., & Slaug, B. (2010). *The housing enabler: A method for rating/screening and analysing accessibility problems in housing* (2nd ed.). Lund and Staffanstorp, Sweden: Veten & Skapen HB and Slaug Enabling Development.

Johansson, K., Lilja, M., Petersson, I., & Borell, L. (2007). Performance of activities of daily living in a sample of applicants for home modification services. *Scandinavian Journal of Occupational Therapy, 14*(1), 44-53.

Johns, C. (2000). *Becoming a reflective practitioner*. Oxford, UK: Blackwell Science.

Katz, S., Ford, A. B., Moskowitz, R. W., Jackson, B. A., & Jaffe, M. W. (1963). Studies of illness in the aged. The index of ADL, a standardized measure of biological and psychological function. *Journal of the American Medical Association, 185*(12), 914-919.

Kielhofner, G., Mallinson, T., Crawford, D., Nowak, M., Rigby, M., Henry, A., & Walens, D. (1998). *A user's manual for the Occupational Performance History Interview—version 2.0 (OPHI-II)*. Chicago, IL: Model of Human Occupation Clearinghouse, University of Illinois at Chicago.

Kielhofner, G., Mallinson, T., Crawford, D., Nowak, M., Rigby, M., Henry, A. & Walens, D. (2004). *The Occupational Performance History Interview-II—version 2.1*. Chicago, IL: Model of Human Occupation Clearinghouse, University of Illinois at Chicago.

Kvale, S. (1996). *Interviews: An introduction to qualitative research interviewing*. Thousand Oaks, CA: SAGE Publications.

Law, M., Baptiste, S., Carswell, A., McColl, M., Polatajko, H., & Pollock, N. (1998). *Canadian Occupational Performance Measure* (3rd ed.). Toronto, ON: CAOT Publications ACE.

Law, M., Baptiste, S., Carswell, A., McColl, M., Polatajko, H., & Pollock, N. (2014). *Canadian Occupational Performance Measure* (5th ed.). Ottawa, ON: CAOT Publications ACE.

Law, M., & Baum, C. (2005). Measurement in occupational therapy. In M. Law, C. Baum, & W. Dunn (Eds.), *Measuring occupational performance: Supporting best practice in occupational therapy* (2nd ed., pp. 1-20). Thorofare, NJ: SLACK Incorporated.

Law, M. C., & Baum, C. M. (2017). Measurement in occupational therapy. In M. Law, C. Baum, & W. Dunn (Eds.), *Measuring occupational performance: Supporting best practice in occupational therapy* (3rd ed., pp. 1-16). Thorofare, NJ: SLACK Incorporated.

Law, M. C., Baum, C. M., & Dunn, W. (Eds.). (2017). *Measuring occupational performance: supporting best practice in occupational therapy* (3rd ed.). Thorofare, NJ: SLACK Incorporated.

Lilja, M. (2002). *Riktlinjer för användning av Client-Clinician Assessment Protocol (C-CAP)*. [*Guidelines for Using the Client-Clinician Assessment Protocol (C-CAP)*]. Karolinska Institutet, Stockholm.

Magasi, S., Gohil, A., Burghart, M., & Wallisch, A. (2017). Understanding measurement properties. In M. C. Law, C. M. Baum, & W. Dunn (Eds.), *Measuring occupational performance: Supporting best practice in occupational therapy* (3rd ed., pp. 29-42). Thorofare, NJ: SLACK Incorporated.

Mattingly, C., & Fleming, M. (1994). *Clinical reasoning: Forms of inquiry in a therapeutic practice*. Philadelphia, PA: Davis Company.

McColl, M. A., & Pollock, N. (2017). Measuring occupational performance using a client-centered perspective. In M. Law, C. Baum, & W. Dunn (Eds.), *Measuring occupational performance: Supporting best practice in occupational therapy* (3rd ed., pp. 83-94). Thorofare, NJ: SLACK Incorporated.

Msall, M. E., DiGaudio, K., Rogers, B. T., LaForest, S., Catanzaro, N. L., Campbell, J., . . . Duffy, L. C. (1994). The Functional Independence Measure for Children (WeeFIM): Conceptual basis and pilot use in children with developmental disabilities. *Clinical Pediatrics, 33*(7), 421-430.

Peloquin, S. M. (1994). Occupational therapy as art and science: Should the older definition be reclaimed? *America Journal of Occupational Therapy, 48*(11), 1093-1096.

Petersson, I., Fisher, A. G., Hemmingsson, H., & Lilja, M. (2007). The Client-Clinician Assessment Protocol (C-CAP): Evaluation of its psychometric properties for use with people aging with disabilities in need of home modifications. *Occupational Therapy Journal of Research: Occupation, Participation and Health, 27*(4), 140-148.

Pierre, B. L. (2001). Occupational therapy as documented in patients' records—Part III. Valued but not documented. Underground practice in the context of professional written communication. *Scandinavian Journal of Occupational Therapy, 8*, 174-183.

Pitrella, F., & Kappler, W. (1988). *Identification and evaluation of scale design principles in the development of the Extended Range Sequential Judgement Scale*. Wachtberg, Germany: Research Institute for Human Engineering.

Pybus, R. (1996). *Safety management: Strategy and practice*. Oxford, UK: Butterworth-Heinemann.

Radomski, M. V. (2008). Planning, guiding and documenting practice. In M. V. Radomski & C. A. Trombly Latham (Eds.), *Occupational therapy for physical dysfunction* (6th ed., pp. 41-64). Philadelphia, PA: Wolters Kluwer/Lippincott, Williams & Wilkins.

Rigby, P., Trentham, B., & Letts, L. (2014). Modifying performance contexts. In B. A. B. Schell, G. Gillen, M. E. Scaffa, & E. S. Cohn (Eds.), *Willard & Spackman's occupational therapy* (12th ed., pp. 364-381). Philadelphia, PA: Wolters Kluwer/Lippincott Williams & Wilkins.

Rogers, J. C., & Holm, M. B. (1991). Occupational therapy diagnostic reasoning: A component of clinical reasoning. *American Journal of Occupational Therapy, 45*, 1045-1053.

Rogers, J. C., & Holm, M. B. (1994). *The Performance Assessment of Self-Care Skills (PASS)—Version 3.1*. Pittsburgh, PA: University of Pittsburgh.

Rogers, J. C., & Holm, M. B. (2009). The occupational therapy process. In E. B. Crepeau, E. S. Cohn, & B. A. Boyt Schell (Eds.), *Willard & Spackman's occupational therapy* (11th ed., pp. 478-518). Philadelphia, PA: Wolters Kluwer/Lippincott Williams & Wilkins.

Rogers, J. C., Holm, M. B., & Chisholm, D. (2016). *The Performance Assessment of Self-Care Skills (PASS)—Version 4.1*. Pittsburgh, PA: University of Pittsburgh.

Sanford, J. A., Pynoos, J., Tejral, A., & Browne, A. (2002). Development of a comprehensive assessment for delivery of home modifications. *Physical & Occupational Therapy in Geriatrics, 20*(2), 43-55.

Schell, B. A. B. (2014). Professional reasoning in practice. In B. A. B. Schell, G. Gillen, M. E. Scaffa, & E. S. Cohn (Eds.), *Willard & Spackman's occupational therapy* (12th ed., pp. 384-397). Philadelphia, PA: Wolters Kluwer/Lippincott Williams & Wilkins.

Schell, B. A., & Cervero, R. M. (1993). Clinical reasoning in occupational therapy: An integrative review. *American Journal of Occupational Therapy, 47*, 605-610.

Shah, S., Vanclay, F., & Cooper, B. (1989). Improving the sensitivity of the Barthel Index for stroke rehabilitation. *Journal of Clinical Epidemiology, 42*, 703-709.

Shotwell, M. P. (2014). Evaluating clients. In B. A. B. Schell, G. Gillen, M. E. Scaffa, & E. S. Cohn (Eds.), *Willard & Spackman's occupational therapy* (12th ed., pp. 281-301). Philadelphia, PA: Wolters Kluwer/Lippincott Williams & Wilkins.

Sonn, U., & Hulter-Åsberg, K., (1991). Assessment of activities of daily living in the elderly. *Scandinavian Journal of Rehabilitation Medicine, 23*, 193-202.

Standards Association of Australia. (2009). *Australian New Zealand Risk Management Standard (AS/NZ ISO 31000)*, Sydney, Australia: Author.

Stark, S. L., Somerville, E. K., & Morris, J. C. (2010). In-Home Occupational Performance Evaluation (I-HOPE). *American Journal of Occupational Therapy, 64*(4), 580-589.

Steinfeld, E. H., & Danford, G. S. (1997). Environment as mediating factor in functional assessment. In S. S. Dittmar & G. E. Gresham (Eds.), *Functional assessment and outcome measures for the rehabilitation health professional* (pp. 37-57). Gaithersburg, MD: Aspen Publishers.

Thomas Jefferson University. (n.d.). Center for Applied Research on Aging and Health. Retrieved from http://www.jefferson.edu/jchp/carah/researchers.cfm

Tickle-Degnen, L. (2002). Client-centered practice, therapeutic relationship, and the use of research evidence. *American Journal of Occupational Therapy, 56*(4), 470-474.

Townsend, E., & Polatajko, H. (2013). Introduction-Intro. 1 Watershed guidelines with a national perspective. In E. Townsend & H. Polatajko (Eds.), *Enabling occupation II: Advancing an occupational therapy vision for health, well-being and justice through occupation* (2nd ed., p. 2). Ottawa, ON: CAOT Publications ACE.

Uniform Data System for Medical Rehabilitation. (1997). *Guide for the Uniform Data Set for Medical Rehabilitation (including the FIM™ instrument)—Version 5.1*. Buffalo, NY: UDSMR, State University of New York at Buffalo.

Uniform Data System for Medical Rehabilitation. (2009). *The FIM system clinical guide—Version 5.2*. Buffalo, NY: UDSMR, State University of New York at Buffalo.

7

Measuring the Person and the Home Environment

*Elizabeth Ainsworth, MOccThy, Grad Cert Health Sci
and Desleigh de Jonge, MPhil (OccThy), Grad Cert Soc Sci*

Having a health condition or impairment can be disabling, limiting a person's capacity to manage everyday tasks in the home or community. A home environment that is not designed for a person's specific needs is more handicapping than one whose design is well suited to the occupant.

This chapter describes the information that needs to be obtained to facilitate goodness of fit of the person with his or her home and discusses the contribution to this of an understanding of anthropometrics, ergonomics, and biomechanics. The chapter describes the characteristics of the home environment, such as the size of spaces, gradients, illuminance, force, and sound, that affect occupational performance and identifies tools for measuring these characteristics. The chapter concludes with information about factors that may influence measurement practice in the home.

CHAPTER OBJECTIVES

By the end of this chapter, the reader will be able to:

✦ Describe measurement and the types needed for home modification

✦ Explain the relevance and limitations of anthropometrics, ergonomics, and biomechanics

✦ Describe methods for measuring people, equipment, and the home environment

✦ Discuss various measures that relate to home design

✦ Describe measuring tools and resources

✦ Describe factors influencing measuring practice

✦ Explain the consequences of not using reliable measuring techniques

THE IMPORTANCE OF MEASUREMENT

Increasingly, occupational therapists are recognizing the importance of measurement in detailing the attributes of clients, their equipment, and caregivers so that they can be incorporated into the redesign of the home environment. The following discussion provides a general overview of measurement and its importance, the types of measurements required for home modification practice, and the consequences of not using sound measurement techniques.

During the home modification process, therapists gather information about the person-occupation-environment fit by taking systematic and accurate measurements of that person's physical characteristics and features in the home environment that

Ainsworth, E., & de Jonge, D. *An Occupational Therapist's Guide to Home Modification Practice, Second Edition (pp. 145-174).*
© 2019 SLACK Incorporated.

affect occupational performance. Measurements are taken of the person, the equipment he or she uses, and the caregiver to determine the environmental characteristics required to support successful completion of a range of occupations in and around the home. The person's height, weight, width, and depth (and those of his or her equipment and caregiver) and the person's visual and hearing capacity are examined to determine the space, load capacity, clearance, size, and placement of features and illumination requirements in the environment. For example, when designing a shower area for a tall, heavy client who uses a customized wheelchair, the therapist takes measurements of the person in his or her wheelchair and observes transfers and movement within the bathroom to determine the circulation spaces required and the load capacity, size, and placement of the drop-down shower seat. A broad range of activities may occur within the different areas of the home, so it is important that therapists talk with the resident to understand how each area of the home is used and how various activities are undertaken in each area.

Therapists also measure aspects of the environment and their impact on occupational performance or the health, safety, independence, quality of life, and participation of people within the home. The features that are commonly examined include lighting, color, space, heights, widths, distances, gradients, force, and sound (Bridge, 2005). For example, a person with age-related vision changes who is experiencing difficulty mobilizing at night and in transition zones (i.e., between the outside and inside of the home) may need lighting levels measured to determine the need for enhanced or consistent lighting.

Good measurement practice is critical to good design. Measurement, rather than assumption or guesswork, enables modifications to be tailored to clients' requirements. Occupational therapists can use these measurements to inform clients and other stakeholders about the functional implications of the various aspects of the design and location of features in the environment. Measurements can be used as a foundation for discussing the limitations of the current situation and how activities or the environment can be changed to support occupational performance. These measurements are especially useful for highlighting the extent to which clients' requirements fall outside of the design and performance criteria in the existing access and design standards.

Several problems can arise when clients and their environment are inaccurately measured. Clients can be unwilling to accept recommended changes if they perceive that these have not been tailored to suit their specific requirements. Inadequate measurement can also result in solutions being poorly designed, which can cause delays, disruption, and extra expense for the service or client as he or she navigates problems and renegotiates alternative options with the client. Further, interventions that have not been adequately tailored to the individual's needs are likely to fail, resulting in an accident or injury, poor health, premature or unnecessary institutionalization, increased reliance on others, and a reduced quality of life.

Effective measurement is informed by an understanding of the relevance and application of anthropometrics, ergonomics, and biomechanics. Each of these fields can contribute to an understanding of the person-environment-occupation fit. Anthropometrics can assist in understanding the dimensions of static postures and dynamic movement and how population data are used to inform design. This field of study informs therapists about the diversity of human body characteristics and the importance of providing individualized measures of people who fall outside of the typical population design range. It has also established standardized methods of measurement, which can be used by therapists when gathering individualized measurement information. Ergonomics provides therapists with an understanding of human task demands, the usability of environments, and the person-environment interaction. Biomechanics enables occupational therapists to appreciate the structural basis for human performance, strength or power capabilities of the human body, and forces generated by the body as people undertake activities (Standards Australia, 1994).

ANTHROPOMETRY AND ANTHROPOMETRIC MEASUREMENT

Anthropometry is the study of the shape, size, and proportion of the human body; the strength and working capacity or abilities; and the variation of these characteristics in populations (Ching, 1995; Paquet & Feathers, 2004; Pheasant, 1996; Pheasant & Haslegrave, 2006; Steinfeld, Lenker, & Paquet, 2002; Steinfeld & Maisel, 2012; Steinfeld, Paquet, D'Souza, Joseph, & Maisel, 2010). Anthropometric data arising from the static and dynamic measurements of the human body are collected on various populations and are used to guide the design of products, spaces, environments, and systems (Australian Safety and Compensation Council, 2009; Baker, 2008; Connell & Sanford, 1999; Cooper, 1998; Pheasant & Haslegrave,

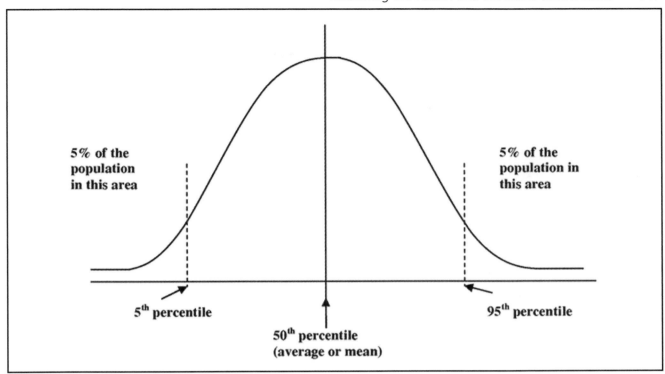

5% of the population in this area

5% of the population in this area

5th percentile

50th percentile (average or mean)

95th percentile

Figure 7-1. The normal distribution represented by the bell-shaped curve.

2006; Steinfeld & Maisel, 2012; Steinfeld et al., 2002, 2010).

Large anthropometric data sets, some of which have been derived from people in the armed forces in various countries, have been compiled and presented in multiple tables with detailed measures for different subgroups (e.g., age and gender; Conway, 2008). When measures of individuals within populations are graphed, they commonly form a normal or bell-shaped curve, with an increasing proportion of the population tending toward the mean near the middle of the curve and a decreasing proportion tending toward the tails of the curve (Diffrient, Tilley, & Bardagjy, 1974), although not all anthropometric measures are symmetrically distributed. It is important that designs sufficiently accommodate anthropometric variability (Pheasant & Haslegrave, 2006). Customarily, measurements for 90% of the population are used for designs; that is, the anthropometric dimensions occurring at either end of or between the 5th and 95th percentiles (Goldsmith, 2000; Pheasant & Haslegrave, 2006; Steinfeld & Maisel, 2012) or at or below the 90th percentile (Figure 7-1). Critics have noted that designs based on the 95th percentile for one dimension, such as height, will not accommodate the 95th percentile for other dimensions such as vision, hearing, and perception (Sanford, 2012). This approach presumes that there are no differences across populations based on gender or other individual attributes that would influence design and, as a result, it can be assumed that no design will suit 90% of all people across all abilities (Sanford, 2012). Some designs that extend beyond the 95th percentile may only cater to one type of ability, which can render the design even more disabling (Sanford, 2012).

Published anthropometric data may be relevant to some people within populations but not to others as the data have historically tended to exclude people with a disability. Published anthropometric data might therefore provide little information about the characteristics of people with a disability (Steinfeld, 2004; Steinfeld & Maisel, 2012). A small number of studies, undertaken in the late 1970s and early 1980s, have provided limited data on the anthropometrics of people with a disability. Many studies on people with a disability are limited in their usefulness because they have tended to focus on specific disability groups rather than on the full range of people with a disability, lack standardized dimensional definitions and measurement methods (Bridge, 2005; Paquet & Feathers, 2004), and do not include or acknowledge the specific requirements of people with more than one disability (Bridge, 2005). Further, the data do not consider the various types of assistive devices used by a range of people with a disability and how and when they are used (Steinfeld, 2004).

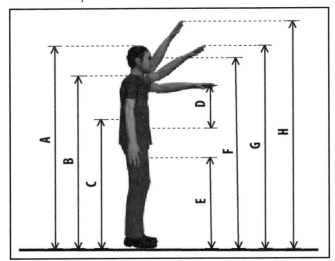

Figure 7-2. Standing anthropometrics. (Adapted from Goldsmith, S. [2000]. *Universal design: A manual of practical guidance for architects.* London: Elsevier.)

Despite the difficulties associated with applying anthropometric data to people with a disability and across subgroups of them, the available data can assist therapists in understanding the complexities of the human form and how it interfaces with the environment (Baker, 2008). Anthropometric data are necessary when the characteristics of individuals are unknown or when establishing initial estimates of measures of the characteristics where the individual is known. Whatever the case, therapists should understand that, when designing for a particular person, it is important that individualized measuring occurs. Without individualized measurements, the suitability of the home modification for the client might be compromised.

Types of Anthropometry and Their Application

Two types of anthropometry are used to guide design: structural (or static) anthropometry and functional (or dynamic) anthropometry (Steinfeld & Maisel, 2012).

Structural (Static) Anthropometry

This form of anthropometry "is the science of measuring length, breadth, and the width of the human population" (Baker, 2008, p. 75). It can include the measurement of size of body parts, stature, and weight (Steinfeld & Maisel, 2012). Static measurements are usually taken with the person sitting, standing, and/or bending (Steinfeld & Maisel, 2012). Human dimensions are always considered in

the sagittal plane (the vertical plane through the longitudinal axis that divides the body into left and right sections) or the coronal plane (the vertical plane through the longitudinal axis that divides the body into front and back sections; Baker, 2008).

The standing posture involves the subjects standing erect and looking straight ahead, with their arms in a relaxed position by their side (Baker, 2008). The seated posture involves the subjects sitting erect and looking straight ahead. Their thighs should be parallel to the floor and their knees bent at a 90-degree angle with feet flat on the floor; the upper arms are to be relaxed and perpendicular to the horizontal plane with the forearm at right angles to the upper arm and parallel to the floor (Baker, 2008). Measurements are taken along imaginary horizontal or vertical lines using specific anatomical landmarks, such as the popliteal crease at the back of the knee, greater trochanter of the femur, and parts of the body, as reference points. For example, a person's stature is determined by measuring the vertical distance from the floor to the vertex (the crown of the head). This measurement is then used to define the vertical clearance required when standing, walking, or wheeling in an area of the minimum acceptable space or with overhead obstructions. The most common static body dimensions to obtain in relation to the design of home interiors include height, weight, sitting height, eye height, buttock to knee and buttock to popliteal lengths, breadths across elbows and hips, seated knee and popliteal heights, and thigh clearance height (Panero & Zelnik, 1979; Figures 7-2 and 7-3).

Measurements to note in Figure 7-2:

+ A = Floor to top of head
+ B = Floor to shoulder
+ C = Floor to elbow
+ D = Waist to hand
+ E = Floor to wrist
+ F = Floor to eye level
+ G = Diagonal reach range—floor to hand
+ H = Diagonal reach range—floor to hand

Measurements to note in Figure 7-3:

+ A = Floor to top of head
+ B = Floor to top of shoulder
+ C = Floor to popliteal area
+ D = Chest to end of hand
+ E = Floor to top of knee
+ F = Floor to eye level
+ G = Diagonal forward reach

Anthropometric data on people with disabilities also include dimensions of people occupying assistive devices. Dimensions of an occupied wheelchair are used to determine the floor space and vertical and horizontal clearance requirements of people using wheelchairs.

Functional (Dynamic) Anthropometry

This form of anthropometry involves the measurement of a subject while in motion to help determine the properties of the body, such as range of motion or reach, grasping, stride, clearance, and space envelopes required for different body movements (Ching, 1995; Cooper, 1998; Steinfeld & Maisel, 2012). This can also include the measurement of the subject during movement associated with certain tasks, such as reaching, using an assistive device to wheel or walk straight ahead or to make a turn, or the measurement of the subject's strength (Steinfeld et al., 2002; Steinfeld & Maisel, 2012). These types of data are more difficult to reliably obtain because of the movement of the subject during the measurement process. However, functional or dynamic anthropometry provides more accurate information about the movement within spaces and during activities. For example, when considering the ability of the body to reach forward, the static measurement that would be used is "arm length" (Australian Safety and Compensation Council, 2009). However, dynamic analysis of a person reaching forward shows that the shoulder joint also moves forward with the arm, thus increasing the person's forward reach capacity beyond the static length of the arm (Australian Safety and Compensation Council, 2009, p. 42).

The size, shape, weight, and movement patterns of people with disabilities vary considerably, requiring the environment to be customized to their unique requirements. Occupational therapists use the principles of anthropometric measurement to position clients and locate anatomical landmarks and parts of the body when establishing clients' specific dimensions. Using an established and standardized approach to measurement, where possible, ensures that practice is accurately and consistently replicated by staff, particularly when there is a range of approaches. Individualizing the measurement process is particularly useful where usability and safety require a close fit between individuals, their equipment and caregivers, and their environment (Steinfeld, Schroeder, Duncan, et al., 1979; Steinfeld et al., 2002; Steinfeld & Maisel, 2012). For example, a bathroom needs to be designed to "fit" an individual's stature and functional reach range to ensure his or her safety and the usability of the fittings. Specifically measuring a person allows therapists to

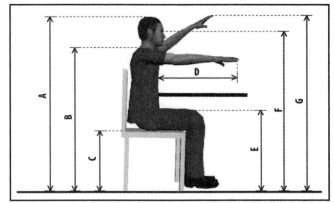

Figure 7-3. Seated anthropometrics. (Adapted from Goldsmith, S. [2000]. *Universal design: A manual of practical guidance for architects*. London: Elsevier.)

collect concrete and scientific information that can be used to analyze why a space is not working and design or redesign spaces to suit the needs of users with specific requirements (Goldsmith, 2000).

BIOMECHANICS

Biomechanics "is effort produced by the human body while moving or resisting force" (Steinfeld & Maisel, 2012, p. 103). It is the study of human movement using mechanical principles (Spaulding, 2008a). It examines movement and equilibrium using the principles of physics to investigate the influence of forces, levers, and torque on performance (Pedretti, 1996). Because the biomechanics of the human body are so complex, no single biomechanical model of the human body currently exists; rather, there are many models from various fields of use to explain movement of the human body (Kroemer, 1987).

Biomechanics can be used to analyze movement in everyday activities to understand the mechanical aspects of the movement. It assists in the examination of the level of effort required to use the environment to accommodate end users' abilities, tolerances, and preferences (Steinfeld & Maisel, 2012, p. 103). In a biomechanical analysis of the sit-to-stand transfer, Laporte, Chan, and Sveistrup (1999) highlight the role of displacement, momentum, velocity, and the relationship between the center of pressure and center of mass throughout the four phases of the sit-to-stand transfer. This type of analysis provides therapists with a detailed understanding of the elements of the movement and how variations in movement may result in performance difficulties.

Using biomechanical principles, therapists systematically observe performance in order to examine the quality of the movement, the effectiveness of performance, the degree of effort involved, and the potential for injury (Kreighbaum & Barthels, 1996; Pheasant, 1987; Steinfeld & Maisel, 2012). By using a qualitative biomechanical analysis, therapists can identify ineffective or problematic aspects of movement. Considerations commonly include:

+ Range of movement: Working outside of safe ranges of motion and/or within extreme ranges

+ Center of gravity: Displacement of the person's center of gravity outside of the base of support

+ Accuracy: Imprecise or uncoordinated movements

+ Speed and momentum: Slow, hesitant, uncontrolled, or impulsive actions

+ Strength: Overexertion or ineffective positioning resulting in poor use of force, levers, and torque

+ Endurance: Limited activity tolerance or excessive energy expenditure (Steinfeld, Schroeder, Duncan, et al., 1979)

Occupational therapists also draw on biomechanical principles to improve movement and make it safer. They identify the most appropriate posture for the performance of a task with a view to maximizing the effect of forces and minimizing muscular effort (Pheasant, 1987). They also advise on strategies to improve the effectiveness and efficiency of movement and reduce the likelihood of discomfort, pain, incidents, accidents, injuries, or disability. For example, occupational therapists use the information on the biomechanical analysis of the sit-to-stand transfer provided by Chan, Laporte, and Sveistrup (1999) to identify a range of strategies to improve the effectiveness and safety of the movement (e.g., the ideal initial body position and the proper use of body mechanics throughout the movement).

Ergonomics

Ergonomics is concerned with shaping environments and tasks to optimize the abilities of individuals to perform activities (Baker, 2008; Conway, 2008; Stein, Soderback, Cutler, & Larson, 2006). It involves measuring and using the dimensions of objects and spaces to examine the human task demands (Conway, 2008; Stein et al., 2006). Though ergonomics emerged from the area of work performance, worker safety, and productivity, it is not solely confined to workplace environments (Berg Rice, 2008). The concepts and principles are derived from research in many fields, including industrial engineering, human factors psychology, occupational medicine, and nursing, as well as occupational therapy (Stein et al., 2006). Like occupational therapy, the field of ergonomics is concerned with the usability of environments and the person-environment transaction (Conway, 2008). The principles of ergonomics can be used to prevent musculoskeletal injures, conserve energy, and use the body in the most efficient way possible when engaging in activity or occupation (Stein et al., 2006).

Two approaches are commonly used in an ergonomic evaluation: task analysis and user trial (Pheasant & Haslegrave, 2006). Task analysis involves examining what the person is doing or needs to do and analyzing the physical movements and information processing involved and the actual or potential environmental barriers or constraints (Conway, 2008). An effective task analysis involves clarifying the person's goals; intended outcome; and potential areas of mismatch between the person, activity, and environment (Conway, 2008). A user trial involves the naturalistic trial of a product or environment to determine its usability (Conway, 2008) and to evaluate whether there is a satisfactory match with the user when considering its comfort, usability, and performance (Pheasant, 1987).

With its user-centered approach and person-environment transactive perspective (Pheasant & Haslegrave, 2006), ergonomics can assist occupational therapists to determine the adequacy of the person-environment fit (Conway, 2008; Stein et al., 2006). Ergonomic principles guide the analysis of the person's posture, movement, and performance and the impact of the environment (Berg Rice, 2008). An ergonomic approach provides therapists with a framework for evaluating and matching the design of the layout, fittings, and fixtures to suit the specific capabilities of the person; additionally, it assists in selecting products, equipment, and designs to improve client or caregiver efficiency, effectiveness, and safety (Berg Rice, 2008).

Measuring the Client, Equipment, and Caregivers

People vary in terms of their body size and movement patterns, the equipment they use, and the assistance they receive; hence, therapists often need to take an individualized approach when measuring clients, their caregivers, and their equipment. Therapists gather this information to alert builders and designers to the specific requirements of clients whose dimensions or abilities fall outside of the population addressed by the access and design standards. Individualized measurement is advisable, particularly for people who vary substantially in terms of height, size, or weight and for those who use equipment other than a standard wheelchair; have impairments that affect their posture, movement, or balance; have limited use of their upper limbs; or require caregiver assistance for various activities.

The challenge for occupational therapists lies in knowing what to measure and how to measure it. By measuring people's size, shape, weight, space requirements (with consideration for their equipment and/or caregiver dimensions), reach, clearance, posture, and strength, the therapist can determine the space they require and the best location for fixtures and fittings.

Individuals' body dimensions might need to be measured in various static or dynamic postures, such as sitting, standing, bending, kneeling, squatting, or lying positions, depending on the nature of the activities they are involved in around the home. Posture relates to the orientation of body parts in space and depends on the dimensions of the body and their relationship with items in the environment. People with poor strength and endurance or visual difficulties might experience change in posture throughout the day or alter their posture for different activities. Posture might vary as a result of natural biological fluctuations. For example, a person's stature can vary approximately 15 mm over 24 hours, being the greatest first thing in the morning when the spine has been relieved of supporting body weight through lying down overnight (Pheasant & Haslegrave, 2006). Shrinkage of the spine tends to occur rapidly within the first 3 hours of rising (Pheasant & Haslegrave, 2006). It may not always be possible to measure clients in seated or standing positions. In these cases, therapists need to choose the posture that best suits the clients' disability, the activities they wish to complete, and the environment in which they will function in that position. For example, if a client needs to reach to operate an intercom while in bed, he or she will need to be measured lying down and reaching to the area on the wall that would best suit the person's capacity to operate the device.

The following diagrams and photos provide an illustration of typical body postures and the location of the body landmarks used as reference points during the measurement process. Pheasant and Haslegrave (2006) provide a detailed description of body dimensions and what these dimensions apply to in relation to the design of the built environment. The examples provided in the following discussion are the measures most commonly taken by occupational therapists.

The Height, Width, and Depth of Parts of the Body

The therapist uses a tape measure to determine height, width, and depth of parts of the person and the equipment above floor level. Pheasant and Haslegrave (2006) provide the following details:

✦ A person's stature is determined by measuring the vertical distance from the floor to the vertex (the crown of the head). This measurement defines the vertical clearance required when standing, walking, or wheeling in an area or the minimum acceptable space of overhead obstructions.

✦ Shoulder height is measured from the floor to the acromion (the bony tip of the shoulder), and it is the reference point for the location of fittings, fixtures, and controls.

✦ Knee height includes the horizontal distance from the floor to the upper surface of the knee (measured to the quadriceps muscle and not the knee cap), and it provides measurement to inform the clearance required beneath the underside of tables.

✦ Popliteal height is the measurement from the floor to the popliteal angle at the underside of the knee where the tendon insertion of the biceps femoris muscle is located. This dimension defines the maximum acceptable height of the seat.

✦ Hip width is the maximum horizontal distance across the hips in the seated position, and this information relates to the minimum width of a seat.

✦ Hand width is measured across the palm of the hand and includes a measurement of the distal ends of the carpal bones to provide information on clearance for hand access to handles or rails.

✦ Depth of the area between the popliteal area at the underside of the knee to the rear of the buttocks provides information to inform the design of the depth of a seat (Figures 7-4 and 7-5).

Measurements to note in Figure 7-4:

✦ A = Shoulder width

✦ B = Seat to the top of the shoulders

✦ C = Seat to the top of the head

✦ D = Width of the buttocks

✦ E = Width of the seat

✦ F = Bottom of buttocks to the elbow

✦ G = Seat to the lumbar area

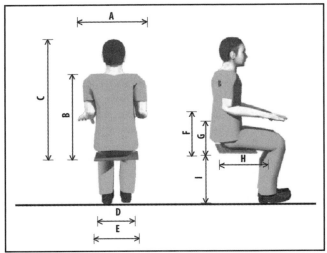

Figure 7-4. Rear and side views of a seated person. (Adapted from Pheasant, S. [1996]. *Bodyspace: Anthropometry, ergonomics and the design of work*. London: T. J. Press.)

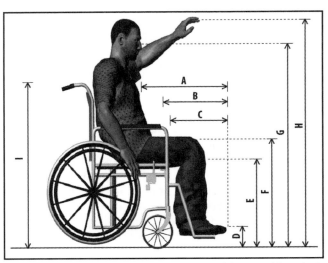

Figure 7-5. Occupied wheelchair. (Adapted from Goldsmith, S. [2000]. *Universal design: A manual of practical guidance for architects*. London: Elsevier.)

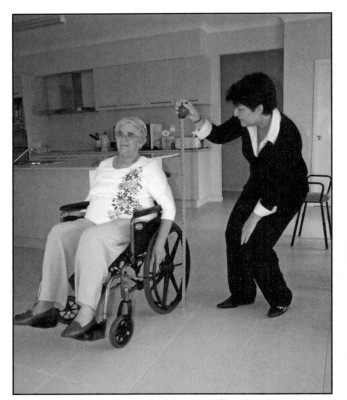

Figure 7-6. Measuring eye height above floor level.

✦ H = Rear of the buttocks to the popliteal area of the leg

✦ I = Floor to the popliteal area

Measurements to note in Figure 7-5:

✦ A = Chest to toe

✦ B = Edge of armrest to end of toe or footplate (whichever protrudes the most)

✦ C = End of armrest to end of toe

✦ D = Floor to toe with foot on footplate

✦ E = Floor to seat of wheelchair (or top of cushion on wheelchair)

✦ F = Floor to knee with foot on footplate

✦ G = Floor to eye level

✦ H = Diagonal forward reach

✦ I = Height of wheelchair

Eye Height

The therapist also measures eye height, which is measured from the floor to the inner canthus (corner) of the eye. This dimension defines the maximum acceptable height for visual obstructions and defines sight lines (Pheasant & Haslegrave, 2006; see Figures 7-2 through 7-6).

Reach Ranges

The measurement of an individual's functional reach ranges, when positioned in various postures, is important in determining the width and height of environmental features, such as storage cupboards, benches, and clotheslines. The therapist considers the location of the features in the environment and asks clients to move and reach either forward or sideways with the arm they are most likely to use. This activity could also be undertaken in a natural environment in which the various features are positioned, or the therapist might need to simulate the location of the various features during the measurement exercise. Refer to Figures 7-2 through 7-12.

Measurements to note in Figure 7-7:

✦ A to G = Side reach

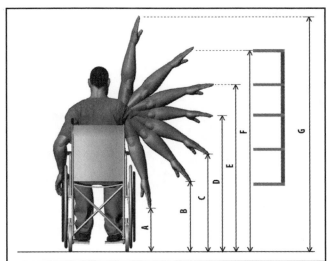

Figure 7-7. Occupied wheelchair. Side reach. (Adapted from Goldsmith, S. [2000]. *Universal design: A manual of practical guidance for architects*. London: Elsevier.)

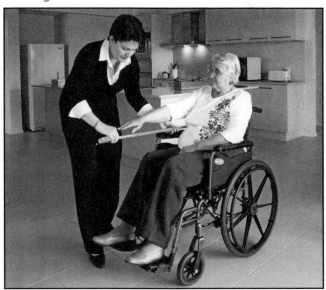

Figure 7-8. Measuring horizontal reach dimension.

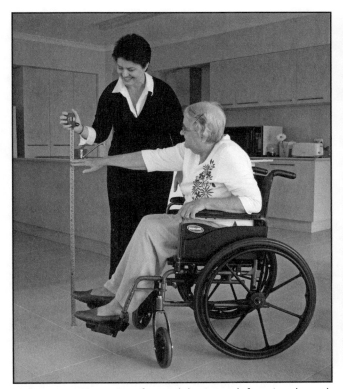

Figure 7-9. Measuring forward horizontal functional reach above floor level.

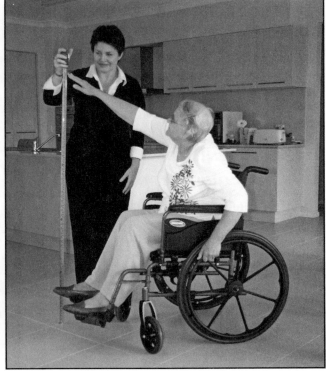

Figure 7-10. Measuring forward diagonal functional reach above floor level.

Determining the Size of Spaces for Transfer and Mobility Equipment

Reflecting the distinction between static or dynamic studies in anthropometrics, two strategies for determining the size of spaces for occupied or unoccupied mobility equipment such as wheelchairs, scooters, or wheeled walking aids can be differentiated, depending upon whether the person is stationary or moving. The distinction is made here because sizes of spaces for stationary equipment can be determined from measurements of the occupied or unoccupied equipment itself, whereas, in practical terms, determining the sizes of spaces

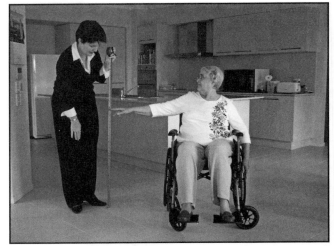

Figure 7-11. Measuring side horizontal functional reach above floor level.

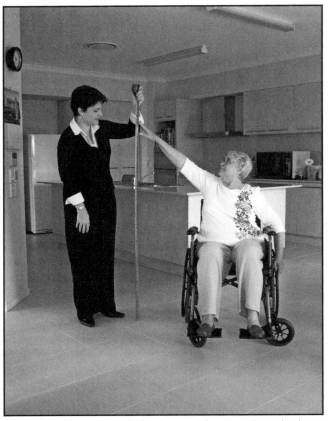

Figure 7-12. Measuring side diagonal functional reach above floor level.

for moving equipment cannot. Spaces to consider when measuring equipment in motion include volumetric (three-dimensional) space and planar (two-dimensional) space traversed on the travel surface (i.e., the ground or floor surface).

Most rooms and spaces in the home will require consideration of the motion of equipment; however, consideration of stationary equipment is necessary for storage and parking spaces and at the start and end positions of their motion.

Measurements for Stationary Mobility Equipment

For the minimum size of spaces to store or park equipment, measurements will be required of at least the overall width, length, and height of the equipment. For more compact storage, such as under bench tops for wheelchairs, the dimensions of foot, back, and arm support assemblies and drive wheels will also be required. For even more compact storage of equipment that can be folded, measurements will be required of them in their folded state.

Occupied and unoccupied wheelchairs and scooters are typically illustrated in plain view as being symmetrical about their longitudinal and lateral axes. However, many unoccupied and especially occupied pieces of equipment are asymmetrical (Hunter, 2009). Asymmetry is attributable to the equipment, the occupant, accessories such as respirators, and loose items such as handbags and walking aids. The need for consideration of loose items in space planning should be confirmed with clients. Figure 7-13 illustrates the typical asymmetry of wheelchairs and scooters.

Measuring unoccupied or occupied wheelchairs and scooters requires measurement of the distance between outermost points on them. These are typically on hand rims, the rear of drive wheels, the ends of handgrips, the tops of back supports, and the ends of armrests and footplates. Outermost points on users of manual or powered wheelchairs include the ends of shoes and elbows, fingers, or wrists on hand rims or controls and the top of users' heads. Outermost points may also be on features or accessories added to the equipment by clients. Outermost points on users do not necessarily occur at the skeletal protuberances commonly used as reference points in biomechanics.

Prior knowledge of key features that typically constitute the two- and three-dimensional outlines of occupied and unoccupied equipment assists in orienting to the measuring task. Of greatest importance, however, is skill in recognizing the features that constitute the envelope of occupied or unoccupied equipment and the relevant outermost points on it.

The number of points is determined by the end use of the measuring. If the end use is to determine the size of a cube for storing equipment, only the

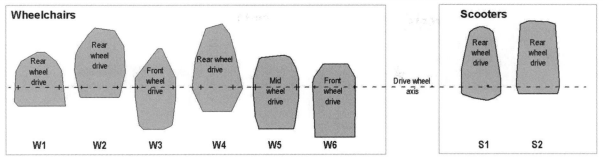

Notes: These outlines are convex hulls (or elastic band outlines) formed by the projection onto the floor of outer-most points at different heights of the occupied wheelchairs and scooters - parts of the actual outline of each occupied wheelchair or scooter therefore occur within the convex hulls (outlines) and are not shown. Only the drive wheels are shown and are indicated by their contact point with the ground.

- Occupied wheelchairs and scooters are typically asymmetrical
- Some wheelchairs are front-wheel drive, some are mid-wheel drive and some are rear-wheel drive (regardless of whether they are manually or electrically propelled).
- Drive-wheel type, size and shape effects the size and shape of manoeuvring space (scooters tend to have a larger turning circle because they are unable to pivot like wheelchairs - their centre of rotation does not occur between their drive wheels).
- Steering control and navigational judgment also affects the manoeuvring space.

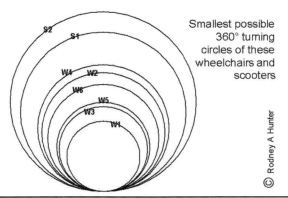

Smallest possible 360° turning circles of these wheelchairs and scooters

© Rodney A Hunter

Figure 7-13. Typical outlines of occupied wheelchairs and scooters. (Reprinted with permission from Rodney A. Hunter.)

pairs of points corresponding with overall width, length, and height of the equipment are required. For space under bench tops and the like for wheelchairs, dimensions of arm support assemblies, legs, and feet positions will also be required.

Methods for recording outermost points include photogrammetry and laser scanning; however, these can be time consuming and costly. Simple, inexpensive, and sufficiently accurate methods for most home modifications are manual ones. The most common and quickest manual method is measuring between outermost points of the equipment with a tape measure.

If only the overall length and width need to be measured, movable panels can be used. Polystyrene is a suitable material for panels; the panels need to have a base that is large and heavy enough to stabilize the panel. For this method, the panels are placed parallel to each other and at each side of the equipment and then moved toward it until they just touch it. The procedure is repeated at the ends of the equipment. There are three advantages of this method:

1. The panels can be easily placed at whatever angle with respect to each other and that most snugly contains the equipment for purpose of storage space that is not rectangular in plan

2. The panels can be used to test for the parking or storing motion of the equipment

3. No prior knowledge of measuring points is required

For mobility equipment with castor wheels, a dimension that may need to be measured is the pivoting radius of the castor wheels. Castor wheels can swing outside of the envelope of equipment, especially if, after the equipment has stopped, it is suddenly moved in the opposite direction. If there is insufficient space for this, the equipment can become jammed in the storage space.

The measured width and length of the stationary equipment will need to be increased to allow for typical imperfect control of the equipment as it is driven or pushed into or out of the parking or storage space. Additional measurement will also be necessary where space is required to transfer in and out of the equipment or if space is required for another person to assist the equipment user (Figures 7-14 through 7-22).

Measurements to note in Figure 7-14:

✦ L = Length of wheelchair

✦ W = Width of wheelchair

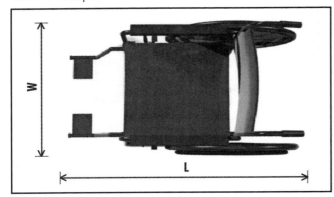

Figure 7-14. Unoccupied wheelchair.

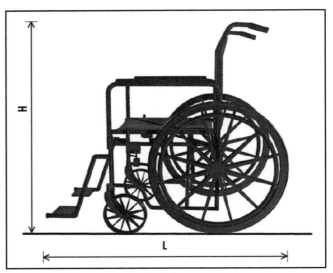

Figure 7-15. Unoccupied wheelchair.

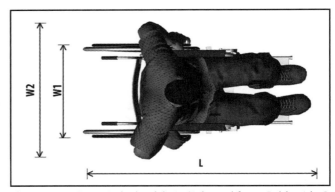

Figure 7-17. Occupied wheelchair. (Adapted from Goldsmith, S. [2000]. *Universal design: A manual of practical guidance for architects*. London: Elsevier.)

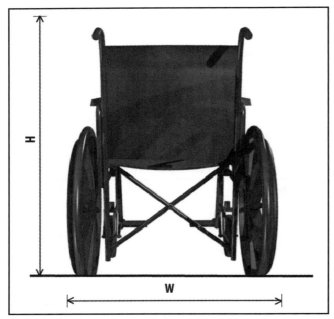

Figure 7-16. Unoccupied wheelchair.

Measurements to note in Figure 7-15:
+ L = Length of wheelchair
+ H = Height of wheelchair

Measurements to note in Figure 7-16:
+ W = Width of wheelchair
+ H = Height of wheelchair

Measurements to note in Figure 7-17:
+ L = Length from back of rear wheel to the front of the footplate or person's toe (edge that protrudes)
+ W1 = Width of the wheelchair without the person's hands on the wheel rims; width from wheel rim to wheel rim
+ W2 = Width of the wheelchair; person's hands on the wheel rims; width measurement to include widest point (knuckles or elbows protruding)

Measurements to note in Figure 7-18:
+ W1 = Width of the wheelchair without the person's hands on the wheel rims; width from wheel rim to wheel rim
+ W2 = Width of the wheelchair; person's hands on the wheel rims; width measurement to include widest point (knuckles or elbows protruding)

It must be noted that some people with a disability have different body shapes, reach, and movement patterns that do not correlate with these diagrams. In such cases, an individualized measurement approach is required.

Measurement for Mobility Equipment in Use

Mobility equipment moves between stationary states corresponding with parked or stored positions; the path between these positions is straight,

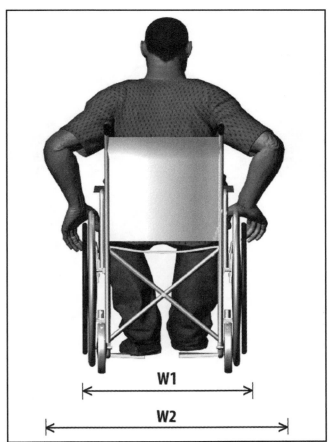

Figure 7-18. Occupied wheelchair. (Adapted from Goldsmith, S. [2000]. *Universal design: A manual of practical guidance for architects.* London: Elsevier.)

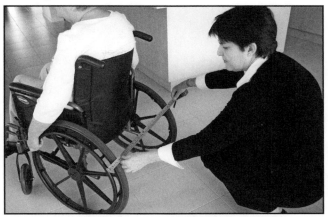

Figure 7-19. Measuring the occupied wheelchair width.

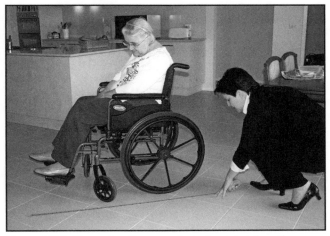

Figure 7-20. Measuring the occupied wheelchair length.

curved, or partly both. Parked positions that typically need to be considered in relation to equipment motion include those in showers and at toilet pans, hand basins, and kitchen sinks.

Measuring for Straight Paths or Curved Paths of Large Diameter

For the cross-sectional dimensions of straight paths or curved paths of large diameter, such as height and width of paths, the minimum required dimensions and the techniques for obtaining them may be the same as those for stationary occupied equipment. Curved paths of large diameter can be treated similarly to straight paths because the relevant outermost points on the occupied equipment will tend to be the same in each case.

Therapists should be aware that even if path widths can be determined from the dimensions of stationary equipment, widths will need to be increased for typical imperfect control of equipment and hence avoidance of damage and injury. The additional width will need to be estimated or measured by trial and error using techniques discussed later. Additionally, for long footpaths and corridors (and for lifts), space might be required for a 180-degree turn, for which the required space will need to be established as discussed later.

Measuring for Maneuvering and Curved Paths of Small Diameter

The term *maneuvering* here denotes motion composed of turns with a very small diameter, including reversing turns that involve alternating forward and backward motion.

Determining the size of spaces from measurements of stationary equipment is much more difficult for maneuvering and for curved paths of small diameter than it is for straight travel or curved paths of large diameter. This is because the relevant outermost points tend to be different between the two cases and different for different maneuvers. This is illustrated in Appendix B. The detail in the appendix illustrates that, for four types of 90-degree clockwise

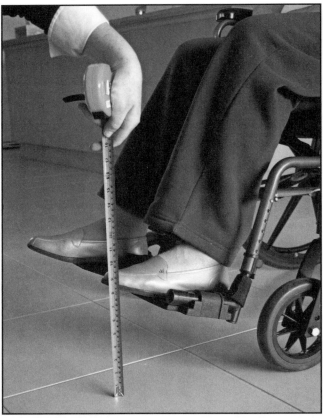

Figure 7-21. Measuring the height of the toe above floor level.

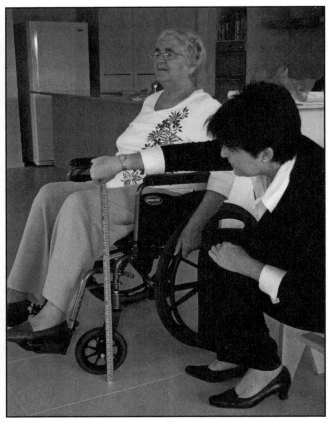

Figure 7-22. Measuring knee height above floor level.

turns, three different pairs of outermost points determine the width of the space.

Because of the complexity of estimating or calculating space for equipment in motion by using measurements of the occupied equipment when they are stationary, it may be much better to measure the spaces occupied by the moving equipment.

Two methods for determining the size of space for maneuvering are recording the space traversed on the floor by the moving equipment and then measuring that space, and using barriers as measuring datums between which to measure dimensions of the space. In this latter method, the barriers act as a large measuring tool with adjustable reference planes (datums).

The first method does not require barriers; however, barriers add greater realism and possibly greater accuracy to path recording. For the second method, the barriers are incrementally positioned closer to or farther away from the occupied equipment until the client reports or it is observed that the maneuver occurs in the least space with reasonable ease and without touching the barriers.

The space traversed by moving equipment can be recorded using a physical scale model fitted with pens (Hunter, 2003a); actual occupied equipment

fitted with pens (Ringaert, Rapson, Qiu, Cooper, & Shwedyk, 2001); sonar or video recording devices; pressure-sensitive mats that record electronically or physically (Hunter, 2003b); or computer simulation (Han, Law, Latombe, & Kunz, 2002; Hunter, 2005). For home modifications, these techniques may be too costly and time consuming. Furthermore, physical scale modeling and computer simulation require additional information for estimates about spatial allowances for steering control and navigational judgments by equipment users and about the space occupied by people assisting the user (this additional information would need to be obtained by one of the other methods using actual equipment).

Barriers as a Measuring Tool

The use of incrementally adjustable barriers as a measuring tool is a simple method suitable for home modifications. The barriers may be simplified ones (Hunter, 2002), replicated or actual barriers (Steinfeld, Schroeder, & Bishop, 1979), or simple panels as previously noted. An advantage of this method is that knowledge of the dimensions of the occupied or unoccupied equipment or of equipment users' steering control or navigational judgments is not required, although the latter may need to be

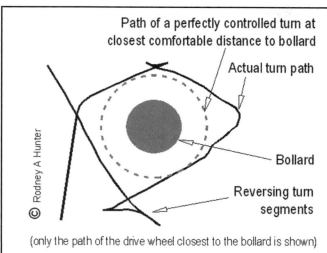

Path of a perfectly controlled turn at closest comfortable distance to bollard

Actual turn path

© Rodney A Hunter

Bollard

Reversing turn segments

(only the path of the drive wheel closest to the bollard is shown)

360° turn around bollard

This diagram of a 360-degree turn around isolated feature is an example of variation between perfectly and imperfectly controlled maneuvers.

The actual path:
- Is not circular
- Is at a distance from the perfect path
- Incorporates two reversing turn segments
- Has a direction of departure misaligned with its direction of approach

The other drive wheel path (not shown) does not necessarily incorporate reversing turn segments.

Figure 7-23. Imperfect turn around bollard. (Reprinted with permission from Rodney A. Hunter.)

specified as part of the testing. The method can also readily incorporate the contribution to space requirements of people assisting the equipment user. Measuring may be easier in premises other than the home but may incur logistical difficulties.

Measuring may be more feasible in homes if chalked or taped lines on the floor are used instead of moveable panels. If the maneuvering overlaps lines, they can be replaced or augmented by lines alongside them. Care is required to identify whether any part of the occupied wheelchair overlaps the lines.

Understanding an Individual's Space Needs

A measuring project for a home is facilitated by first learning how clients move about in their homes, in particular, how areas are approached, activities in them carried out, and the areas departed. For example, when examining the space requirements of a wheelchair user during toileting, observations need to be made of the client's capacity to wheel to the room, negotiate the doorway, wheel beside or in front of the toilet, transfer on and off the toilet, access and use the hand basin, and then depart from the area. Movement must be possible without having to move furniture or inflicting damage to walls and doorways and other fittings and fixtures.

Consideration may also need to be given to the circumstance where more than one wheelchair is used in the home and whether a wheelchair may be changed in size or type after a period. The equipment that requires the greatest space will therefore probably have to take priority over the others in determining space requirements.

The Geometry of Curvilinear Travel

Understanding the basic geometry (shapes) of curvilinear travel can be useful for measurement projects. The geometry of curvilinear travel is infinitely variable, but some generalizations are possible.

In terms of geometry of travel, common types of wheelchairs and scooters are rear-, mid-, and front-wheel-drive wheelchairs and three- and four-wheel scooters. The geometry of scooter travel is similar to tricycles. The type, size, and shape of wheelchairs determines the least possible space required for them; that is, the space required by them as if they were perfectly driven. There can be a pronounced variation between the spaces traversed by different wheelchairs in terms of sizes and shapes and the location of the spaces in relation to the physical feature with which the turn is associated.

Curvilinear travel and maneuvers are typically composed of circular turns and noncircular turns such as hyperbolic-shaped turns (the diameter of the turn path becomes successively bigger or smaller throughout the turn). Each of these turn types may be performed as a single motion in the one direction (clockwise or counterclockwise) or as several motions in different directions as occurs in reversing turns. Most maneuvers involve reversing turns of varying complexity. A predominantly single-motion turn can also incorporate a very small reversing turn (Figure 7-23 shows an imperfect turn around a bollard).

Motion at a feature can be regarded as a single maneuver, with start and end stationary positions (even though the equipment may be stationary for a barely measurable period). Approach and departure travel paths also need to be considered to this maneuver because of their contribution to the overall size of space required at the feature and, importantly, because of their influence on the type and therefore size and shape of the space traversed by the maneuvering.

Of relevance to the conventional incorporation of right-angled room layouts in buildings is categorization of compact turns of wheelchairs and scooters in terms of a small number of fundamental types. These are 360-, 180-, and 90-degree turns about the midpoint between the drive wheels of wheelchairs; 90-degree turns about either of the drive wheels of wheelchairs; 360-, 180-, and 90-degree turns about the center of the smallest turning circle of scooters (or tricycles); and noncircular turns. Reversing turns can be categorized as 180-degree turns, of which two types can also be differentiated, although reversing turns are really just successive 90-degree turns. Examples of these fundamental types of turns are indicated and further explained in Appendix B. In reality, the variety of turns employed by wheelchair and scooter users, knowingly or otherwise, is infinite. Nevertheless, knowledge of the fundamental types of turns allows an approximation or initial estimation of maneuvering space requirements.

Turns of 360 degrees are applicable to general living areas or other spaces in which there is no predominant direction of travel. Spaces for 180-degree turns are smaller than spaces for 360-degree turns and may be acceptable to clients. Turns of 90 degrees apply to doorways and corners of corridors or footpaths.

The fundamental turns should not be regarded as absolute bases for determining sizes and shapes of spaces for equipment use. Rather, they should be used as initial approximations in designing, or for the initial setup of panels or floor lines for maneuvering trials. Whether the size of spaces should be determined with reference to any one of the fundamental turns will be a matter of trial and error and collaboration with the client.

Procedures for Measuring Maneuvering Spaces

360-Degree Turn Test

The occupied equipment is positioned in a corner formed by fixed panels or the walls of a room; two relocatable panels or other barriers or floor lines are placed parallel and opposite these walls to enclose the occupied equipment. Starting from a position facing one of the fixed elements, the person operating the equipment then performs a 360-degree turn. If space is insufficient or excessive, the moveable elements are gradually and successively positioned until the turn can be performed without the equipment or the person's body touching the walls or overlapping the barriers (International Organization for Standardization, 2005) as per Figure 7-24.

180-Degree Turn Test

A fixed panel or wall of a room is used as one side of a corridor, and a moveable panel or other barrier or line marking is placed parallel with it as the other side. Starting from a position between the panels and facing along the corridor, the person operating the equipment performs a 180-degree turn. If space is insufficient or excessive, the moveable element is gradually and successively positioned until the turn can be successfully performed.

Two trial procedures should be conducted: one where the 180-degree turn is performed as a single turn in a clockwise or counterclockwise direction or both, and the other as a reversing turn as illustrated in Appendix B. Two reversing turn trials should also be undertaken: one where the initial motion is forward and one where the initial motion is backward as shown in Diagrams 9 and 10 in Appendix C.

90-Degree Turn Test

Two types of 90-degree turns should be tested: around the corner of a corridor (or through a doorway into a corridor) or from a corridor through a doorway. Instead of or as well as the corridor corner test, turns around the outside and inside of wall corners (that is, not in a corridor) will yield additional information. The procedures are similar to those for 360- and 180-degree turns. For the outside and inside corner tests, the wheelchair users should be asked to stay as close to the corner as possible. There are a large number of other configurations and maneuvers that might also need to be tested.

Specifying Circular or Noncircular Turns

Though it is easy to distinguish between circular and noncircular turns on a drawing for 180-degree reversing turns and 90-degree turns, actually testing separately for these turns will probably be impracticable. What is important is that clients employ whatever strategy is most effective for them in performing turns in as little space as comfortably possible.

Weight

The weight of the person and his or her equipment can be measured using specifically designed

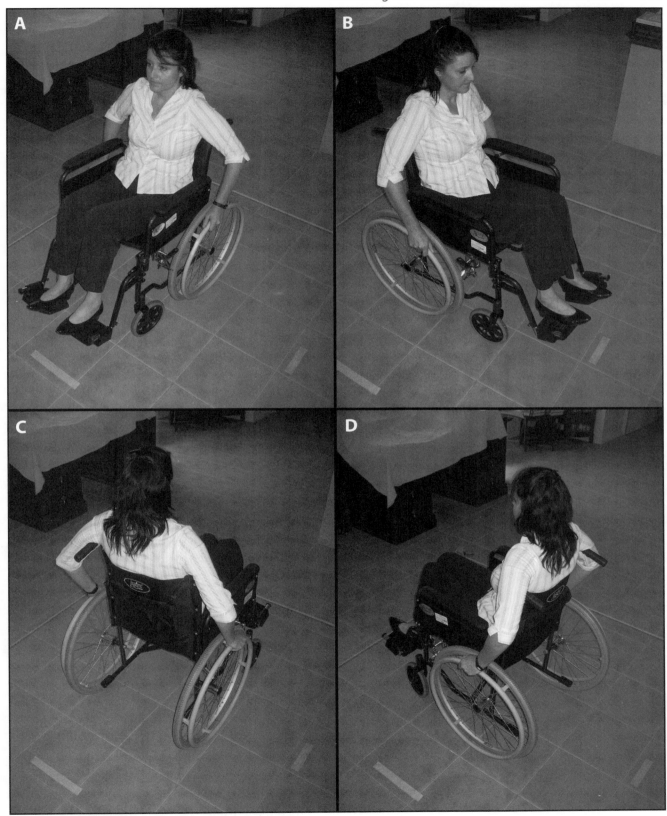

Figure 7-24. Commencing a 360-degree turn.

weight scales. Alternatively, the client might be able to report his or her own weight at the time of the home visit, and the weight of the equipment may be documented in the technical specifications available from medical equipment suppliers. This information is important in designing ramps and other structures that need to take the load of the person and his or her equipment, and these weights can be particularly important if the client has bariatric equipment requirements.

Recording Measurement Information

The measurement information can be recorded in a form similar to Table 7-1, which has been compiled from figures and information from Goldsmith (1976, 2000); Pheasant and Haslegrave (2006); Steinfeld, Maisel, and Feathers (2005); and Steinfeld et al. (2010).

Measuring Features in the Built Environment

The aspects measured in the environment depend on the nature of the environmental barrier or issue that is presented at the time of the home visit. Therapists measure the observable aspects of the home environment to gather information to assist in the redesign of the area. Environmental features typically measured include the length and width of rooms and the height and location of fixtures and fittings. Distances and gradients can also be measured when the person's ability to mobilize around the property needs to be addressed. In addition, therapists may wish to establish noise and lighting levels throughout the home and the force required to open and close doors and drawers.

At times, it might be necessary for a technical specialist to visit the home to undertake more formal and specific measurement activities, particularly in cases where major modifications are to be undertaken or the therapist does not have the skill, training, and technical expertise in specific measurement techniques. For example, a builder can be engaged to measure the levels of external areas around the home in order to design a ramp, or an acoustic engineer might be required to measure the sound levels of a household.

The following section provides information on the various tools and resources used to measure features in the built environment.

Dimensions

Dimensions include measures of length, width, and height and are taken using key reference points within the built environment. These reference points

are conventions documented in publications such as access standards for consistency and to establish the start and finish of a measure. For example, the reference point for measuring dimensions of walls is the finished face of the wall (i.e., the plaster sheeting or tiling, which can be placed on the face of the plaster sheet). The reference points for doorways are in the inside face of the door jamb on the latch side of the doorway and the face of the door leaf in the 90-degree open position. The top of the hand rail or grab bar is the reference point for measuring their height above the nosing of the stair or floor. The center of the operable part of the power or light switch is the reference point for measuring the height above the bench or floor. The center line of the toilet is the reference point for measuring the distance of the toilet from the side wall. Figures 7-25 through 7-28 provide examples of reference points in the built environment that are used during the measurement process.

A number of resources are available to guide therapists in measuring specific features in the built environment and identifying specific reference points. Illustrations of the location of reference points and corresponding dimension lines can guide measurement practice, and they can be found in resources such as the Comprehensive Assessment and Solution Process for Aging Residents (Extended Home Living Service, n.d.), which provides detailed illustrations of the essential measurements for a range of architectural features important to home modifications, such as stairs at entrances and within the home (Figures 7-29 through 7-32).

A range of tools are used to measure dimension as illustrated in Figure 7-33. The most commonly used tools to measure dimensions are the tape measure, distance meter (Figure 7-34), and stud finder (Figure 7-35).

A tape measure should:

+ Be at least 16-ft (5,000-mm) long to measure features in the residential environment, such as the length and width of the room and the height of the ceiling

+ Be made of metal rather than plastic or woven plastic to ensure that this does not stretch, twist, buckle, or sag and result in inaccurate measurements

+ Have markings that can be clearly understood and recognized (Bridge, 1996)

+ Have a wide tape blade so it can be aligned to a feature in the home without sagging

When measuring:

+ A tape measure is easier used on flat surfaces and in an environment that is well lit.

Table 7-1. Measuring a Person and His or Her Mobility Equipment

FEATURE	MEASUREMENT	HOUSING FEATURES (EXAMPLES)	BUILT ENVIRONMENT DIMENSION REQUIRED
General Measurements of the Person—Seated or Standing			
Height		Clearance below overhead obstructions	
Width		Width of doors, hallways	
Depth		Depth of shower seat	
Height above floor level standing—Head height		Height of window awnings	
Height above floor level seated—Head height		Height of window sills, mirror above the vanity	
Height above floor level standing—Shoulder height		Height of fittings, fixtures	
Height above floor level seated—Shoulder height		Height of fittings, fixtures	
Height above floor level seated—Knee height		Height to the underside of sink	
Popliteal height—Seated		Height of toilet, shower seat	
Hip width		Width of shower seat	
Hand width		Diameter of rails	
Popliteal crease to back of buttocks		Depth of shower seat	
Height above floor level standing—Eye height		Height of window sills, mirror above the vanity	
Height above floor level seated—Eye height		Height of window sills, mirror above the vanity	
Functional Reach Range Measurements of the Person—Seated or Standing			
Distance between chest and edge of fingertips—Horizontal reach		Width of counters	
Height above floor level—Forward horizontal reach		Height of power point above bench, door handles, light switches, shelving, towel rails	
Height above floor level—Side horizontal reach		Height of power point above bench, height of shelving, width of laundry hub, height of door handles, height of window latches	
Height above floor level—Forward diagonal (up) reach		Height of hanging rail, clothesline, power points, or cupboards, etc., with straight-on approach	
Height above floor level—Forward diagonal (down) reach		Height of power points or cupboards, etc., with side-on approach	
Height above floor level—Side diagonal (up) reach		Height of hanging rail, clothesline, power points, or cupboards, etc., with straight-on approach	
Height above floor level—Side diagonal (down) reach		Height of power points or cupboards, etc., with side-on approach	

(continued)

Table 7-1. Measuring a Person and His or Her Mobility Equipment (continued)

FEATURE	MEASUREMENT	HOUSING FEATURES (EXAMPLES)	BUILT ENVIRONMENT DIMENSION REQUIRED
Unoccupied and Occupied Equipment Measurements			
Unoccupied Device			
Width of device (unfolded)		Space for storing device	
Width of device (folded)		Space for storing device	
Length of device		Space for storing device	
Height of device		Space for storing device	
Occupied Device			
Width of device (unfolded)		Circulation space required at doorways off corridors, corridor width, ramp width, path width, area required between kitchen counters and in front of appliances	
Length of device (unfolded)		Circulation space required at doorways off corridors and on ramps that turn 90 to 180 degrees; area required between kitchen counters and in front of appliances	
Height above floor level—Floor to toe with foot on wheelchair or shower chair footplate		Height and depth of toe recesses on cupboards	
Height above floor level—Floor to knee or thigh (highest point) with foot on wheelchair or shower chair footplate		Under sink clearance (bathroom and kitchen) or under breakfast bar clearance	
Height above floor level—Wheelchair or shower chair seat height		To compare to toilet seat height (for side- or front-on transfers)	
Height above floor level—Floor to wheelchair or shower chair armrest		Under counter clearance	
Height above floor level—Floor to hand on wheelchair control on armrest		Under counter clearance	
Height of hoist legs		Under bath clearance	
Width of hoist legs with legs closed		Under bath clearance	
Turning circles: 90-degree turn 180-degree turn 360-degree turn		Circulation space required at doorways off corridors and on landings on ramps that turn 90 or 180 degrees; area required between kitchen counters, within a bathroom and bedroom, in front of appliances and cupboards, and at mailbox, clothesline, and garden shed areas	
Weight			
Weight of person		Weight load for lift capacity	
Weight of device		Structural weight load for ramps	
Other			

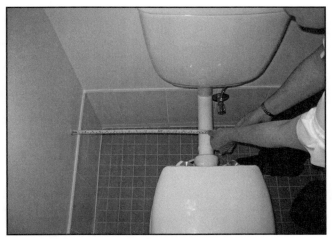

Figure 7-25. Measuring the center line of the toilet.

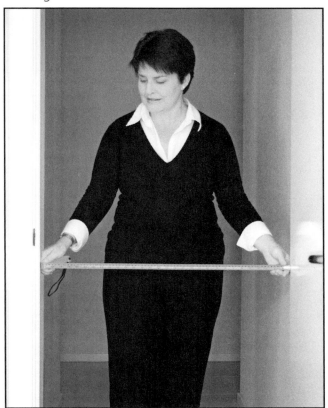

Figure 7-26. Measuring the clearance of the doorway.

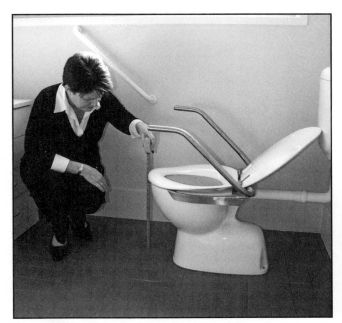

Figure 7-27. Measuring the datum point of the toilet.

✦ The area should be measured at least two or three times to ensure the information is accurate and to establish the average measurement.

✦ Wall lengths should be measured at floor level and at 35.5 in/900 mm above floor level because walls are not always straight (Bridge, 1996).

A battery-powered distance meter can be used to measure horizontal or vertical distances in rooms. The distance meter is particularly useful when measuring distances greater than 197 in/5 m (e.g., example, a vertical clearance such as floor to ceiling or between two walls in a large room). Many distance meters incorporate a laser pointer to assist in accurately positioning the beam for measurement.

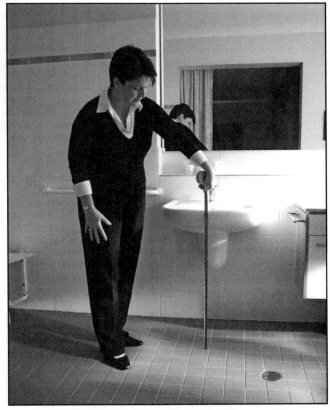

Figure 7-28. Measuring the datum point of the vanity basin.

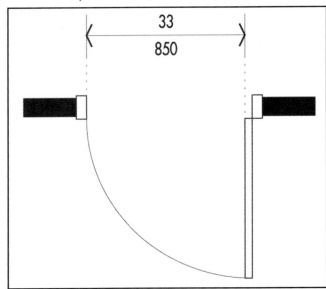

Figure 7-29. Measuring the clearance of a doorway with a swing door. The measurement on top of the line is in inches (imperial measurement), and the measurement below the line is in millimeters (metric measurement).

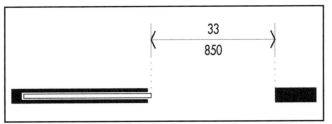

Figure 7-30. Measuring the clearance of a doorway with a sliding door. The measurement on top of the line is in inches (imperial measurement), and the measurement below the line is in millimeters (metric measurement).

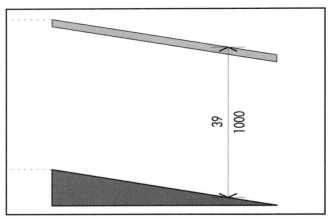

Figure 7-31. Measuring the height of a handrail above the surface of a ramp. The measurement on the top of the line is in inches (imperial measurement), and the measurement below the line is in millimeters (metric measurement).

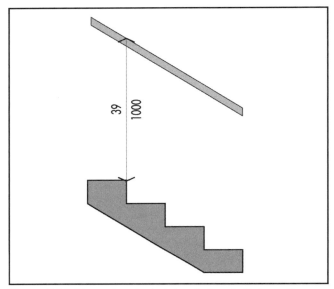

Figure 7-32. Measuring the height of a handrail above the nosing of a step. The measurement on the top of the line is in inches (imperial measurement), and the measurement below the line is in millimeters (metric measurement).

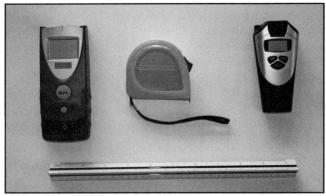

Figure 7-33. Tools to measure dimension.

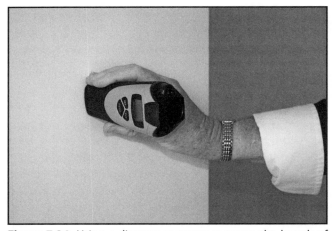

Figure 7-34. Using a distance meter to measure the length of a room.

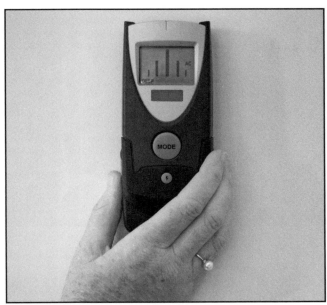

Figure 7-35. Tool used to locate studs.

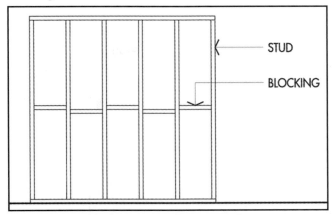

Figure 7-36. Diagram showing studs on a wall.

When using a distance meter, ensure:

✦ The tool sits squarely on a wall or floor surface.

✦ The beam is aimed at a solid feature, such as a wall or ceiling, and no plants, windows, wall furnishings, lights, or other floating matter interfere with the line of sight.

✦ Three sets of measurements are taken and an average established to ensure the accuracy of the data (Bridge, 1996).

Locating Structural Framing

The safe use of load-bearing aids in the home such as grab bars and hoists typically requires that they be fixed to wall or ceiling structural members, such as wall studs or ceiling joists. Wall studs are vertical structural framing members that occur at intervals of typically 18 in (450 mm) or 24 in (600 mm) and to which the wall lining or sheeting is fixed (Figure 7-36). Where such members do not occur or are structurally inadequate for the aid, a new structural member will need to be installed within the framing or on the face of the wall or ceiling lining but fixed to the underlying structure.

Therapists may wish to determine the feasibility of soundly fixing load-bearing aids in the preferred locations for the client and therefore to identify the location of framing members. Though this can assist in designing the recommendation, it is preferable that the tradesperson undertake an accurate assessment of the position and integrity of the structural supports behind the wall facings. For this reason,

therapists might locate the position of studs but not include this information in their drawings so that the builder retains responsibility for determining the capacity of the wall structure to support the grab bar in the recommended location.

Framing members can be found by:

✦ Looking for joints in wall or ceiling linings that indicates the direction of the framing members (they will typically run at right angles to the joints)

✦ Looking for lines of nails or screws

✦ Tapping along wall or ceiling linings to hear changes from hollow to solid knocking sounds (this may be ineffective for dense linings)

✦ A magnetic or electronic stud finder (for timber studs)

✦ A magnet (for steel studs)

Greater accuracy can be achieved by using two or more of these methods. A knowledge of the era in which the home building occurred and the typical spacing and thickness of framing members will expedite finding the framing members.

Electronic stud finders may be much more useful than magnetic ones. There are several different types of electronic stud finders, including ones that can be used for timber or metal framing and that identify the presence of electrical wiring and metal piping.

Tapping and stud finders should be employed along a line at right angles to the direction of the framing member. This will also confirm responses of the stud finder to electrical wiring and metal piping. For example, to find a wall stud, the stud finder should be moved horizontally until a stud is found. The method should continue past the stud or else be repeated in the opposite direction so that the thickness and hence midline of the stud can be

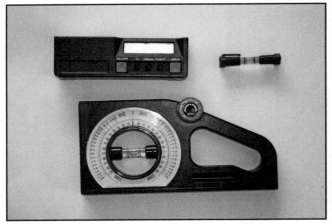

Figure 7-37. Tools to measure gradient.

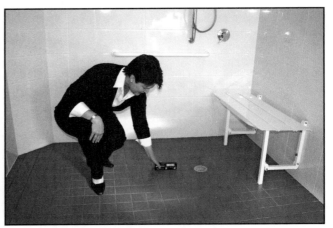

Figure 7-38. Measuring the gradient of the shower floor.

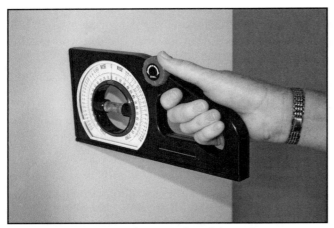

Figure 7-39. Measuring the verticality of the wall.

established. The procedure should be repeated at two or more heights above the floor because the wall studs will not be perfectly parallel with each other or at right angles to floor and to avoid false readings from noggings between studs and electrical wiring or metal piping. Noggings are short horizontal members located between and at approximately the midheight of studs; they impart greater rigidity to framed walls.

For ceilings, care is required to ensure that ceiling battens are not detected instead of ceiling joists. Ceiling joists are small-sectioned members that are fixed to the underside of ceiling joists to achieve, among other things, greater planarity of the ceiling lining (the ceiling lining is fixed to the ceiling battens, not the joists).

Therapists should bear in mind that noggings and ceiling battens are unlikely to be adequate for fixing load-bearing aids. It would be prudent for therapists to seek confirmation from design or construction professionals about the suitability and load-bearing capacity of wall and ceiling structures for the fixing of grab bars, hoists, and other aids.

Gradient

The gradient, or slope, of surfaces influences the ability of a person to walk or wheel around the home and whether water will accumulate on the surfaces. Obtaining measurements of gradients of ramps, paths, landings, or shower floors enables comparison with design guides and standards and thereby the determination of the suitability of the inclined surfaces for ease and safety of movement and the stationary positioning of equipment.

Two methods for determining gradients can be differentiated by trigonometric calculation and by use of a gradient measuring device (Figures 7-37 through 7-39). To determine gradients by trigonometric calculations, at least two dimensions are required: the horizontal and vertical dimension or either of the horizontal or vertical dimensions plus the inclined length. Part of the horizontal or inclined length and the corresponding vertical dimension can be used to calculate the gradient, but this will tend to be less accurate than using the whole length of the inclined surface. Similarly, for greater accuracy, using the vertical dimension with either the horizontal or inclined length is preferable for calculations than use of the horizontal and inclined lengths.

A gradient measuring device indicates the angular difference of a surface with respect to the vertical. Using a gradient measuring device is generally quicker and may be more convenient to determine gradients than by trigonometric calculation. Measuring devices are available in various forms and are called by a variety of names, including *clinometers*, *slope gauges*, and *gradient meters*. Two commonly available devices are the clocklike device whereby the gradient is indicated by a pointer with respect to

Table 7-2. Conversion of Angle Data to Gradient Ratios

(Using trigonometric calculations - tan = opposite/adjacent)

INCLINE IN DEGREES	GRADIENT RATIO OF 1:X	EXAMPLES OF USE OF GRADIENTS IN RELATION TO ARCHITECTURAL FEATURES (MINIMUM GRADIENT)
7.13	1:8	Ramp
5.71	1:10	
4.76	1:12	Ramp
4.09	1:14	Ramp
2.86	1:20	Path
1.91	1:30	
1.43	1:40	Landing, sideways slope of a path, ramp, car park area, or landing
1.15	1:50	1:50 to 1:60 shower recess floor
0.95	1:60	
0.82	1:70	1:70 to 1:80 bathroom floor to the edge of the shower recess
0.72	1:80	
0.64	1:90	
0.57	1:100	
0.27	1:200	

Adapted from "A cheat sheet for converting angle data to gradient ratios": Trigonometric calculations provided by Tanner, D., Senior Mechanical Engineer of ABB Engineering, 1996 (as cited by Bridge, C. (1996). In *Environmental measurement: A handbook for the subject OCCP 5051*. The University of Sydney, School of Occupational Therapy and Leisure Sciences, Faculty of Health Sciences, Cumberland Campus, Lidcombe, Australia. (Chapter 7, pp. 32).

a perimeter scale and, increasingly commonly, the electronic digital gradient indicator. The former device is commonly smaller and may therefore need to be used with a straight edge; it is also prone to inaccurate readings from parallax error.

Units of measure of these devices are degrees, percentage, or both. Interconversion of degrees and percentages, or of either of these and ratios (e.g., 1 in 20 or 1:20), is readily obtainable from websites or by using published tables such as that in Table 7-2.

Measurement procedure:

✦ Take at least three sets of measurements to ensure they are accurate and to gain an average reading.

✦ Ensure the measuring devices are well illuminated and that they are appropriately aligned on the surfaces whose gradients are to be measured. For example, to determine the verticality of walls, the device should be aligned vertically; to determine the gradient of a ramp, the device should be aligned in the direction of travel (or the intended or most common direction of travel) and at right angles to it to establish the cross-fall; to establish the gradient of a four-sided shower floor with four facets sloping to a drainage outlet, the device should be aligned along the shortest distance between the drain and each of the sides (i.e., along a line from the center of the outlet and at right angles to each side).

Irregularity of surface gradient is not uncommon and needs careful consideration. Obtaining several measurements and using a straight edge enables an average or overall gradient to be determined. However, any localized gradients should also be measured because gradient irregularities can impede travel on inclined surfaces. Moreover, two relevant lengths, or scale, of localized gradient might need to be considered: that over which a wheel has to travel in, say, part of its revolution, or the length corresponding with the wheel base of wheeled equipment (the distance between the ground contact points of front and rear wheels). Three gradients may therefore need to be obtained: that of the steepest "small" irregularity on the inclined surface, that of the steepest "medium" irregularity on the inclined surface, and the overall or average gradient.

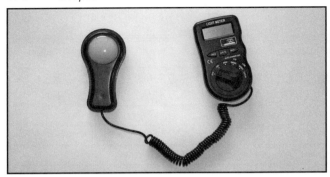

Figure 7-40. Tool to measure lighting levels.

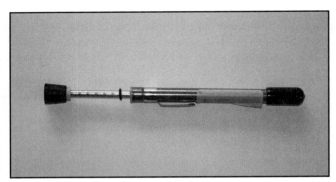

Figure 7-41. Tool used to measure force.

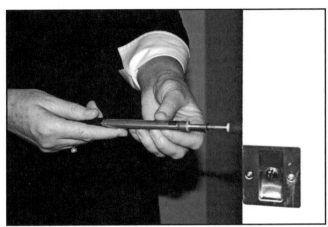

Figure 7-42. Measuring door force.

Gradient is particularly relevant in the design of ramps. Instructions on how to determine the location and configuration of external ramps can be found in Appendix D.

Light

Lighting can facilitate a person's ability to see. However, if it is not set at the correct level, it can impede function and eventually damage vision (Spaulding, 2008b). In an indoor environment, lighting is provided by both ambient and artificial light. Ambient light can vary, depending on the season of the year and the time of day. It generally comes from outside through windows, whereas artificial light is emitted from fittings such as light bulbs (Spaulding, 2008b).

Lighting must be provided, by natural and/or artificial light sources, so that there is sufficient illumination of the activity area but without causing glare. People vary in their requirements for levels of illumination and in their sensitivity to glare.

To determine whether lighting levels are adequate, therapists examine lighting levels in different areas of the home where people mobilize and undertake specific tasks. Measurements are generally taken on stairs and ramps; in entries and hallways; and in kitchens, living areas, bathrooms, and bedrooms. A light meter is used to measure the level of lighting, and this is recorded in lux (Figure 7-40). Recommended lux measures for various areas of the home may be found in design guides and standards. Further information on suitable lighting conditions for people with specific vision impairments should be sought from vision impairment experts or organizations such as Lighthouse International (www. lighthouse.org).

When measuring:

+ Take three readings to ensure data are reliable and to establish an average measurement.

+ Take readings at different times of the day when activities are more likely to occur in the area to ensure a true reading of variation in lighting.

+ Be aware that the accuracy of these readings can vary as a result of daylight and adjacent reflective surfaces or if the batteries are low.

+ Place the light meter on the work or viewing surface. For example, if the task was writing at a desk, the light meter would be placed flat on the desk. Where the task is viewing an item on the wall, the light meter would be placed vertically on the wall (Bridge, 1996).

Force

Force is required to open, hold, or swing features such as doors, drawers, and windows. Although door-force gauges are mainly used to measure forces required to push moving features in the public access arena, they can also be used in the home environment if people are experiencing difficulty with specific features (Figures 7-41 and 7-42). Spring-load measures are used to measure the amount of force required to open features such as drawers. These gauges measure force in newtons and/or pounds.

When measuring push force:

✦ Place the device at the point on the door where the force is to be applied.

✦ Move the feature using force uniformly and slowly, in a consistent horizontal/vertical/oblique direction as required.

✦ Take three sets of measurements to ensure reliability and to get an average measurement (Bridge, 1996).

When measuring pull force:

✦ Position the hook in the middle of the handle on the drawer where pull force is applied.

✦ Use a perpendicular line of action to gain a reading at the point of maximal force to stretch the load measure.

✦ Take measurements three times to ensure reliability and to get an average reading (Bridge, 1996).

Sound

Sound is a combination of either simple or complex waveforms (Spaulding, 2008b) and, when unwanted (now called *noise*), can interfere with how a person manages in the home environment. Factors affecting the individual's response may relate to sound level, duration of exposure, or frequency of the sound (Spaulding, 2008b). Sound-level meters are used to measure noise levels. The formal testing of sound in the home environment is usually completed by an ergonomist or acoustic engineer rather than a therapist.

Recording Measurements of the Home Environment

Occupational therapists can develop specific forms to record the information gathered using tools to measure the built environment or add the information into existing forms such as the Comprehensive Assessment and Solution Process for Aging Residents (Extended Home Living Service, n.d.).

General Considerations in Measurement Practice

There may be changes in a person's measurements and capacity as he or she ages, which might affect his or her posture, height, hand/arm and leg strength, body breadth, visual acuity, and weight. Over time, people might experience changes in their health and capacities and alterations in the type or dimensions of the equipment or level of caregiver support they use. Therapists need to anticipate possible changes, accommodate variability in individual performance and household structure, and adjust measurements accordingly. In some situations (e.g., with a growing child) therapists will need to plan regular reviews as the situation changes and new equipment is required.

Factors Influencing Accuracy of Measurement

A range of factors influence occupational therapy measurement practice, including the following:

✦ The competence of the person taking the measurements

✦ Tool selection use and training

✦ Time allocated for the visit

✦ The nature of the measure or feature

✦ The condition of the measurement tools

✦ The timing of measurement

The Competence of the Person Taking the Measurements

Measurement error is described as having four components: error in the measuring equipment itself, error in locating the landmark or reference point, error in standardizing the posture of the person or positioning of the measuring tool, and error in the client's understanding or response to instructions on adopting the required posture or obstacles in the environment (Pheasant & Haslegrave, 2006).

To prevent measurement error, occupational therapists need to be competent and well trained in measurement practice. This includes understanding measurement practice, knowing how to take accurate measurements, and recording measurements in a meaningful format. Therapists should ensure that the measurement process generates consistent, quality information by using reliable tools and being comprehensive when gathering and documenting data.

Tool Selection, Use, and Training

Therapists can use various sophisticated devices and techniques to measure body dimensions, including calipers, tape scales, weight scales, protractors, and computer-aided anthropometric tools. Occupational therapists generally do not have access to such equipment and will need to observe the client and use a tape measure to measure basic body dimensions, reach range, and clearances. For analysis, therapists could also take digital footage of the client reaching and moving. Alternatively, therapists might want to undertake training in specific measurement techniques to enhance their competencies in the area.

The environmental measurement tools selected by therapists generally provide operating instructions. Although this information might be included when tools are first purchased, it is important that the therapist checks with people providing any technical design or building advice on how they measure features in the environment as there is variation in practice within the design and construction industry. For example, a tape measure is used to check the height and size of the light switch plate, but the therapist needs to confirm the reference point for light switches with an electrician, designer, or building professional.

Time Allocated for the Visit

Therapists must allocate sufficient time for taking measurements during the visit. This includes time for measuring the client, their equipment, and carer, as well as the environment. The therapist will need to allocate 1 to 2 hours to observe and measure the client, the equipment, their carer, and the environment depending on the extent of modifications required. If time is limited at the initial visit, a subsequent appointment might be required to complete the measurement process. If there are insufficient resources such as time and money to undertake repeated measures, therapists are to make sure the method chosen is valid, has been tested rigorously, and compares with other measures (Steinfeld & Danford, 1997). This requires an understanding of which tool and technique to use in relation to the factors to be measured in the person-environment fit. It can be time consuming to measure all dimensions of the existing room, person, caregiver, and all equipment used in the house; however, taking thorough measurements at the initial visit can reduce the need for a repeat visit and avoid the difficulties faced when working with incomplete information.

The Nature of the Measure or Feature

The type of measurements taken by therapists can include, for example, static measurements of the client standing and using various postures to reach or bend or dynamic measurements of the client completing a movement to determine the space or clearance required for the activity. Some features, such as the diameter of grab bars or handrails or the width of lips on baths, are difficult to measure accurately due to the round surface.

The Condition of the Measurement Tools

For accuracy and ease of use, measurement tools need to be kept in good working order, be regularly cleaned or calibrated, and, for battery-powered devices, batteries regularly checked or replaced.

Timing of the Measurement

A person's performance can vary between different times of the day, week, or season, depending upon factors such as fatigue, temperature, and the level and type of illuminance of the environment. Variance in posture can also occur (Pheasant & Haslegrave, 2006). Measurements of performance and posture may therefore also vary, and this should be considered in deciding upon the time and/or frequency of home visits for measuring purposes. For example, it may be preferable to visit the client at the beginning of the day when they have the most energy for activities, or the therapist may choose to visit when the client requires considerable assistance during performance of activities and to gather measurements. There may be variation in space requirements for the client, their equipment, and carer during activities with these two circumstances that need to be considered in planning the home modification.

Variations in measurement may need to be recorded, with specific reference to those factors influencing the data (Dunn, 2005; Law & Baum, 2005; Law, Baum, & Dunn, 2005). Knowledge of this variation can lead to an enhanced understanding of the individual's specific situation and ensure that the modification is designed to work for the client at all times (Dunn, 2005).

CONCLUSION

This chapter has provided the reader with information on the role of measurement in improving the person-environment fit. The contribution of anthropometrics, biomechanics, and ergonomics to measurement practice has been described in addition to how each is used by occupational therapists to inform home modification practice. The value of taking an individualized approach to measuring clients and their home environment has been emphasized, and the range of tools and resources that are available to assist this process has been described. Also discussed is the importance of considering the range of factors that can affect the measurement process.

Although occupational therapists need to work collaboratively with building industry stakeholders to understand the building industry's approach to measurement of the environment, it is recognized that design and construction professionals do not have the expertise to undertake such a technical and detailed approach in isolation from therapists. Occupational therapy training in the use of various tools and measurement techniques continues to be required for therapists working in home modifications to ensure that clinical reasoning about changes to the home environment is based on sound evidence rather than guesswork and to ensure an optimal home modification solution for the client.

REFERENCES

Australian Safety and Compensation Council. (2009). Sizing up Australia: How contemporary is the anthropometric data Australian designers use. *Commonwealth of Australia*. Retrieved from http://www.safeworkaustralia.gov.au/NR/rdonlyres/95EED167-56D7-41EA-9E17-51A0121F8EC9/0/Sizing_up_Australia_report.pdf

Baker, N. A. (2008). Anthropometry. In K. Jacobs (Ed.), *Ergonomics for therapists* (pp. 73-93). St. Louis, MO: Mosby Incorporated.

Berg Rice, V. J. (2008). Ergonomics and therapy: An introduction. In K. Jacobs & C. M. Bettencourt (Eds.), *Ergonomics for therapists* (pp. 1-16). Newton, MA: Butterworth-Heinemann.

Bridge, C. (1996). *Environmental measurement: A handbook for the subject OCCP 5051.* Lidcombe, Australia: The University of Sydney, School of Occupational Therapy and Leisure Sciences, Faculty of Health Sciences, Cumberland Campus.

Bridge, C. (2005). Computational case-based redesign for people with ability impairment: Rethinking, reuse and redesign learning for home modification practice (Unpublished thesis). University of Sydney, Sydney, Australia.

Chan, D., Laporte, D. M., & Sveistrup, H. (1999). Rising from sitting in elderly people, part 2: Strategies to facilitate rising. *British Journal of Occupational Therapy, 62*(2), 64-68.

Ching, F. D. K. (1995). *A visual dictionary of architecture.* New York: Van Nostrand Reinhold.

Connell, B. R., & Sanford, J. A. (1999). Research implications of universal design. In E. Steinfeld & G. S. Danford (Eds.), *Enabling environments: Measuring the impact of the environment on disability and rehabilitation* (pp. 35-57). New York: Kluwer Academic/Plenum Publishers.

Conway, M. (2008). *Occupational therapy and inclusive design: Principles for practice.* Oxford, UK: John Wiley & Sons.

Cooper, R. A. (1998). *Wheelchair selection and configuration.* New York: Demos Medical Publishing.

Diffrient, N., Tilley, A. R., & Bardagjy, J. (1974). *Humanscale 1-3.* Cambridge, MA: MIT Press.

Dunn, W. (2005). Measurement issues and practices. In M. Law, C. Baum, & W. Dunn (Eds.), *Measuring occupational performance: Supporting best practice in occupational therapy* (pp. 21-32). Thorofare, NJ: SLACK Incorporated.

Extended Home Living Service. (n.d.). CASPAR: Comprehensive assessment and solution process for aging residents. Retrieved from http://www.ehls.com/CASPAROverview.pdf

Goldsmith, S. (1976). *Designing for the disabled.* London: RIBA Publications.

Goldsmith, S. (2000). *Universal design.* Oxford, UK: Architectural Press.

Han, C. S., Law, K. H., Latombe, J. C., & Kunz, J. C. (2002). A performance-based approach to wheelchair accessible route analysis. *Advanced Engineering Informatics, 16*(1), 53-71.

Hunter, R. A. (2002). Testing wheelchair driving skills: The slalom. Retrieved from http://www.hunarch.com.au/Articles/The%20slalom.pdf

Hunter, R. A. (2003a). *Review of Bails's A80 Wheelchair Research and its application to AS1428.* Balwyn, Australia: Hunarch Consulting.

Hunter, R. A. (2003b). Vehicle tracking with corrugated paper. Retrieved from http://www.hunarch.com.au/Articles/Veh%20tracking%20wi%20Corrug%20Paper.pdf

Hunter, R. A. (2005). Automated reconfiguration of path boundaries for wheelchair access. Paper presented at Include 2005 Conference, Royal College of Art, April 5-8, 2005; London, UK.

Hunter, R. A. (2009). Asymmetry of occupied wheelchairs and scooters. Retrieved from http://www.hunarch.com.au/Articles/Shapes%20of%20occupied%20wheelchairs%20and%20scooters.pdf

International Organization for Standardization. (2005). ISO 7176-5:2008 Wheelchairs—Part 5: Determination of dimensions, mass and manoeuvring space. Retrieved from https://www.iso.org/standard/46429.html

Kreighbaum, E., & Barthels, K. M. (1996). *Biomechanics: A qualitative approach to studying human movement.* Needham Heights, MA: Allyn & Bacon.

Kroemer, K. H. E. (1987). Biomechanics of the human body. In G. Salvendy (Ed.), *Handbook of human factors* (pp. 169-181). New York: John Wiley & Sons.

Laporte, D. M., Chan, D., & Sveistrup, H. (1999). Rising from sitting in elderly people, part 1: Implications of biomechanics and physiology. *British Journal of Occupational Therapy, 62*(1), 36-42.

Law, M., & Baum, C. (2005). Measurement in occupational therapy. In M. Law, C. Baum, & W. Dunn (Eds.), *Measuring occupational performance: Supporting best practice in occupational therapy* (pp. 3-20). Thorofare, NJ: SLACK Incorporated.

Law, M., Baum, C., & Dunn, W. (2005). *Measuring occupational performance: Supporting best practice in occupational therapy.* Thorofare, NJ: SLACK Incorporated.

Panero, J., & Zelnik, M. (1979). *Human dimension and interior space: A sourcebook of design reference standards.* London: Architectural Press Ltd.

Paquet, V., & Feathers, D. (2004). An anthropometric study of manual and powered wheelchair users. *International Journal of Industrial Ergonomics, 33*, 191-204.

Pedretti, L. W. (1996). Occupational performance: A model for practice in physical dysfunction. In L. W. Pedretti (Ed.), *Occupational therapy: Practice skills for physical dysfunction* (pp. 3-12). St. Louis, MO: Mosby.

Pheasant, S. (1987). *Ergonomics—Standards and guidelines for designers.* Suffolk, UK: Richard Clay Ltd.

Pheasant, S. (1996). *Bodyspace: Anthropometry, ergonomics and the design of work.* London: T. J. Press.

Pheasant, S., & Haslegrave, C. M. (2006). *Bodyspace: Anthropometry, ergonomics and the design of work* (3rd ed.). London: Taylor & Francis Group.

Ringaert, L., Rapson, D., Qiu, J., Cooper, J., & Shwedyk, E. (2001). *Determination of new dimensions for universal design codes and standards with consideration of powered wheelchair and scooter users.* Manitoba, CA: Universal Design Institute.

Sanford, J. A. (2012). *Universal design as a rehabilitation strategy.* New York: Springer Publishing Company.

Spaulding, S. J. (2008a). Basic biomechanics. In K. Jacobs (Ed.), *Ergonomics for therapists* (pp. 94-102). St. Louis, MO: Mosby.

Spaulding, S. J. (2008b). Physical environment. In K. Jacobs (Ed.), *Ergonomics for therapists* (pp. 137-150). St. Louis, MO: Mosby.

Standards Australia. (1994). *Glossary of building terms.* Sydney, Australia: Author.

Stein, F., Soderback, I., Cutler, S. K., & Larson, B. (2006). *Occupational therapy and ergonomics: Applying ergonomic principles to everyday occupation in the home and at work.* Chichester, West Sussex, UK: Whurr Publishers, Inc.

Steinfeld, E. (2004). Modeling spatial interaction through full scale modeling. *International Journal of Industrial Ergonomics, 33,* 265-278.

Steinfeld, E., & Danford, S. (1997). Environment as a mediating factor in functional assessment. In S. S. Dittmar & G. E. Gresham (Eds.), *Functional assessment and outcome measures for the rehabilitation health professional* (pp. 37-56). Gaithersburg, MD: Aspen Publishers.

Steinfeld, E., Lenker, J., & Paquet, V. (2002). The anthropometrics of disability. Retrieved from http://www.ap.buffalo.edu/idea/anthro/the%20anthropometrics%20of%20disability.pdf

Steinfeld, E., & Maisel, J.L. (2012). *Universal design: Creating inclusive environments.* Hoboken, NJ: John Wiley and Sons.

Steinfeld, E., Maisel, J., & Feathers, D. (2005). Standards and anthropometry for wheeled mobility. Buffalo, NY: Center for Inclusive Design and Environmental Access (IDEA), School of Architecture and Planning, University of Buffalo. Retrieved from http://www.ap.buffalo.edu/idea/Anthro/FinalAccessReport.pdf

Steinfeld, E., Paquet, V., D'Souza, C.., Joseph, C., & Maisel, J. (2010). Anthropometry of wheeled mobility: Final report. Buffalo, NY: IDEA Center. Retrieved from http://www.udeworld.com/documents/anthropometry/pdfs/AnthropometryofWheeledMobilityProject_FinalReport.pdf

Steinfeld, E., Schroeder, S., & Bishop, M. (1979). *Accessible buildings for people with walking and reaching limitations.* Washington, DC: U.S. Department of Housing and Urban Development.

Steinfeld, E., Schroeder, S., Duncan, J., Faste, R., Chollet, D., Bishop, M., . . . Cardell, P. (1979). *Access to the built environment: A review of literature* (pp. 98-128). Washington, DC: US Department of Housing and Urban Development, Office of Policy Development and Research.

8

Drawing the Built Environment

Elizabeth Ainsworth, MOccThy, Grad Cert Health Sci
and Desleigh de Jonge, MPhil (OccThy), Grad Cert Soc Sci

Measuring the built environment is an important part of the home modification process to ensure that there is detail for the planning of environmental interventions. Once measurements have been taken of the existing home environment, this information needs to be put into a format that can be understood by the person approving the recommendations, developing the architectural drawings, or undertaking the modification work. Occupational therapists need to know how to read and use drawings and have an understanding of their basic components in order to communicate effectively with others in the home modification field. Therapists need to know the different stages of plan development and the alternative types of plan views and be familiar with the technical drawing conventions used in the design profession in order to communicate with construction personnel. An understanding of how and when to draw to scale and being familiar with the various types of drawing tools and technologies can enhance the professionalism and credibility of therapists as they work with others in the design and building profession.

CHAPTER OBJECTIVES

By the end of this chapter, the reader will be able to:

✦ Describe the purpose of drawings and concept drawing requirements for occupational therapy home modification reports

✦ Recognize the value of knowing how to read drawings and draw using various tools and technologies

✦ Describe the range of tools and resources available for developing concept drawings

✦ Recognize the importance of clear documentation to inform the work of the design and/or construction professional

RECORDING ENVIRONMENTAL MEASUREMENT INFORMATION

The Purpose of Drawings

Drawings are a means of communicating ideas to all parties involved in the planning, design, and construction of the building represented. These ideas are set out in a pictorial format that incorporates spaces filled with shapes and objects (Housing Industry Association & Illaring Pty Ltd., 2006). Being the language of the building design and construction industry, drawings are used to visualize possibilities, study alternatives, and present design ideas about

Ainsworth, E., & de Jonge, D. *An Occupational Therapist's Guide to Home Modification Practice, Second Edition (pp. 175-194).*
© 2019 SLACK Incorporated.

the form and spaces of a building (Ching & Eckler, 2013). To be useful for this purpose, they need to be clear, consistent, easy to comprehend, and free of ambiguity for the reader.

Occupational therapy drawings are not architectural drawings because therapists do not have professional training in this field. Rather, therapists develop concept drawings to clearly detail what is required for the home modification and to complement the individual's background information and the proposed scope of works in their report. Concept drawings describe the basic design and modification elements and approximate dimensions in the current and proposed home environment using basic technical drawing conventions. Depending on the type and complexity of the home modification work, concept drawings can be drawn by hand or developed using basic computer software. Concept drawings differ from architectural drawings, which are more precise and detailed and adhere to strict technical drawing conventions. Concept drawings do not contain the same level of detail, but rather provide an overview of the basic layout of spaces, fittings and fixtures and their associated dimensions.

Concept drawings are used to communicate with a broad range of people from a variety of backgrounds and interests in the home modification process. These people include clients, other health professionals, people involved in the design and construction industry, and staff in organizations providing funding for the modifications. Primarily, these drawings are used by occupational therapists to describe clients' requirements; however, they are often used as the basis of the tendering and quoting process for home modifications where the work is small in size and able to be installed by people who may or may not be registered tradespersons, or for the development of more detailed architectural drawings where home modifications are complex and need to be installed by registered building professionals. Concept drawings can provide a foundation for the following:

+ Communicating the intent of the building work

+ Discussing design and modification proposals and issues

+ Illustrating proposed changes or variations to the building work

When minor changes are required to be made to the design, these alterations can be put in writing in a report and noted directly on the drawing; however, if major changes are needed, a new set of drawings is usually developed. This allows the design to evolve and the final option to be documented clearly. Concept drawings also serve as a useful audit tool during and after the home modification works have been completed to ensure that the work has been done as planned by the design and/or building professional.

Resources to Assist Drawing Practice

Organizations such as the International Organization for Standardization, American National Standards Institute (ANSI), Standards Australia, the British Standards Institution, and the Canadian Standards Association establish common practice across the industry and contribute to the development of rules or manuals for the preparation and presentation of drawing documents. These standards describe the technical drawing conventions used in drawings to denote the overall layout of the design and the various features in the built environment.

Textbooks by Bielefeld and Skiba (2013); Ching (2015); Ching and Eckler (2013); Clutton, Grisbrooke, and Pengelly (2006); Thorpe (1994); and Yee (2012) and online resources can also be used to guide occupational therapy drawing practice. These books and online resources include recommendations for drawing practice relating to dimensioning, lines, symbols, abbreviations, scales, layout of drawing sheets, orientation of drawings, architectural conventions for cross-referencing drawings, coordinates, grids, and material representation. They also provide architects, building designers, contractors, and occupational therapists with information about methods of presenting drawings before, during, and after the modification of a building.

READING AND UNDERSTANDING DRAWINGS

Development of Architectural Drawings

Reading and understanding the different types of architectural drawings enables occupational therapists to communicate more efficiently and effectively with design and construction professionals. Once therapists learn the language and practice of the design and construction industry, they can critically appraise plans to assess their suitability in relation to the design needs of their clients (Ashlee, Clutton, Pengelly, & Cowderoy, 2006). This ensures the person-environment fit as described in previous chapters.

There are three types of architectural drawings in home modification practice that therapists are likely to encounter and need to be able to read and understand: sketch design drawings, developed design drawings, and working drawings.

Sketch Design Drawings

Sketch design drawings are simple or quickly executed drawings representing the essential features of an object or scene. Lacking detail, they are often used as a preliminary study (Ching, 2015). In outline form, these drawings depict the designer's general intention. They give an overall picture of the scheme but do not show constructional details and are usually prepared early in the development of a design with the aim to give those involved some general information on how things ultimately go together in the bigger picture. These plans indicate space but do not provide significant detail or dimensions. An occupational therapist, architect, or builder might do a range of sketch drawings of a room or area of the house to show the client how the various features might be laid out (Figure 8-1). This type of drawing can stimulate discussion about different design layouts to create the best possible option for the area being built or modified.

Developed Design Drawings

Developed design drawings are more complex than sketch design drawings and are usually completed by an architect or licensed building contractor. These drawings provide detailed information about the overall layout of the built environment and the relationships of the spaces within and around the building. They can include, for example, illustrations of furniture placement and other features within and around the home and equipment turning circles using specific technical design conventions. The plans include specific illustrations and technical design conventions but are not as developed as those used at the working drawing stage. They are more pictorial than technical in nature and are less likely to feature the drawing conventions of the working drawings that are produced for construction or modification work.

Sketch designs and developed design drawings are often done freehand or, if computer generated, are presented to appear freehand. The reader may feel more comfortable offering feedback if drawings are "only" freehand than if they have the "firmed up" look of technically drafted drawings.

Working Drawings

Working drawings show, in graphical or pictorial form, the design, location, dimensions, and

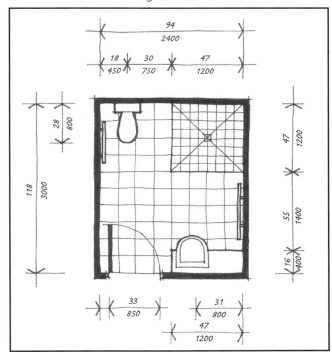

Figure 8-1. Sketch drawing of a bathroom floor plan, not to scale. The measurement on top of the line is in inches (imperial measurement), and the measurement below the line is in millimeters (metric measurement).

relationships of elements of a building (Ching, 2015). They describe the constituent parts of a building, articulate their relationships, and reveal how they go together (Ching & Eckler, 2013). Using different technical drawing conventions than those of developed drawings, working drawings are usually developed by the architect or licensed building designer and are used to guide contractors as they undertake the building work (Figure 8-2). For example, developed drawings might show an illustration of a bathroom in pictorial form using simple lines, whereas working drawings would be more technical and use specific lines to represent the features in this area in more detail on the plan.

There are usually various sets of drawings at this stage, each describing in detail different aspects of the design, such as site plans, floor plans, elevations, sections, and drainage plans. Such complex drawings are usually drawn using drafting equipment or computer software rather than freehand.

Plan Documentation Process for Home Modification Work

Drawings can be documented and classified according to the type of information presented. A design process for home modifications might include

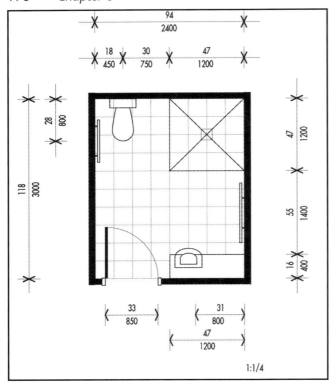

Figure 8-2. Working drawing of a bathroom floor plan. The measurement on top of the line is in inches (imperial measurement), and the measurement below the line is in millimeters (metric measurement).

the development of sketch and/or working drawings for the tender, quoting, and construction processes (Wang, 1996).

Because home modification work can be extensive, costly, and time consuming to draw to scale, it is preferable that occupational therapists and clients rely on an architect or building designer for these complex drawings. The completion of drawings by an architect or building designer may be a mandatory requirement under legislation, depending on the nature and extent of work to be completed. This practice needs to be checked with local authorities to ensure that therapists who choose to do their own drawings are not operating outside their area of professional expertise or beyond the extent of their qualifications.

TYPES OF VIEWS USED IN DRAWINGS

Various types of views can be incorporated into the drawings to understand and depict the total 3D configuration of the built environment. The most common drawing types designers use to communicate their design ideas are plans, elevations, and sections (Wang, 1996). These are the drawings through which most buildings can be read, and they make up one part of a whole series of documentation that describes a building in detail (Dernie, 2014).

Occupational therapists use plan, elevation, and section views in their concept drawings, depending on the size and complexity of the home modification work to be undertaken and the amount of detail to be provided for design or construction professionals. For example:

+ An elevation might be drawn for the installation of a grab bar beside the toilet.
+ An elevation and floor plan view might be drawn for a bathroom undergoing extensive home modifications.
+ A section might be drawn of a set of stairs or a vanity to illustrate the location of the shelving in the cupboard.

Site Plan

The site plan is a view looking down on a site from above, illustrating location and orientation of the building on a parcel of land, and providing information about the site's topography, landscaping, utilities, and site work (Ching & Eckler, 2013). The site plan also details site boundaries and the location of the street, paths, and existing and adjacent buildings. There are various styles of lines used in drawings (e.g., thick lines to denote the external walls of the home and covered outdoor areas; thinner lines to represent the planted areas, pavements, and driveways; and dotted lines to indicate the line of the roof of the building).

From the site plan, a reader can glean the indoor/outdoor relationship between the landscape and the building and the orientation of the building in relation to the direction of the sunrise and sunset and the prevailing breezes, as well as location in relation to structures or features on the site and adjacent to the site (Figure 8-3). Features on the site may include trees and permanent structures such as separate car parking facilities, storage facilities, and boundary fencing. Structures adjacent to the site may include trees and buildings occupied by neighbors and local council structures such as electricity poles and paths.

Floor Plan

Of all of the working drawings, the floor plan is one of the most important because it includes the

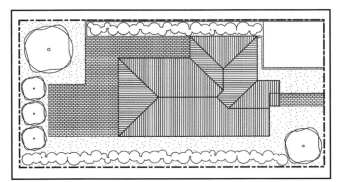

Figure 8-3. Site plan.

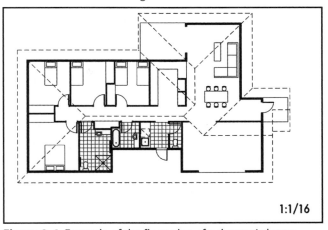

1:1/16

Figure 8-4. Example of the floor plan of a domestic home.

Elevation

An elevation is a horizontal or side view of a building's interior or exterior, usually taken from a point of view perpendicular to the principal vertical surfaces. It illustrates the size, shape, and materials of the interior or exterior surfaces, as well as the size, proportion, and nature of the door and window openings in the design (Ching & Eckler, 2013). Elevations show distance, length, width, and height dimensions of areas and features and are named by the direction they face (e.g., a north elevation faces north). Internal elevations may be cross-referenced and named through a diagram on the floor plan (e.g., four arrows labeled A to D in the center of the floor plan can each point to four internal walls represented in the corresponding elevation view; Figures 8-5 through 8-10).

Section

A building section is a cross-sectional or horizontal view after a vertical plane is cut through a building and the front portion is removed. It reveals the vertical and, in one direction, the horizontal dimensions of a building's spaces and can illustrate the thickness of floors, roofs, and walls. Sections can also include exterior and interior elevations seen beyond the plane of the cut (Figure 8-11; Ching & Eckler, 2013).

Overall, sections add depth and meaning to the drawings, as well as interest. These types of drawings can take on a variety of appearances due to the evolutionary nature of the design process (Wang, 1996).

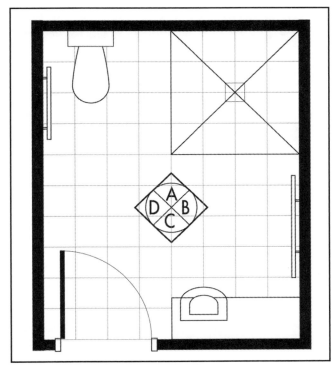

Figure 8-5. Bathroom floor plan.

greatest amount of information. It is a sectional drawing obtained by passing an imaginary cutting plane through the walls above the floor, usually at a height that allows windows to be located. The floor plan is a view looking down from above, and it illustrates the dimensions of a building's spaces, as well as the thickness and construction of the vertical walls and columns that define these spaces (Figure 8-4). Among other features, it will show the building layout, room sizes, door and window placement, and bathroom and kitchen design (Ching & Eckler, 2013). The floor plan illustrates distance, circulation space, width, depth, length of areas, and features (see Figure 8-4).

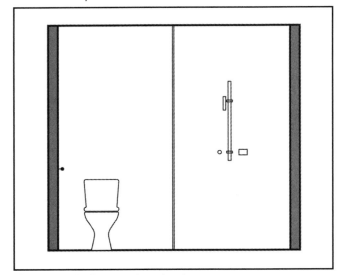

Figure 8-6. Bathroom, elevation A.

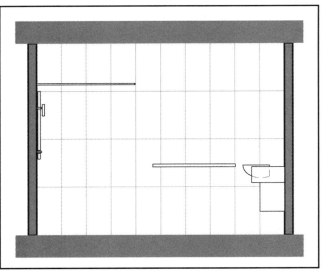

Figure 8-7. Bathroom, elevation B.

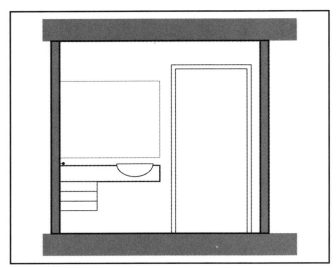

Figure 8-8. Bathroom, elevation C.

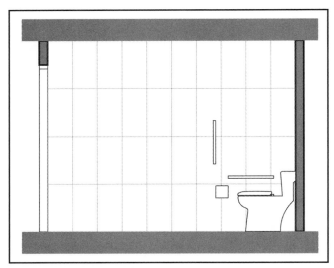

Figure 8-9. Bathroom, elevation D.

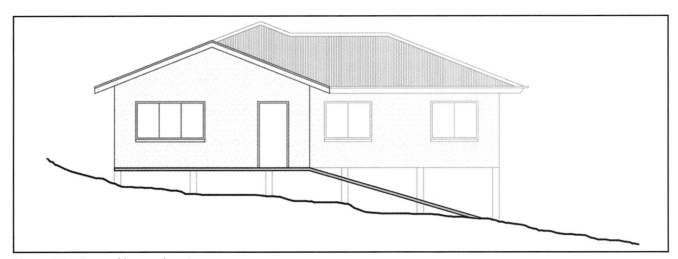

Figure 8-10. External house elevation.

SPECIFICATIONS

Once finalized, plans form the basis from which the agreed building work is undertaken. They can be used with, or as an alternative to, a written specification (Ashlee et al., 2006). Because drawings in themselves might not convey all of the information, written specifications can be developed to provide a detailed description of the technical nature of the materials, standards, and quality of execution of the work. The specifications are a business document, a contract document, and a working document, and they serve a diversity of readers (Standen, 1995). They provide the following:

+ Evidence to the person paying for the construction or modification that the building will include his or her requirements

+ Information on items to be priced that are not indicated on the drawings

+ A record of what has been built or modified

+ A reference during inspections to check that the correct products, designs, and features have been incorporated into the design or modification (Standen, 1995)

The drawings should be used to show whatever is best displayed by the drawings, and the specification should be used to communicate information that is best described by words (Standen, 1995). By way of example, a drawing might indicate the need for tiles in a bathroom and the pattern in which they are to be laid. A specification will identify the tile manufacturer, the color, the slip resistance when wet or dry for pedestrians walking on the product, the method of installation, and the type and color of the grout. The specification can be prepared by a builder, engineer, architect, or licensed building designer to advise a contractor about the materials and workmanship that is expected and that cannot be displayed on the plans.

Access standards can be referred to in a specification to direct the reader to review the most appropriate section of the standards when completing the construction or modification. It is essential that occupational therapists and the reader of the specification understand the application and intent of the access standards to ensure that they are referenced appropriately during the design and modification process. If the therapist is requesting complex or extensive home modifications, a design or construction professional might be required to develop a detailed building specification to provide the required level of technical detail for quoting and construction purposes. If required, therapists

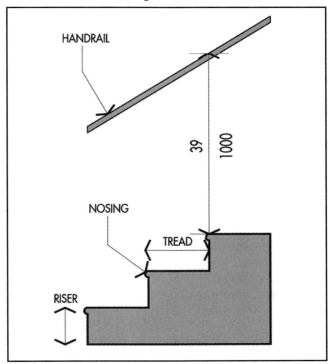

Figure 8-11. Stairs. Section view. The measurement on top of the line is in inches (imperial measurement), and the measurement below the line is in millimeters (metric measurement).

should refer the design and construction professional to specific figures or clauses in the access standards that describe the specific performance criteria for products and building work.

UNDERSTANDING SCALE

The aim of scale drawings are to prevent confusion and to ensure consistent documentation of information for use by design and construction professionals. They are drawn to conventions, with design features such as walls, doors, windows, and stairs, that will look the same on different plans for different buildings.

Scale drawings allow therapists to examine the layout, dimensions, and spaces in the drawing to determine whether the person (the caregiver and/or the equipment he or she uses) can move between buildings and external areas or into and within the home and utilize the space, fittings, and fixtures effectively. It is a means of transferring or reducing information from actual size to a more convenient size with which to work and represent on a suitably proportioned piece of paper (Ashlee et al., 2006).

Scales are used to accurately reproduce a large object on a sheet of paper in its correct proportions.

Table 8-1. Common Scales Used in Architectural Plans

TYPES OF DRAWINGS	IMPERIAL	METRIC
Site or dwelling floor plan	3/16" = 1'0"	1:100
	1/4" = 1'0"	1:50
Floor plan of a room (for example, a bathroom, kitchen, or bedroom)	1/2" = 1'0"	1:20

Scale uses a ratio to show the size of a real object in relation to the size of the drawn object. A full-size drawing is one with a scale ratio of 1:1 (International Organization for Standardization, 1979). The scale chosen for the drawn object depends on the size of the real object, the amount of detail required, the complexity of the object, the purpose of the presentation (International Organization for Standardization, 1979), and the size of the piece of paper being used (Ashlee et al., 2006).

Drawings will indicate both scale and unit of measurement in either imperial or metric language. For example, 1/4 in equals 1 for 12 in (1/4" = 1'0" indicates that the real object is 48 times larger [1:48] than the drawn object, or in metric 1:50 indicates that the real object is 50 times larger than the drawn object).

Architectural scales used in the United States are generally grouped in pairs using the same dual-numbered index line, including the following:

3" = 1'0" (ratio equivalent 1:4)	1 1/2" = 1'0" (1:8)
1" = 1'0" (1:12)	1/2" = 1'0" (1:24)
3/4" = 1'0" (1:16)	3/8" = 1'0" (1:32)
1/4" = 1'0" (1:48)	1/8" = 1'0" (1:96)
3/16" = 1'0" (1:64)	3/32" = 1'0" (1:128)

In the United Kingdom, Canada, and Australia, the architectural scales are as follows:

+ 1:1/1:10
+ 1:2/1:20
+ 1:5/1:50
+ 1:100/1:200

Scale changes might occur between section and elevation drawings. Table 8-1 shows common scales used in architectural plans.

Small or detailed objects, such as a door sill or door furniture, are often drawn to a larger scale ratio (e.g., 1 1/2" = 1'0" [1:10] or larger). The detail on the larger scale drawing takes precedence or overrides the detail on the smaller scale drawing of the same area or object. For example, the detail in the floor plan area of the bathroom (1/2" = 1'0" or 1:20) overrides the detail provided for the same bathroom as drawn in the floor plan of the house or apartment (3/16" = 1'0" or 1:100). The scale 1/2" = 1'0" or 1:20 is a "larger" scale than 3/16" = 1'0" or 1:100 because the drawing itself is larger than the same object (Figures 8-12 and 8-13).

TECHNICAL DRAWING CONVENTIONS

To read a plan, occupational therapists need to understand how objects are illustrated and labeled. This involves understanding the technical drawing conventions and symbols that are used by the design or construction professional to describe the building design (Weidhaas, 2002). Technical drawing standards contain specific information about the conventions and symbols, and they are used by the building and construction industry. Ensuring that design and construction professionals use the same terminology and symbols assists in establishing common design and construction practice. The technical drawing standards are not a mandatory requirement for architectural drawings, but they are a useful guide. Publications such as International Organization for Standardization standards, access standards (e.g., ICC/ANSI A117.1 [ANSI, 2009]) or architectural books (Bielefeld & Skiba, 2013; Ching, 2015; Ching & Eckler, 2013) and online resources set out examples of technical drawing conventions and symbols that occupational therapists can use as a guide when they develop concept drawings. In many instances, design and building professionals might further stylize the basic elements described in the technical drawing standards to increase the readability and attractiveness of the image.

Technical drawing standards may contain basic conventions (e.g., dimension lines [Table 8-2] and symbols for architectural features [Figure 8-14]). These conventions and symbols vary because there is no set requirement for them to be drawn a specific way.

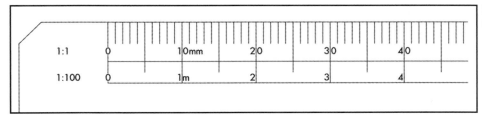

Figure 8-12. Example of scales (metric).

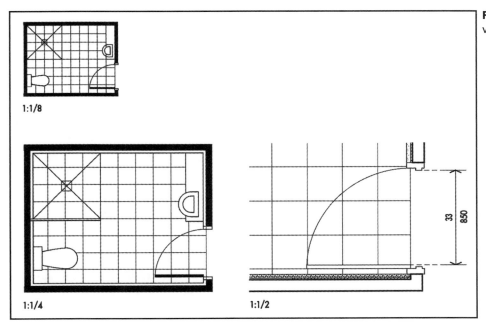

Figure 8-13. Examples of floor plan views drawn at different scales.

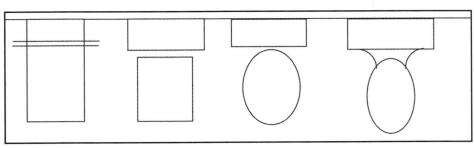

Figure 8-14. Examples of symbols for toilets.

Lines

The basic graphic symbol for all drawings is the line, which defines spatial edges, renders volume, creates textures, and connects to form words and numbers (Wang, 1996). Creating lines is a major element of a drawing, and good line work is critical to the development of an accurate and neat drawing (Bielefeld & Skiba, 2013; Housing Industry Association & Illaring Pty Ltd., 2006). Line work in plan, elevation, and section views should be sharp, dense, of uniform width, and consistent for the purpose of legibility (Wang, 1996). The specific types and thickness of each line and their application are often set out in technical drawing standards or textbooks. There are common line and dimensioning standards for home design (Figure 8-15).

Six major types of lines are used in drawings that have specific meanings:

1. Visible object line: A solid line representing the contour of an object or the visible edges

2. Hidden object line: Hidden or unseen objects below or in front of the reader

3. Dimension: A line terminated by arrows, short slashes, or dots indicating the extent or magnitude of a part or whole along which dimensions are scaled and indicated

Table 8-2. Examples of Conventions

CONVENTION	DESCRIPTION
Min	Minimum
Max	Maximum
>	Greater than
≥	Greater than or equal to
<	Less than
≤	Less than or equal to
- - - - - - - - - - -	Boundary of clear floor space or maneuvering clearance
—·—·—·—·— ℄	Center line
⇨	Direction of travel or approach
▨	Location zone of element, control, or feature

Graphic convention for figures from American National Standards Institute. (2009). *ICC/ANSI A117.1-2009: Accessible and usable buildings and facilities.* New York: Author.

4. Center line: A broken line with relatively long segments separated by single dashes and dots to represent the axis of a symmetrical element or composition

5. Break line: Broken line segments joined by short zigzag strokes to show a portion of the drawing that has been cut off

6. Overhead line: Hidden or unseen objects behind or above the observer (Ching, 2015)

Dimensioning

Dimensions are used on drawings in conjunction with dimension lines to denote the length, height, or width of the object being represented. Although the imperial system of measurement is commonly used in the United States, a combination of metric and imperial measurements is generally noted in various U.S. design standards. When imperial dimensions are used, they are expressed as feet and inches, whereas metric dimensions are expressed in millimeters (mm), never centimeters (cm). In some instances, dimensions may be written in meters (e.g., 1.50 m), particularly at the sketch and developed design stages. The actual dimension number is conventionally written along the lines and placed above it (Figures 8-16 and 8-17; Bielefeld & Skiba, 2013).

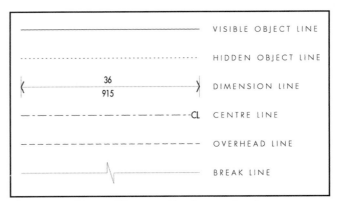

Figure 8-15. Types of lines used in plans or drawings.

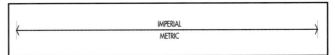

Figure 8-16. Dimension line that shows imperial and metric measurements.

Creating Concept Drawings

Design or construction professionals undergo specific technical drawing training to develop the skills to create drawings that are technically sound and provide significant construction detail. These drawings have a technical detail and accuracy that cannot be achieved by therapists who have not had formal technical drawing training.

Therapists can create preliminary or concept sketch drawings to develop design ideas for home modifications in advance of an architect or building designer's more detailed drawings. If therapists want to incorporate more developed drawings into their reports, they should refer the work to a design professional. If they would like to become skilled in any of these forms of drawing, they need to undertake formal training in architectural drawing.

CONCEPT DRAWING INFORMATION PROVIDED TO DESIGN AND CONSTRUCTION PROFESSIONALS

Concept drawings provide more detail to the written wording that is contained in the occupational therapy report. If home modification work is simple and straightforward to undertake, such as the installation of grab rails, handrails, stairs, or small ramps,

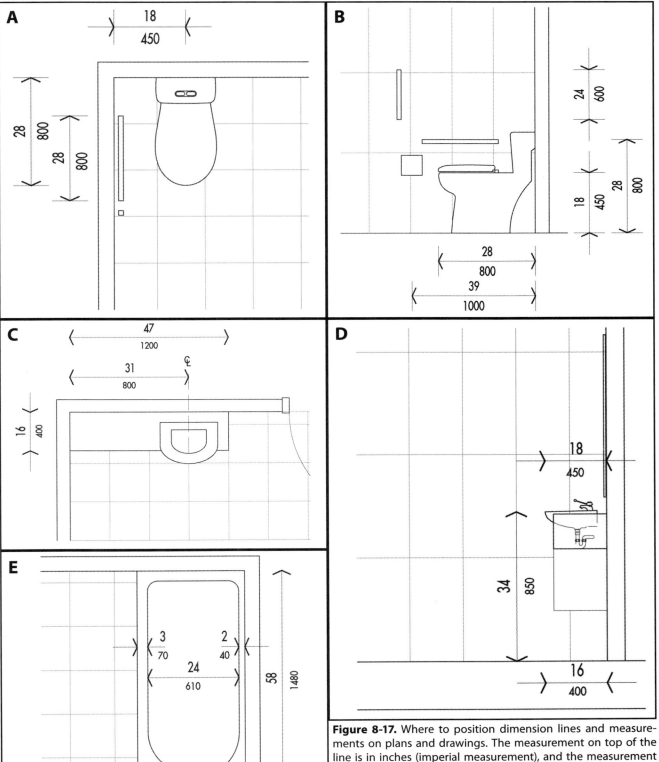

Figure 8-17. Where to position dimension lines and measurements on plans and drawings. The measurement on top of the line is in inches (imperial measurement), and the measurement below the line is in millimeters (metric measurement). (A) Toilet floor plan; (B) toilet elevation; (C) vanity floor plan; (D) vanity elevation; (E) bath floor plan; (F) bath elevation; (G) stairs elevation. *(continued)*

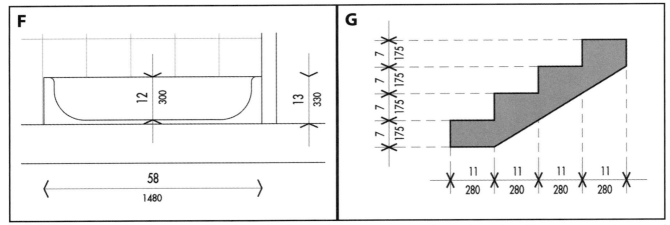

Figure 8-17 (continued). Where to position dimension lines and measurements on plans and drawings. The measurement on top of the line is in inches (imperial measurement), and the measurement below the line is in millimeters (metric measurement). (A) Toilet floor plan; (B) toilet elevation; (C) vanity floor plan; (D) vanity elevation; (E) bath floor plan; (F) bath elevation; (G) stairs elevation.

a concept drawing may be sufficient to guide the builder. This concept drawing needs to have a written scope of works to accompany the illustration to ensure there is sufficient information for the modification. If the home modification work is complex, such as the renovation of the bathroom or kitchen or the installation of a lift, lengthy ramp, or additional room, the concept drawing may be used as the basis for a more detailed technical drawing and written specification that is completed by the design or construction professional. It is sometimes helpful to include photos and drawings of the existing areas to be modified as well as the drawing of the proposed changes to provide the design or construction professional with a more comprehensive picture of the area, particularly if they are developing a more detailed technical drawing for the proposed home modifications. The provision of photos and drawings ensures that the design or construction professional is able to clearly visualize the area to be modified and use these illustrations for ongoing reference during the drawing and modification stages of the work.

When to Draw to Scale

Drawings of minor modifications, such as grab bar installations and handrails on stairs, do not generally need to be drawn to scale. If they are not drawn to scale, this should be noted on the drawing. However, the figures should always be proportionate to ensure that the reader has a good understanding of the relationship of items and areas in relation to one another. When developing drawings for a major modification, scale drawings enable occupational therapists to determine which fittings, fixtures, equipment, or furniture can reasonably fit into a room and whether the space is adequate for items to be placed and for the circulation of individuals with and without their equipment. Scale drawings can also be used to indicate the precise location and assess the ease of access to, and use of, existing fixtures, such as doors and windows. However, drawing to scale is time consuming because it requires that relevant dimensions of the person, their caregiver and equipment, and the existing home environment are accurately measured and then translated into a scale drawing.

Drawing on Photographs

Drawings may be done on a photograph of an area or feature by hand or by computer, and it is advisable that occupational therapists complete an accompanying concept drawing that is either to scale or not to scale depending on the complexity of the work. The provision of the photo and line drawing for the one area ensures that the building professional has adequate information for completion of the home modification that is not open to interpretation. Drawings on a photo may be problematic if the photo is not clear or if the photo has been taken at an angle.

DRAWING BY HAND

Although drawing can be completed with the assistance of computer technology, therapists can make concept drawings by hand quickly and easily if they are skilled in drawing. They can translate measurements of clients, their equipment and caregiver, and the home environment into a simple concept drawing, particularly if computer technology is unavailable. However, drawings developed by hand using pencils, rulers, scale rulers, pens, and paper are often labor intensive and take significant time. These drawings can also vary in quality, depending on the skills of the person completing the drawings and the type of equipment used. They cannot be edited, saved, or adjusted as easily as computer-assisted drafting (CAD) or computer-assisted drawings (e.g., Microsoft Word, PowerPoint, Visio, Idapt Planning [www.idapt-planning.co.uk], or OT Draw [www.OTdraw.com] drawings).

Tools for Drawing by Hand

Hand drawing can be completed with the aid of drafting equipment, such as a drafting board, squares, rulers, scale rulers, and other tools, for the systematic representation and dimensional specification of architectural features in the home (Bielefeld & Skiba, 2013; Ching, 2015). Quality equipment and materials make the act of drawing a more enjoyable experience, and the achievement of quality work becomes much easier in the long term (Ching, 2015). The equipment and materials need to be good quality, clean, and appropriate to the task. The following items can be used by therapists when hand drawing, including paper, pencils, pens, templates, scale ruler, set square, or T-square.

Paper

Various types of paper can be used when doing concept drawings: plain paper, graph paper, and drafting film. Although plain paper is the medium most regularly used by occupational therapists, they might need to talk to representatives from local drawing and drafting companies about the most appropriate paper for their drawing requirements. Sketch-grade paper is suitable for quick sketches and overlays on drawings where alternative layouts are being developed. For a quality finish to a concept drawing, drafting film is used. It is translucent and has a matte textured surface on one side and a plain, smooth textured surface on the other. It resists humidity that can affect the sheet size because it is made of a plastic that is more dimensionally stable. Although it is more expensive and resists tearing, it is also "harder" on equipment (e.g., pens wear out more quickly). Grid paper is also useful if drawings are being done to scale, as the grid can come in various scale sizes. It provides therapists with a good visual guide during drawing. The grid paper has the disadvantage of having extra lines compared to the drafting film, making concept drawings look "busy" when drawn directly onto this grid paper. The drafting film can be placed on top of the drafting paper and the concept drawing done on the film to create a less cluttered drawing.

Pencils

The most common pencils used for drawing are 2H and H (hard), F or HB (medium), and B (soft). Often, 2B (or even softer) pencils are used for sketches (the B stands for black). The choice of pencil depends on the user's preference and drawing skills. Sharp pencils or propelling (clutch) pencils using a narrow lead are ideal for drafting. These enable the user to continue drawing without having to stop and sharpen the tool. A soft eraser is also essential to clean markings off of the drawing sheets.

Pens

Final concept drawings should always be in ink or pen. Although pencil may be used initially to draw the lines, once complete, they should be drawn over in ink or felt pen. Felt-tipped technical drafting pens are available in various thicknesses and are generally used to draw specific line widths. Ballpoint pens are not appropriate for drawing work because the lines produced by these types of pen are not clean and clear on paper.

Templates and Other Drawing Tools

Templates and a compass can save time when drawing. Templates are generally made of plastic and have geometric shapes and shapes of plumbing fixtures and furnishings. They also have lettering, numerals, and other symbols, all of which can provide a guide for drawing objects accurately and to scale. Circles are drawn with a pair of compasses.

Scale Ruler and Set Square or T-Square

Scale rulers are used to draw in a precise ratio to the original (Housing Industry Association & Illaring Pty Ltd., 2006). These rulers vary in style, quality, and scale. There are common scales used for specific plans. As indicated previously, common scales used by therapists when drawing include 3/16" = 1'0" (1:100); 1/4" = 1'0" (1:50) for site or dwelling floor plans; and 1/2" = 1'0" (1:20) for floor plans of rooms or for internal elevations. Scale rulers also vary in style (Figures 8-18 and 8-19).

Scale rulers need to be kept clean by washing with a mild soap and water. Ideally, they should only be used to measure drawings and not to draw lines because scale rulers become worn and the divisions of the scale can affect the quality of the line drawn. Routinely, a set square or T-square is used to rule lines. Scale rulers should not be used as a cutting edge or be used with color markers because these will destroy the edge and markings.

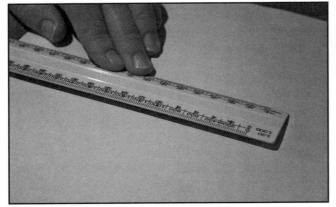

Figure 8-18. A flat scale ruler does not hold to the paper tightly unless the user tilts the ruler to the paper.

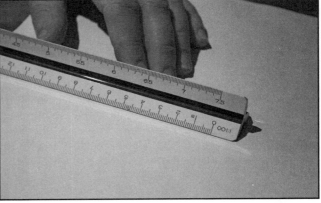

Figure 8-19. A different type of scale ruler that grips the paper tightly.

Drafting Board

This is a flat working surface to which paper can be secured with clips or tape. Drafting boards vary in size but should be at least 25% larger than the largest piece of paper that will be regularly used on the board (Housing Industry Association & Illaring Pty Ltd., 2006). The paper is attached to the board so that it sits squarely to a T-square or straight-edge or, if preprinted, the border is used to square up the paper (Housing Industry Association & Illaring Pty Ltd., 2006). Plastic drafting boards with parallel rules will generally suit occupational therapists' drawing needs.

Square

The T-square is held firm on one edge of the drafting board (e.g., to the left) and can move up and down on the page to draw horizontal lines. The T-square can also be used as a surface against which to place set squares to create vertical and angled lines. Most drafting boards have sliding rulers in place of the T-square (Housing Industry Association & Illaring Pty Ltd., 2006). The clear plastic T-square enables the user to see through to the paper.

Set Squares

Set squares are manufactured from clear plastic, and the most commonly used in home modification drawing are those that are 45/45/90 degrees and 60/30/90 degrees to assist with drawing angled and horizontal or vertical lines.

The Drawing Process

The process for completing a concept drawing includes the following:

+ Selecting the view(s) to be drawn
+ Choosing the paper type and size
+ Drawing the view(s)
+ Checking that all information included in the concept drawing is accurate
+ Providing the title block on the right side or bottom of the page
+ Dating and signing the drawing

The concept drawing might need to include a range of different views of the area to be modified (e.g., the floor plan to show distance, circulation space, width, depth, and length and the elevation view to show distance, heights, width, and length). Occupational therapists should ensure that each different view, or plan, of the same area contains consistent information. In particular, the measurements need to be compared to ensure that there are no discrepancies between the drawings. For example, the location of the grab bar beside the toilet—the distance from the back wall (e.g., cistern wall)—in the floor plan view needs to be identical to its location in the elevation view.

Before starting their final scale concept drawings, occupational therapists might sketch them out roughly on a piece of paper first. This allows them to get a clear picture in their mind of what they want to draw. For concept drawings that are not drawn to scale, they can draw directly onto white paper, using a black pen to build on the final pencil drawings. All lines should be drawn using a ruler, and figures should be recognizable using conventional symbols, be clearly labeled, and be in proportion. If drawing to scale, therapists need to select an appropriately sized scale for the area being drawn, as per the earlier discussion on scale. For example, a floor plan of a bathroom may be drawn 1/2" = 1'0" or 1:20.

There are three different ways of completing the scale concept drawing using the pens or pencils and various types of paper (Figure 8-20):

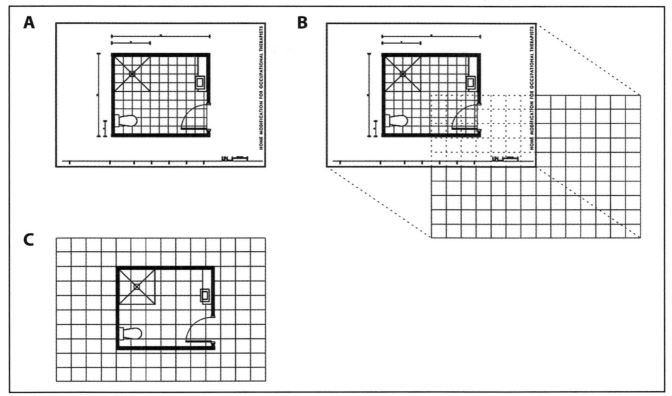

Figure 8-20. Paper options for concept drawings. (A) Using drafting paper for drawings. (B) Combining drafting paper on top of grid paper for drawings. (C) Using grid paper for drawings.

1. Therapists can draw directly onto white paper or drafting film using a pencil or pen. The drafting film illustration can be photocopied onto white paper when finished.

2. Therapists can lay drafting film over grid paper, which has been set out according to a scale, to guide their drawings, using pencil and pen and a scale ruler as described previously. The grid paper provides therapists with an inbuilt reference scale during the drafting process. It helps correct alignment of features within the drawing and the whole drawing itself, and guides them as they use their ruler (International Organization for Standardization, 1979). A cross-check of the scale ruler against the grid paper that is positioned under the drafting film can be done during the drawing process. Space needs to be left around the drawing for listing lines and measurements, which requires that the drafting film be offset from the grid paper.

3. Therapists can draw directly onto grid paper.

When drawing a room, therapists first outline the overall shape of the area (e.g., the walls, windows, and doors). All permanent fixtures or fittings are then drawn in their respective locations using appropriate conventions and symbols, starting with the larger items and working down to the smaller. For example, a drawing of a bathroom would include bath/shower, vanity, toilet, taps, spouts/shower roses, soap/toilet roll holder, light switches, electrical fittings, and power outlets. Dimension lines are then drawn on the outside of the drawing in line with the items they are representing. This ensures that the inside of the drawing remains uncluttered and clear. The smaller dimensions are usually recorded closest to the outside of the drawing, with dimensions increasing incrementally away from the drawing. This creates a hierarchy of dimensions. The area drawn can be divided horizontally and vertically to guide the set of the dimension lines (Figure 8-21). When divided horizontally, dimension lines with measurements are to match the items in the top and bottom halves of the drawing and located either above or below the drawing to match the half of the drawing they reference. When divided vertically, the dimension lines with measurements are to match the right and left halves of the drawing and located either to the right or left of the drawing the measurements reference. Further, the dimension lines should be written in such a way that the page is turned only once (e.g., clockwise) to read the figures on the dimension lines along the top, bottom, and sides of the drawing (see Figure 8-21).

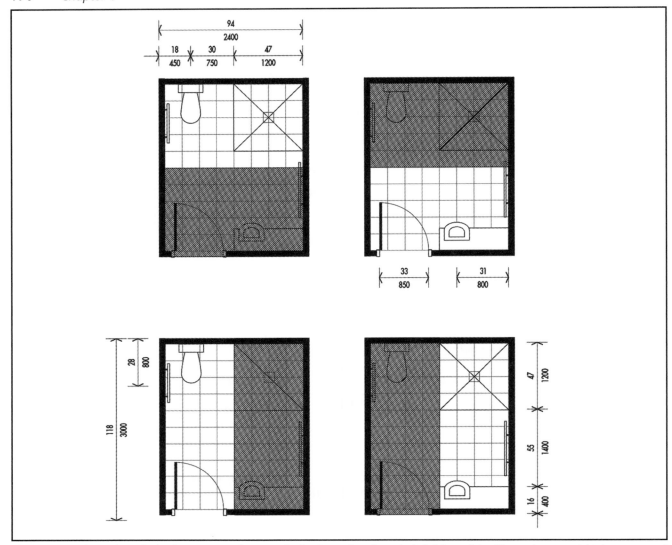

Figure 8-21. Floor plan of a bathroom area showing the horizontal and vertical division of the illustration to guide the set-out of measurements and dimension lines. The measurement on top of the line is in inches (imperial measurement), and the measurement below the line is in millimeters (metric measurement).

Drawings are initially developed using pencil. Once the drawing has been finalized, pencil lines are built on using a felt-tip pen, and the pencil lines are removed with a soft rubber eraser.

When developing a drawing, therapists should be mindful to include all of the required information in the drawing, such as the permanent fittings and fixtures and accompanying recommendations. For example, in an elevation of a grab bar on a wall, essential elements include the following:

+ Configuration of bar
+ Diameter of bar
+ Length of bar
+ Height of bar above floor level

+ Wall the bar is to be located on
+ Distance of end of the bar from the back wall (e.g., distance on the wall next to the toilet adjacent cistern wall)
+ Structure/surface of mounting wall
+ Whether studs have been located
+ Other elements described in the standards that are relevant to the client's specific requirements

A title block may be included at the side or bottom of the page to enable all relevant details about the drawing to be recorded, including the client's name and address, project name/type, the name of the area, the type of view, whether the drawing has been drawn to scale and the size of the scale, the page number or set total, the date of drawing, the review date and/or number, and the name of the designer/draftsman/occupational therapist (Housing Industry Association & Illaring Pty Ltd., 2006). Other information can include the name of the area drawn, the type of view (e.g., the floor plan view or elevation), the scale, and whether measurements are in feet and inches or millimeters if the abbreviation for these measurements is not included with the dimensions. A title block at the bottom of the page or on the right side of the page allows large sheets to be folded into sections and clipped to the left, and the drawing remains easy to read. For future reference, the occupational therapist should sign and date plans to provide evidence of the authorship and the date they were finalized.

Lettering on Hand Drawings

Therapists are required to incorporate neat lettering into their drawings to ensure that items are clearly labeled and the document is professionally presented. Some of the most important characteristics of a lettering style are readability and consistency in both style and spacing (Ching, 2015). Skillful lettering enhances the appearance and clarity of the drawing, whereas poor lettering can be difficult to read and can detract from the drawing. Lettering needs to be consistent, dark, crisp, and sharp for the best presentation. It can be in pencil, spaced equally to the height of letters, and finished in pen. Lettering must be neat, brief, straight, and completed horizontally on drawings. It is not to be placed over part of a space or a drawn object. Numerals are to be placed outside the view shown to ensure the drawing remains uncluttered.

Therapists can find more information on the placement of lettering and lines from local architects or building designers, through completing an architectural drawing course, or by referring to texts such as books by Ching (2015) or by checking resources online.

DRAWING USING COMPUTER TECHNOLOGY

In order to anticipate expected changes, home modification documents need to be flexible, time efficient to create, and inexpensive to revise (Wang, 1996). To accommodate minor changes and to avoid redrawing the entire sheet of documentation, Wang (1996) notes that computer technology has become popular in preparing drawings.

Computer Tools for Drawing

Once these tools are mastered, drawings using computer technology are faster to draw, store, and retrieve. They can be created using drawing features in existing business software, such as Microsoft Word and Microsoft PowerPoint; general drawing programs such as Paint and VisioPro; dedicated CAD software of varying levels of sophistication (e.g., AutoCad, Autosketch, SmartDraw, and Google Sketch-Up); or specific software for use by health and other professionals such as Idapt Planning, and OT Draw (Figure 8-22). Items drawn using computer technology can be edited, saved, copied, resized, colored, and manipulated in a range of ways. Templates for areas around the home can be created that can be easily modified through the use of drawing tools to add more detail to the illustration. For example, therapists might create templates of bathroom or toilet areas for quick and easy retrieval to add in illustrations of grab rails. Further, photos, cut-outs, photocopies, and other documents can be uploaded and manipulated using software tools. Software packages provide a variety of tools, including pens, airbrushes, drafting tools, and texture maps (Montague, 2005).

Drawings developed using CAD programs or specific software for use by health professionals appear professional and stylish and make it easier to achieve accuracy of scale (see Figure 8-22). These programs have additional desirable features, including the ability to draw to scale and to import symbols that adapt to the scale. Further, some CAD programs allow scaled drawings to be converted to two- and three-dimension images with walk-through views. However, to be able to make full use of such computer software, therapists require training. The more sophisticated the program, the more features and drawing options provided, and the greater the level of skill and expertise required to operate them. Experienced draftspeople and architects are the main users of this technology, although industry training and packages are available that range from simple to complex that can be used by occupational therapists. Further, these packages usually contain training tutorials. It is often assumed that CAD-based drawings have been developed for use by people with building and design knowledge and expertise. Bearing this in mind, therapists who use CAD to develop concept drawings should state that they are to provide an overview of the area only and do not provide the specific technical detail required for building works. They should be careful to clarify that they do not have professional knowledge and expertise in design and construction.

Figure 8-22. Occupational therapist's drawings of the bathroom using (A) Word, (B) CAD, (C) OT Draw, (D) (i, ii, iii, iv, v) Idapt Planning (Reprinted with permission from Idapt LLP, Acton Turville, UK); and (E) photos of bathroom features after modification *(continued).*

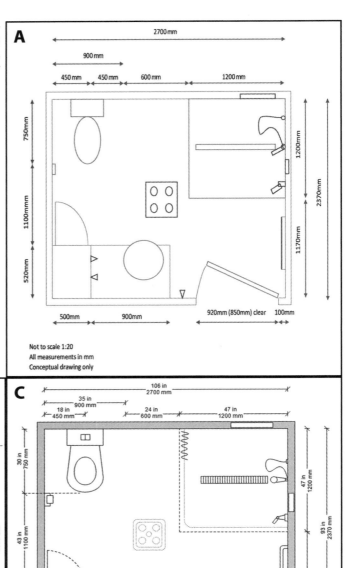

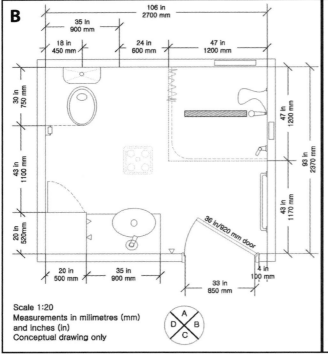

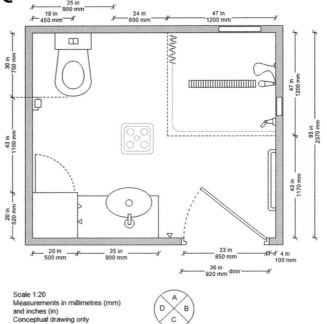

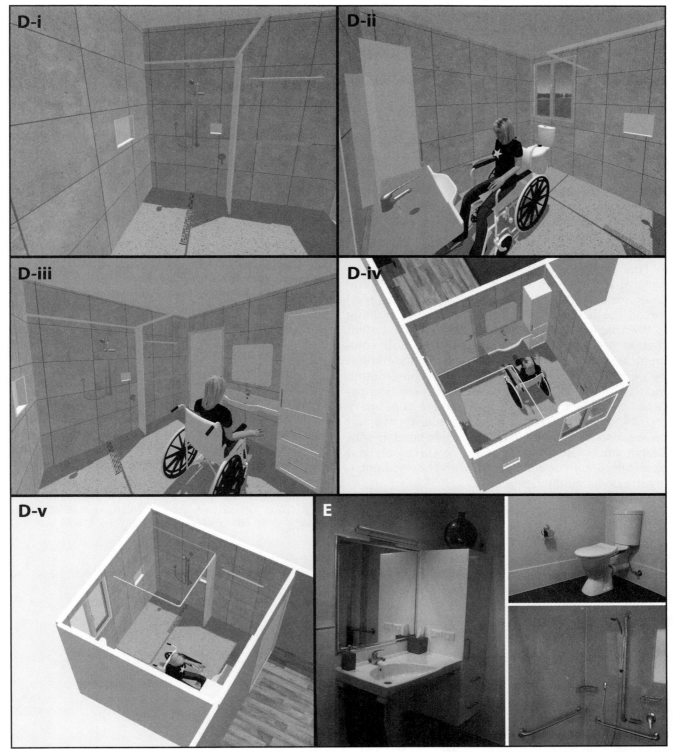

Figure 8-22 (continued). Occupational therapist's drawings of the bathroom using (A) Word, (B) CAD, (C) OT Draw, (D) (i, ii, iii, iv, v) Idapt Planning (Reprinted with permission from Idapt LLP, Acton Turville, UK); and (E) photos of bathroom features after modification.

CONCLUSION

This chapter discussed how a client's home modification requirements can be represented in concept drawings that complement photos and other information that has been put in writing in the occupational therapy report. Though occupational therapy concept drawings are not architectural drawings, they can become the basis for the development of more detailed technical drawings by design or construction professionals. This chapter has described the resources to guide occupational therapy drawing practice, the basic requirements for drawings, and tools and technology that can provide further information to guide knowledge and skill development in the area.

This chapter has not sought to provide comprehensive information to ensure occupational therapists are competent in drawing. Rather, it has reinforced the need for therapists to consider training in the area to ensure that home visit documentation that is produced is clear and concise and communicates information that is easily understood by people working in the design and construction industry. This chapter has discussed how occupational therapists should take advantage of industry training courses and review available hard-copy and online resources in the field to become familiar with design and construction industry requirements and to ensure good communication with those completing the home modification work.

REFERENCES

American National Standards Institute. (2009). *ICC/ANSI A117.1-2009: Accessible and usable buildings and facilities.* New York, NY: Author.

Ashlee, P., Clutton, S., Pengelly, S., & Cowderoy, J. (2006). Conveying information through drawing. In S. Clutton, J. Grisbrooke, & S. Pengelly (Eds.), *Occupational therapy in housing: Building on firm foundations* (pp. 83-108). London: Whurr Publishers.

Bielefeld, B., & Skiba, I. (2013). *Basics: Fundamentals of presentation. Technical drawing.* Boston, MA: Birkhauser.

Ching, F. D. K. (2015). *Architectural graphics.* Hoboken, NJ: John Wiley and Sons.

Ching, F. D. K., & Eckler, J. F. (2013). *Introduction to architecture.* Hoboken, NJ: John Wiley & Sons.

Clutton, S., Grisbrooke, J., & Pengelly, S. (2006). *Occupational therapy in housing: Building on firm foundations.* London: Whurr Publishers.

Dernie, D. (2014). *Architectural drawing* (2nd ed.). London: Lawrence King Publishing Ltd.

Housing Industry Association & Illaring Pty Ltd. (2006). *Introduction to drafting: Participant guide.* Brisbane, Australia: Author.

International Organization for Standardization. (1979). *International Standard ISO 5455.* West Conshohocken, PA: ASTM International.

Montague, J. (2005). *Basic perspective drawing: A visual approach.* Hoboken, NJ: John Wiley & Sons.

Standen, D. (1995). *Construction industry specifications.* Victoria, Australia: The Royal Australian Institute of Architects.

Thorpe, S. (1994). *Reading and using plans.* London: Center for Accessible Environments.

Wang, T. C. (1996). *Plan and section drawing.* Hoboken, NJ: John Wiley & Sons.

Weidhaas, E. R. (2002). *Reading architectural plans for residential and commercial construction* (5th ed). Upper Saddle River, NJ: Prentice Hall.

Yee, R. (2012). *Architectural drawing: A visual compendium of types and methods* (4th ed). New York: John Wiley & Sons.

9

Developing and Tailoring Interventions

Desleigh de Jonge, MPhil (OccThy), Grad Cert Soc Sci;
Melanie Hoyle, BSc (Psych), MOccThySt, Grad Dip Health Sci, Post Grad Dip Psych;
and Elizabeth Ainsworth, MOccThy, Grad Cert Health Sci

Occupational therapists address a variety of occupational performance issues in the home using a range of interventions. Based on an analysis of the person-environment-occupation transaction and the home environment, occupational therapists identify alternative strategies, assistive devices, social supports, and modifications to the environment to promote occupational performance. In developing an intervention strategy, the occupational therapist collaborates with the client to find the solution that best fits with the person and the way he or she engages in occupations in the home environment. This chapter will outline the various approaches occupational therapists use to enhance occupational performance in the home and provide a structure for analyzing the suitability of various interventions. The role of clinical reasoning in determining the most suitable intervention will also be discussed. In addition, the chapter will introduce occupational therapists to architectural elements of the built environment that might be considered when tailoring interventions to suit the person-environment fit and will present a framework for developing and tailoring environmental interventions.

CHAPTER OBJECTIVES

By the end of this chapter, the reader will be able to:

✦ Describe the typical occupational performance issues faced by people in the home

✦ Describe the range of interventions that occupational therapists use to enhance occupational performance in the home

✦ Describe a systematic approach to identifying potential interventions

✦ Discuss the potential interaction between interventions and the person, the nature of the occupation, and the environment

✦ Discuss the use of clinical reasoning in determining the most suitable intervention option

✦ Describe the use of architectural elements in developing environmental interventions

Ainsworth, E., & de Jonge, D. *An Occupational Therapist's
Guide to Home Modification Practice, Second Edition (pp. 195-223).*
© 2019 SLACK Incorporated.

Box 9-1. Problems Reported by Older People in the Home

- External access: Walking on uneven pavements, dealing with slopes, steps, clutter, and ground surfaces
- Entry: Getting in/out of the house, managing stairs, locks, keys, and doorknobs
- Internal mobility: Mobilizing inside the house, negotiating stairs, clutter, obstacles, level changes, slippery surfaces
- Interior (general): Poor lighting, managing control and outlets, hearing doorbell, and using telephone
- Living room: Getting up from chairs
- Bathroom: Getting into and out of tub, completion of bathing and showering, dressing from waist down, transferring to toilet (toilet too low), completion of toileting, difficulty with faucets
- Kitchen: Cabinets too high, too low, difficulty using appliances, trash disposal
- Bedroom: Getting in and out of bed

Adapted from Connell & Sanford, 1997; Gitlin et al., 2001, 2006; Johansson et al., 2007, 2009; and Mann et al., 1994.

IDENTIFYING OCCUPATIONAL CHALLENGES IN THE HOME

Occupational therapists commonly address occupational challenges that result from a poor fit between the person's capacities, what he or she needs or wants to do, and the demands of the environment where the performance takes place. Occupational challenges can arise as a consequence of the following:

- ✦ Changes in a person's functional capacities as a result of aging, injury, impairment, or a health condition
- ✦ Variations in occupational demands or the way activities are undertaken
- ✦ Barriers or challenges presented by the environment

When evaluating occupational performance of various valued and required activities in and around the home, occupational therapists analyze the person-environment-occupation transaction to identify a specific cause for any difficulties experienced and determine how occupational performance can be further enabled. From this analysis, occupational therapists are able to develop a number of alternative intervention options to address the identified concern and to further enhance performance.

Traditionally, occupational therapists have focused on the impact of various impairments and functional deficits on daily activities and sought to maintain or enhance health, safety, and independence by recommending assistive devices or alternative methods of undertaking activities. Increasing focus is now being given to the environment and the demands it places on people. Conventional housing design creates a number of challenges for older people and people with disabilities as they go about their daily activities. Houses with stairs, narrow doorways and corridors, inaccessible toilets and bathrooms, and limited space "create" disability (Heywood, 2004a; Oldman & Beresford, 2000) and can compromise a person's health, safety (Stone, 1998; Trickey, Maltais, Gosslein, & Robitaille, 1993), independence (Frain & Carr, 1996), and well-being (Heywood, 2004a). Studies undertaken by Connell and Sanford (1997); Gitlin, Hauck, Winter, Dennis, and Schulz (2006); Gitlin, Mann, Tomita, and Marcus (2001); Johansson, Josephsson, and Lilja (2009); Johansson, Lilja, Petersson, and Borell (2007); Mann, Hurren, Tomita, Bengali, and Steinfeld (1994); and other authors have identified a number of problems experienced by older people in the home environment that would be equally relevant for people with various impairments and health conditions (Box 9-1).

The design of the residence can:

- ✦ Place people at risk of incidents or accidents resulting in injury
- ✦ Make it difficult for people to carry out daily activities in and around the home
- ✦ Place unnecessary demands on people in terms of managing and maintaining the environment

People need to feel well supported by their home environment. When the home provides too many challenges, it can place people at risk of injury arising from incidents or accidents. A challenging home environment can undermine confidence and make people apprehensive and even fearful as they go about routine activities in the home and community. Poorly designed environments may also affect relationships (Heywood, 2004a, 2005; Tanner, Tilse, & de Jonge, 2008), interactions with family and cohabitants (Granbom, Taei, & Ekstam, 2017; Heywood, 2004b), and the capacity of people to get out of the home to participate in community activities (Bedell, Khetani, Cousins, Coster, & Law, 2011; Gillespie et al., 2009; Heywood, 2004b; Law, Di Rezze, & Bradley, 2010; Pettersson, Löfqvist, & Malmgren Fänge, 2012).

People need to be able to manage their home environment—open windows, operate controls, answer the telephone and doorbell (Connell & Sanford, 1997), and maintain the home in order to feel comfortable and safe. Older people and people with disabilities often experience difficulties cleaning and maintaining their homes (Peace & Holland, 2001). Homes that are unkempt and poorly maintained can create further hazards and can expose the occupants to increased risk of home invasions when passers-by realize that residents may be vulnerable and may not be able to defend themselves (Jones, de Jonge, & Phillips, 2008).

INTERVENTIONS USED TO ADDRESS OCCUPATIONAL PERFORMANCE ISSUES

In the home environment, occupational therapists aim to assist people to find ways to perform routine activities of daily living and household tasks that, however inconsequential they might seem, can be integral to leading a full and satisfying life (Crepeau, Schell, Gillen, & Scaffa, 2014). Interventions can address a presenting problem by establishing or restoring the person's capacities, altering the way the task is undertaken, or adapting or modifying the existing environment (Dunn, Brown, & McGuigan, 1994). Alternatively, the person-environment-occupation fit can be altered (Dunn et al., 1994; Iwarsson et al., 2016; Wahl, Fänge, Oswald, Gitlin, & Iwarsson, 2009) by moving the person to a more supportive environment or providing additional support in the way of informal or formal assistance. In some cases, occupational therapists support other people in caring for or assisting people with severe or degenerative conditions (Rogers & Holm, 2009). This type of intervention is referred to as a *palliative intervention* (Rogers & Holm, 2009). Occupational performance difficulties can also be prevented by anticipating potential problems before they occur (Dunn et al., 1994). Furthermore, occupational performance can be enriched by creating enabling environments that promote activity engagement and well-being (Dunn et al., 1994). When providing interventions in the home, occupational therapists need to not only address identified problems, but also be mindful of preventing future problems and creating environments that enrich occupational performance and the experience of home.

Interventions can be focused on the person, task, or environment (Rogers & Holm, 2009).

Person-oriented interventions attempt to remediate the person's capacity or manage his or her performance difficulties when undertaking activities by:

+ Maintaining or restoring functions such as muscle strength, endurance, attention, concentration, and visual scanning

+ Managing issues such as reduced vision, pain, fatigue, and short-term memory difficulties

+ Establishing habits and routines for activities that need to be undertaken regularly

These interventions usually require education, training, and, in some cases, regular involvement with an occupational therapist. Consequently, they are mostly recommended for clients who can modify their usual approach to tasks, follow a prescribed program independently, or regularly access a rehabilitation program. In contrast, environment-focused interventions, such as home modifications, recognize the person's existing capacities and seek to optimize occupational performance by eliminating barriers in the home and creating a more supportive environment.

CONCEPTUAL FRAMEWORK FOR DEVELOPING INTERVENTIONS

Everyday activities are commonly undertaken using a combination of strategies, tools, and social and physical supports in the environment (Dunn et al., 1994; Enders & Leech, 1996). Each individual uses a unique blend of these resources to carry out activities in a preferred way. Changes in the person's capacities, the demands of the activity, or the resources available usually prompt people to modify their approach to the task (the strategy), the tools they use, or the way they use the social and physical elements in the environment. For example, there is substantial variation in the way people undertake a simple activity such as cooking scrambled eggs:

+ First, the activity is guided by the preferred outcome; that is, whether the individual prefers eggs light and fluffy, creamy, firm, with a natural flavor, lightly salted, spicy, etc.

+ How the task is undertaken is governed by the person's cooking skills, experience, and knowledge and how he or she was shown to scramble eggs.

+ The nature of tools available, such as whisk, pans, microwave, and cook-top, dictates how the tasks will be performed.

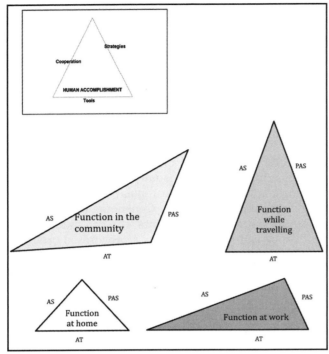

Figure 9-1. Generic support system for human accomplishment. (Reprinted with permission from Albrecht, G. L., Seelman, K. D., & Bury, M. [2001]. *Handbook of disability studies*. Thousand Oaks, CA: Sage Publications.)

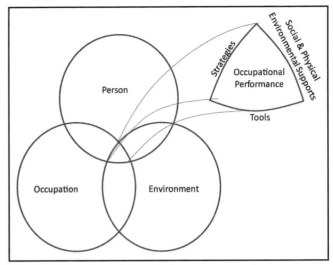

Figure 9-2. Framework for developing interventions.

✦ Finally, the people available to help and the space and layout of the kitchen will shape the way the necessary tasks are undertaken.

If the person is cooking for a number of guests with varying preferences, has an injured hand, breaks the whisk, is offered assistance, or is cooking in a different kitchen, he or she will need to alter the strategy, reconsider the tools, or structure the social and physical environment differently.

Litvak and Enders (2001) described a generic support system for human accomplishment as including strategies, tools, and cooperation and described the function of people with disabilities as being variously supported by adaptive strategies, assistive devices (tools), and personal assistance or social support (Figure 9-1).

This is a useful framework for thinking about ways in which occupational performance can be supported when people encounter difficulties. As highlighted in the ecological models, such as Person-Environment-Occupation-Performance (Baum & Christiansen, 2005; Baum, Christiansen, & Bass, 2015; Christiansen & Baum, 1997) and the Person-Environment-Occupation (Law et al., 1996), discussed in Chapter 3, occupational performance is a function of the dynamic and reciprocal interaction between the person, occupation, and environment.

Therapists seek to optimize occupational performance by improving the fit between the person and his or her occupations and roles and pertinent environments. Working with the unique capacities, skills, preferences, and experiences of each individual, therapists examine how strategies, tools, and the social and physical environment are currently working to support occupational performance and how they might be modified to optimize that performance.

To illustrate the relationship between the person-environment-occupation transaction and these supports, Litvak and Ender's (2001) model of support systems has been modified and superimposed on the Venn diagram of the person-environment-occupation interaction (Figure 9-2).

The curved/Reuleaux triangle created by the intersection of the person, occupation, and environment represents occupational performance. Each side of this triangle represents the resources that support occupational performance—namely, strategies (the way the person approaches the occupation), tools (the devices in the environment used to support the occupation), and the social and physical environmental supports (the resources the person avails him- or herself of in the environment). This simple graphic representation provides therapists with a mechanism for examining and acknowledging the current supports available and exploring alternative ways of supporting and enhancing occupational performance. It also recognizes the role of occupational analysis in evaluating the person-environment-occupation transaction and the contribution of strategies, tools, and social and physical environmental supports to occupational performance.

Strategies or Adaptive Approaches to Enhance Occupational Performance

Occupational therapists have a long tradition of making activities more manageable by altering the way they are undertaken. Activities can be done a different way using energy conservation or work simplification techniques to reduce the physical demands on the person. People can sit to undertake parts of a task or take regular rest breaks to conserve energy. Rescheduling activities to another time when the person is more energetic and mobile (e.g., in the morning) can also enhance performance. Activities can also be scheduled at specific time intervals to remove the complexity or urgency of performance (e.g., establishing regular times for toileting to reduce accidents and the need to rush to the toilet). Sometimes, activities can be simplified and broken into a number of tasks to reduce the cognitive load. They can also be reordered or relocated to make them easier to perform. For example, during bathing, it might be easier to sit in the bedroom when undressing and dressing rather than attempting this task while standing in what might be the cluttered and slippery environment of the bathroom.

People often develop their own alternative strategies to address difficulties in occupational performance. For example, when getting up from a low toilet, many people grab hold of fixtures and fittings in the room such as the toilet roll holder, towel rail, or door handle to assist. Though it is important to acknowledge people's resourcefulness in solving everyday problems, some of these strategies are not safe, practical, or sustainable and can place the person at risk of injury. Occupational therapists might suggest a range of alternative strategies to keep the person safe during such a transfer, such as placing hands on knees to assist with lift-off or "keeping nose over toes" to maintain the center of gravity over the base of support (Chan, Laporte, & Sveistrup, 1999; Deane, Ellis-Hill, Dekker, Davies, & Clarke, 2003). However, it is often difficult to change entrenched patterns of behavior. Many occupations in the home are undertaken using individual and unique approaches that have been honed over many years and have become habitual and almost instinctive. Because people are often unable or unwilling to change the way they undertake tasks, therapists need to work closely with them to find alternative methods that are comfortable and acceptable. Alternatively, therapists can explore the use of other supports such as tools or environmental interventions such as home modifications, which can promote a change in approach and decrease reliance on unsafe methods.

Tools or Assistive Devices to Enhance Occupational Performance

Tools or assistive devices are another intervention strategy used by occupational therapists to address occupational performance issues in the home. This intervention strategy is often easiest for therapists to use because myriad devices are available to address a variety of performance and troublesome task components. Information on specialized devices is readily available through catalogues and equipment databases. For a number of health conditions, assistive devices are viewed as a routine element in treatment protocols. Assistive devices are frequently funded through a range of schemes because they are generally more affordable and more readily available than environmental interventions. However, assistive devices can often change the way tasks are undertaken and, in some cases, can increase the complexity of the task. For example, tub transfer benches and shower chairs require people to sit to shower. This changes the nature of the task, possibly removing the relaxation experienced when standing under a showerhead and having warm water spraying down the back. Sitting to shower may create difficulties in washing the perineal area. Tub transfer benches are frequently removed because they get in the way of others who use the bathroom. The task of then replacing the bench and fitting it safely can often prove challenging for the user.

Assistive devices are not always easy to use. For example, it might be easier for some people to walk through the house leaning on the walls for support rather than to navigate a wheeled walker through narrow hallways and doorways. Useful devices are not always at hand when needed. Reachers are very useful for retrieving items out of reach; however, they need to be nearby when required. This means keeping a reacher in each room of the house or carrying it around in case it is needed. With abandonment of assistive devices a major concern (Batavia & Hammer, 1990; Hocking, 1999; Mann & Tomita, 1998; Phillips, 1993; Scherer, 2005), it is evident that many people are receiving devices they do not need or are unable or unwilling to use long term.

Social Supports to Enhance Occupational Performance

People with significant physical, psychological, social, sensory, or cognitive difficulties often receive formal and informal personal assistance to help them successfully complete activities. Support can be provided in the form of organizational assistance, verbal prompting, or physical support or assistance. Assistance might be required prior to, during, or after the activity is completed. For example, a family member could prepare the area for the activity, supervise performance, verbally prompt the person through the tasks, or physically assist the person at various stages or throughout the entire activity. Where he or she is no longer able to undertake the activity, another family member or a paid caregiver/service provider might assume complete responsibility for completing the task (e.g., doing the laundry or mowing the lawn).

Therapists need to understand what informal supports are available to assist the person and determine whether caregivers are willing, or have the capacity, to provide the required assistance. If appropriate support is available, therapists need to ensure that assistance is provided in a way that maintains the person's autonomy and safety and, wherever possible, that the meaning of the occupation to the person is retained. For example, people might bathe before bed to relax. When a caregiver is assisting with this task, the focus often shifts to cleaning the person as efficiently as possible rather than providing a routine with activities focused on comfort and relaxation. The activity can become centered on the availability and needs of the caregiver rather than the needs of the person being bathed. This is understandable, but when someone is always dependent on others for assistance, the loss of control over daily routine and the relaxing pre-bed routine (or the routine of that whole day) can be distressing and might even have implications for the person's long-term health and well-being.

Therapists are also concerned with the health and well-being of caregivers, especially when they are providing support over an extended period. This is a particularly important consideration as it has been identified that a significant portion of primary carers have a health condition/disability themselves (Australian Bureau of Statistics, 2013). The occupation of caring can also become a focus of intervention, with alternative strategies, assistive devices, and environmental modifications used to minimize the demands on the caregiver and reduce the risk of injury (Aplin, de Jonge, & Gustafsson, 2015; Heaton & Bamford, 2001; Heywood, 2004a; Stark, Keglovits, Arbesman, & Lieberman, 2017).

Formal caregiver assistance can also be used to support the completion of a range of activities; however, the amount and type of assistance available can vary from one location to another. Therapists need to be aware of the resources available within the local community and use these effectively. Formal assistance removes the demands on the family and frees the client from being dependent on family members for his or her daily needs. When clients receive assistance with routine tasks, such as bathing, it allows them to invest their limited time and energies in more highly valued occupations, such as parenting or work.

However, these formal caregiver services can be costly and often determine when and how activities are completed. Caregivers can also intrude on personal spaces and disrupt personal routines. Formal support can disrupt social relationships and routines in the household and extended family. For example, a client once declined the offer of a formal service to do the weekly washing of her bed linen and larger items. The client was able to manage washing her smaller items but had her daughter wash the bed linen when she visited each week. She was concerned that if she removed the daughter's reason for visiting, she may not visit as regularly or might cease to visit at all. This task provided an opportunity for the client to prepare a snack for her daughter while she stripped the bed and put the linen in the washing machine. She could then watch television with her while they waited for the washing to dry. Further, it allowed the daughter to do something concrete and meaningful for her mother. The mother-daughter relationship required the structure of these activities because the client appeared to be a very practical and matter-of-fact woman who did not engage easily in general social chatter.

Environmental Supports to Enhance Occupational Performance

Occupational performance can also be enhanced by modifying the environment. Spaces can be reallocated, expanded, rearranged, remodeled, or redesigned to allow the client to perform activities more effectively. In addition, fixtures and fittings can be removed, relocated, replaced, or added to enhance performance. Sometimes, a room on the first floor—a study, for example—can be reassigned as a bedroom so that the client does not have to climb the stairs to go to bed. Further, a separate and adjacent toilet and bathroom may be combined by removing the dividing wall to allow greater circulation space for both activities. The orientation or position of furniture or fixtures and fittings can also be changed to facilitate access and performance in the room. For example, vanity units may be relocated, baths may be removed, and the inward swing of the door into the toilet may be reversed to increase circulation space.

Home modifications can include repairs, maintenance, nonstructural or structural modifications, and the integration of smart technologies. Generally, nonstructural modifications are referred to as *minor modifications* and structural modifications are termed *major modifications*. For a review of the differences between minor and major modifications and an in-depth discussion of modification complexity and associations with situational complexity, see Chapter 5. Repairs and maintenance are essential to ensuring the ongoing integrity of the environment and the safety and well-being of the occupants. Common repairs and maintenance tasks include the following:

+ Mending stairs, handrails, paths, and flooring

+ Removing clutter and trip hazards

+ Installing and/or replacing lighting, locks, security screens, smoke alarms and carbon monoxide detectors, and faucets

Minor modifications may involve installing items that incorporate nonstructural changes to the home and include the following:

+ Installing grab bars, rails, shower hoses, door wedges, stair climbers, and privacy screens

+ Fitting shower seats into shower recesses

+ Altering door swings and window openings

+ Replacing faucets and door handles

+ Installing slip-resistant adhesive strips in baths and showers and on stairs

+ Installing slip-resistant flooring

+ Inserting solid risers between open treads

+ Repainting walls, door frames, and stair edges

+ Repositioning fixtures and fittings

+ Introducing specialized shelving, drawers, and hanging rails into storage cupboards and closets

+ Adding and/or relocating controls, light fittings, and power and telephone outlets

Major modifications are structural changes to the home that incorporate changes to the fabric of the dwelling and include the following:

+ Widening doorways and passages

+ Moving or removing walls and combining spaces

+ Redesigning bedrooms, laundries, bathrooms, toilets, and kitchens

+ Installing ramps, pathways, roll-in shower recesses, and elevators

+ Replacing toilets with accessible pans and cisterns

+ Removing shelving and cupboards under sinks and hotplates

+ Installing additional height-adjustable pantries and shelving

+ Lowering countertops, cupboards, and windows

+ Raising flowerbeds

+ Adding or reassigning rooms

Increasingly, smart technologies are being used to help people maintain their health and well-being, supporting them to remain living safely and independently in their own homes. These technologies may or may not require structural work or changes to the home's plumbing and electrical systems. Security and home automation systems provide older people and people with disabilities with improved safety and security and an efficient means of managing their home environment. Environmental and remote control systems and devices allow people to manage their environment and the fixture and fittings within it (e.g., automatic door openers, keyless entry, remote window and curtain opening, automated lighting sensors, etc.). Mobile phones can also be used to regulate the temperature, lighting, electrical outlets, air conditioning, and security of homes and to answer and open front doors through connection with intercoms. A growing number of home entertainment options, including smart televisions, accessible/online computing and gaming systems, etc. afford people many different ways of enjoying their time at home. Mobile phones, video chat, and telepresence allow people to maintain contact with friends and relatives. Alarms, automated detectors (e.g., falls and seizure), and emergency call devices/systems ensure that people are able to access assistance as required. Those who need to monitor the whereabouts or safety of a loved one at home can use technologies such as remote cameras, sensors, and wearable devices to oversee or monitor movement and activity remotely. Various devices, sensors, administration aids, and apps also assist people and their health care teams to manage complex health conditions, monitor vital signs, identify changes in performance and/or behavior, or record or predict an adverse event within the home. A range of high- and low-technology assistive devices enable people to undertake their daily activities with greater ease by facilitating movement, reducing the impact of conditions/symptoms, enabling participation, augmenting the senses, and/or supporting caregivers to assist in the completion of activities. Reminder and scheduling technologies can also be used to assist people to manage their routines by prompting them through various tasks such as their self-care routine in the bathroom, cooking, and collecting the mail.

Modifications to the environment can make it easier and safer for people to engage in valued occupations and to participate actively in family and community life. They can remove the burden of using an unfamiliar strategy and specialized devices or relying on others to be available for support. However, on the negative side, they can be disruptive and change the way the home is used by other household members and visitors. They may also change the look and feel of spaces in the home, the associated memories, and the personal identity derived from the design and décor (Aplin, 2013; Aplin et al., 2015). Modifications can also be costly. People mostly rely on social services or their own personal resources to fund modifications, so therapists need to be familiar with the building and funding resources available within the community to access environmental interventions effectively (Rigby, Trentham, & Letts, 2014).

DEVELOPING INTERVENTION STRATEGIES

Identifying a range of suitable interventions to address occupational performance difficulties is a complex task. Each person has unique capabilities, expectations, preferences, and experiences and has a distinctive way of undertaking activities. In addition, as outlined in Chapter 1, the home environment, including the physical, personal, social, temporal, occupational, and societal dimensions, needs to be considered when proposing and developing any type of intervention (Aplin, de Jonge, & Gustafsson, 2013). Therapists traditionally use occupational analysis, professional reasoning, and problem solving in developing their understanding of occupational performance difficulties and the range of possible interventions. Additionally, they tailor interventions to suit each situation, drawing on their knowledge of strategies, assistive devices, products, and design, as well as their professional experience.

USE OF OCCUPATIONAL ANALYSIS

Therapists use occupational analysis to develop a clear and detailed understanding of the occupation and the specific way it is performed; to identify where task breakdowns occur; and to analyze factors that contribute to the breakdown. They then generate a list of alternative strategies, assistive devices, social support, and modification options that have the potential to address the identified occupational performance difficulty. Building on the example of going to the toilet discussed earlier in this chapter and in Chapter 6, Table 9-1 details a range of alternative interventions for breakdowns at each stage of the activity. Note that this is a theoretical analysis and, as such, does not claim to be comprehensive or account for the variation that may occur in the way the activity is undertaken by an individual or the unique characteristics of a home environment.

When analyzing activities, therapists are encouraged to consider the whole activity within the context of the relevant area of the home (i.e., access to and egress from the activity area and all the stages or elements of the activity from start to finish). Occupational therapists sometimes restrict analysis to select parts of the activity, for example, focusing exclusively on the transfer on and off the toilet. Problems can arise when designing a support, such as a grab bar, to assist with only one stage of the activity. For instance, the therapist is likely to overlook the impact of this support when the person is attending to personal hygiene while seated on the toilet. The grab bar might not provide the person with the support he or she requires when shifting his or her weight while seated and, more importantly, could be an obstruction to the person when performing this action.

The type of intervention used is, in part, dependent on the nature of the identified problem. Experienced occupational therapists can often generate a number of alternative solutions for any one difficulty. This provides the client with the opportunity to select the interventions that best fit his or her style and preferences, the way he or she completes the activity, and the demands of the environment. Therapists with limited knowledge of alternative options can have difficulty problem solving unique situations and responding to the specific requirements of the individual and household. Because occupational therapists have traditionally used alternative strategies or assistive devices to address occupational performance issues, they are less familiar with the range of ways the environment can be modified to support performance.

Table 9-1. Interventions to Address Breakdowns in Going to the Toilet

TASK	STRATEGY	ASSISTIVE DEVICE	ENVIRONMENTAL MODIFICATION
Register need to go to the toilet	Set at regular intervals	Use an alarm to remind or register moisture	Have a clock visible with marker
Locate and find way to toilet	Feel way along the wall	Install sensor lights	Use lighting or colored line to illuminate way
Open the door	Leave the door open	Install sensor opener	Install lever handle or reverse opening
Enter the room	Leave mobility device outside of toilet	Place threshold ramp at doorway	Widen doorway / Remove level change
Turn lights on and off at night	Leave light on permanently	Install sensor light or timer on light (i.e., turns off at same time each night)	Large switch
Close the door	Leave the door open		Install self-closing hinge
Travel, turn, and position at front of pedestal	Use cues or markers on the floor	Use walking frame	Increase circulation space
Undress		Wear pants with elastic waist	Hold onto grab bar
Sit down onto toilet	Use supportive lowering technique	Use raised toilet frame	Raise pedestal / Install grab bar
Reach for toilet paper/ release sheet	Use pretorn sheets	Use extend-a-hand	Install automatic sheet dispenser
Transfer weight for wiping	Stand to wipe		Lean onto grab bar
Attend to personal hygiene		Use toilet duck or other wiping aid	Bidet
Move from sitting to standing	Push up on knees	Use toilet frame	Push up on grab bar
Don and adjust clothing	Pull up to thighs while seated	Use easy reacher	Hold onto grab bar
Turn and flush toilet	Leave unflushed	Modify button/lever	Auto flush
Clean toilet bowl		Brush with extended handle	
Open door	Leave door open	Install sensor opener	Install lever handle or reverse opening
Negotiate doorway	Leave mobility device outside of toilet	Place threshold ramp at doorway	Widen doorway / Remove level change
Find way to sink to wash hands	Feel way along the wall	Install sensor lights	Use lighting or colored line to illuminate way
Turn on faucets		Use faucet turner	Level handles
Wash hands	Use moist wipes/antiseptic hand wash		
Dry hands			Use electric hand dryer
Please note potential for collapse or assistance need	Education for independent getting up the floor	Emergency call system	Widen circulation space and doorway to enable assistance/attention / Lift off hinges

USE OF REASONING

The nature of the intervention chosen is dependent on a range of factors. First, the person is likely to have specific skills and abilities, past experiences, and preferences that influence how receptive he or she is to an intervention. Second, although some tasks are more conducive to a change in strategy, others are better supported by an assistive device, social support, or home modification. Third, other people within or external to the home environment are likely to influence decisions when interventions affect how they perceive and/or use the home environment. Finally, the home environment might also constrain what can be achieved as a result of the design and physical structure of the house, including building materials.

Therapists rely on professional reasoning to determine the potential effectiveness and impact of proposed interventions by using a combination of scientific, narrative, pragmatic, ethical, and interactive reasoning to design acceptable, effective, and workable home modifications. Refer to Chapter 6 for a definition of each of these reasoning styles and the contribution each makes to the evaluation process. A description of the role reasoning styles play in developing interventions follows.

Occupational therapists use scientific reasoning to identify a range of suitable interventions and tailor them to each client's specific requirements. Knowledge of interventions and their effectiveness—derived from databases, professional literature, education and training events, and professional experience—guides therapists in selecting suitable options. Therapists also review research to ascertain the level of support for proposed interventions and the applicability of this information to each client's situation (Chapter 10 has further information on the use of evidence in designing interventions). In addition, therapists are able to design individualized solutions using their expertise in anthropometrics, biomechanics, and ergonomics; knowledge of health conditions, impairments, and aging, including associated impacts; and an understanding of occupational performance and various aspects of the environment.

Working within a person-environment-occupation theoretical framework, therapists examine the potential impact of each option on the associated interaction. For each alternative strategy, assistive device, social support, or environmental intervention, the therapist asks the following questions:

+ Person
    + Can the client manage the alternative strategy, device, or approach to the occupation?
    + Is he or she willing or able to do the activity in a different way?
    + Is he or she satisfied with the recommended changes?
+ Occupation
    + How will the recommended option affect the nature of the occupation?
    + Is the recommended option well suited to the unique way the person undertakes the occupation?
    + In what way does the recommended option alter the occupation procedure, meaning, or routine?
+ Environment
    + How well will the environment support the recommended option?
    + Are resources available in the environment to support the recommended option?
    + How does the recommended option affect other people in the environment?
    + How does the recommended option affect the physical, personal, social, temporal, occupational, and societal dimensions of the home?

Therapists use narrative reasoning to explore each client's story, particularly their preferences and perceptions of the effectiveness of the recommended options in addressing the identified problem and the potential impact of each solution on the identified goal, the meaning of the occupation, and the various dimensions of the home environment. It is essential that therapists also discuss the proposed interventions with all household members to fully explore the impact of these on the household.

Therapists use pragmatic reasoning to examine the relative costs and availability of resources to implement each option. The physical design and materials of the house and immediate environment can often define the suitability of interventions, particularly modifications. The focus and policies of services can also affect what, and how, resources are made available. However, because clients retain the right to decline the options on offer, they can also access their own resources or an alternative service to address their needs in their preferred way. It is also important to remember that installation or construction might disrupt the household temporarily and that the potential impact of these disturbances on the household needs to be considered when deciding on the most suitable option.

Therapists also use ethical reasoning to evaluate the potential value of options and to identify the most suitable solution for each situation. Although therapists have a duty of care to deliver the best possible intervention, they frequently use ethical reasoning when working with inadequate resources to determine how to proficiently implement an effective solution. When clients and therapists differ in their understanding of the effectiveness and impact of various solutions, therapists seek to fully understand the person's perceptions of each option and provide him or her with a deeper understanding of their professional perspective. An exchange of information and understanding may result in the establishment of a workable solution that meets the person's goals and preferences and addresses the therapist's concerns, or the development of a plan to achieve an appropriate solution. Ultimately, clients have the right to do what they think is best in their own homes, but therapists also have a responsibility to inform them of the potential risks in choosing a less-than-ideal option. See Chapter 12 for further discussion of managing ethical decisions.

Throughout the development of intervention strategies, it is vital that the occupational therapist and client work in collaboration and that the therapeutic relationship remains strong and intact to enable the continuation of the necessary working alliance. To this end, interactive reasoning is used by the therapist in order to consider the client's preferences and implement particular automatic and conscious communication skills and interpersonal behaviors that engage and motivate the client. This allows the therapist to maintain a continued allied relationship based in trust. This relationship is essential for gaining the information necessary for the other reasoning types to occur successfully and for the client to have confidence in the value and intention of the therapist's intervention recommendations.

DETERMINING AND NEGOTIATING SUITABLE OPTIONS

There are usually any number of potentially useful alternative solutions to occupational performance problems in the home; however, there are several issues that can affect decision making, including economic, architectural, and social barriers (Rigby et al., 2014). Cost is often a consideration when designing environmental interventions. It is important to work responsibly within a budget, but therapists should also be mindful of the potential long-term costs of interventions. For example, some assistive devices, such as a tub transfer bench for the bath or an over-toilet frame, initially cost less to install than a shower recess or an accessible toilet with grab bars. However, these interventions can prove to be more costly in the long term if the client deteriorates and cannot manage sit-to-stand transfers. In addition to possible further costs associated with additional strategies, tools, and/or modifications to meet the new needs, the client may require additional supervision or assistance to complete the task, or he or she could sustain an injury from being incapable of using the assistive device safely. It is well recognized in the occupational health and safety arena and in the area of workplace accommodations that there is a hierarchy of interventions that vary in terms of anticipated effectiveness. It is proposed that environmental interventions are among the most effective in managing risk and reducing incidents and accidents (Peek-Asa & Zwerling, 2003) as it can be difficult for people to change entrenched behaviors in familiar environments.

The design and structure of the home also pose a number of challenges when designing environmental interventions (Rigby et al., 2014). Therapists need to understand the constraints presented by the built environment in order to determine what is feasible. Because this is not an occupational therapist's area of expertise, it is advisable to consult a design or construction professional to provide technical building advice on the suitability of the home for modification. Further information will be provided later in this chapter to assist therapists in understanding the complexities they are likely to encounter when working with the built environment.

Although home visits provide therapists with an enriched understanding of clients and their home environment, therapists, in reality, experience only a snapshot of people's lives at the time of these visits. It is therefore critical to examine solutions thoroughly with clients to ensure that they will fit well with them and their families, routines, lifestyles, and home environments. Collaboration is required if interventions are to be effectively designed to suit the goals and preferences of clients and their families.

The nature of interventions considered is also likely to be influenced by factors related to therapists' knowledge, experiences, models of practice, and the service and information resources available. Each therapist tends to have a particular scope of knowledge and expertise, which will likely affect the options identified. Therapists who have worked with particular products or designs are likely to favor these over less familiar options. The models of practice therapists employ also predispose them to using some interventions in preference to others. For example, therapists using a rehabilitation framework are likely to focus on remediating function before compensating for lost function by using assistive devices or removing barriers in the environment to accommodate specific impairments and activity limitations. On the other hand, therapists using a Person-Environment-Occupation model would focus primarily on enabling occupational performance by ensuring that the environment was designed to promote engagement in personally meaningful activities in the home and community.

Therapists might work within a particular service with its own specific focus, policy, procedures, or protocols that dictate the resources therapists have readily available to them. Some services and agencies fund assistive devices more readily than environmental interventions, which define the intervention options available. The availability of technical advice can also vary between services, which affects therapists' capacity to consider modifications that require structural changes or building expertise. Though research and industry standards provide information on the safety and effectiveness of some interventions, there can be limited information on other options. This can result in options such as exercise, education, and assistive devices being favored in the absence of evidence on environmental interventions. Further, the detail provided in the access standards on the design requirements of independent adult manual wheelchair users often predominates because little is known about the design requirements of people with severe and multiple impairments who use other devices and rely on caregiver support to complete activities in areas of the home.

Tailoring Interventions

Environmental interventions in the home need to be practicable and acceptable to the client and other household members and accommodate everyone who lives in or visits the home regularly. They should not only address the identified problem but should also promote occupational performance and ensure that the essential qualities and meaning of activities and the home environment are retained. Therapists should also ensure that the interventions will not cause any unexpected stress or discomfort and will not create new issues for the person in the home environment.

Therapists generally tailor the intervention to the specific requirements of the person, the occupation, and the environment, giving consideration to the following:

✦ The characteristics of the person

✦ The way the activity is undertaken and, specifically, where performance breakdowns or difficulties occur and/or where the activity could be further supported

✦ Whether the environment can accommodate an intervention or places any constraints on its availability, usefulness, or location

Characteristics of the Person

When tailoring an intervention for a specific situation, therapists consider the person's goals; preferences; specific impairments and occupational performance difficulties; ability to cope with the intended change; and general skills, abilities, and capacities that include the anthropometrics of the person(s) likely to use the intervention. People have preferred ways of approaching activities and also personal experiences and likes/dislikes that can affect their decisions. Some people find it difficult to approach a task in a different way, so it is important that therapists acknowledge this and devise therapeutic interventions that work with the client's preferred approach. Other household members using the space will also be affected by the changes and will need to be consulted during the planning process.

Therapists determine whether the individual has specific impairments in his or her sensory, motor, cognitive, or psychosocial function that may present additional difficulties and ensure these are accommodated in the design of the solution. For example, when recommending the installation of a grab bar to assist during toileting, the therapist would consider the following:

✦ Static balance in the seated and standing positions and dynamic balance when moving to ascertain the amount and type of support required

✦ Strength and coordination of the upper limbs and condition of the joints and muscles to determine whether the grab bar can be used for pushing or pulling during sit-to-stand or side-on transfers

✦ Sensation to establish whether additional slip resistance is required

✦ Vision and visual perception to determine the degree of color contrast required

✦ Cognition to establish whether the person requires any training, prompting, supervision, or assistance in using the grab bar

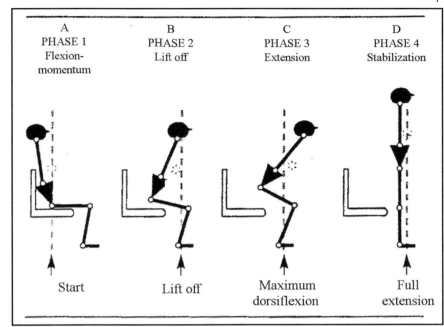

A PHASE 1 Flexion- momentum	B PHASE 2 Lift off	C PHASE 3 Extension	D PHASE 4 Stabilization
Start	Lift off	Maximum dorsiflexion	Full extension

Figure 9-3. Phases of rising. (Reprinted from Laporte, D. M., Chan, D., & Sveistrup, H. [1999]. Rising from sitting in elderly people, part 1: Implications of biomechanics and physiology. *British Journal of Occupational Therapy, 62*[1], 36-42.)

+ The person's confidence and self-efficacy during the activity

Anthropometrics, which uses standardized methods of measurement, can also assist therapists in determining the most suitable configuration and position for a grab bar. Chapter 7 provides a detailed description of this methodology. Therapists often use anthropometrics to tailor the intervention to suit each client. They assess the person's:

+ Body weight to choose a rail that has been load tested to manage the person's weight (downward and sideward force)

+ Location of key body landmarks and reach range when seated and standing to determine the required height of the bar above the floor

+ Length of forearm to establish the preferred length of the grab bar

+ Hand size to guide the size of the diameter of the grab bar

+ Grip strength to guide the size of the diameter of the grab bar and the finish on the surface of the bar

+ Right- or left-hand dominance to determine the side of the toilet on which the bar should be placed (influenced by the side of the body affected by the person's health condition or disability, his or her presentation, and how he or she completes activities)

Characteristics of the Activity and Occupation

Therapists customize solutions to support clients through troublesome aspects of activities while ensuring that other aspects of the activity are not disrupted. For example, when designing a grab bar to assist an individual to transfer on and off the toilet, the therapist observes the client's posture, movement, and center of gravity in relation to his or her base of support and notes specific aspects of the transfer that are problematic. With an understanding of the biomechanical factors that affect the sit-to-stand transfer, the therapist determines whether the client is experiencing difficulty with flexion momentum, lift-off, extension, and stabilization (Laporte, Chan, & Sveistrup, 1999; Figure 9-3) and recommends the grab bar configuration accordingly. If a client is having difficulty bending forward, the therapist might provide a vertical grab bar that he or she can pull on to move forward. If lift-off is problematic, the therapist might provide a horizontal grab bar to push up on. To assist the client in the extension or stabilization stage of the transfer, the therapist might provide a diagonal or vertical bar that the client can hold on to while transitioning into standing and to arrest the movement to maintain a static standing posture. If a client stands for toileting rather than sitting, a vertical grab bar may be required to provide stability in this position. A vertical or diagonal grab bar may also assist as the client moves from standing to sitting on the toilet, as these configurations allow the hand to move down the rail. It is important to note that if the client experiences difficulty at each stage of the transfer, the grab bar configuration would need to incorporate each of these elements.

The therapist would also determine other aspects of the activity where the client could benefit from grab bar support and ensure that the solution is adequate for these aspects of the activity. For example, clients might require support when shifting their weight while seated to attend to their hygiene or when standing to adjust clothing. In addition, the therapist would need to ensure that the proposed design does not interfere with other actions or tasks the person performs during this activity (e.g., that the person will not knock his or her elbow on the grab bar when doffing or donning his or her clothes). The therapist would also remain mindful of the value of the activity to the person and, in particular, the unique elements and methods he or she should aim to retain when tailoring the intervention to the occupation (e.g., a modification to create a solid backrest may be required to allow the client to lean back and relax during toileting, particularly on an accessible toilet where the distance between the bowl and cistern is usually greater than a standard toilet).

Characteristics of the Environment

The physical, personal, social, temporal, occupational, and societal dimensions, discussed previously in Chapter 1, require careful consideration when designing and determining interventions. Each of these dimensions affects how modification recommendations are accepted, used, or rejected by the clients, their families, and other householders (Aplin et al., 2015).

The physical environment poses considerable challenges to intervention planning. Often, the environment can constrain the design of a solution because there is insufficient space or structural support for the proposed modification. For example, therapists are commonly interested in maximizing circulation space in the bathroom, which is often achieved by removing other fixtures, such as the bath, or annexing spaces adjacent to the bathroom, such as the toilet, and incorporating this space into the bathroom. If the wall between the bathroom and toilet is load bearing (i.e., supporting the roof or upper floor), costly structural work can preclude this option. The positioning of grab bars can also be limited by the location of studs (vertical supports in the wall) because grab bars need to be anchored directly into studs that sit behind the wall sheeting or onto solid blocking mounted onto the studs to

ensure the grab bars do not come out of the wall when used (Adaptive Environment Center, 2002).

Therapists should consult with building and design professionals if they are uncertain about whether the environment can support the proposed intervention. This consultation is vital as there is often a range of different ways to modify spaces and provide additional structural support, and the expertise, insight, and advice of these professionals can be invaluable in discerning the best potential option. For example, Figure 9-4 shows a number of alternatives to securing grab bars directly into studs:

+ Using special fasteners
+ Fixing a backing board onto the studs
+ Installing blocking between studs
+ Replacing the wall sheeting with plywood that is at least 3/4 in (19 mm) or more in thickness

Therapists are encouraged to develop an understanding of the physical structure of the built environment so that they have knowledge of the possibilities and constraints for designing environmental interventions and can effectively discuss alternatives with building and design professionals.

Outside of the structure of the home, there are further physical aspects that can influence design and decision making. The ambient conditions of the home is one consideration that requires careful review. For example, people are often reluctant to install lifts or alter the placement of windows or walls if it means they lose a view or natural sources of light in the home (Aplin et al., 2013). Other considerations might be ensuring people are protected from weather conditions when entering and leaving the house by providing roofing to landings and pathways (Aplin et al., 2013). Therapists also need to be mindful of the impact of changing light conditions that occur across the day/night and how these might affect things like safety, ambience, and associated modification decisions. The location of the home can also influence decision making. For example, the topography and geology of an area can influence the design and placement of ramps and whether earthworks can be used to enhance access to entryways, a mailbox, or clotheslines. Further, proximity to public transport, access to shops and other services, and family and friends are important considerations when deciding whether to modify the existing home or to relocate.

Although it is often easy to understand the physical dimensions of the home that affect home modification decisions, it can be challenging for therapists to develop sufficient understanding of the personal, social, temporal, occupational, and societal dimensions of the home during a home visit. The impact

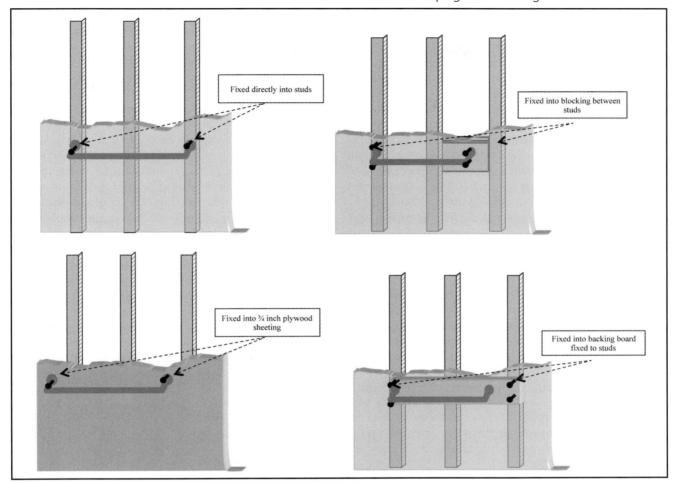

Fixed directly into studs

Fixed into blocking between studs

Fixed into ¾ inch plywood sheeting

Fixed into backing board fixed to studs

Figure 9-4. Alternative ways to secure grab bars.

of these dimensions often comes to light when discussing alternative options and therapists encounter clients' reluctance to modify the home, and in some cases, active resistance to modification recommendations. During these discussions, therapists come to understand the clients' concerns and negotiate solutions that respect their experience of home.

The personal dimension, the emotional connection with home, has been found to strongly influence home modification decision making (Aplin et al., 2013) and requires sensitivity dedicated to the client's perspective. Having control over one's home is key to a positive experience of home, so consequently having choice and control in the home modification process is paramount. The literature consistently reports that successful home modifications result from consultation and affording clients control in the home modification process (Aplin et al., 2013, 2015; Hawkins & Stewart, 2002; Johansson, Borell, & Lilja, 2009; Kruse et al., 2010; Tanner et al., 2008). The amount of control clients wish to have over their modification(s) can vary from making choices about

simple aspects such as color or style of fittings to full control of the project. With the latter, clients are able to project-manage their modification(s) with a service, choosing their own materials, products, and tradespeople/building professionals to complete the work. In this approach, occupational therapists, building and design professionals, and other service providers are viewed as consultants to the client rather than leading the process.

The appearance is often an aspect of home that is of importance to clients as it reflects their identity and promotes their connection to the home. This aspect of home can be challenging for therapists as it is not easily observable and can therefore take time to understand and appreciate. Some clients fear that modifications will make their home "look disabled" or "like a hospital" and want to ensure the modifications match the current style of the home (Aplin et al., 2013). Ensuring that the design of modifications is aesthetically pleasing and consistent with the look and feel of the home will often reduce these concerns, and the implementation of resources such as pictures and videos of potential modifications can be very useful in assisting clients to visualize proposed changes. Further, although costs are often a consideration for many clients, it is important to not make assumptions as sometimes clients are willing to pay significant additional costs to ensure modifications match their home or provide a less "clinical" look (Aplin et al., 2013). Further to aesthetics, safety and security considerations can also affect clients' willingness to consider or undertake a modification. For example, a ramp can improve accessibility and safety when entering or leaving the home; however, people may be reluctant to have one installed at the front of the home as it potentially identifies the resident as having a disability and portrays a potential image of vulnerability to people passing by the home. Consequently, the therapist might negotiate to have the ramp installed at the rear entrance. Reducing the visibility of modifications from the street also protects a person's privacy as some clients may prefer to conceal their disability from others' awareness or knowledge. Additionally, some clients are reluctant to have modifications in the toilet or family bathroom because visitors will potentially be made aware of the difficulties the client is experiencing. Furthermore, an en suite bathroom may be a preferred choice to a main bathroom for modification so the client can bathe and dress in a private space rather than mobilizing or being transported through public areas of the home.

Independence is generally the primary goal of home modifications; however, freedom within the home is equally important. For example, parents of a child with a disability often seek to involve the child in all household activities and may require access and circulation in spaces such as the kitchen to allow the child to watch or participate in the preparation of dinner. Further, although parents might currently be assisting the child with various activities, they may want to ensure spaces, fixtures, and fittings are accessible so they can encourage the child's independence as he or she develops. Understanding these aspects of the personal dimension help to create solutions that are inclusive and promote future independence.

Social connections and relationships with the people whom we share and invite into our home are an important aspect of life. Therapists often consider the requirements of a partner when making changes in a space. This is most apparent when placing a grab bar in the toilet for an older couple who differ in height and experience different challenges rising from the toilet. When designing modifications, therapists also consider the caregiver(s) and the demands placed on them when supporting the client in activities. Clients are also often mindful of the impact of modifications on people who may visit regularly. For example, an older grandmother may be reluctant to remove a bath to make a shower recess if it affects the ability of her grandchildren to use the bathtub when they stay over. When other people and relationships are not considered, tension can result, especially when the needs of one member are prioritized over others (Heywood, 2005). Consequently, it is critical that therapists consider the social dimension of the home, such as other people who also use the area (e.g. partners and family), visitors, and any caregivers involved in the completion of home-based activities when making recommendations.

Considering the temporal dimension of home is also important in home modification decision making as many modifications are costly and fixed or permanent. The daily routines and cycles of activities in the home are not always evident to a therapist during a brief home visit. Similarly, the number of people in the environment and the range of activities that occur vary considerably from day to day and across the week. People may be resistant to modifications that disrupt the familiar rhythms of the household. For example, if the bathroom has been the same for 20 years, people may be uncomfortable with or reject the modification simply because it is different from what is known and may disrupt the order of their home and routine (Aplin, 2013). Furthermore, clients may be concerned about the disruption to the home and routine resulting from modification works, especially those that extend over a number of weeks. It is important to recognize that objection or rejection of suggested modifications may be about the change to the home itself rather than issues of identity, cost, or lack of control in the process. In these circumstances, it is important to work with the client to come up with solutions that will allow him or her to keep some of the aspects that are important to them, such as keeping a particular cabinet, reusing tiles, or painting in the same color. It is also important that clients are given the opportunity to process the information provided and consider alternative options before making a decision, even if it means that modifications need to be delayed.

Anticipating changes over time, such as growth in children or deterioration or improvement in health, can also ensure that the modifications address client needs long term. One recurring preoccupation for clients and families is the impact of modifications on the resale value of the home (Aplin, 2013). In these situations, clients can be reassured by information on the removal of minor modifications such as grab bars. However, if the future needs and wants of occupants are not considered, clients can be left with unsuitable modifications and wasted resources

(Aplin, 2013). In some circumstances, people may need to consider whether it might be better to move to a more suitable home rather than modify their existing home. Occupational therapists support families facing this decision by providing information about key considerations, such as the implications of moving or remaining in the same location, considering proximity to family and services and their connectedness to their current home. Working with families to discuss these issues may help to create solutions that avoid costly errors, both financially and emotionally, for families.

The meaning of everyday activities within the home and the roles the client wishes to undertake (the occupational dimension) also influences home modification decision making. The way an individual completes an occupation is important and can affect design, particularly if different from standard expectations (Aplin et al., 2013). For example, the aforementioned recommendation for the grandmother to install a shower recess to replace a bath may be declined if she herself prefers to bathe rather than shower. Within the home, people participate in a range of occupations, including but not limited to personal activities of daily living, that are meaningful to them. For example, access to the garden or shed may be necessary to participate in meaningful leisure occupations or be important to maintaining a role of home maintenance (Aplin et al., 2013). Although many services focus on personal activities of daily living, it is important that therapists recognize that clients may have other priorities for modifications and associated resources (i.e., money) and choose to focus on occupations that are considered more important. When using a client-centered approach, therapists are mindful of meaningful occupations and the positive impact these can have on clients' health and well-being. Consequently, therapists seek to promote safety and independence in these activities and ensure continued engagement in these valued occupations.

The societal dimension can have a substantial influence on home modification decision making as it shapes the scope of practice of occupational therapists and what they offer to their clients, and consequently determines the amount of control and choice people have over their home modifications. Occupational therapists are often bound by service restrictions and guidelines, but they are also responsible for upholding professional ethics and adhering to professional frameworks that seek to enhance independence and well-being. For example, a service might only fund home modifications that improve safety and independence in personal activities of daily living and not be concerned about the client's safety when gardening, which is a meaningful occupation for the client and therefore important to their health and well-being. Additionally, services may restrict options by only making a small range of faucet fittings, grab bar styles, or tiles available (Aplin, 2013), limiting client choice and control. Changes to standard products, materials, and design can lead to additional expenses for clients; however, the freedom to choose modifications increases acceptance and enhances the enjoyment and use of the home. The competing demands between dimensions can make home modification decision making complicated and solutions difficult to negotiate with clients. Chapter 12 provides a framework for dealing with dilemmas that inevitably arise from these complexities in home modification practice.

Another societal influence is building codes and design standards. Modifications that require structural, building, plumbing, or electrical work are likely to be subject to building regulations and require consultation with a contractor or designer. Although not required in private dwellings, accessible design standards are often a key consideration for home modification design and can have an oppressive impact on modification decision making as some services may not install modifications unless they meet access standards (Aplin, 2013). Clients have spoken of their frustrations with service providers who rigidly apply access standards when designing home modifications and their frustration with therapists who prioritize standards over the needs, requirements, and specifications of the person (Aplin et al., 2013, 2015; Tanner et al., 2008). It is important that therapists have a solid understanding of the access design standards and their application in residential settings when negotiating with clients and services. The appropriate use of access standards in domestic dwellings is discussed in further detail in Chapter 11.

DEVELOPING ENVIRONMENTAL INTERVENTIONS

As noted earlier in this and other chapters, the capacity and potential of the environment to support occupational performance are well recognized. Changes to the environment can reduce demands on the person; enhance health; increase safety, independence, and effectiveness of performance; improve the quality of life and experience; and promote further occupational engagement. Environmental changes can also reduce the need to learn new ways of performing activities and can limit reliance on assistive devices and on other people.

Although therapists are experts in promoting occupational performance, they tend to be less familiar with home modification options and the architectural and technical aspects of the built environment. Consequently, they can feel uncomfortable proposing environmental recommendations, seeing themselves as ill equipped to assess the viability of an environmental solution. Therapists can address this in a number of ways by:

+ Liaising with specialists who can advise them on environmental solution options, including appropriate products and designs

+ Using resources targeted specifically at common occupational performance problems in the home and typical environmental interventions

+ Using tools that direct them to specific environmental problems and how these can be addressed

+ Familiarizing themselves with general resources about designing safe and accessible environments

+ Developing expertise in the technical aspects of the built environment

+ Using a framework for considering the various elements in the built environment

Liaising With Specialists

Occupational therapists can refer clients to specialist services for an environmental intervention or seek advice from other experts, such as more experienced therapists, design and building professionals, or suppliers of home modification products. When referring clients to a specialist service, it is important to provide them with appropriate information and liaise with them about alternative strategies and assistive devices that have been recommended.

It is often necessary for occupational therapists to access the expertise of an experienced colleague, building or design professional, or supplier of home modification products when designing an environmental intervention. Ideally, it is useful for the therapist, builder/designer, and supplier of products (such as vertical lifts) to review the property together because there are often constraints when attempting to modify an existing structure. The most suitable solution is often achieved when the therapist, builder/designer, and product supplier collaborate with the client to identify the environmental intervention that will achieve the best person-environment-occupation fit. Remote strategies such as video teleconferencing have also been used by therapists with building and design specialists to observe direct measurement of the client and environment and examine activity participation in key areas of the home (Sanford & Butterfield, 2005). This technology allows the therapist, client, and specialists to discuss concerns in real time without everyone being physically present at the home and to draw on the experience and expertise of all parties in negotiating an acceptable solution in a cost-effective and efficient way.

If it is not possible to visit the property with the building and design professional or negotiate a remote consultation, tools such as the Comprehensive Assessment and Solutions Process for Aging Residents (CASPAR; Sanford, Pynoos, Tejral, & Browne, 2002) can guide therapists to measure aspects of the environment that designers and builders need to be cognizant of in order to redesign or modify the area (Figure 9-5).

Targeted Resources

Targeted resources are generally aimed at assisting clients in identifying problems in the home and informing them of potential solutions. For example, the Adaptive Environments Center (2002) has developed the *Consumer's Guide to Home Adaptation*, which can be used by a client, community care worker, or building and design professional to evaluate needs, identify solutions, plan, and undertake environmental modifications (Figure 9-6).

Similarly, the Canada Mortgage and Housing Corporation (CMHC) has developed a number of useful publications to assist with making homes accessible and safe, including *Accessible Housing by Design Series* (CMHC, 2016a) and *Maintaining Seniors' Independence Through Home Adaptation: A Self-Assessment Guide* (CMHC, 2016b).

Box 9-2 provides an extract from the *Maintaining Seniors' Independence Through Home Adaptation: A Self-Assessment Guide* (CMHC, 2016b) publication, detailing recommendations for people who experience difficulty stepping into or out of the bathtub.

These publications introduce therapists to the broad range of environmental interventions available to address specific occupational performance difficulties in the home for older people and for people who mobilize using wheelchairs.

Tools for Identifying and Addressing Specific Environmental Problems

Tools such as the Housing Enabler (HE; Iwarsson & Slaugh, 2010) assist therapists in identifying and

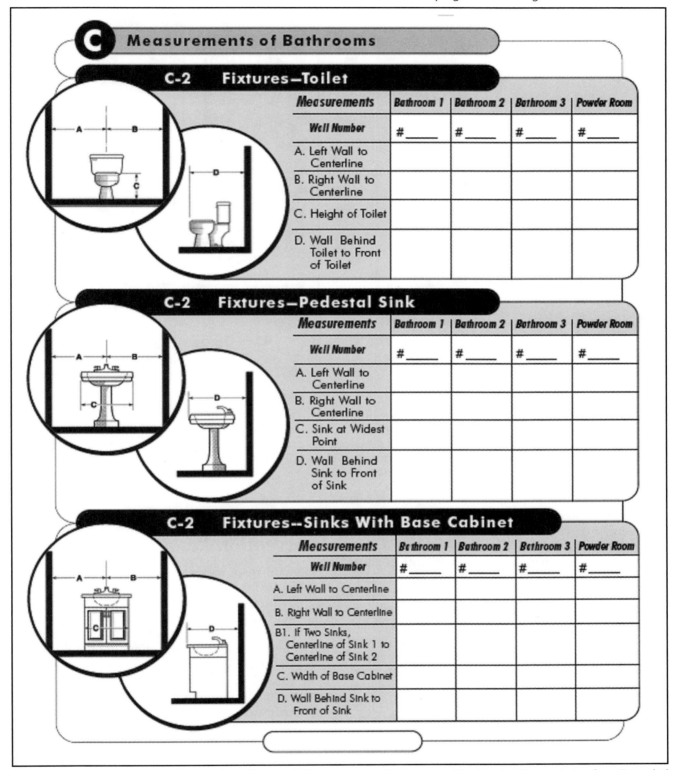

Figure 9-5. CASPAR Part 5, Description of the Home—C, Measurement of Bathrooms. (Reprinted with permission from Extended Home Living Services, Wheeling, IL.)

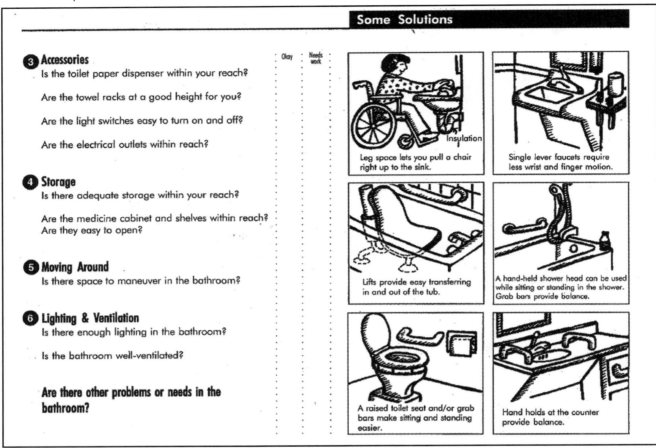

Figure 9-6. Consumer's Guide to Home Adaptation—Bathroom Solutions. (Reprinted with permission from Adaptive Environments Center. [2002]. *Consumer's guide to home adaptation*. Boston, MA: Author.)

measuring problematic design elements in the built environment. The HE provides therapists with details of environmental design elements that interfere with the performance of people with a range of identified functional and mobility impairments. It also provides the minimum design requirements according to Swedish accessibility standards. As noted in Chapter 6, the HE alerts therapists to elements in the physical environment that present challenges to people with varying functional and mobility impairments, such as difficulty interpreting information, severe loss of sight, complete loss of sight, severe loss of hearing, prevalence of poor balance, incoordination, limitations of stamina, difficulty in moving head, difficulty in reaching with arms, difficulty in handling and fingering, loss of upper extremity skills, difficulty bending or kneeling, reliance on walking aids, reliance on wheelchair, and extremes of size and weight (see Figure 6-3). Once potential barriers have been identified, therapists can focus on removing or modifying the environment to be more accessible (Figure 9-7).

General Environmental Intervention Resources

General resources on accessible design, such as the Americans With Disabilities Act (ADA; 1990) and Architectural Barrier Act (ABA: 1968), accessibility guidelines (United States Access Board, 2004/2014), and *The Accessible Housing Design File* (Barrier Free Environments Incorporated, 1991), assist therapists in understanding the design requirements for people with disabilities and, in particular, people with mobility impairments. Therapists often refer to the standards to identify the recommended specifications for particular design elements (e.g., the circulation spaces around various fixtures and fittings, heights of power points and light switches, and grab bar specifications, such as diameter, wall clearance, load capacity, and clearance from the centerline of the toilet). However, these standards were designed for public buildings and were aimed to suit the majority of users. Based on the anthropometrics of young adults who mobilize independently using

Box 9-2. Maintaining Seniors' Independence Through Home Adaptation: A Self-Assessment Guide Item— Canada Mortgage and Housing Corporation

CMHC has developed *Maintaining Seniors' Independence Through Home Adaptation: A Self-Assessment Guide*, which is designed to assist older people in addressing specific problems in the home environment. This guide details a range of activities that older people typically experience difficulties with in the home and describes adaptations to address these difficulties. Activities addressed include getting in and out of the home, using the stairs, moving around the home, using the kitchen, using the bathroom, getting out of a bed or chair, using closets and storage areas, doing laundry, using the telephone or answering the door, and controlling light and ventilation. This tool does not attempt to diagnose the specific cause of the difficulty but provides a range of environmental interventions aimed at reducing difficulty in performing the tasks such as removing, moving, modifying, replacing, or adding various fixtures and fittings. Example of *Maintaining Seniors' Independence Through Home Adaptation: A Self-Assessment Guide* item:

5.3 Do you have any difficulty stepping into or out of the bathtub?

☐ **NO** >> If no, go to the next question.

☐ **YES** >> If yes, check off the adaptations below that would help you.

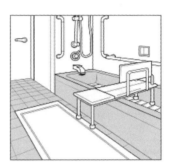

> ☐ Install vertical and horizontal grab bars in locations that will best assist you in entering and exiting the tub.
>
> ☐ Ensure the grab bars are well secured.
>
> ☐ Install nonslip flooring throughout the bathroom.
>
> ☐ Ensure floor mats have nonslip backing.
>
> ☐ Install a nonslip surface in the bathtub.
>
> ☐ Install a commercial or custom-made transfer bath bench, so that the tub can be entered from a seated position.
>
> ☐ Replace the bathtub with a shower stall or wheel-in shower if stepping over the tub wall is too difficult or unsafe.
>
> ☐ Install a separate shower stall or wheel-in shower if the difficulty is severe.
>
> ☐ Modify the tub with a custom cut-out to eliminate the need to lift legs over the side of the tub.
>
> ☐ Install a ceiling track or other lift system for use by caregivers to transfer individuals with serious disabilities into the tub with the appropriate bath seat.
>
> ☐ Other (describe).

A vertical grab bar provides support when entering the tub, while a horizontal (or angled) bar helps you to complete the entrance and lower yourself onto a shower seat or to the bottom of the tub.

a wheelchair, the specifications in these standards are not always appropriate for occupational therapy clients, many of whom do not fit the profile on which these standards were founded. Further discussion on how the standards are used in home modification practice is provided in Chapter 11.

There are also a number of resources dedicated to designing for specific groups; some examples include the following:

✦ Aging:

　✦ *Residential Design for Aging in Place* (Lawlor & Thomas, 2008)

✦ Alzheimer's and dementia:

　✦ *Adapting Your Home to Living With Dementia: A Resource Book for Living at Home and Guide to Home Adaptations* (CMHC, 2009)

　✦ *Alzheimer's and Related Dementias Homes That Help: Advice From Caregivers for Creating a Supportive Home* (Olsen, Ehrenkrantz, & Hutchings, 1993)

　✦ Dementia Centre: Design for Dementia (HammondCare, 2017)

　✦ *Design Innovations for Aging and Alzheimer's: Creating Caring Environments* (Brawley, 2006)

C. Indoor environment General (p. 128)	A	B1	B2	C	D	E	F	G	H	I	J	K	L	M	N	NOTES
																Note that the indoor assessment is linked to "necessary housing functions" (in particular stairs, door widths).
1. Stairs/thresholds/differences in level between rooms/floor spaces (more than 25 mm).		3	3		3	3	1						3	4		
2. Complicated/illogical circulation routes (p. 129).	3	3	3				4						1	1		
3. Narrow passages/corridors in relation to fixtures/design of building (less than 1.3 m, p. 131).													3	4	1	*Note the difference between C3 and C9.*
4. Narrow doors (clearance less than 0.80 m, pp. 146–47).													4	4	1	
5. Slippery walking surface (hygiene rooms are rated separately) (pp. 96–97).		3	3		3	3	1						3		1	
6. High-pile/loose-weave/soft floor covering (pp. 96–97).							1						1	3		
7. Loose small mats.					3	2	1						2	3		
8. Loose cables etc. on the floor.					3	2	1						2	3		
9. Insufficient manoeuvring areas in relation to movable furnishings (pp. 26–27)	2	3			3	3							3	4	1	*Note the difference between C3 and C9.*

Figure 9-7. HE Environmental Assessment. (Reprinted with permission from Iwarsson, S., & Slaug, B. [2010]. *The Housing Enabler: A method for rating/screening and analysing accessibility problems in housing* [2nd ed.]. Lund & Staffanstorp, Sweden: Veten & Skapen HB and Slaug Enabling Development.)

+ *Designing for Alzheimer's Disease: Strategies for Creating Better Care Environments* (Brawley, 1997)

+ The Dementia Centre: Design Resource Centre (The Dementia Services Development Centre, 2012)

+ *Occupational Therapy and Dementia Care: The Home Environmental Skill-Building Program for Individuals and Families* (Gitlin & Corcoran, 2005)

+ *Universal Design Guidelines Dementia Friendly Dwellings for People With Dementia, Their Families and Carers* (Grey, Pierce, Cahill, & Dyer, 2015)

+ Visual impairments:

+ *Making Life More Livable: Simple Adaptations for Living at Home After Vision Loss* (Duffy, 2002)

+ Young people with significant disability:

+ New Housing Options for People With Significant Disability: Design Insights (Ryan & Reynolds, 2015)

+ Other country/locality-specific web-based/electronic resources include examples such as:

+ Australia: Guide to Planning Bathrooms and Kitchens 2015 (Independent Living Centre NSW, 2015)

+ Australia: Livable Housing Design (Livable Housing Australia, 2015)

+ Hong Kong: Universal Design Guidebook for Residential Development in Hong Kong (Hong Kong Housing Society, 2014)

+ New Zealand: Lifemark (Lifemark, 2017)

+ United States of America: Better Living Design (Better Living Design Institute, 2014)

+ United Kingdom: Housing LIN (Housing LIN, n.d.)

+ United Kingdom: Lifetime Homes (Lifetime Homes, n.d.)

Increasingly, there is an emphasis on designing homes using a universal approach. Universal design ensures that features in the home are usable, comfortable, and convenient for everyone in the home, regardless of ability or life stage. A growing number of resources describe universal design features for residential buildings and community environments, including:

+ *Practical Guide to Universal Home Design* (Wilder Research Center, 2002) is a 19-page booklet that illustrates essential universal design features for various areas of the home, including entrance, kitchen, bathroom, laundry, bedrooms, living and dining rooms, storage, garage, doorways and hallways, floors, windows, and stairs.

+ *Design for the Ages: Universal Design as a Rehabilitation Strategy* (Sanford, 2012) is a book written for building, design, and health professionals interested in the use of universal design for the promotion of participation and performance. It considers the influence of universal design on social and health movements and demonstrates a focus on reducing segregation and stigma that has traditionally been associated with many previous design strategies.

+ *Universal Design: Creating Inclusive Environments* (Steinfeld & Maisel, 2012) is a text that provides a comprehensive overview of practices and solutions in universal design. It examines the difference between accessibility and universal design and the associated relationships with active living and sustainable design.

It is important to note that these resources provide therapists with a vision of what is possible and an understanding of specific design requirements. However, they do not generally assist the therapist in determining the specific design requirements for an individual or whether the existing environment is able to accommodate the proposed design elements.

In addition to the aforementioned text and web-based resources, social media and social networking are means of communication that are widely being used to share and disseminate information relevant to environmental interventions and provide support for therapists and professionals working within applicable fields. These "online interactions" enable electronic communications through which a wide range of information related to home modifications can be shared through web-based media and online groups, including videos, blogs, forums, chats, networking sites (e.g. Facebook, Twitter), etc. It is important to consider these as a potential resource when sourcing information, examining options and alternatives, and seeking training and support when working in the field of home modification. However, it is also vital to be critical of the source and quality of the information that is provided, as the nature of the internet enables a vast range of people with varying backgrounds and experience to make claims and recommendations.

Some examples of current social networking opportunities include:

+ Association of Consultants in Access Australia, available via Facebook and Twitter

+ Australian Network for Universal Housing Design, available via Facebook and Twitter

+ Centre for Universal Design Australia, available via Facebook, Twitter, and LinkedIn

+ HomeMods4OT, available via Facebook

+ Home Design for Living, available via Facebook, Twitter, and LinkedIn

Developing Expertise in the Technical Aspects of the Built Environment

Some therapists find it useful to invest time reading or studying the technical aspects of the built environment to assist them in understanding building structures and systems that affect modification design. Additional knowledge assists therapists to communicate more effectively with building and design professionals and enables them to identify whether a solution is viable before referring to a builder/architect for a work design or quote. For example, if the therapist knows that the existing wall in the toilet is unable to support the installation of grab bars in the required location, he or she can discuss alternative options with the client or prepare the client with information about the structural work required to install the grab bars. It is, however, unwise for therapists who do not have formal building qualifications to provide advice that is outside of their area of expertise. Occupational therapists understand the person-environment-occupation transaction but do not necessarily have knowledge of specific products, design and construction techniques, systems and structures, or building legislation. It is always advisable for therapists to seek further advice when environmental interventions require building or design expertise.

Framework for Dealing With Elements in the Built Environment

A deeper understanding of the built environment will assist therapists to appreciate the impact of the environment on the person-environment-occupation transaction. Therapists have a sound understanding of body structures and functions that allows them to understand the impact of impairments on function. They also possess a deep understanding

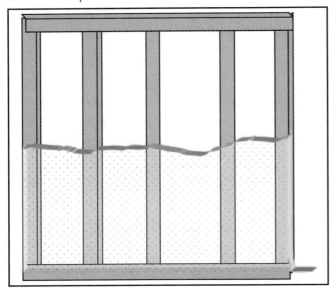

Figure 9-8. Structure of a stud wall.

of occupational performance that allows them to analyze the value and elements of various activities. A richer understanding of the environment and the elements within an occupational performance space and their associated structure will help therapists recognize the limitations of the existing environment. This assists in determining what can be altered and how it can be improved to support occupational performance. This understanding will also enable therapists to collaborate with builders and designers in developing modifications that fit with the person, the occupations he or she undertakes in the space, and the realities of the built environment.

Elements in the built environment that need to be considered when designing modifications include:

+ Building structures
+ Service systems
+ Spaces and places
+ Products, devices, and technologies
+ User interfaces

Building Structures

Therapists need to appreciate the importance of structures in the built environment when developing environmental interventions. The structure of a house is found in the framework, which is composed of four basic parts: floors, walls, ceiling, and roof.

In modification work, therapists are mostly interested in moving or removing walls or adding, modifying, or repositioning fixtures and fittings on walls, so it is important to understand how they are constructed and the functions that walls perform.

In most houses, walls are constructed using 2-in × 4-in (50-mm × 75-mm) timber. They consist of a frame with studs or vertical lengths every 16 in (450 mm) to 24 in (600 mm) along the length of the wall. This frame is then covered with some type of sheeting, such as plywood, particleboard, fiberboard, plasterboard, or some other drywall material (Figure 9-8).

Increasingly, stud walls are being constructed from steel rather than timber, which has implications for whether fixtures and fittings can be attached and what extra reinforcement or fixings are required. Walls can also be constructed of concrete blocking or masonry (brickwork), which is more difficult to remove or modify and requires special tools and fasteners to install fittings and fixtures. When items such as grab bars are installed on a wall, they need to be secured into the studs or other structural supports in the wall. The nature and location of these structures can determine whether a grab bar can be safely attached and where it or other accessories can be located. Alternative structural supports can be put in place if the wall structure is inadequate or if the studs are not located in the required positions; however, the advice of a suitably qualified building contractor or designer should be sought if there are concerns about the capacity of the wall to support these fittings.

Although walls are mostly used to divide up interior spaces, some walls are load bearing and serve the additional function of supporting an upper floor, ceiling, and/or roof. Therapists need to be aware that a supporting or load-bearing wall cannot be removed without being replaced by a suitable support structure. This type of alteration requires the expertise of a building or design professional and can be costly.

When considering any structural modification, it is advisable to employ a building or design professional to inspect the building to ensure that it is in good repair and able to accommodate the recommended changes. It is also essential to know what is behind the surfaces of walls, floors, and ceilings before work begins to avoid damage to service systems such as electrical wiring, plumbing, and ducting.

Service Systems

The service systems within a home include plumbing; wiring or the electrical system; and the heating, ventilation, and air conditioning system. Plumbing in residential structures involves the water supply system as well as the drainage system. The home's electrical system is made up of wiring, outlets, and switches and has many circuits, each of which starts from a main service panel. The heating, ventilation, and air conditioning system includes the heating or

Table 9-2. Common Attributes of Physical Environment Features Proposed by Sanford and Bruce (2010)

SPACES AND PLACES	PRODUCTS, DEVICES, AND TECHNOLOGIES	USER INTERFACES
• Entry • Circulation/level changes • Orientation cues • Configuration/layout • Location of products, devices, and technologies • Location of environmental controls • Ground/floor and wall materials/finishes • Ambient conditions	• Product type • Dimensions • Weight • Location of user interfaces • Materials/finishes	• Type of interface • Minimum approach • Distance and angle • Dimensions • Activation force required • Operational attributes • Materials/finishes • Feedback mechanisms

Reprinted with permission from Sanford, J., & Bruce, C. (2009). Measuring the physical environment. In E. Mpofu & T. Oakland (Eds.), *Rehabilitation and health assessment* (pp. 207-228). New York: Springer.

cooling unit as well as a series of ducts leading to and from various rooms in the house. Each of these systems has lines (pipes, wiring, and ducts) that run through the wall, floor, and ceiling cavities, which need to be considered when proposing changes.

Due to the potential for service systems to be housed in walls, it necessary that care is taken when securing fixtures and fittings to the wall. Furthermore, it is important to note that these systems will also need to be relocated if the wall is being moved or removed. In some buildings, it is extremely costly or impossible to relocate systems, such as electrical wiring, power outlets, water pipes, and sewage and waste outlets. For example, relocating a toilet or a waste outlet in the bathroom would require the drainage pipes and outlets in the floor to be repositioned. Where this is possible, it can be costly, and in some constructions, such as a slab-on-ground construction, it is difficult to undertake such changes. Consequently, when looking to remodel a bathroom, for example, it is advisable to note the location of existing fixtures and fittings and plan to keep them in those locations or to account for the cost in relocating them when discussing the relative merit of designs and installations.

Though therapists are not required to possess this building knowledge, it is important that they are aware of some of the limits to what is possible and seek the advice of a suitably qualified builder, designer, or contractor when investigating modifications that require changes to the building structures or systems.

When working within the existing structure of a home, a number of design elements can affect occupational performance. These elements, or attributes, of the physical environment have been identified as spaces and places; products, devices, and

technologies; and user interfaces (Table 9-2; Sanford & Bruce, 2009).

Spaces and Places

When considering the impact of the environment on occupational performance, it is useful to examine the spatial elements of the environment and whether these elements need to be altered to promote performance. Sanford and Bruce (2009) identify key spatial considerations to include the following:

✦ Entry: Can the person approach the entry and negotiate the clearance through the doorway safely and efficiently?

✦ Circulation/level changes: Is there adequate room for the person to move, approach, reach, and use various fixtures and fittings in the room? Are there any changes in levels to negotiate between areas?

✦ Orientation cues: Is signage clear and appropriately located? Are key landmarks well lit, visible, and located in a logical position?

✦ Configuration/layout: Is the layout logical in terms of the way the person uses the space? Does the size of the spaces, configuration, or layout allow the person and/or caregivers to maneuver equipment? Do these allow flexibility in use of space?

✦ Location of products, devices, and technologies: Are the switches, outlets, and fixtures visible, accessible, and located in a logical place?

✦ Location of environmental controls: Are the controls visible, accessible, and located in a logical place? Can they be operated or adjusted easily?

+ Ground/floor and wall materials/finishes: Are the floor materials appropriate for the activities being undertaken and the people using the space? Do the materials used create a suitable look and feel? Do the materials used assist in differentiating spaces for different purposes? Do the wall materials provide flexibility in supporting future fixtures and fittings?

+ Ambient conditions: Is the lighting adequate for the tasks being undertaken, and is it located in the appropriate area? Is the room a comfortable temperature for the activity being undertaken?

Products, Devices, and Technologies

Products such as fixtures, appliances, and building elements (e.g., flooring, doors, and windows) have characteristics that affect ease of use. Considerations identified by Sanford and Bruce (2009) include the following:

+ Product type: What products does the user need to interact with?

+ Dimensions: Do the fixtures fit into the space or location available (leaving adequate room for approach and operation)?

+ Weight: Can the fixtures and fittings be moved if required?

+ Location and size of user interfaces: Can the controls on the fixture be reached and operated easily? Are they visible and well lit? Can they be easily read?

+ Materials/finishes: Do the materials and finishes provide appropriate contrast, friction, or resistance? Can the fixtures and fittings be operated using limited force/dexterity? Do the fixtures and fittings provide adequate auditory and/or visual information to the user? Are they comfortable to use (temperature and texture of the surface against the skin, etc.)? Will materials and finishes stand up to the anticipated wear (to suit heavy equipment use or impact by equipment)?

User Interfaces

User interfaces include controls and hardware such as handles, knobs, faucets, locks, and handrails and grab bars. Electronic and mechanical controls and dispensers also affect use. Key considerations identified by Sanford and Bruce (2009) include the following:

+ Type of interface: What controls and hardware does the user need to interact with?

+ Minimum approach distance and angle: Can the controls/hardware be accessed easily?

+ Dimensions: Do the controls fit into the space and location available (leaving adequate room for approach and operation)?

+ Activation force required: Can the controls/hardware be operated using limited force/dexterity?

+ Operational attributes: What is the direction and distance that controls/hardware need to be moved? Can they be easily read and operated?

+ Materials/finishes: Do the controls/hardware provide adequate contrast/friction? Are they comfortable to use (temperature and texture of the surface against the skin, etc.)? Will they tolerate the way they are likely to be used?

+ Feedback mechanisms: Do the controls/hardware provide adequate auditory and/or visual information to the user?

The number of design elements that require consideration can be overwhelming for new therapists. Consequently, checklists and frameworks for considering these elements systematically are quite useful. However, when attempting major modifications, the expertise of a designer or builder is essential. Therapists should not take responsibility for determining the suitability or integrity of the existing building for modification. They should, however, have sufficient understanding of the built environment to be alert to its limitations to enable them to collaborate effectively with builders and designers and to ensure that their recommendations are reasonable, the needs of the client are adequately addressed in the redesign, and the modifications do not present any unanticipated difficulties or complexities for the people living in the home.

Conclusion

This chapter has described the range of performance issues that older people and people with disabilities experience in the home and the range of intervention strategies occupational therapists use to address these issues. It has introduced a framework for analyzing the resources used during activities and identifying ways in which alternative strategies, assistive devices, social supports, and environmental modifications can address occupational performance concerns and further facilitate the person-environment-occupation transaction. The role of occupational analysis and clinical reasoning in designing client-centered interventions has also been examined. In particular, this chapter described considerations in determining the most suitable intervention and tailoring it to the specific needs of the person, activity, occupation, and environment. Finally, this chapter has detailed the range of environmental interventions used to address occupational performance issues in the home and provided therapists with mechanisms for developing their understanding of the built environment.

REFERENCES

Adaptive Environment Center. (2002). *Consumer's guide to home adaptation*. Boston, MA: Author.

Aplin, T. (2013). Development and psychometric analysis of the dimensions of home measure (DOHM): A measure of the home environment for home modification practice (Doctoral dissertation, The University of Queensland, Australia). Retrieved from http://espace.library.uq.edu.au/

Aplin, T., de Jonge, D., & Gustafsson, L. (2013). Understanding the dimensions of home that impact on home modification decision making. *Australian Occupational Therapy Journal, 60*, 101-109.

Aplin, T., de Jonge, D., & Gustafsson, L. (2015). Understanding home modifications impact on clients and their family's experience of home: A qualitative study. *Australian Occupational Therapy Journal, 62*, 123-131.

Australian Bureau of Statistics [ABS]. (2013). 4430.0 - Disability, ageing and carers, Australia: Summary of findings, 2012. Retrieved from http://www.abs.gov.au/ausstats/abs@.nsf/Lookup/D9BD84DBA2528FC9CA257C21000E4FC5?opendocument

Barrier Free Environments Incorporated. (1991). *The accessible housing design file*. New York: Van Nostrand Reinhold.

Batavia, A. I., & Hammer, G. S. (1990). Toward the development of consumer-based criteria for the evaluation of assistive devices. *Journal of Rehabilitation Research and Development, 27*(4), 425-436.

Baum, C. M., & Christiansen, C. H. (2005). Person-environment-occupational performance: An occupation-based framework for practice. In C. H. Christiansen, C. M. Baum, & J. Bass-Haugen (Eds.), *Occupational therapy: Performance, participation and well-being* (3rd ed., pp. 243-266). Thorofare, NJ: SLACK Incorporated.

Baum, C. M., Christiansen, C. H., & Bass, J. D. (2015). The person-environment-occupational performance (PEOP) model. In C. H. Christiansen, C. M. Baum, & J. D. Bass (Eds.), *Occupational therapy: Performance, participation and well-being* (4th ed., pp. 49-55). Thorofare, NJ: SLACK Incorporated.

Bedell, G. M., Khetani, M. A., Cousins, M., Coster, W. J., & Law, M. (2011). Parent perspectives to inform development of measures of children's participation and environment. *Archives of Physical Medicine and Rehabilitation, 92*, 765-773.

Better Living Design Institute. (2014). Better Living Design. Retrieved from http://betterlivingdesign.org/

Brawley, E. C. (1997). *Designing for Alzheimer's disease: Strategies for creating better care environments*. Hoboken, NJ: John Wiley & Sons.

Brawley, E. C. (2006). *Design innovations for aging and Alzheimer's: Creating caring environments*. Hoboken, NJ: John Wiley & Sons.

Canada Mortgage and Housing Corporation. (2009). *Adapting your home to living with dementia: A resource book for living at home and guide to home adaptations*. Ottawa, ON: CMHC. Retrieved from https://www.cmhc-schl.gc.ca/odpub/pdf/66495.pdf

Canada Mortgage and Housing Corporation. (2016a). *Accessible housing by design series*. Ottawa, ON: CMHC. Retrieved from https://www.cmhc-schl.gc.ca/en/hoficlincl/hoficlincl_002.cfm

Canada Mortgage and Housing Corporation. (2016b). *Maintaining seniors' independence through home adaptations: A self-assessment guide*. Ottawa, ON: CMHC. Retrieved from https://www.cmhc-schl.gc.ca/odpub/pdf/61087.pdf

Chan, D., Laporte, D. M., & Sveistrup, H. (1999). Rising from sitting in elderly people, part 2: Strategies to facilitate rising. *British Journal of Occupational Therapy, 62*(2), 64-68.

Christiansen, C., & Baum, C. (Eds.). (1997). *Occupational therapy: Enabling function and well-being* (2nd ed.). Thorofare, NJ: SLACK Incorporated.

Connell, B. R., & Sanford, J. A. (1997). Individualizing home modification recommendations to facilitate performance of routine activities. In S. Lanspery & J. Hyde (Eds.), *Staying put: Adapting the places instead of the people* (pp. 113-131). Amityville, NY: Baywood.

Crepeau, E. B., Schell, B.A.B., Gillen, G., & Scaffa, M. E. (2014). Analyzing occupations and activity. In B.A.B. Schell, G. Gillen, M. E. Scaffa, & E. S. Cohn (Eds.), *Willard & Spackman's occupational therapy* (12th ed., pp. 234-248). Philadelphia, PA: Wolters Kluwer Lippincott Williams & Wilkins.

Deane, K. H. O., Ellis-Hill, C., Dekker, K., Davies, P., & Clarke, C. E. (2003). A Delphi survey of best practice occupational therapy for Parkinson's disease in the United Kingdom. *British Journal of Occupational Therapy, 66*(6), 247-254.

Duffy, M. A. (2002). *Making life more livable: Simple adaptations for living at home after vision loss*. New York: AFB Press.

Dunn, W., Brown, C., & McGuigan, A. (1994). The ecology of human performance: A framework for considering the impact of context. *American Journal of Occupational Therapy, 48*, 595-607.

Enders, A., & Leech, P. (1996). Low-technology aids for daily living and do-it-yourself devices. In J. C. Galvin & M. J. Scherer (Eds.), *Evaluating, selecting and using appropriate assistive technology* (pp. 30-39). Gaithersburg, MD: Aspen Publishers, Inc.

Frain, J. P., & Carr, P. H. (1996). Is the typical modern house designed for future adaptation for disabled older people? *Age and Ageing, 25*(5), 398.

Gillespie, L. D., Robertson, M. C., Gillespie, W. J., Lamb, S. E., Gates, S., Cumming, R. G., & Rowe, B. H. (2009). Interventions for preventing falls in older people living in the community. *Cochrane Database of Systematic Reviews*, (2), CD007146. doi: 10.1002/14651858.CD007146.pub3

Gitlin, L. N., & Corcoran, M. A. (2005). *Occupational therapy and dementia care: The home environmental skill-building program for individuals and families*. Bethesda, MD: American

Gitlin, L. N., Hauck, W. W., Winter, L., Dennis, M. P., & Schulz, R. (2006). Effect of an in-home occupational and physical therapy intervention on reducing mortality in functionally vulnerable older people: Preliminary findings. *Journal of the American Geriatrics Society, 54*, 950-955.

Gitlin, L. N., Mann, W., Tomita, M., & Marcus, S. M. (2001). Factors associated with home environmental problems among community-living older people. *Disability and Rehabilitation, 23*(17), 777-787.

Granbom, M., Taei, A., & Ekstam, L. (2017). Cohabitants' perspective on housing adaptations: a piece of the puzzle. *Scandinavian Journal of Caring Sciences, Advance online publication*, 1-9.

Grey, T., Pierce, M., Cahill, S., & Dyer, M. (2015). *Universal design guidelines dementia friendly dwellings for people with dementia, their families and carers*. Dublin, Ireland: Centre for Excellence in Universal Design & National Disability Authority. Retrieved from http://universaldesign.ie/Web-Content-/UD_Guidelines-Dementia_Friendly_Dwellings-2015-full-doc.pdf

HammondCare. (2017). Dementia Centre: Design for dementia. Retrieved from http://www.dementiacentre.com.au/shop/design-for-dementia

Hawkins, R., & Stewart, S. (2002). Changing rooms: The impact of adaptations on the meaning of home for a disabled person and the role of occupational therapists in the process. *British Journal of Occupational Therapy, 65*(2), 81-87.

Heaton, J. & Bamford, C. (2001). Assessing the outcomes of equipment and adaptations: Issues and approaches. *British Journal of Occupational Therapy, 64*(7), 346-356.

Heywood, F. (2004a). The health outcomes of housing adaptations. *Disability and Society, 19*(2), 129-143.

Heywood, F. (2004b). Understanding needs: A starting point for quality. *Housing Studies, 19*(5), 709-726.

Heywood, F. (2005). Adaptation: Altering the house to restore the home. *Housing Studies, 20*(4), 531-547.

Hocking, C. (1999). Function or feelings: Factors in abandonment of assistive devices. *Technology and Disability, 11*, 3-11.

Hong Kong Housing Society. (2014). Universal design guidebook for residential development in Hong Kong. Retrieved from https://www.hkhs.com/eng/wnew/udg.asp

Housing LIN. (n.d.). Housing LIN. Retrieved from https://www.housinglin.org.uk/

Independent Living Centre NSW. (2015). Guide to planning bathrooms and kitchens 2015. Retrieved from https://at-aust.org/home/publications/publications#pub_bkGuide

Iwarsson, S., Löfqvist, C., Oswald, F., Slaug, B., Schmidt, S., Wahl, H., . . . Haak, M. (2016). Synthesizing ENABLE-AGE research findings to suggest evidence-based home and health interventions. *Journal of Housing for the Elderly, 30*(3), 330-343.

Iwarsson, S., & Slaug, B. (2010). *The housing enabler: A method for rating/screening and analysing accessibility problems in housing* (2nd ed.). Lund & Staffanstorp, Sweden: Veten & Skapen HB and Slaug Enabling Development.

Johansson, K., Borell, L., & Lilja, M. (2009). Older persons' navigation through the service system towards home modification resources. *Scandinavian Journal of Occupational Therapy, 16*(4), 227-237.

Johansson, K., Josephsson, S., & Lilja, M. (2009). Creating possibilities for action in the presence of environmental barriers in the process of 'ageing in place.' *Ageing & Society, 29*(1), 49-70.

Johansson, K., Lilja, M., Petersson, I., & Borell, L. (2007). Performance of activities of daily living in a sample of applicants for home modification services. *Scandinavian Journal of Occupational Therapy, 14*(1), 44-53.

Jones, A., de Jonge, D., & Phillips, R. (2008). The role of home maintenance and modification services in achieving health, community care and housing outcomes in later life (research report). Melbourne, Australia: Australian Housing and Urban Research Institute.

Kruse, R. L., Moore, C. M., Tofle, R. B., LeMaster, J. W., Aud, M., Hicks, L. L. . . . Mehr, D. R. (2010). Older adults' attitudes toward home modifications for fall prevention. *Journal of Housing for the Elderly, 24*(2), 110-129.

Laporte, D. M., Chan, D., & Sveistrup, H. (1999). Rising from sitting in elderly people, part 1: Implications of biomechanics and physiology. *British Journal of Occupational Therapy, 62*(1), 36-42.

Law, M., Cooper, B., Strong, S., Stewart, D., Rigby, P., & Letts, L. (1996). The person-environment-occupation model: A transactive approach to occupational performance. *Canadian Journal of Occupational Therapy, 63*, 9-23.

Law, M., Di Rezze, B., & Bradley, L. (2010). Environmental change to improve outcomes. In M. Law & M. A. McColl (Eds.), *Interventions, effects and outcomes in occupational therapy: Adults and older adults* (pp. 155-182). Thorofare, NJ: SLACK Incorporated.

Lawlor, D., & Thomas, M. A. (2008). *Residential design for aging in place*. Hoboken, NJ: Wiley & Sons.

Lifemark. (2017). Lifemark. Retrieved from http://www.lifemark.co.nz/

Lifetime Homes. (n.d.). Lifetime Homes. Retrieved from http://www.lifetimehomes.org.uk/

Litvak, S., & Enders, A. (2001). Support systems: The interface between individuals and environments. In G. L. Albrecht, K. D. Seelman, & M. Bury (Eds.), *Handbook of disability studies* (pp. 711-733). Thousand Oaks, CA: Sage Publications.

Livable Housing Australia. (2015). Livable Housing Design. Retrieved from http://www.livablehousingaustralia.org.au/library/SLLHA_GuidelinesJuly2015-3.pdf

Mann, W., Hurren, D., Tomita, M., Bengali, M., & Steinfeld, E. (1994). Environmental problems in homes of elders with disabilities. *Occupational Therapy Journal of Research, 14*(3), 191-211.

Mann, W. C., & Tomita, M. (1998). Perspectives on assistive devices among elderly persons with disabilities. *Technology and Disability, 9*, 119-148.

Oldman, C., & Beresford, B. (2000). Home sick home: Using housing experiences of disabled children to suggest a new theoretical framework. *Housing Studies, 15*(3), 429-442.

Olsen, R., Ehrenkrantz, E., & Hutchings, B. (1993). *Alzheimer's and related dementias homes that help: Advice from caregivers for creating a supportive home.* Newark, NJ: Njit Press.

Peace, S. M., & Holland, C. (2001). *Inclusive housing in an ageing society: Innovative approaches.* Bristol, UK: Policy Press.

Peek-Asa, C., & Zwerling, C. (2003). Role of environmental interventions in injury control and prevention. *Epidemiologic Reviews, 25*, 77-89.

Pettersson, C., Löfqvist, C., & Malmgren Fänge, A. (2012). Clients' experiences of housing adaptations: A longitudinal mixed-methods study. *Disability and Rehabilitation, 34*(20), 1706-1715.

Phillips, B. (1993). Technology abandonment from the consumer point of view. *NARIC Quarterly, 3*(2-3), 4-91.

Rigby, P., Trentham, B., & Letts, L. (2014). Modifying performance contexts. In B. A. B. Schell, G. Gillen, M. E. Scaffa, & E. S. Cohn (Eds.), *Willard & Spackman's occupational therapy* (12th ed., pp. 364-381). Philadelphia, PA: Wolters Kluwer Lippincott Williams & Wilkins.

Rogers, J. C., & Holm, M. B. (2009). The occupational therapy process. In E. B. Crepeau, E. S. Cohn, & B. A. Boyt Schell (Eds.), *Willard & Spackman's occupational therapy* (11th ed., pp. 478-518). Philadelphia, PA: Wolters Kluwer Lippincott Williams & Wilkins.

Ryan, S., & Reynolds, A. (2015). New housing options for people with significant disability: Design insights. Melbourne, Australia: Summer Foundation Ltd. Retrieved from file:///C:/Users/uqmhoyle/Documents/Book%20Chapters/Home%20Mods%202017/Resources/Chapter%209/nho_design_report.pdf

Sanford, J. A. (2012). *Design for the ages: Universal design as a rehabilitation strategy.* New York: Springer Publishing.

Sanford, J., & Bruce, C. (2009). Measuring the physical environment. In E. Mpofu & T. Oakland (Eds.), *Rehabilitation and health assessment* (pp. 207-228). New York: Springer.

Sanford, J. A., & Butterfield, T. (2005). Using remote assessment to provide home modification services to underserved elders. *Gerontologist, 45*(3), 389-398.

Sanford, J. A., Pynoos, J., Tejral, A., & Browne, A. (2002). Development of a comprehensive assessment for delivery of home modifications. *Physical and Occupational Therapy in Geriatrics, 20*(2), 43-55.

Scherer, M. J. (2005). *Living in a state of stuck: How technology impacts on the lives of people with disabilities* (2nd ed.). Cambridge, MA: Brookline Books.

Stark, S., Keglovits, M., Arbesman, M., & Lieberman, D. (2017). Effect of home modification interventions on the participation of community-dwelling adults with health conditions: A systematic review. *American Journal of Occupational Therapy, 71*(2), 1-11.

Steinfeld, E., & Maisel, J. L. (2012). *Universal design: Creating inclusive environments.* Hoboken, NJ: John Wiley & Sons, Inc.

Stone, J. H. (1998). Housing for older persons: An international overview. *Technology and Disability, 8*(1-2), 91-97.

Tanner, B., Tilse, C., & de Jonge, D. (2008). Restoring and sustaining home: The impact of home modifications on the meaning of home for older people. *Journal of Housing for the Elderly, 22*, 195-215.

The Dementia Services Development Centre. (2012). The Dementia Centre: Design Resource Centre. Retrieved from http://dementia.stir.ac.uk/information/design-resource-centre

Trickey, F., Maltais, D., Gosslein, C., & Robitaille, Y. (1993). Adapting older persons' homes to promote independence. *Physical and Occupational Therapy in Geriatrics, 12*(1), 1-14.

United States Access Board. (2004/2014). Americans with Disabilities Act and Architectural Barriers Act (ADA-ABA) Accessibility Guidelines - July 23, 2004. Retrieved from https://www.access-board.gov/attachments/article/412/ada-aba.pdf

Wahl, H., Fänge, A., Oswald, F., Gitlin, L. N., & Iwarsson, S. (2009). The home environment and disability-related outcomes in aging individuals: What is the empirical evidence? *The Gerontologist, 49*(3), 355-367.

Wilder Research Center. (2002). *Practical guide to universal home design: Convenience, ease, and livability.* Saint Paul, MN: East Metro Seniors Agenda for Independent Living [SAIL] & Minnesota Department of Human Services. Retrieved from http://mngero.org/downloads/homedesign.pdf

10

Sourcing and Evaluating Products and Designs

Desleigh de Jonge, MPhil (OccThy), Grad Cert Soc Sci and
Melanie Hoyle, BSc (Psych), MOccThySt, Grad Dip Health Sci, Post Grad Dip Psych

Therapists use a wide range of mainstream and specialized products and design solutions to address a variety of occupational performance concerns and difficulties. Consequently, they need access to a number of different information systems to locate information on what is available. They also need to be able to evaluate the relative benefits of each option to determine the best solution for each client and his or her household. The first section of this chapter overviews the information systems therapists can use to gain an understanding of environmental interventions and then examines the nature of information provided by each of these systems. Therapists can use these resources to locate suitable options for individual clients, to enable them to remain informed about developments in the area, and to build a body of knowledge about the range of interventions available.

The second section of this chapter outlines a systematic process for reviewing and comparing products and designs and details considerations when evaluating the relative merits of various options. It identifies the information therapists require to undertake a thorough comparison of options and discusses the unique perspective clients bring to the decision-making process. It also highlights the benefits of drawing on the experiences of other therapists, designers, builders, and clients to understand the advantages and disadvantages of various products and designs. The role of evidence and standards in reviewing the suitability of options is also discussed, as are the evolution and principles of good design, which strive to ensure that products and designs used for older people and people with disabilities are aesthetic, flexible, and functional in the long term.

CHAPTER OBJECTIVES

By the end of this chapter, the reader will be able to:

✦ Identify and discuss the benefits and limitations of various information systems used to gather information on products and designs

✦ Describe a systematic process for reviewing products and designs

✦ Identify key issues in evaluating the potential value and effectiveness of product and design solutions

✦ Describe the development of design and the implications of design approaches for older people and people with disabilities

Ainsworth, E., & de Jonge, D. *An Occupational Therapist's*
Guide to Home Modification Practice, Second Edition (pp. 225-246).
© 2019 SLACK Incorporated.

Sourcing and Evaluating Product and Design Options

When developing environmental interventions, therapists draw from a broad range of products and design solutions, including specialized and mainstream options. Consequently, they need access to information on specialized assistive devices for people with various functional impairments as well as the many generic building products on the market. They also need to understand various design approaches and be able to evaluate their suitability for each situation. Because there is an ever-increasing number and range of options and information on these is scattered across industries, information systems, and suppliers, it is often difficult for therapists to feel confident that they have a good understanding of all the options available.

Information on Products and Designs

To develop effective interventions, therapists need to actively develop their understanding of the broad range of specialized and mainstream options available. They need to know where to find information on products and designs and how to search for solutions suited to the unique requirements of each client. It is therefore important that therapists are aware of the information systems available and can use these effectively to locate suitable options for individual clients.

When searching for potential options, these questions come to mind:

+ What products and design options exist?
+ Where are they available?
+ Who were they designed for?
+ How well will they suit the person's identified needs?
+ How long have they been tested and available in the marketplace?
+ Why choose one product over another?

Therapists need a good understanding of the range of options available and their specifications, such as size, shape, weight, and finish. They need to know where they are available and how much they cost. It is also important to be familiar with who the product was designed for because this gives therapists an indication of its potential strengths/limitations and the situations it best suits. Therapists should also have knowledge of how the product can be adjusted or customized as well as understand its installation, maintenance, and service requirements. Ultimately, therapists need to be able to specify performance criteria of the recommended product type and explain why these specifications are best suited to the situation. In the case of a legal challenge, therapists need to be able to defend their recommendations. To answer these questions, therapists need to access a range of resources to gather information. These include the following:

+ Company catalogues
+ Trade exhibits or information and display centers
+ Databases
+ Online resources: Dedicated home modification websites, as well as building, government, and community websites concerned with home renovation, modification, repair, and maintenance (e.g., checklists, buyers' guides, renovation guides, and product reviews)
+ Professional publications and resources: Books, journals, and newsletters
+ Conferences and workshops
+ People with experience: Clients, professional colleagues, builders, and designers

A list of some potential online resources is available in Appendix E.

Company Catalogues

Many specialist and mainstream building suppliers provide catalogues of their products, either in hard copy or online. These resources answer the "what" and "where" questions well because they can provide good graphics and specifications of the products in their range. They can also provide an up-to-date price list and the contact details of suppliers in various locations. Generally, companies supply a defined range of goods, which means that therapists need to access a number of companies' catalogues to understand the full range of options available. The clear photos or drawings of each product generally provided can be used when describing alternatives to clients. Sales representatives might also be able to provide a sample of the product to view or test in various situations. It is important to remember that sales representatives are paid to promote their products, so they will be able to describe the features and identify all of the advantages of their products. A discussion with representatives from a number of companies is usually required to develop a full understanding of the relative strengths and limitations of all options on the market. Company representatives may also be able to provide information on whom the product was specifically designed for or situations where it is best suited. Additionally, they usually have knowledge of legislative requirements regarding installation such as council requirements, access standards and/or work health and safety compliance. Therapists would then need to ascertain whether the product would meet the specific requirements of each client and meet his or her particular needs. Catalogues are useful for therapists who have a clear understanding of the requirements of the client and his or her situation and well-developed professional reasoning skills that allow them to filter and analyze the information provided. Therapists with a good knowledge of the range of options should also ensure that they access catalogues from all relevant suppliers and not limit themselves to a restricted range of alternatives. It is also advantageous to have some experience with the application of the products or access to people who have used them so that sales information can be balanced with an understanding of how well products work in various situations.

Trade Exhibits or Display Centers

Trade exhibits or information and display centers are an excellent way for therapists to develop an overview of the range of products available and to keep up to date with recent developments. These resources provide therapists with similar benefits and challenges; however, having a number of companies and products co-located makes it easier to gather information on a range of options and to view and compare alternatives. It should be noted that, although these exhibits and display centers have many products on display, they might not be comprehensive or representative of all the products available on the market. They are likely, however, to showcase local suppliers and contractors, which is advantageous to people who are unfamiliar with resources in the area or who live in more remote areas where such resources are often scattered.

Databases

There are many specialist and mainstream databases that allow therapists to search for specific products. Most of these are now available online; however, some require subscription or membership. The advantage of using a database is that many of them feature consistent fields to describe the various products they have on file. This allows therapists to quickly access information on a range of options and compare specifications and costs. It is sometimes possible to search for products with specific features, thus allowing therapists to define their search and locate suitable products quickly. The amount of information and graphics provided varies, and the currency of the information depends on how regularly the database is updated. Some of the information provided may be location specific, so it is important to use databases that have information on products from the appropriate region. Therapists with sound clinical skills and a clear idea of what they want from products are well placed to maximize the use of these resources. The volume of information available can be overwhelming for therapists who are new to the area. Once again, it is advantageous to have some experience with the application of the products or access to people who have used them so that information can be augmented with an understanding of how well the products work in various situations.

Online Resources

There are many dedicated home modification and building websites, as well as government and community websites that display a variety of resources related to home renovation, modification, repair, and maintenance. With the increase in the aging population, and disability and aged care reforms occurring in many countries, there has been an explosion of resources designed to assist older people and people with disabilities in identifying and addressing their home modification and maintenance needs. Many checklists, buyers' and renovation guides, and product reviews can be uncovered with an online search engine. Several of these resources have been written specifically to assist the target population to identify and address their safety and function in the home as they age. In addition, a number of resources outline how to make homes accessible for people using wheelchairs or manageable when caring for someone with dementia. These resources can be particularly useful for clients and therapists because they provide an overview of issues and an introduction to potential solutions, especially low-cost options. They may or may not provide details of specific solutions or products and, if they do, the information may be location-specific. These resources can be useful for clients and novice therapists; however, it is important that therapists check the authority of these sites by confirming, against other resources, the expertise of the authors and the validity of the information provided. It is also advisable to be aware of the domain of the website and to interpret the information accordingly. For example:

+ .com is a commercial site

+ .org is a community organization

+ .edu is an educational institution

+ .gov is a government site

Further, there are also a range of social media and social networking sites (refer to Chapter 9) that enable clinicians to disseminate and review information and connect to share and discuss issues and gain collegial support respectively. Each of these site types has a function and perspective that need to be considered when assessing the authority and validity of the information provided. Therapists need to dedicate time to becoming familiar with, and regularly reviewing, resources on the internet. Experienced therapists are well placed to piece together these scattered resources and direct new therapists and clients to the best resources available.

Professional Publications and Resources

There are an increasing number of books, journals, newsletters, and websites that provide information related to home modifications. Books written by occupational therapists and other industry-related professionals on home modifications provide therapists with an understanding of a range of solutions; however, the qualifications and experience of the authors, the frames of reference from which they operate, and the focus of the book can define the range of options presented. For example, occupational therapists will generally seek to define the specific needs of the client before detailing the potential options. They also see environmental interventions as part of a suite of interventions and will, therefore, discuss these in conjunction with alternative strategies, assistive devices, and supports. On the other hand, books written by building and design specialists will provide details of alternative designs without necessarily identifying who they best suit or alternatives to costly renovations. However, these texts allow therapists to develop their understanding of the range of options and necessary considerations when designing environmental solutions. Books do not generally refer to specific products but might provide a list of suppliers relevant to the location of the publication. It is important, however, to be aware that the information may be dated, given that books generally are not frequently revised. A range of books has been written on aspects of home design for people with specific requirements, including older people, people with dementia or vision impairment, or wheelchair users. Some books focus exclusively on low-cost modifications to existing premises and others describe design elements that need to be incorporated into the design of a new home or in extensive renovations of an existing home.

Journals and newsletters might also discuss and evaluate various intervention approaches or provide reviews of products. Several websites are dedicated to home design, construction, and modification.

These sites are a repository for publications, reviews, and information on training and education opportunities, and they often provide links to other relevant sites.

By monitoring these information resources, therapists can develop a broader understanding of the effectiveness or usefulness of various interventions and products and can search for more specific details when relevant situations arise. Therapists who need an overview of the area and an understanding of the range of possible solutions available will find such resources invaluable; however, they would also need to ensure they are well informed about current products and design approaches in their local area.

Conferences and Workshops

Conferences and workshops are useful in assisting therapists to understand the range of interventions, approaches, and products available and in helping to develop an awareness of existing services and expertise. The location of the conference or workshop and the background and experience of the presenters might be considerations in applying the information directly to clinical practice. Therapists might need to evaluate whether the approach, products, or designs are well suited to the needs of their client group and location. These resources provide therapists with benefits and challenges like those provided by professional publications and resources; however, novice therapists might find workshops a more efficient way of getting the basic knowledge and skills they require because the expert presenters often collate current information from a range of resources and tailor it to the background and level of experience of the workshop participants. More experienced therapists are well equipped to use information presented at conferences and will benefit from having access to the range of home modification experts and exhibitors who attend international, national, and regional conferences.

Specialist Education and Training

Home modification practice requires therapists to develop specialist skills and knowledge. In addition to identifying occupational performance difficulties in the home and addressing these using alternative strategies, assistive devices, and social supports, therapists are required to understand how and when the environment can be modified. Many therapists seek additional training or courses to extend their knowledge of the built environment. These courses introduce therapists to building practices, various design approaches, products, and finishes and show how to navigate funding systems and modification services and manage building processes. This understanding complements the clinical knowledge therapists have and the reasoning they use to address occupational performance difficulties and concerns in the home. Additionally, it enables them to work more effectively with designers and builders in developing effective home design solutions.

People With Experience

Clients, professional colleagues, builders and designers, and suppliers with experience designing, supplying, or using home modifications can be invaluable in assisting therapists to identify alternatives or select and tailor environmental interventions to individuals' needs. With the explosion of social networking, social media, and communication technologies, therapists have ready access to a diverse group of people with expertise and experience. Discussing situations with professional colleagues or building and design professionals can help clarify issues and solve problems associated with difficult scenarios. People with specialist skills and knowledge or experience using products and designs over extended periods can provide insights into what does and does not work well in different situations. They often have extensive knowledge of the products and designs that can be supported locally and the quality of after-sales and maintenance services for various products. Older people and people with disability who have experience with negotiating environments and living with products and designs also have a wealth of valuable experience and knowledge from which to draw. These resources are of value to novice and experienced therapists alike, allowing them to make use of the experience of others to complement their own skills and knowledge and develop the best possible solution for their clients.

Reviewing Product and Design Alternatives

Once the range of alternative products and designs has been identified and located, each option must be evaluated to determine the best one for each situation. When evaluating the suitability of designs or products, therapists need to ask the following:

+ For whom has the product/design been developed?

+ How well will the product/design meet the client's specific requirements?

+ How long has the product/design been tested and available in the marketplace?

+ Why choose one product/design over others?

There are many considerations when examining the origin of products and designs. First, design and product requirements can vary between countries and regions. Therapists need to ensure that designs and products they recommend meet the requirements of their national and local standards or building codes. For example, design standards or building codes for a region with a low-density population, high winds, or low rainfall might not reflect the standards of a region with a high-density population and heavy snowfall. Second, commercially available products are generally designed for the mainstream market and might not acknowledge the diversity of function in the broader population. Therapists therefore need to be mindful of the needs of their client group and individual circumstances when assessing the suitability of various mainstream products and designs. For example, many fittings require fine motor control that can be problematic for older people and people with disabilities. In addition, labels or indicators are often difficult to see or read, and even specialized products or designs can be developed with one disability group in mind. For example, products and designs developed to address the needs of wheelchair users with full upper limb function might not readily address the needs of people with other disabilities.

When choosing the most suitable product for a client or situation, therapists need to think about the client's specific situation and consider the strengths and limitations of each option in relation to their requirements. Each product or design should be evaluated in terms of how well they will:

+ Be used by the client, given his or her physical, cognitive, sensory, and emotional capacities

+ Enable the client to complete the occupation in his or her preferred manner

+ Fit with the physical, personal, social, temporal, occupational and societal dimensions of the environment.

In addition, each option needs to be compared in terms of the following:

+ Product features and specifications

+ Clients' priorities and preferences

+ Experience of the product or design

+ Existing evidence of the benefits of the product or design

+ Conformity with design or product standards or building code requirements

+ Good design practice

Furthermore, it is beneficial to know how long the products and designs have been available in the marketplace. This will provide information about whether the product, for example, has been tried and tested extensively, whether there is likely to be service support for setup and maintenance/servicing, whether parts are available, and whether there are people who can comment on its suitability for their circumstance. Such knowledge will guide practice decisions about a product's application and use.

Product Features and Specifications

When reviewing products and designs, it is useful for therapists to gather information on the features, specifications, and cost of each option so that they can be systematically compared. Therapists often develop templates that allow them to gather all the information they need when considering the suitability of options. These templates can include:

+ Name of product and a description

+ Models

+ Appearance, a graphic

+ Specifications

+ Price range

+ Warranty

+ Construction (what the product is made of)

+ Installation requirements

+ Care and maintenance requirements

+ Advantages and limitations

+ Compliance with relevant standards or building codes

+ Suppliers and services able to fit and maintain the product

+ Notes regarding supply (e.g., availability and after-sales support)

When considering the cost of interventions, as well as the original purchase price, it is also important to consider the installation, maintenance, and replacement costs (Andrich, 2002). Further, the social cost of various options also needs to be examined (Andrich, 2002). For example, the cost of formal or informal support as an alternative to the product or design can be prohibitive. Although the cost of formal support can be readily calculated, the cost of informal support can be overlooked. Therapists need to be mindful that it might be more cost-effective to employ a product or design rather than recommend the provision of formal or informal support as an alternative (Chiatti & Iwarsson, 2014; Heywood & Turner, 2007; Scottish Government, n.d.). These issues are important considerations when comparing options and ensure that the comparisons account for the long-term impact of solutions as well as immediate expenses.

Consumers' Priorities and Preferences

Clients are often not afforded sufficient choice and control over the home modification process, which can result in them feeling disempowered (Aplin, de Jonge, & Gustafsson, 2015; Hawkins & Stewart, 2002; Heywood, 2004; Sapey, 1995) and dissatisfied that their priorities and preferences are not reflected in the outcome. Professionals often have knowledge of and experience with a range of products and designs and have assessed their functional suitability. However, clients are best placed to evaluate how suitable the products or designs would be for his or her situation and how well they will fit with the look and feel of the home, the people who live there, and the many activities that are undertaken in it. Clients can often have quite different views of their homes and needs to service providers, and this can impact on how they value advice and their willingness to proceed with recommendations (Aplin et al., 2015; Auriemma, Faust, Sibrian, & Jimenez, 1999). It is therefore crucial that the client's experience of home is valued during this decision-making process.

When clients are evaluating products and designs, they are most often concerned with the following:

+ Appearance

+ Cost

+ Longevity (including suitability over time and accommodation of future needs)

+ Safety

+ Privacy

+ Support meaningful activities and routines

+ Availability

+ Functionality or usability

+ Independence

+ Impact on other household members or visitors

+ Adaptability and suitability

+ Installation or construction requirements

+ Care requirements

+ After-sales support

+ Anticipated lifespan

Modifications can sometimes have a clinical appearance, which might not fit well in the home environment (Duncan, 1998). Complying with design standards or building codes designed for public buildings and spaces can also result in modifications having an institutional appearance, which is not generally in keeping with residential environments (Lund & Nygard, 2004). Furthermore, clients report frustration when service providers adhere to building codes which can result in modifications that do not suit his or her preferences and needs (Aplin et al., 2015). It is important that products and designs are well suited to a domestic situation, are in keeping with the style and décor of the client's home and reflect personal preferences. When deciding on modification designs, in the forefront of clients' minds is often their wish for enhanced safety, privacy, and independence (Aplin, de Jonge, Gustafsson, 2013). Modifications, therefore, must provide safety and consider the need for privacy. This includes both the privacy needs for private activities such as toileting and bathing, but it also extends to having a private space of one's own in the home.

Though clients are often mindful of the costs associated with home modifications, they are also likely to want quality products, designs, and finishes in their home. Many therapists can let the expectations and restricted financial resources of the subsidizing organization determine their choice of products and designs (Rousseau, Potvin, Dutil, & Falta, 2001). However, the cheapest option is not always the best value. Additionally, the future is an important consideration for clients where, for example, deteriorating health or the growth of the child should be accommodated in designing modifications (Aplin et al., 2013). Modifications that do not fully satisfy the current and anticipated needs of the household can result in wasted expenditure (Home Adaptations Consortium, 2013). Householders often have pragmatic concerns when reviewing alternative options. Once they decide to proceed with the modification, they want to ensure minimal delay and disruption. Consequently, they might show a preference for products that are readily available and choose designs that have been used locally, especially if they can view the finished product prior to confirming choice.

Another important consideration is usability, or the extent to which an individual's performance and activity patterns can be fulfilled in an environment (Bernt & Skar, 2006). Potential usability is best judged by the individual who will be using the product or space and is likely to be influenced by his or her experiences and expectations (Steinfeld & Danford, 1999). Because performance and activity patterns can vary from day to day or throughout the day, it is important to consider the capacity of the product to support or to be adjusted to account for these variations. Further, clients will seek modification designs that will provide the most opportunity for independence and freedom in the home (e.g.,

freedom of movement and ability to have choice in what activities they do at home; Aplin et al., 2013). When there are a number of people using the product or space, its ability to accommodate all users needs to be examined. This includes the potential impact of the product or design on other household members as well as regular visitors.

The installation or construction requirements might also be a matter for consideration when reviewing alternatives. Some clients find it difficult to tolerate major disruptions to their routines or households and might prefer an option that is less intrusive in the short term. It is therefore important that they are made aware of potential disturbances associated with product and design choices. In addition, the care requirements may prove problematic for some clients. For example, although textured flooring provides good grip and reduces the risk of slipping, it is more difficult to clean, especially for people with reduced mobility and upper limb strength. Over time, the buildup of soap and grime can make these floors more hazardous.

The availability of after-sales support for products or the construction is also of interest to clients, who are often responsible for the repair and replacement of the modification to his or her home. Clients wanting value for money will also be concerned with the lifespan of the product. Selecting a product with a longer lifespan, even if it costs more initially, might be preferable and less expensive in the long term.

Experience of the Product or Design

Therapists, designers, and builders with extensive experience in home modifications can draw on this wealth of knowledge when selecting products and designs. They usually know how well a product or design works in various situations and the range of people who have used the intervention successfully. These professionals may also be aware of difficulties encountered in acquiring, installing, adapting, or getting approval for a solution in a variety of situations or locations. Experienced therapists, designers, and builders can, similarly, have a good understanding of the lifespan of products and designs that have been used over time. This information assists in anticipating how well certain materials and finishes can stand up to wear and tear in a range of situations.

Follow-up with clients provides therapists with information on the usability of interventions, care requirements, and the responsiveness of after-sales support. Seeking feedback from clients and monitoring their experience over variable periods is an effective way of accumulating experience of various products and designs. This enables therapists to gain a richer understanding of the application of products and designs in a range of situations. It is especially valuable in identifying any unexpected issues in relation to the following:

+ Acceptance

+ Cost

+ Functionality or usability

+ Adaptability and suitability

+ Installation or construction

+ Care and repair

+ After-sales support

+ Lifespan

As noted previously, these issues are also important considerations for clients.

Therapists often encounter challenging situations that require products or designs with specific features and functions. Those with limited experience can benefit greatly from discussing options with their more experienced colleagues. Listservs and social networking sites where people come together online to discuss issues can be an effective medium for therapists seeking information and opinions from a wide range of experienced people. Useful information can also be gained from examining products and designs in public environments that receive extensive use. Products and designs commonly used in the building industry can also give an indication of their reliability and cost-effectiveness.

Existing Evidence of the Benefits of the Product or Design

Therapists draw on a range of evidence when designing interventions and evaluating the suitability of various products and designs. Evidence-based practice requires that the best available information or evidence is integrated with clinical experiences and expertise and with due consideration of the clients' priorities and preferences (Sackett, 2000; Turpin & Higgs, 2009). It is therefore important that therapists review the nature of evidence they are accessing and consider its dependability and generalizability carefully in light of their own experience and expertise and the priorities and preferences of their clients.

There are various types of evidence, including the following:

+ Anecdotal material (e.g., home modification listservs)

+ Expert opinion or theoretical/unsystematic literature reviews or standards

+ Case (i.e., case series and case comparative)

+ Observational (i.e., cohort studies, pre- and post-test studies, and cross-sectional and longitudinal studies)

+ Quasi-experimental (i.e., no randomization)

+ Randomized controlled trial (RCT)

+ Systematic review (Bridge & Phibbs, 2003)

Each of these types of evidence provides a different type of information, which varies in terms of its applicability to specific situations, level of dependability, and ability to demonstrate the benefits of a particular intervention (Turpin & Higgs, 2009). Anecdotal information and expert opinion can be based on accumulated experience and often provides the detailed and practical information required when considering specific situations and local products and designs. Therapists should be aware, however, that these sources are prone to bias; the information is likely to be shaped by personal preferences and unique experiences. Similarly, case-based, observational, and quasi-experimental studies can provide detailed information about interventions, the contexts in which they have been applied, and the changes that resulted from these. It is important to note, however, that the observed changes might also be attributable to other variables that have not been controlled for. RCTs and systematic reviews provide dependable information about the outcomes of interventions because they are structured to control for confounding variables and to minimize potential bias. For example, a 2011 RCT reviewed the effectiveness of an environmental assessment and modification intervention in the prevention of falls in older people (Pighills, Torgerson, Sheldon, Drummond, & Bland, 2011). However, to date, these types of studies have tended to examine the impact of home modifications generally and in combination with a range of other interventions, and research on specific home modification interventions and their relative impact in a variety of situations is limited. Table 10-1 reviews the advantages and disadvantages of various types of evidence as described by Bridge and Phibbs (2003).

Although applied research comparing the effectiveness of various environmental interventions for populations is limited, research on home modifications is increasing (Box 10-1 includes current evidence on grab bars). Literature about many traditional occupational therapy interventions is in the category of health; however, home modification and related literature can also be found in other fields of study, such as social sciences and architecture. Chapter 14 provides more detailed information on home modifications research.

Table 10-1. Advantages and Disadvantages of Various Types of Evidence

TYPE OF EVIDENCE	ADVANTAGES	DISADVANTAGES
Anecdotal material	• May assist in reconceptualization of problem area • May add to knowledge in terms of scoping variables or measurement methods	• May be based on hearsay • May not clearly indicate assumptions or method • May be faulty or inaccurate
Expert opinion/ theoretical/ unsystematic literature review/standards	• May assist in reconceptualization of problem area • May add to knowledge in terms of scoping variables or measurement methods	• May be based on hearsay • May not clearly indicate assumptions or method • May be faulty or inaccurate
Case (i.e., case series and case comparative)	• May generate hypotheses • Less expensive than other research designs • Can have large sample sizes	• No statistical validity • Hard to control for confounders as no controls • Subject to recall bias as retrospective • Difficult to demonstrate causality
Observational (i.e., cohort studies, pre- and posttest studies, cross-sectional and longitudinal studies)	• Most reliable observational data are cohort studies because there is no recall bias and can ensure baseline similarities between groups • More reliable answers and less statistical problems than case control	• Can take a long time • Can be an expensive, large-scale undertaking • Useful when randomized studies are inappropriate • External factors can change over time with panel or longitudinal data
Quasi-experimental (i.e., no randomization)	• Remains experimenter controlled • Most reliable when variables of interest and controls for these made explicit	• Because variables not fully controlled may exhibit selection, performance, and measurement bias
RCT	• Provides evidence with causality • Considered "gold standard" in health research • Random allocation balances known, unknown, and unmeasurable confounding variables • Greater confidence that conclusions are attributable solely to intervention manipulation • Reduces selection bias • Blinding reduces measurement and performance bias • Provides evidence of causality	• Assumes variables can be controlled and groups appropriately matched • Assumes randomized blind allocation of intervention is given ethical clearance by relevant human ethics review board • Very expensive in terms of time and money • May be compliance and participant attrition problems • Blinding and random allocation can be problematic
Systematic review	• Attempts to answer a particular research question in an evidence-based manner • Provides policymakers with a summary of available evidence • Effectively maps the inputs and outcomes under review	• Cutoffs for inclusion may be too high or too low • Question under consideration may not be specified properly (i.e., it may be too broad or too specific) • Results capture a snapshot of published research at a particular time interval so results must be interpreted in relation to currency of information and change in the body of knowledge being reviewed

Reprinted with permission from Bridge, C., & Phibbs, P. (2003). *Protocol guidelines for systematic reviews of home modification information to inform best practice.* Sydney, Australia: Home Modification Information Clearinghouse, University of New South Wales (UNSW): Sydney. Retrieved from https://www.homemods.info/about/administrative-publications/protocol-guidelines-for-systematic-reviews-of-home-modification-information-to-inform-best-practice#main-content. Table 4: Study design definitions.

Box 10-1. Grab Bars—Current Evidence

Grab bars are commonly installed to compensate for age-related deficits (impaired balance, range of motion, strength, and endurance) and to enable safe and independent transfers on and off toilets and in and out of baths and showers (Axtell & Yausda, 1993; Struyk & Katsura, 1988; Tideiksaar, 1997). Evidence is emerging that they may assist in preventing falls (Sattin, Rodriguez, DeVito, & Wingo, 1998). They are a common fitting in people's homes with seniors installing two grab bars on average, (Clemson & Martin, 1996; Plautz, Beck, Selmar, & Radersky, 1996). Although some studies report that community-dwelling individuals commonly own grab bars (Parker & Thorslund, 1991; Sonn & Grimby, 1994; Trickey, Maltais, Gosselin, & Robitaille, 1993), others suggest that they may not always use them. In one study, only one participant reported using the grab bars present at the time of the fall; most participants did not use grab bars because the grab bars felt awkward or unsafe to use (Aminzadeh, Edwards, Lockett, & Nair, 2000). Such findings highlight the need for occupational therapists to be careful about grab bar recommendations in relation to other options such as equipment.

WHICH CONFIGURATION IS BEST?

Multiple grab bar configurations may be used by people who present with a diverse range of health conditions or disabilities (Kennedy, Arcelus, Guitard, Goubran, & Sveistrup, 2015). It is important to use clinical reasoning to determine the most appropriate configuration of grab bar. Current literature discusses a range of options for positioning of grab bars including, for example, options for people who are seated on toilets and who engage in sit-to-stand transfers. These ideas include:

- Positioning the horizontal grab bar 4 cm above the person's greater trochanter when he or she is in the seated position (Bridge, 2003; McDonald, 1997; McDonald, Bridge, & Smith, 1996; Ongley, 1999; Roland, 1996). This recommendation needs to be treated with caution as a small sample size was used in the original research and the findings cannot be generalized
- Positioning the shoulder at 90 degrees flexion and elbow at 150 to 180 degrees flexion to determine the location of the grab bar (Woodson, 1981). This recommendation needs to be treated with caution as not all people like to pull on a grab bar when moving from sitting to standing.
- Aligning the grab bar on the nonaffected side of body (O'Meara & Smith, 2006)

Other research indicates the following findings:

- Vertical grab bars are suited to stage 1 and 4 of sit-to-stand transfers (Chan, Laporte, & Sveistrup, 1999; Laporte, Chan, & Sveistrup, 1999); they require a pull-up action; they reduce total range of motion at hip, hip extension torque, movement needed at knees; they reduce perceived pain levels; and higher rails reduce biomechanical load.
- Angled grab bars suit stages 1 and 4 of the sit-to-stand transfers and allow for flexible hand placement as the person moves (Chan et al., 1999; Laporte et al., 1999).
- Horizontal grab bars require a push-up action, assist weightbearing, and support the forearm, but if they are too high or too low, they will not assist momentum and postural stability; they also require larger forces and kinetic and kinematic outcomes observed (Bridge, 2003; O'Meara & Smith, 2002, 2005, 2006).
- Unilateral grab bars
  - » Suit stages 2 and 3 of sit-to-stand transfers (Chan et al., 1999; Laporte et al., 1999)
  - » Suit people with lower limb weakness and asymmetrical conditions
  - » Need to be placed ipsilateral for hip and ankle conditions or contralateral for knee joint problems (O'Meara, 2003)
- Bilateral grab bars
  - » Suit people with kyphosis, lordosis, back pain
  - » Ensure symmetry of body position, the alignment of center of mass and center of pressure (Chan et al., 1999; Laporte et al., 1999)
  - » Allow the alternating of hands and bilateral hand use (e.g., when someone needs to stand to adjust his or her clothes)

Most international access standards for countries such as the United States, Canada, and Australia recommend multidirection rails in public bathrooms. Occupational therapists are choosing to use this information to guide their practice and some nongovernment and government organizations are making it mandatory for their services to install grab bars to match this information in domestic homes rather than tailor the installation to suit the clinical requirements of the person (refer to Chapter 4 for a discussion about the relevance and intent of access standards for home modification work).

(continued)

Box 10-1. Grab Bars—Current Evidence (continued)

Sanford, Arch, and Megrew (1995) found that toilet grab bar configurations preferred by most nonambulatory older adults did not comply with either American or Canadian building code regulations (Kennedy et al., 2015). Sanford and Bosch (2013) also compared an American With Disabilities Act Accessibility Guidelines (ADAAG)–compliant design with alternative designs for people needing assisted toileting. The ADAAG is a set of prescriptive requirements for accessible design in public facilities. Findings indicated that caregivers preferred the largest of the tested configurations, where there were two fold-down grab bars provided and the center line of the toilet was 30 in from the sidewall rather than the 18 in required by the ADAAG.

Caregivers perceived the grab bar locations as better for helping them safely transfer subjects in a modified (non-ADAAG) configuration, and also that the grab bar style in a modified (non-ADAAG) configuration improved safety when transferring subjects. Although not statistically significant, there was a general downward trend in the number of incidents with the fold-down grab bars compared to the side-mounted grab bar, and fewer incidents associated with an increase in the amount of space provided adjacent to the toilet.

These international access standards can provide some helpful information to guide grab bar recommendations (such as detail on how to describe, measure, and draw grab bars in different environments), but they should not be used as the starting point for clinical reasoning. Occupational therapists need to be mindful that the grab bar configurations for ambulant or wheelchair users may not suit the specific needs of their clients. For example, this is particularly relevant if clients are of short stature, have shoulder pain or limited reach and grasp, are in the bariatric range, and/or take pain medication affecting their toileting. Further, the home environment may not have a shower or toilet configuration matching those described in the access standards for the location of the grab bar. Equipment that is not described in the access standards (such as mobile shower commodes) and the presence of a carer with their specific access requirements also need to be considered when determining the best grab bar product and location.

WARNING!

There are specific situations where grab bars should not be installed. For example, occupational therapists need to check with design and construction professionals about whether it is appropriate to install any type of grab bar that may pierce the waterproof lining on the bathroom floor. This may include grab bars that are swing-away (mounted to a post that fastens to the floor), wall-to-floor, or floor-to-ceiling grab bars. Occupational therapists should not encourage clients to use suction rails as these are not designed for weightbearing. Similarly, if builders wish to use toggle bolts to fasten rails to walls rather than securing them into studs, the grab bars may not hold on the wall, depending on the thickness of the wall material and the weight placed on the grab bar by the user.

The following databases can be useful for locating literature on home modifications and environmental design:

+ Health-related databases: Pubmed (www.ncbi.nlm.nih.gov/pubmed/), OTseeker (www.otseeker.com), OTDbase (www.otdbase.org), and Cinahl (https://health.ebsco.com/products/the-cinahl-database)

+ Social-sciences databases: Social Services Abstracts, Sociological Abstracts, and Ageline (aging-related information in psychological, health-related, social, economics, public policy, and the health sciences)

+ Architectural databases: The Avery Index to Architectural Periodicals, and Architectural Publications Index

These databases access literature on theoretical frameworks, literature reviews, and research published in refereed journals and can be searched using keywords or broad search terms. In areas of practice with vast quantities of research, it can be useful to confine searches using specific terms related to the problem, intervention, client group, and outcome (PICO). For example, if searching for research on grab bars to assist older people into and out of the bath, the search would be defined as follows:

+ P—Problem: Getting in and out of the bath

+ I—Intervention: Grab bar

+ C—Client group: Older people

+ O—Outcome: Increased safety and independence

Other terms would also need to be included in the search to ensure that all relevant literature was identified. For example, the bath might be referred to in some studies as a *tub*; older people are also referred to as *elders*; grab bars are called *grab rails* in some countries; and some studies might also identify outcomes as *reduced falls* or *hospitalizations*. It is useful to seek the assistance of a librarian when developing a list of search terms because they are aware of alternative terms and terms used in different databases, such as the Medical Subject Headings terms. Some databases also provide advanced search strategies that allow the user to define the age range of the subjects and nature of the studies (e.g., RCTs).

Using specific PICO search terms assists in narrowing the search to the most relevant studies; however, targeted research is limited in many areas of occupational therapy practice. In home modification practice, it is advisable to use broad terms to ensure that all relevant literature is located.

Systematic reviews of research can be located in the Cochrane Collaboration (www.cochrane.org/reviews). Cochrane reviews examine the evidence for and against the appropriateness and effectiveness of a range of interventions in specific circumstances based on the best available information. For example, reviews have examined the impact of home modifications on the reduction of injuries (Lyons et al., 2006) and interventions for preventing falls in older people (Gillespie et al., 2009).

The Home Modification Information Clearing House (www.homemods.info) is also a valuable resource, providing evidence-based reviews on a range of home modification-related interventions, such as coatings for tiled floors (Whitfield, Bridge, & Mathews, 2005), designing home environments for people who experience problems with cognition and who display aggressive or self-injurious behavior (Hodges, Bridge, Donelly, & Chaudhary, 2007), and selecting diameters for grab bars (Oram, Cameron, & Bridge, 2006).

Additionally, the genHOME project (https://www.rcot.co.uk/about-us/specialist-sections/housing-rcot-ss/genhome) is a collaboration between academics, practitioners, researchers and members of the public supported by the Royal College of Occupational Therapists, United Kingdom (RCOT), which seeks to raise the quality and impact of research related to housing design and home modifications (RCOT, 2017). This project aims to achieve this goal by identifying research priorities, building evidence, facilitating interdisciplinary research, promoting efficient use of research resources, influencing policy and legislation, and providing a means for creating and sharing information between health professionals (RCOT, 2017).

There is also a wealth of information of relevance to home modification practice in legislative and regulatory documents and on the internet and, in particular, on websites and social media dedicated to home design and modification, and in the grey literature such as non-refereed publications posted on the internet, social media sites, industry newsletters, and manufacturers' specifications (Bridge & Phibbs, 2003). It is important that therapists carefully evaluate information for its relevance, dependability, and generalizability and consider their own experience and expertise and the priorities and preferences of their clients before applying it in practice.

Conformity With Standards, Guidelines, and Codes

Legislative and regulatory documents are particularly important when selecting and designing environmental interventions and evaluating the suitability of various options. Many products and designs are governed by design and installation requirements detailed in various standards, guidelines, and codes. Therapists need to be aware of these documents and ensure that proposed products or designs meet the appropriate requirements of their region or country.

The three national standards that guide the accessible design of buildings in the United States are the following:

1. Americans With Disabilities Act and Architectural Barriers Act (ADA-ABA) Accessibility Guidelines (United States Access Board, 2004/2014)

2. The Fair Housing Accessibility Guidelines (U.S. Department of Housing and Urban Development, 1990)

3. American National Standards Institute [ANSI] ICC A117.1-2009—Accessible and Usable Buildings and Facilities (ANSI, 2010)

Because the specifications in these standards relate specifically to the design of public buildings and multifamily dwellings and units, they do not apply directly to the design of single-family houses, except where elements are included in local building codes. Model building codes that serve as a basis for local codes might include accessibility requirements for specific building projects within their jurisdiction.

Elements of these standards can sometimes be used in the design of new homes or the modification of existing homes to promote access and mobility within the dwelling. Designers can depart from technical and scoping requirements in these guidelines when they can demonstrate that alternative designs and technologies can provide equivalent or greater access to, and usability of, the facility. In addition, variations to the specifications detailed in building standards are often required in residential settings when residents have particular requirements or when design is limited by existing topography of the land, building structures, service systems, and space restrictions.

There are several design elements specified in these standards, which include the following:

+ Dimensions (e.g., the height, width, depth of clearances and spaces, and size and location of various fixtures and fittings)

+ Features of fixtures and fittings (e.g., level handles on doors and drawers or taps)

+ Structural and technical requirements (e.g., sheer forces, maximum slope, maximum length of ramps, minimum height of edgings, minimum space between rail and wall)

+ Materials and finishes (e.g., the nature of surfaces and edges)

Dimensions and the features of fixtures and fittings detailed in these accessibility standards allow adults with disabilities to function in buildings. The standards are designed to ensure adult wheelchair users can independently move into and through the structure and use various controls. These specifications provide a useful reference when designing modifications for individuals similar in stature, size, and functional ability who are using similar assistive technologies to those for whom the standards were designed. However, many young clients with multiple and severe impairments and older clients with comorbidities and secondary conditions do not fit this profile and require dimensions and features to be tailored to their specific requirements (Sanford, 2012; Steinfeld & Shea, 1993). Additionally, it is important that therapists are aware that many standards are based on research from past periods and that changes in user demographics and advances in technology can and will likely impact on the suitability for applying standards to specific situations or client circumstances in current times (Steinfield, Maisel, Feathers, & D'Souza, 2010).

Therapists are often well placed to assist in customizing designs to the specific requirements of an individual because they can determine the circulation space each person requires to move throughout the home and maneuver in various areas. They are also able to measure each individual and his or her equipment to determine the best location for various fixtures and fittings. Therapists' understanding of function and occupational performance allows them to define and identify design features that promote better performance. In addition, their observations of daily routines assist them in understanding how spaces and controls are used and when and where people are provided with assistance. Because most standards do not consider the requirements of people who rely on assistance (Sanford, 2012), dimensions detailed in these documents often need to be modified to accommodate the spatial requirements of caregivers during tasks and the equipment they might use in their routine with the client.

The structural and technical specifications in the standards ensure the safety of people using the building. Engineering evaluations have determined the structural strength requirements of fixtures and fittings, such as grab bars, tub and shower seats, fasteners, and mounting devices, under regular use by people within the average weight range. It is inadvisable to select products or design modifications that do not meet these requirements without the advice of an engineer or suitably qualified consultant. Therapists should check that products have been certified as meeting these specifications and that contractors are aware of the requirements when installing these fixtures and fittings. Promotional materials produced by suppliers that make a general statement that their products meet accessibility standards are not sufficient proof. Therapists should seek supporting documentation and ensure that the product meets all the specifications. For example, some products might meet the requirements in terms of dimensions but may not meet, or only partially meet, the structural strength requirements. In the ADA-ABA, specifications relating to the structural strength of shower "compartment" seats state that "allowable stresses shall not be exceeded for materials used where a vertical or horizontal force of 250 pounds (1,112 Newton) is applied at any point on the seat, fastener mounting device, or supporting structure" (ANSI, 2010, p. 62). For example, therapists would want to ensure that shower seats under consideration are able to substantiate their claims for meeting both the vertical and horizontal force requirements. Further, therapists working with people who are outside of the average weight range would need to select products that have been designed to withstand the additional forces to which they are likely to be subjected.

It is particularly important that any imported products meet the legislative building requirements of the country where they are to be installed. For example, many grab bars made in the United States designed to meet the ADA-ABA would withstand a lateral load of 250 pounds (1,112 Newton). However, these would not meet the requirements set out in Australia where the accessibility standards require grab bars to withstand 1,100 Newton in all directions. It is important that therapists are aware of the specific building and plumbing legislation for the area(s) in which they are making recommendations as these are often region specific and variations between regions are not uncommon. For example, slip resistant surfaces must be provided on any ramp or set of stairs as per the requirements of building legislation in specific countries. Further, some legislation refers to access standards for large external modifications that must be installed in domestic homes, but others do not.

Regarding access standards, the gradient or slope and maximum height and length of ramps detailed in these documents have been determined as being functionally appropriate for most adults with disabilities (Sanford, Story, & Jones, 1997). It is therefore advisable to design ramps to these requirements unless it is determined that the client or the attendant is unable to manage a ramp with these specifications. In these situations, therapists can recommend that the ramp be designed to specifications greater than the minimum required by the standards if this is practicable in the environment and if there is no legislative requirement to comply with the standard. In some situations, the ramp might need to be made steeper or the length shortened due to environmental constraints. In these situations, the therapist would need to demonstrate that the client has the capacity to traverse a steeper or shorter ramp and provide justification for deviating from the standard (Canada Mortgage and Housing Corporation, 2005, 2016). Support for varying from the standard might include a description of the existing environmental limitations, a statement of intended usage and potential users, and a report on the user's performance when trialing a ramp of the proposed gradient, or research evidence on the effect of ramp slope on performance, such as that undertaken by Sanford and colleagues (1997). Though it is reasonable to tailor an environmental intervention to the specific needs of the current resident, therapists should also be mindful of the person's long-term capacities, visitors to the property, and future residents when designing permanent modifications and the requirements of their local authorities with respect to installing modifications that comply with local or state/provincial planning laws.

Design elements, such as the presence and height of edging to ramps or the space between grab bars or handrails and the adjacent wall, also improve people's safety and promote effective use of the built environment. It is important that these elements or suitable alternatives are reflected in product choices and are incorporated into the design of modifications. Materials and finishes might also have safety and/or functional implications; for example, insulating exposed pipes or removing sharp and abrasive surfaces under sinks or recommending ceramic

shrouds covering the pipework ensures that wheelchair users' knees and thighs are not injured when they wheel under sinks. Grab bars that rotate in their fittings can also be hazardous to users. The recommended level of slip resistance for walkways and ramps is also an important consideration when designing modifications for the home environment to ensure the safety of householders walking or wheeling on the surface.

By understanding the specifications in the accessibility standards and their intent, therapists can ensure that elements relating to safety are incorporated into the design of modifications. However, where a client's age, stature, size, functional abilities and equipment type, and dimensions lie outside of those covered by the standards, the dimensions and functional elements of the product and design should be reviewed considering the functional requirements of each individual. Therapists also need to be mindful that there are many standards governing the design of domestic dwellings that need to be adhered to when redesigning areas of the home, and they will need to liaise closely with designers and building professionals to ensure that designs and products conform to these. In some instances, these standards might impede the design of accessible features, resulting in therapists having to work closely with building and design professionals to negotiate a mutually acceptable outcome if possible. Further information on these is provided in Chapter 11.

Evolution of Design and Good Design Practice

Over time, the thinking and approaches to design have changed in response to population changes and the recognition of the rights of all people in society (Persson, Ahman, Yngling, & Gulliksen, 2015). This has resulted in an evolution of design and building practice (Figure 10-1; Ainsworth & de Jonge, 2008). With the population aging, the associated influence on rates of disability, and many people's desire to remain living independently as long as possible, there is an increased need for housing design that accommodates the needs of all people over the lifespan (Smith, Rayer, & Smith, 2008).

Initially, the design approach used for people with specific housing needs was purpose-built design. This approach, design, and building practice centered on the specific conditions and needs of the individual for whom the design was primarily for. This saw the inclusion and consideration of specialized equipment and products that were necessary to support the individual's function, particularly in activities of basic self-care. In this first stage of evolution, the environment was a prosthetic and the features of the design and associated modifications

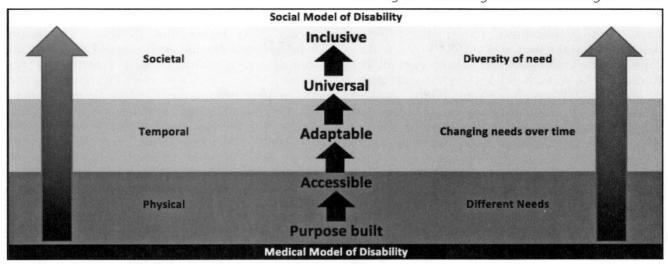

Figure 10-1. Evolution of design and building practice (Ainsworth & de Jonge, 2008).

were fixed in place and noticeable. To this end, homes and modifications were designed to meet the specific needs of individuals and the emphasis was on designing and modifying to enable and improve the access for people using wheelchairs. To achieve purpose-built design, occupational therapists would often assess the individual's function and make the relevant recommendations and suggestions for modification, which would be summarized into reports for architects to interpret and design. This approach perpetuated people with disabilities being defined in terms of their dysfunction (e.g., "a paraplegic" and as being "sick" and dependent on care). It provided a fragmented view of the person and offered little recognition of the person's needs beyond that of basic self-care (Ainsworth & de Jonge, 2008).

Purpose-built design was followed by accessible design. This stage of evolution was primarily focused on design features for access and mobility associated with public buildings and meeting the requirements of the relevant standards. In many countries, accessible design standards were established and these formed the foundation for many recommendations for home modification and design for people with disabilities (see Chapter 11 for a detailed description of the development, benefits, and limitations of accessible design standards). Access standards were established using a generalized view of the needs of the population of people with disabilities and were based on the capabilities of young people who mobilize independently in standard manual or electric wheelchairs. To this end, clearances, circulation spaces, and reach zones in the home were based on dated and restricted data and the associated specifications. Accessible design stresses the application of minimum standards to design and

modification while maintaining the consideration of client specific needs, with emphasis on designing for wheelchair access. It incorporated and considered the spatial requirements and dimensions of the base building; however, design and modifications solutions were often prescriptive and lacked creativity and the fixtures often continued to be permanently fixed and noticeable. This often resulted in home designs and modifications that were clinical, oversized, and inelegant. This approach to design continued to view the person in terms of their functional ability, dimensions (anthropometrics), and how they fit the relevant standards. The emphasis remained on activities of daily living, extending beyond that of just basic self-care to include mobility and access within and around the home, however, did not consider the person's roles in the home or community. The needs of the individual were interpreted by the occupational therapist and were communicated through and between professionals, often with little input from the client, which created and reinforced an information gap between people with disabilities and the industry (Ainsworth & de Jonge, 2008).

Both purpose-built design and accessible design were more traditional approaches to design and modifications that originated from the medical model of disability. In these approaches, therapists focused on achieving independence using alternative strategies and devices designed within a medical context. Many of these are made of metal and plastic with cold, hard surfaces and have a clinical appearance. Similarly, early home modifications tended to have an institutional appearance (Sanford & Butterfield, 2005). Such devices and modifications often do not fit well with the ambience of a home environment where soft surfaces and warm colors often predominate. Further, when the appearance of devices and modifications provoke strong negative reactions from the user and visitors to the home, it can influence acceptance and use (Aplin et al., 2013; Hocking, 1999; Wessels, Dijcks, Soede, Gelderblom, & De Witte, 2003; Wielandt & Strong, 2000).

After these more traditional approaches came adaptable design (referred to as *lifetime homes* in some countries). This stage in evolution offered greater choice, flexibility, and market appeal than its predecessors, while maintaining previous consideration of accessible features including clearances, circulation spaces, and reach zones. Adaptable design demonstrated an appreciation of diversity of function across the lifespan. People were seen to have a variety of needs and to interact with the social and physical environment. Additionally, there was an increased recognition of the person's role in the home and community and their need to be able to access and socialize with friends and family. These led to an improved understanding of the intent of design elements, enabling more creativity in approaches to design and modifications. Furthermore, the traditional focus on one individual shifted and designs and modifications were developed to suit a range of individuals and could often be adjusted to be fully accessible with adjustments frequently possible using unskilled labor. This stage of evolution resulted in designs and modifications in homes that remained centered on access requirements, but also included:

+ All essential elements and some desirable elements

+ Enhanced measurements and additional residential features

+ Space for carers, security, and color contrast (Ainsworth & de Jonge, 2008)

To this end, while some public design elements persisted (e.g. large open bathrooms), designs and modifications usually made good design sense and had an increased focus on safety, climate, aesthetics, flow, and affordability (Ainsworth & de Jonge, 2008). This resulted in environments appearing less institutional and the solutions being more elegant overall (Ainsworth & de Jonge, 2008). The designs and modifications of this design approach created housing that provided greater choice for people with a variety of abilities and that was useable across the life span (Ainsworth & de Jonge, 2008). This enabled people to age in place, remain in the community, and maintain natural support networks (Balandin & Chapman, 2001).

With the emergence of universal design (UD) there has been an increased emphasis on designing products, environments, and systems for the broader community rather than designing specifically for people with disabilities or special requirements (Connell and Sanford, 1999). UD recognizes the diversity of capabilities of users (Wylde, 1995) and aims to make products, environments, and systems inclusive, spanning age, gender, and ability while reducing the need for accommodations and specialized assistive devices (The Center for Universal Design, 1997; Steinfeld & Maisel, 2012). It does not, however, remove the need for standards that outline the legal limits for minimum accessibility (Steinfeld & Maisel, 2012).

Traditionally, UD has been defined as "the design of products and environments to be usable by all people, to the greatest extent possible, without the need for specialized design" (Mace, 1985 p. 147; RL Mace Universal Design Institute, 2017).

However, due to concerns regarding specificity and impracticality, further terms and definitions have been posited, including:

> Design for All—design for human diversity, social inclusion, and equality. Design for All aims to enable all people to have equal opportunities to participate in every aspect of society. To achieve this, the built environment, everyday objects, services, culture and information—in short, everything that is designed and made by people to be used by people—must be accessible, convenient for everyone in society to use and responsive to evolving human diversity (European Institute for Design and Disability, 2004)

and, more recently,

> Universal design is a process that enables and empowers a diverse population by improving human performance, health and wellness, and social participation. (Steinfeld & Maisel, 2012, p. 29)

Despite the evolution of the terms and definitions, consensus is yet to be established on the specifics of a definition. It is clear, however, that benefit to the broader community and inclusion are common themes (Steinfeld & Maisel, 2012).

This approach to design required a fundamental shift in thinking from previous stages of evolution (i.e., progressing from removing environmental barriers to designing to ensure inclusion of all people to the greatest possible extent, regardless of age or ability; Ainsworth & de Jonge, 2008). It addresses the design of products, buildings and information system and requires:

+ An understanding of the broad range of human abilities

+ An appreciation of changes that occur across the lifespan

+ A creative approach to design

+ Consideration of shape, adjustability, and placement of features

However, if successfully achieved, it promotes social mobility and integration for persons of all abilities (Ainsworth & de Jonge, 2008). This allows all people, regardless of ability, to be part of society and ensures that people with disabilities or special requirements are no longer viewed as being different. UD provides a range of choices that enables designs and products to be elegant and suitable for the home environment while promoting safety and ease of use for everyone living in or visiting the home (Ainsworth & de Jonge, 2008). Further, attention to the design ensures that modifications continue to be useful as the needs of clients and other householders change over time without the need to modify the product or design. Universally designed products and environments have also been found to be considered more functional, accessible, safe, and attractive by users and less visible than specialized options (Park, 2006). Moreover, while there are often additional immediate costs for designs, products, and systems, there are frequently persisting cost benefits in the long term (Ainsworth & de Jonge, 2008).

When examining universally designed products and environments, it is noted that like the definition of UD, there has been a variety of descriptions proposed over time. These descriptions have also often guided the development of subsequent methods of UD evaluation in clinical practice.

One such description was outlined by Wylde (1995), who described universally designed products and environments as being:

+ Usable and useful: Can be used successfully to perform the intended function simply and expediently

+ Neutral: Do not demand right- or left-handed performance

+ Inclusive: Built to include a diverse population of users (i.e., of differing sizes and abilities)

+ Visible: Provide clear, visible clues as to how they are to be used

+ Elegant: Are aesthetically pleasing

+ Redundant: Provide additional cues to the user (e.g., acoustic, tactile, and visual information)

+ Simple: Avoid superfluous controls, ornamentation, and embellishments

+ Accessible, adaptable, and adjustable: Accessible to individuals of varying abilities and designed to be adjusted or adapted for those whose abilities fall beyond the ranges of practical design considerations

+ Logical: Built purposefully with each component and feature, and placement and function consistent with expectations

This set of descriptors forms the basis for the *Enabling Products Sourcebook 2* (Wylde, 1995), which provides a "head-to-toe" evaluation of products using the following criteria:

+ The head: Cognition, vision, audition, and olfaction

+ The upper body: Manual dexterity

+ The lower body: Strength and stamina

+ Overall safety features

+ Product features related to cleaning and maintenance

While not every criterion will be relevant to every product, the criteria assist in evaluating the range of users who will be able to use the product effectively (Wylde, 1995). For example, when reviewing the visual demands of a product, Wylde (1995) examines whether:

+ Functions with a visual output are accompanied by audible and/or tactile output

+ The surface of the product has a non-glare finish in areas where vision is required

+ All graphics, signage, and coding are legible under adverse viewing conditions

+ The print and symbols provide color contrasting with the background

+ Use of colors as indicators is purposeful and visible

+ Indicator lights relate directly to the function they control

+ An integral light source is provided where vision is required for safe operation

+ Raised lettering is used where possible

+ Where audible and tactile cues are not feasible, the product accommodates Braille overlays on functions requiring vision

Despite the presence of other descriptions, such as that of Wylde (1995), the most well-known and possibly popular description is that of the Seven Principles of Universal Design proposed by The Center for Universal Design (1997). These principles were developed to promote products and

Universal Design Performance Measures for Products

VERSION 1.0

PRINCIPLE ONE	EQUITABLE USE	Not Applicable	Strongly Disagree	Disagree	Neutral	Agree	Strongly Agree	Comments
1A.	All potential users could use this product in essentially the same way, regardless of differences in their abilities.							
1B.	Potential users could use this product without feeling segregated or stigmatized because of differences in personal capabilities.							
1C.	Potential users of this product have access to all features of privacy, security, and safety regardless of personal capabilities.							
1D.	This product appeals to all potential users.							

PRINCIPLE TWO	FLEXIBILITY IN USE							
2A.	Every potential user can find at least one way to use this product effectively.							
2B.	This product can be used with either the right or left hand alone.							
2C.	This product facilitates (or does not require) user accuracy and precision.							
2D.	This product can be used at whatever pace (quickly or slowly) the user prefers.							

Figure 10-2. Universal Design Performance Measures for Products. (Reprinted with permission from Center for Universal Design. [2000]. *Evaluating the universal design performance of products.* Raleigh, NC: The Center for Universal Design, North Carolina State University. Retrieved from https://www.ncsu.edu/ncsu/design/cud/pubs_p/docs/UDPMD.pdf)

environments consistent with the original definition of UD, provided on page 242.

The principles encourage designers to develop products and environments that allow the following:

+ Equitable use: Useful and marketable to people with diverse abilities

+ Flexibility in use: Accommodates a wide range of individual preferences and abilities

+ Simple and intuitive use: Easy to understand, regardless of the user's experience, knowledge, language skills, or current concentration level

+ Perceptible information: Communicates necessary information effectively to the user, regardless of ambient conditions or the user's sensory abilities

+ Tolerance for error: Minimizes hazards and the adverse consequences of accidental or unintended actions

+ Low physical effort: Can be used efficiently and comfortably and with a minimum of fatigue

+ Size and space for approach and use: Appropriate size and space for approach, reach, manipulation, and use regardless of user's body size, posture, or mobility (The Center for Universal Design, 1997)

Further to the principles, The Center for Universal Design (2000) also developed the Universal Design Performance Measure (Figure 10-2), which designers and therapists can use to evaluate the design characteristics of options and compare the universality of various products and designs being considered in home modification practice. The measure is not intended to replace user evaluation or experience with a product or design but assists therapists and designers in evaluating the broader usability of interventions.

Although these principles appear to be simple, people vary enormously in terms of height, weight, endurance, strength, balance, mobility, and visual and hearing acuity (Conway, 2008). When considering the suitability of design, therapists need to draw on their understanding of this diversity and aim to maximize the usability of the product and environment for as many people as possible while ensuring that they continue to support clients' occupational performance. To this end, it is vital that therapists have a comprehensive understanding of diversity to enable them to design universally. As a profession, occupational therapy encourages its members to develop and consistently expand upon their knowledge of diversity, and this can be invaluable in reviewing the potential of product and design solutions. Furthermore, this expertise allows therapists to make a significant contribution to the development of products and designs. Notwithstanding the well-intentioned nature and the benefits of UD, this approach does continue to experience challenges to successful implementation. Some of these include:

+ Confusion with accessibility using a "template" approach

+ Association with disability design (Maisel, 2005)

+ Overemphasis on physical aspects (Calkins, Sanford, & Proffitt, 2001)

+ Lack of understanding of sensory, cognitive, psychological, and social diversity

+ The perception that UD restricts creativity and employs a "one size fits all" approach (e.g., a "McDesign" approach; Ainsworth & de Jonge, 2008; Sanford, 2012)

+ Concern about additional immediate costs

+ Principles that are incomplete, complex, and ambiguous (Steinfeld, 2006).

However, of the challenges that exist, probably the most noteworthy is the absence of consensus on the definition. This challenge has seen the creation of terminology, often used interchangeably, which has been created in a similar fashion but in different areas of the world (Persson et al., 2015; The Norwegian Centre for Design and Architecture, 2010). While some of these terminologies, associated definitions, and accompanying concepts are very similar (e.g., UD and Design for All), there is another: inclusive design, evolved from product design rather than design of the built environment, which offers a slightly different focus (University of Cambridge, 2017a).

Inclusive design has been defined as "the design of mainstream products and/or services that are accessible to, and usable by, as many people as reasonably possible … without the need for special adaptation or specialized design" (British Standards Institution, 2005). While this concept displays similarities with the others previously mentioned, one primary difference is the presence of the phrase "reasonably possible" (Persson et al., 2015). The presence of this phrase has been criticized in the literature as possibly impeding the rights of inclusion of people with disabilities, contrary to documentation, such as the United Nations' Convention on the Rights of Persons With Disabilities, if it is too costly or difficult (Persson et al., 2015). However, this approach to design aims to give greater acknowledgement to the existing diversity in the population, identifying that it is not always feasible or appropriate to design one product that meets the needs of the entire population (University of Cambridge, 2017a). It proposes that every decision related to design has the potential to include or exclude people and highlights the necessity for understanding diversity to make informed decisions to include as many people as possible (University of Cambridge, 2017a). To respond to diversity in the population, this approach directs design through:

+ "Developing a family of products and derivatives to provide the best possible coverage of the population

+ Ensuring that each individual product has clear and distinct target users

+ Reducing the level of ability required to use each product, in order to improve the user experience for a broad range of customers, in a variety of situations" (University of Cambridge, 2017a)

Furthermore, this approach, while not outlining a specific set of criteria, does offer a more pragmatic approach to acknowledging and responding to diversity as it offers an actionable process for decision making at the concept stage of design development. This process includes the following four phases:

1. Manage: Review the evidence to decide "What should we do next?"

2. Explore: Determine "What are the needs?"

3. Create: Generate ideas to address "How can the needs be met?"

4. Evaluate: Judge and test the design concepts to determine "How well are the needs met?" (University of Cambridge, 2017b)

Further details about these phases can be found in the Inclusive Design Toolkit (University of Cambridge, 2017b). Approaches to design and building practice have evolved over many years in response to society's growing awareness of population diversity and the rights of people to be included in all aspects of society regardless of age or disability. This has influenced the modifications, products, and services that have been available and offered to people as the perspectives have moved from seeing people as "different" and requiring specialized features to recognizing that all design should be able to accommodate all people regardless of their abilities. While this evolution has occurred in a positive trajectory overall, there is still room for further improvement and standardization of current approaches to design, particularly at the international level.

CONCLUSION

There is a range of resources available to assist therapists in locating and sourcing products and designs. Each of these contributes different information and allows therapists to develop a portfolio of products and designs suited to the needs of an individual in a range of situations. Initially, therapists need to establish a broad understanding of the diverse range of options available. They can then build on this solid foundation to undertake a targeted search of resources to identify products and designs suited to the specific needs of each client. It is often difficult for therapists who are new to the field or only undertake modifications as a small part of their work to establish and maintain the expertise required to do modifications well. In these situations, therapists need to consult with colleagues with greater expertise to ensure the best outcomes for their clients.

To determine the best solution in each case, therapists review and evaluate options by comparing the features and specification of each, with due consideration to client priorities and preferences. Therapists also draw on available evidence and use professional reasoning to collect and interpret different types of information to determine the best option for each situation, assessing the quality and relevance of information and applying it judiciously. Therapists also need to be conscious of the standards when selecting and evaluating products and designs while remaining mindful of the specific needs of each client and his or her situation. Finally, therapists need to ensure that products and designs incorporated into modifications are aesthetic and recognize the diverse and changing abilities of all residents of the household while reflecting the expectations of society in terms of what a home should look and feel like.

REFERENCES

Ainsworth, E. & de Jonge, D. (2008). Architectural design influences on outcomes for older people and people with disabilities. Paper presented at the International Conference on Aging, Disability and Independence, St Petersburg, FL.

American National Standards Institute. (2010). *ICC A117.1-2009—Accessible and Usable Buildings and Facilities.* Retrieved from https://law.resource.org/pub/us/code/ibr/ansi.a117.1.2009.pdf

Aminzadeh, F., Edwards, N., Lockett, D., & Nair, R. (2000). Utilization of bathroom safety devices, patterns of bathing & toileting and bathroom falls in a sample of community living older adults. *Technology and Disability, 13*, 95-103.

Andrich, R. (2002). The SCAI instrument: Measuring costs of individual assistive technology programmes. *Technology and Disability, 14*, 95-99.

Aplin, T., de Jonge, D. & Gustafsson, L. (2013). Understanding the dimensions of home that impact on home modification decision making. *Australian Occupational Therapy Journal, 60*, 101-109.

Aplin, T., de Jonge, D. & Gustafsson, L. (2015). Understanding home modifications impact on clients and their family's experience of home: A qualitative study. *Australian Occupational Therapy Journal, 62*, 123-131.

Auriemma, D., Faust, S., Sibrian, K., & Jimenez, J. (1999). Home modifications for the elderly: Implications for the occupational therapist. *Physical and Occupational Therapy in Geriatrics, 16*(2-4), 135-144.

Axtell, L. A., & Yausda, Y. L. (1993). Assistive devices and home modifications in geriatric rehabilitation. *Geriatric Rehabilitation, 9*, 803-821.

Balandin, S., & Chapman, R. (2001). Aging with a developmental disability at home: an Australian perspective. In W. F. E. Preiser, & E. Ostroff (Eds.), *Universal design handbook* (pp. 38.1-38.16). New York, NY: McGraw-Hill Inc.

Bernt, N., & Skar, L. (2006). A pilot study of the activity patterns of five elderly persons after a housing adaptation. *Occupational Therapy International, 13*(1), 21-34.

Bridge, C. (2003). *Basic biomechanical and anatomical principles underpinning grabrail prescriptions for sit-to-stand transfers.* Sydney, Australia: Home Modification Clearinghouse. Retrieved from http://www.homemods.info/publications-by-hminfo/occasional/basic-biomechanical-and-anatomical-principles-underpinning-grabrail-prescription-for-sit-to-stand-transfers#main-content

Bridge, C., & Phibbs, P. (2003). *Protocol guidelines for systematic reviews of home modification information to inform best practice.* Sydney, Australia: Home Modification Information Clearinghouse, University of New South Wales. Retrieved from https://www.homemods.info/about/administrative-publications/protocol-guidelines-for-systematic-reviews-of-home-modification-information-to-inform-best-practice#main-content

British Standards Institution. (2005). *BS 7000-6:2005—Design management systems. Managing inclusive design: Guide.* London: Author.

Calkins, M., Sanford, J., & Proffitt, M. (2001). Design for dementia: Challenges and lessons for universal design. In W. F. E. Preiser & E. Ostroff (Eds.), *Universal design handbook* (pp. 22.21-22.24). New York, NY: McGraw-Hill Inc.

Canada Mortgage and Housing Corporation. (2005). *Measuring the effort needed to climb access ramps in a manual wheelchair. Research highlight—Socio-economic series 05-011, (1-4).* Ottawa, ON: Author. Retrieved from www.cmhc-schl.gc.ca/odpub/pdf/63916.pdf?fr=1495674159007

Canada Mortgage and Housing Corporation. (2016). *Ramps: Accessible housing by design, (1-13)*. Ottawa, ON: Author. Retrieved from www.cmhc-schl.gc.ca/odpub/pdf/65023.pdf

Chan, D., Laporte, D. M. & Sveistrup, H. (1999). Rising from sitting in elderly people, part 2: Strategies to facilitate rising. *British Journal of Occupational Therapy, 62*(2), 64-68.

Chiatti, C., & Iwarsson, S. (2014). Evaluation of housing adaptation interventions: integrating the economic perspective into occupational therapy practice. *Scandinavian Journal of Occupational Therapy, 21*(5), 323-333.

Clemson, L. & Martin, R. (1996). Usage and effectiveness of rails, bathing and toileting aids. *Occupational Therapy in Health Care, 10*(1), 41- 59.

Connell, B. R., & Sanford, J. A. (1999). Research implications of universal design. In E. Steinfeld & S. Danford (Eds.), *Enabling Environments: Measuring the impact of environment on disability and rehabilitation* (pp. 35-57). New York, NY: Springer US.

Conway, M. (2008). *Occupational therapy and inclusive design: Principles for practice*. Oxford, UK: Blackwell Publishing Incorporated.

Duncan, R. (1998). Blueprint for action: The National Home Modifications Action Coalition. *Technology and Disability, 8*(1-2), 85-89.

European Institute for Design and Disability. (2004). The EIDD Stockholm Declaration 2004.Retrieved from http://dfaeurope. eu/what-is-dfa/dfa-documents/the-eidd-stockholm-declaration-2004/

Gillespie, L. D., Robertson, M. C., Gillespie, W. J., Lamb, S. E., Gates, S., Cumming, R. G., & Rowe, B. H. (2009). Interventions for preventing falls in older people living in the community. *Cochrane Database of Systematic Reviews*, (2), CD007146. doi: 10.1002/14651858.CD007146.pub2

Hawkins, R., & Stewart, S. (2002). Changing rooms: The impact of adaptations on the meaning of home for a disabled person and the role of occupational therapists in the process. *British Journal of Occupational Therapy, 65*(2), 81-87.

Heywood, F. (2004). The health outcomes of housing adaptations. *Disability and Society, 19*(2), 129-143.

Heywood, F., & Turner, L. (2007). *Better outcomes, lower costs: Implications for health and social care budgets of investment in housing adaptations, improvements and equipment: a review of the evidence*. Leeds, England: Office for Disability Issues, Department for Work and Pensions. Retrieved from http:// www.wohnenimalter.ch/img/pdf/better_outcomes_report.pdf

Hocking, C. (1999). Function or feelings: Factors in abandonment of assistive devices. *Technology and Disability, 11*, 3-11.

Hodges, L., Bridge, C., Donelly, M., & Chaudhary, K. (2007). *Evidence based research bulletin: Designing home environments for people who experience problems with cognition who display aggressive or self-injurious behaviours*. Sydney, Australia: Home Modification Information Clearinghouse, University of New South Wales: Sydney. Retrieved from https://www. homemods.info/resources/hminfo-research-publications/evidence/designing-home-environments-for-people-who-experience-problems-with-cognition-and-who-display-aggressive-or-self-injurious-behav#main-content

Home Adaptations Consortium. (2013). Delivering housing adaptations for disabled people: A detailed guide to related legislation, guidance and good practice. Retrieved from http:// careandrepair-england.org.uk/wp-content/uploads/2014/12/ DFG-Good-Practice-Guide-30th-Sept-131.pdf

Kennedy, M. J., Arcelus, A., Guitard, P., Goubran, R. A., & Sveistrup, H. (2015). Toilet grab-bar preference and center of pressure deviation during toilet transfers in healthy seniors, seniors with hip replacements, and seniors having suffered a stroke. *Assistive Technology, 27*(2), 78-87.

Laporte, D. M., Chan, D. & Sveistrup, H. (1999). Rising from sitting in elderly people, part 1: Implications of biomechanics and physiology. *British Journal of Occupational Therapy, 62*(1), 36-42.

Lund, M. L., & Nygard, L. (2004). Occupational life in the home environment: The experiences of people with disabilities. *Canadian Journal of Occupational Therapy, 71*(4), 243-251.

Lyons, R. A., John, A., Brophy, S., Jones, S. J., Johansen, A., Kemp, A., . . . Weightman, A. (2006). Modification of the home environment for the reduction of injuries. *Cochrane Database of Systematic Reviews, 18*(4), CD003600. doi: 10.1002/14651858. CD003600.pub2

Mace, R. L. (1985). Universal design, barrier-free environments for everyone. *Designers West, 33*(1), 147-152.

Maisel, J. L. (2005). *Visitability as an approach to inclusive housing design and community development: A look at its emergence, growth, and challenges*. Buffalo, NY: Center for Inclusive Design and Environmental Access (IDEA)—School of Architecture and Planning, University at Buffalo. Retrieved from http://www.townofpinedale.us/DocumentCenter/Home/ View/71

McDonald, G. (1997). *An investigation into vertical grabrail use and grabrail grasp height for older women with bilateral knee osteoarthritis*. Unpublished Honour Thesis, University of Sydney, Sydney Australia.

McDonald, G., Bridge, C., & Smith, R. (1996). *Osteoarthritis, grabrail use and positioning: What are the implications*. Paper presented at the Proceedings of the NSW AOT 10th Annual State Conference, Sydney Australia.

O'Meara, D. M. (2003). *Properties of manual support fixtures*. Unpublished PhD Thesis. Sydney, Australia: University of Sydney.

O'Meara, D. M., & Smith, R. M. (2002). *The effects of grabrail position and orientation on body motion and handle force*. Melbourne, Australia: ABC4, La Trobe University; 28-29.

O'Meara, D. M., & Smith, R. M. (2005). Differences between grab rail position and orientation during the assisted sit-to-stand for able-bodied older adults. *Journal of Applied Biomechanics, 21*(1), 57-71.

O'Meara, D. M., & Smith, R. M. (2006). The effects of unilateral grab rail assistance on the sit-to-stand performance of older aged adults. *Human Movement Science, 25*, 257-274.

Ongley, J. (1999). *An investigation of the sit-to-stand transfer in healthy older women when standing up from different toilet pan heights, with and without grabrail assistance*. Unpublished Honors Thesis. Sydney, Australia: University of Sydney.

Oram, L., Cameron, J., & Bridge, C. (2006). *Diameter: Evidence based research: Selecting diameters for grabrails*. Sydney, Australia: Home Modification Information Clearinghouse, University of New South Wales: Sydney. Retrieved from http:// www.homemods.info/resources/hminfo-research-publications/evidence/diameter-evidence-based-research-selecting-diameters-for-grabrails#main-content

Park, D. (2006). Universal design in aging in place senior housing: A pilot study of residents' perspectives. In W. C. Mann & A. A. Helal (Eds.), *Promoting independence for older persons with disabilities* (pp. 193-203). Fairfax, VA: IOS Press.

Parker, M. G., & Thorslund, M. (1991). The use of technical aids among community based elderly. *American Journal of Occupational Therapy, 36*(8), 507-508.

Persson, H., Ahman, H., Yngling, A., & Gulliksen, J. (2015). Universal design, inclusive design, accessible design, design for all: Different concepts—one goal? On the concept of accessibility—historical, methodological and philosophical aspects. *Universal Access in the Information Society, 14*, 505-526.

Pighills, A., Torgerson, D., Sheldon, T., Drummond, A., & Bland, M. (2011). Environmental assessment and modification to prevent falls in older people. *Journal of the American Geriatric Society, 59*(1), 26-33.

Plautz, B., Beck, D., Selmar, C., & Radersky, M. (1996). Modifying the environment: A community-based program for elderly residents. *American Journal of Prevention, 12*, 33-38.

RL Mace Universal Design Institute. (2017). What is universal design? Retrieved from http://www.udinstitute.org/whatisud.php

Roland, M. (1996). *Effectiveness of grabrails during sit to stand transfers.* Unpublished Masters Thesis. Sydney, Australia: University of Sydney.

Rousseau, J., Potvin, L., Dutil, E., & Falta, P. (2001). A critical review of assessment tools related to home adaptation issues. *Occupational Therapy in Health Care, 14*(3-4), 93-104.

Royal College of Occupational Therapists. (2017). genHOME. Retrieved from https://www.rcot.co.uk/about-us/specialist-sections/housing-rcot-ss/genhome

Sackett, D. L. (2000). *Evidence based medicine: How to practice and teach EBM.* Edinburgh, UK: Churchill-Livingstone.

Sanford, J. A. (2012). *Design for the ages: Universal design as a rehabilitation strategy.* New York, NY: Springer Publishing.

Sanford, J. A., Arch, M., & Megrew, M. B. (1995). An evaluation of grab bars to meet the needs of elderly people. *Assistive Technology, 7*, 36-47.

Sanford, J., & Bosch, S. J. (2013). An investigation of non-compliant toilet room designs for assisted toileting. *HERD, 6*(2), 43-57.

Sanford, J. A., & Butterfield, T. (2005). Using remote assessment to provide home modification services to underserved elders. *The Gerontologist, 45*(3), 389-398.

Sanford, J. A., Story, M. F., & Jones, M. L. (1997). An analysis of the effects of ramp slope on people with mobility impairments. *Assistive Technology, 9*(1), 22-33.

Sapey, B. (1995). Disabling homes: A study of the housing needs of disabled people in Cornwall. *Disability and Society, 10*(1), 71-85.

Sattin, R. W., Rodriguez, J. G., DeVito, C. A., & Wingo, P. A. (1998). Home environmental hazards and the risk of fall injury events among community-dwelling older persons: Study to Assess Falls Among the Elderly (SAFE) group. *Journal of the American Geriatrics Society, 46*, 669-676.

Scottish Government. (n.d.). Spend now. Save for the future. A social return on investment study of adaptations. Retrieved from https://envoypartnership.files.wordpress.com/2016/05/sroi_adaptations.pdf

Smith, S., Rayer, S., & Smith, E. (2008). Ageing & disability: Implications for the housing industry and housing policy in the United States. *Journal of the American Planning Association, 74*(3), 289-306.

Sonn, U., & Grimby, G. (1994). Assistive devices in an elderly population studied at 70 and 76 years of age. *Disability and Rehabiliation, 16*(2), 85-92

Steinfeld, E. (2006). *Position paper: The future of universal design.* Buffalo, NY: Inclusive Design and Environmental Access [IDEA] Center.

Steinfeld, E., & Danford, G. S. (1999). Theory as a basis for research on enabling environments. In E. Steinfeld & G. S. Danford (Eds.), *Enabling environments: Measuring the impact of environment on disability and rehabilitation* (pp. 11-33). New York, NY: Kluwer Academic/Plenum Publishers.

Steinfeld, E., & Maisel, J. L. (2012). *Universal design: Creating inclusive environments.* Hoboken, NJ: John Wiley & Sons, Inc.

Steinfeld, E., Maisel, J., Feathers, D., & D'Souza, C. (2010). Anthropometry and standards for wheeled mobility: An international comparison. *Assistive Technology, 22*, 51-67.

Steinfeld, E., & Shea, S. (1993). Enabling home environments: Identifying barriers to independence. *Technology and Disability, 2*(4), 69-79.

Struyk, R. J. & Katsura, H.M. (1988). *Aging at home: How the elderly adjust their housing without moving.* New York, NY: The Haworth Press, Inc.

The Center for Universal Design. (1997). *The principles of universal design version 2.0.* Raleigh, NC: Author. Retrieved from https://www.ncsu.edu/ncsu/design/cud/about_ud/udprinciplestext.htm

The Center for Universal Design. (2000). *Evaluating the universal design performance of products.* Raleigh, NC: Author. Retrieved from http://www.design.ncsu.edu/cud/pubs_p/docs/UDPP.pdf

The Norwegian Centre for Design and Architecture. (2010). *Inclusive design—A people centered strategy for innovation: Definitions.* Retrieved from http://www.inclusivedesign.no/practical-tools/definitions-article56-127.html

Tideiksaar, R. (1997). *Falling in old age: Prevention and management* (2nd ed.). New York, NY: Springer.

Trickey, F., Maltais, D., Gosselin, M. A., & Robitaille, Y. (1993). Adapting older persons' homes to promote independence. *Physical & Occupational Therapy in Geriatrics, 12*(1), 1-14.

Turpin, M., & Higgs, J. (2009). Clinical reasoning and evidence-based practice. In T. Hoffman, S. Bennett, & C. Del Mar (Eds.), *Evidence-based practice across the health professions* (pp. 300-317). Melbourne, Australia: Elsevier.

University of Cambridge. (2017a). Inclusive design toolkit: What is inclusive design? Retrieved from http://www.inclusivedesigntoolkit.com/whatis/whatis.html

University of Cambridge. (2017b). Inclusive design toolkit: Concept design process: Overview. Retrieved from http://www.inclusivedesigntoolkit.com/GS_overview/overview.html

U.S. Access Board. (2004/2014). Americans With Disabilities Act and Architectural Barriers Act (ADA-ABA) Accessibility Guidelines—July 23, 2004. Retrieved from https://www.access-board.gov/attachments/article/412/ada-aba.pdf

U.S. Department of Housing and Urban Development. (1990). The Fair Housing Accessibility Guidelines: Adoption of final guidelines. Retrieved from https://portal.hud.gov/hudportal/HUD?src=/program_offices/fair_housing_equal_opp/disabilities/fhguidelines/fhefha1

Wessels, R., Dijcks, B., Soede, M., Gelderblom, G. J., & De Witte, L. (2003). Non-use of provided assistive technology devices: A literature overview. *Technology and Disability, 15*, 231-238.

Whitfield, K., Bridge C., & Mathews, S. (2005). *Coatings: Evidence based research: Selecting coatings for tiled floors.* Sydney, Australia: Home Modification and Maintenance Information Clearinghouse, University of New South Wales: Sydney. Retrieved from http://www.homemods.info/resources/hminfo-research-publications/evidence/coatings/coatings-evidence-based-research-selecting-coatings-for-tiled-floors#main-content

Wielandt, T., & Strong, J. (2000). Compliance with prescribed adaptive equipment: A literature review. *British Journal of Occupational Therapy, 63*(2), 65-75.

Woodson, W. E. (1981). *Human factors design handbook.* New York, NY: McGraw Hill.

Wylde, M. (1995). *Enabling products sourcebook 2.* Hackettstown, NJ: National Kitchen and Bath Association and Promatura. Retrieved from http://www.homemods.org/resources/pages/enabling.shtml

11

Access Standards and Their Role in Guiding Interventions

Elizabeth Ainsworth, MOccThy, Grad Cert Health Sci;
Desleigh de Jonge, MPhil (OccThy), Grad Cert Soc Sci;
and Bronwyn Tanner, BOccThy, Grad Cert Occ Thy, Grad Cert Soc Planning, MPhil

There is much confusion and debate about the relevance and application of access standards to home modification practice. Although access standards were created in response to public access requirements in the community, occupational therapists in home modification practice use them as a reference and in some instances, comply with them, particularly major modifications. The primary focus of occupational therapy home modification practice is a thorough understanding of the needs of the individual and the unique fit between the individual and his or her home environment. However, sound practice also requires an understanding of the relevance and the appropriateness of the application of access standards when recommending modifications to the home environment. This chapter seeks to inform occupational therapists about access standards (how they are developed, their benefits and limitations, and their use in the design of public buildings) as well as their applications to home modification practice. Therapists will find this information useful with working with other stakeholders involved in the home modifications process as there can be confusion about the application of access standards to modification of domestic homes.

CHAPTER OBJECTIVES

By the end of this chapter, the reader will be able to:

✦ Describe access standards, their development, and how and when they are to be used as a guide or when they need to be adhered to in home modification practice

✦ Describe the benefits and limitations associated with the application of access standards in home modification practice

INTRODUCTION

The following discussion includes general information on standards, their development, their general benefits for society, and the specific benefits for people with disabilities.

Standards are described as documents that define best practice. Information provided by standards include dimensions, ratings, terminology, symbols, test methods, and performance and safety requirements for personnel, products, systems, and services in a wide range of industries (American National Service Institute [ANSI], 2009).

Ainsworth, E., & de Jonge, D. *An Occupational Therapist's Guide to Home Modification Practice, Second Edition (pp. 247-257).*
© 2019 SLACK Incorporated.

Specifications and procedures are detailed in standards with the objective of ensuring that a material, product, method, or service is fit for its purpose and consistently performs in the way that it was intended (ANSI, 2009). These documents are generally established by consensus and are approved by a recognized body, such as ANSI, the British Standards Institution (BSI), or Standards Australia (SA). They provide a common language to describe criteria for safety, reliability, and consistency of products, services, and systems (SA, 2017a) and define terms to ensure that there is no misunderstanding among those using the standard (ANSI, 2009).

Standards are based on industrial, scientific, and consumer experience and are regularly reviewed to ensure they keep pace with new technologies (SA). There are three kinds of standards:

1. International standards are developed by the International Organization for Standardization, The International Electrotechnical Commission (SA). Countries can adopt these standards directly for their national use (SA).

2. Regional standards are prepared by a specific region, such as the European Union, which develops European standards. Similarly, joint Australian/New Zealand standards can be considered regional standards.

3. National standards can be developed by a national standards body (like ANSI, SA) or other accredited bodies. Standards developed under the brand of Australian Standard are developed within Australia or are adoptions of international standards.

There are also other technical documents that provide guidance and assistance on implementing standards, including handbooks and technical reports (SA).

Standards can be voluntary or mandatory. While voluntary standards by themselves impose no obligations regarding use, mandatory standards are generally published as part of a code, rule, or regulation by a regulatory government body and impose an obligation on specific parties to conform to them (Breitenberg, 1987). Specifications detailed in the standards are either prescriptive or performance based. Prescriptive standards detail or prescribe specifically what is required (e.g., the location of the center line of the toilet from the side wall; International Code Council [ICC] & ANSI, 2009). Performance-based standards identify a function or an operation that needs to be met (e.g., the grab bar to be installed must be able to take 1112 Newton of force; ICC & ANSI, 2009).

Standards cover consumer products and services, construction, engineering, business, information technology, human services, energy and water utilities, the built environment, and other areas (SA). Some of these govern the safety, amenity, and integrity of public and residential built environments as well as the consistency and quality of products that may be used in these environments.

Standards relating to the built environment are specific technical guidelines that encompass the entire process of construction and assembly of buildings; structural, plumbing, electrical, and mechanical systems; and fire protection and energy conservation and consumption within and around commercial and residential buildings (Lawlor & Thomas, 2008). Standards related to public buildings detail the design requirements to address wind resistance; structural load; fire safety and egress; and electrical, plumbing, and mechanical systems. Depending on the jurisdiction and type of construction, standards may also address safety, accessibility, and indoor quality (Lawlor & Thomas, 2008).

Residential buildings are governed by similar standards relating to the structure and safety of the building, but these are tailored to the specific building type, geographic location, and use of various areas within the building. For example, there are a range of standards that govern the design and construction of domestic dwellings, including standards having to do with electrical and wiring installation, slip resistance in wet areas, and waterproofing requirements. Various standards also guide the design of fixtures and fittings and materials used within the home. Many of these standards are mandatory, especially when they are incorporated into building legislation, such as national construction codes. Consequently, there are several standards that can influence the outcome of the home modification process. For example, compliance with plumbing and electrical standards is a requirement when undertaking modification work in a bathroom area. Further, products and equipment such as mobile shower commodes, scooters, wheelchairs, and stair and platform lifts are generally required to meet specific standards. Therapists therefore need to be aware of the range of standards that exist; their influence on design, construction products, and equipment; and the requirements of their local councils or national building codes with respect to their use for home modification work.

DEVELOPMENT OF STANDARDS

Nearly all countries have standards, which are developed by specific standards organizations consisting of expert committees set up and supported by government (Bridge & Kendig, 2005). These organizations seek to serve the interests of a range of industry sectors, as well as government, individuals in the community, employees, and society in general. They aim to ensure the various standards are useful, relevant, and authoritative in their country (BSI, 2017).

There are various benefits of having standards to guide practice. They can:

+ Provide protection for businesses and consumers to ensure that goods and services are safe and reliable and will do the intended job

+ Provide a yardstick for the measurement of public health, safety, and environmental policies

+ Provide a platform on which to build new and innovative ideas relating to the latest technologies and industry practices

+ Boost production and productivity to save businesses time and money and to foster new technologies

+ Enhance the competitive nature of businesses nationally and internationally

+ Provide linkages with international markets and enhance international competition through reducing technical barriers to international trade, increasing the size of potential markets and positioning firms to compete in the world economy through guiding the manufacturing of products to suit other countries

+ Complement laws and regulations and enhance consistency of these across the marketplace (SA, 2017a)

Various countries have bodies that develop standards, which include the following:

+ United States: ANSI

+ Australia: SA

+ Canada: Standards Council of Canada

+ Finland: Finnish Standards Association

+ France: Association Française de Normalization

+ Germany: Deutsches Institut fur Normung

+ Italy: Ente Nazionale Italiano di Unificazione

+ Japan: Japanese Industrial Standards Committee

+ Malaysia: Standards and Industrial Research of Malaysia

+ Netherlands: Nederlands Normalisatie-instituut

+ Norway: Norwegian Standards Association

+ Philippines: Bureau of Product Standards

+ United Kingdom: BSI

These organizations can be a useful resource for therapists. Further information on these organizations can be found in Appendix F.

Expert committees that operate on national, continental, or international levels develop standards in response to a defined market need (BSI, 2012; SA, 2017b). Some standards committees use a consortium model, where consultation involves steering groups, review panels, and standing committees to fast-track the development of standards, while others use a model of consensus whereby national committees form to develop documents (BSI, 2012). Most standards committees rely on expertise from a wide range of sources, including researchers, experts from design disciplines, code officials, and other interested parties, such as consumer groups. Standards are researched, developed, and revised by committees made up of people from the government, business and industry, the community, and academia (SA, 2017a). For example, committee members involved in the development of standards related to access and mobility within public buildings include representatives from the design and construction industry, the disability sector, and health professionals. To provide their professional perspective, occupational therapists sit on committees related to the design of buildings, products, and fixtures and fittings for people with disabilities. Standards are under continuous review, being updated regularly to take account of changing technology, industry practices, and community expectations (Bridge & Kendig, 2005). Amendments may be issued between editions (SA, 2009), and they may also be withdrawn from circulation as required (BSI, 2012).

There are specific processes associated with the development and ongoing revision of standards. Formal British, European, and international standards are developed according to strict rules to ensure they are transparent and fair. This involves a technical committee proceeding through the following stages:

+ Proposal for new work or revision of existing standard

+ Project acceptance

+ Preparation or drafting

+ Committee stage

+ Public consultation period

+ Comment resolution

+ Approval stage

+ Publication

+ Review (BSI, 2012)

Such stages are similar in other countries, such as the United States and Australia. The central body responsible for the identification of a single consistent set of voluntary standards in the United States is ANSI, a non-profit organization. ANSI accredits organizations that develop standards, publishes procedures for standards development, and approves standards according to its procedures (Steinfeld & Levine, 1998). ANSI specifically indicates that it has a positive role in enhancing the global competitiveness of U.S. business and quality of life by promoting and facilitating voluntary consensus standards and conformity assessment systems and safeguarding their integrity (ANSI, 2017).

In the United States, standards can develop in three ways: through an accredited committee, accredited organization, or community group (Steinfeld & Levine, 1998). Discussions at the committee level are documented, which assists in tracing the rationale and decision-making process in relation to items proposed for inclusion in the standards. The various organizations that develop standards have the main role of preparing these documents and reviewing them on a regular basis to keep up to date with industry requirements. It is estimated that there are more than 200 accredited ANSI bodies that develop consensus standards in different sectors, with more than 10,000 American National Standards (ANSI, 2017).

LANGUAGE OF STANDARDS

A list of terminology is usually provided in the introduction to a standard. This acts as a reference for various people using the documentation to guide design practice. A review of this list will ensure clear understanding of the industry wording and language and design requirements because there are differences between standards in various countries in terms of terminology and measurement conventions (imperial/metric; Steinfeld, Maisel, & Feathers, 2005). For example, the U.S. standard ICC/ANSI A117.1 (ANSI, 2009) describes a ramp as having "a running slope greater than 1:20 and not steeper than 1:12" (p. 22). In the comparative Australian standard AS 1428.1 (SA, 2009), a ramp is described as "an inclined surface on a continuous accessible path of travel between two landings with a gradient steeper than 1 in 20 but not steeper than 1:14" (p. 7).

In access standards, there are words used to describe various design features that might not be explained in the terminology guide. For example, it would be assumed that people reading the access standards would be familiar with standard building terms such as *riser* or *tread on stairs*. To ensure there

is clear understanding of the meaning of the terms used in the access standards, it is useful to refer to a glossary of building terms (ICC & ANSI, 2003).

Some words have a very specific meaning when used in the standards. For example, the U.S. standards use terms such as *shall* when referring to an essential or mandatory requirement. With respect to grab bars, for example, "grab bars shall be provided on the rear wall and on the side wall closest to the water closet" (ANSI, 2009). Other standards use additional terminology such as *should*, which refers to a desirable requirement, and *may*, which indicates an option to guide the reader. It is important for occupational therapists to check the definitions of the various terms used in the standards to ensure that they understand how they are being used to direct designers and others using these documents.

ACCESS STANDARDS FOR PUBLIC BUILDINGS

The creation and use of access standards grew out of the recognition that the design and construction of much of the built environment is inaccessible to a significant sector of the population and that people with disabilities are "entitled to have their special needs taken into consideration at all stages of economic and social planning" (United Nations, 1975). Access standards for public buildings or federally funded buildings, therefore, have been created to improve access for people with disabilities in the general community and to provide the greatest access for the greatest number of people.

In countries where access standards exist, such as the United States, public buildings such as libraries, hospitals, office spaces, meeting halls, schools, and retail areas are designed to provide external and internal wheelchair access. Design features include accessible paths of travel within and outside of a building, ramp designs, car parking, bathroom design, circulation space for access to and through doorways and within rooms, grab bar and handrail installation, electrical switch location, the location of blocking or reinforcement behind walls for supporting grab bars, and other features. These standards might also provide information on spatial requirements and reach ranges relating to the person in a wheelchair or ambulant people with mobility impairment who sit and stand during activities (Steinfeld et al., 2005; Steinfeld, Maisel, Feathers, & D'Souza, 2010, Steinfeld, Paquet, D'Souza, Joseph, & Maisel, 2010). In the United States, access standards have emerged that govern accessible design, such as ICC & ANSI A117.1 (ANSI, 2009).

ACCESS STANDARDS FOR RESIDENTIAL PREMISES

Until recently, developing and implementing access standards in most countries had little to do with residential building design and construction. The increasing proportion of older people and people with disabilities within populations across the world has heightened awareness of the need for housing construction that is adaptable, accessible, visitable, or universally designed. In general, however, the creation of design standards relating to adaptable, accessible, visitable, or universal design for newly constructed domestic premises to create inclusive housing and residential communities has not been well supported by local, state, and federal governments (Ward, Franz & Adkins, 2014). This is in part due to the perception that monitoring compliance by the construction industries with these standards would be problematic, and that the cost of building in specific housing features would be considered quite expensive (Ward et al., 2014). Additionally, the perspective that private homeowners have a right to choose how they wish to spend their own money and design their own homes has contributed to a lack of legislative action regarding the construction of accessible residential housing (Imrie, 2006a).

However, a few countries have developed standards or design guidelines for accessible and adaptable residential premises that people can refer to. These include the Fair Housing Accessibility Guidelines (United States), the Adaptable Housing Standard (Australia), and Lifetime Homes Standard (United Kingdom). The United States is one of the few countries to have a requirement for residential design in the Fair Housing Amendment Act (1988); however, this does not require full accessibility and is only mandatory in select building types. The ICC/ANSI A117.1 Standard on Accessible and Usable Buildings and Facilities is the consensus standard in the United States for defining the details of accessible construction and is referenced by most building codes in the country (Centre for Inclusive Design and Environmental Access [IDEA Centre], 2009–2013). In 2008, the ICC committee that develops the A117 Standard developed a new section with technical design criteria for visitability based on a document developed by disability rights advocates for the Inclusive Home Design Act (IDEA Centre, 2009–2013). This Act (H.R. 1408) has not yet been passed by the U.S. Congress (IDEA Centre, 2009–2013).

In England, the Greater London Authority developed the London Plan 2004, requiring that new homes (including houses and flats of varying sizes in both the public and private sectors) adopt the Lifetime Homes Standard (Lifetime Homes, 2017). Currently, all public-sector housing is being built to the Lifetime Homes Standard (Rooney, Hadjri, & Craig, 2013). The Interim London Housing Design Guide, developed on behalf of the mayor by the London Development Agency, has integrated the Lifetime Homes design criteria into its guidance on general needs housing (Lifetime Homes, 2017). In Wales and Northern Ireland, the Welsh Assembly and the Northern Ireland Housing Executive require the Lifetime Homes Standard in their funded developments (Lifetime Homes, 2017). The Lifetime Homes Standard is generally higher than that required by Part M of the Building Regulations, which deals with accessibility, although some elements of Part M are equal to the Lifetime Homes requirements or need relatively minor changes to comply (Lifetime Homes, 2017).

BENEFITS OF ACCESS STANDARDS

Access standards describe the performance criteria for access and mobility and establish design expectations for the building industry (Harrison, 2004). They contain agreed-upon solutions that have already been time-tested and proven (Breitenberg, 2009). Standards provide detailed diagrams and minimum performance criteria that can be used by designers and builders, thus saving money, time, and effort in design and construction and reducing costly errors and poor design and construction outcomes (Harrison, 2004; Imrie, 2006a). By providing clear and precise specifications, access standards reduce uncertainty in expectation about accessible design and make it easier and less costly for developers to create accessible environments (Harrison, 2004).

A product or design's conformance with accepted standards allows the manufacturer or designer to efficiently convey complex information on the product or design (Breitenberg, 1987). It also affords consumers with certainty about the product and its performance, quality, safety, and suitability.

Standards provide several benefits, namely:

+ A description of the minimum requirements for equipment, appliances, products, finishes, and designs
+ Criteria relating to the level of quality, safety, reliability, and functionality of equipment, appliances, products, finishes, and designs to ensure the health and safety of people using them

+ Detail on the technical aspects of equipment, appliances, products, finishes, and designs

+ A degree of legal certainty regarding quality for all parties, especially if they are referred to in legislation

Access standards are publicly available and are a practical tool to facilitate access and mobility in the built environment. Access standards, particularly those referred to in legislation, are regularly reviewed in response to research, the introduction of new equipment onto the market, and the change in design approaches over time.

Standards also stimulate the innovation of products, services, and systems, just as innovation stimulates standardization (Breitenberg, 2009). They foster innovation by establishing a baseline for design and performance that will satisfy user requirements. The performance criteria and minimum standards outlined allow suppliers or manufacturers some creativity and flexibility to vary features, function, or price, which means they can establish their own niche in the marketplace (Breitenberg, 2009). Standards are the baseline for improvements and can help elevate the expectation of users who then demand improvements to current practice (Breitenberg, 2009).

Limitations of Access Standards

The specifications in access standards from a range of countries have largely been based on limited research that, in some instances, dates back to the 1970s. For example, the anthropometric research on wheeled mobility users that underlies the technical requirements of the ICC and ANSI A117.1 (2003) Accessible and Usable Buildings and Facilities and the Americans With Disabilities Act Accessibility Guidelines were generated from research completed from 1974 to 1978 on a sample of 60 individuals who used wheelchairs (Steinfeld, Schroeder, & Bishop, 1979; Steinfeld et al., 2005; Steinfeld, Maisel, et al., 2010; Steinfeld, Paquet, et al., 2010).

Research informing many of the prescribed standards of physical dimension and performance has been criticized as being poorly designed and using small sample sizes that are not representative of the population of older people and people with disabilities in terms of age range, type of disability, stature, and other factors that impact on design (Harrison, 2004; Imrie & Hall, 2001; Imrie & Kumar, 1998; Steinfeld, Maisel, et al., 2010; Steinfeld, Paquet, et al., 2010). Various access standards around the world

have been developed on anthropometric data of populations of people where their bodies have been reduced to a universal type or standard, characterized by fixed body parts (Imrie & Hall, 2001).

The standards have been developed using a generalized view of the needs of the population of people with disabilities rather than a view that acknowledges the true diversity of the population (Imrie, 2006a; Imrie & Kumar, 1998). Concerns have also been raised about the profile of the people used as a basis to create the dimensions and performance criteria of the access standards. It has been argued that access standards have been based on the capabilities of young people who mobilize independently in standard manual or electric wheelchairs and thus do not reflect the requirements of children, many young people with multiple and severe impairments, or older people with comorbidities and secondary conditions (Czaja, 1984; Faletti, 1984; Sanford, 2001; Sanford, Echt, & Malassigné, 1999; Steinfeld, Schroeder, & Shea, 1993). In addition, standards do not consider the requirements of people who rely on caregiver assistance (Sanford, 2001; Sanford & Bosch, 2013).

Though some information in standards might have been considered accurate at a moment in time, there has been little attention to advances in wheeled mobility technology that influences the accuracy of the current standards (Steinfeld et al., 2005; Steinfeld, Maisel, et al., 2010; Steinfeld, Paquet, et al., 2010). New wheelchair technology for manual and electric wheelchairs is resulting in different performance characteristics and new environmental design requirements (Steinfeld, Lenker, & Paquet, 2002). Further, different styles of mobility devices are affecting the design requirements for environments (e.g., motorized scooters and floor-based and ceiling track hoists), which have not been included in the design of the access standards.

Research methods also have not been clearly documented, leading to questions about the reliability and validity of studies (Steinfeld et al., 2005; Steinfeld, Maisel, et al., 2010; Steinfeld, Paquet, et al., 2010). Furthermore, studies across various countries have not always used the same terms, definitions, standards, or variables in the respective countries (Steinfeld et al., 2005; Steinfeld, Maisel, et al., 2010; Steinfeld, Paquet, et al., 2010). This limits the likelihood of combining findings from around the world into a single database for generalization (Steinfeld et al., 2002). An international approach to access design would be advantageous in assisting people as they travel and interact in different communities around the world (Steinfeld et al., 2005; Steinfeld, Maisel, et al., 2010; Steinfeld, Paquet, et al., 2010). This would require the development of an international consensus on standards and research methods and the use of terminology, definitions, and measurements to prevent divergent approaches during the review of standards, as well as consideration of differences in body size, wheeled mobility technology, and cultural differences in economic development and expectations for independence in populations between various countries (Rapoport & Watson, 1972; Steinfeld et al., 2005; Steinfeld, Maisel, et al., 2010; Steinfeld, Paquet, et al., 2010). There also needs to be improvement and thorough documentation of research methods to ensure transparency of the quality of the methods used to gather data (Steinfeld, Maisel, et al., 2010; Steinfeld, Paquet, et al., 2010). This will then ensure that the standards from the Western world are not automatically applied to societies without determining whether they are appropriate for use (Steinfeld, Maisel, et al., 2010; Steinfeld, Paquet, et al., 2010).

Finally, access standards can constrain design (Imrie, 2006b). Minimum access standards tend to be about "building down to something" rather than maximum standards, which are about "building to the highest quality" (Imrie & Kumar, 1998). Imrie and Hall (2001) indicate that design professionals rarely exceed the legislative minimum in providing access and regard the provision of access as a significant cost. Adherence to access standards can, therefore, result in a design solution that is only minimally acceptable but viewed, incorrectly, as best practice and perhaps the only solution possible (Imrie, 2006a). Access standards that are conservative in their design tend to be rigid and incomplete (Steinfeld et al., 2002). Designers tend to over-rely on these documents to define access requirements rather than creatively designing to optimize access and utility, and incorporate flexibility and options within designs.

ACCESS STANDARDS AND HOME MODIFICATION PRACTICE

Though the design information contained in access standards can be useful to the design of home modifications, there are several issues related to the use of such standards in a residential setting. There is continued debate in the literature over the use of access standards as the basis of home modification design (Danford & Steinfeld, 1999; Pynoos & Regnier, 1997; Pynoos, Sanford, & Rosenfelt, 2002; Steinfeld et al., 1993; Tanner, Tilse, & de Jonge, 2008).

The debate centers on the relevance of standards developed for public access and intended to provide the greatest access for a range of people (i.e., a faceless population) to the unique and individual home environment. Accessibility standards are typically designed to determine minimal legal guidelines and have very little to do with the needs, aspirations, desires, and uniqueness of an individual (Danford & Steinfeld, 1999). A danger in approaching home modifications from a public access agenda is that the meaning of home as a private, personalized space can be undermined, and the individual's needs can become compromised. Using access standards in residential settings has also resulted in a physical or technical approach to building design (Imrie, 2006a). Within access standards, there is little emphasis on or information about domestic design and, where it does exist, there is little consideration about using flexible features, such as demountable walls, smart technologies, and design of multifunctional rooms with integrated elements, such as bathing or sleeping areas (Imrie, 2006b).

Because the building sector operates in an environment governed by regulations, codes, and standards, contractors are required to comply with a range of national, state, or local codes and standards in many aspects of their work. When any remodeling work is being undertaken, additional maintenance or repair work may be required to address noncompliance, such as old electrical wiring and replumbing old pipe work. This additional work can add substantially to the cost (Jones, de Jonge, & Phillips, 2008; Steinfeld, Levine, & Shea, 1998). In addition, building contractors often mistakenly apply public access standards to the remodeling of domestic premises, which can impact the nature and overall cost of a solution (Steinfeld et al., 1998) and the considerable expense of reverting the work when the house is sold (Balandin & Chapman, 2001). Further, inappropriate adherence to the standards, which were not created with the older person in mind, can result in inadequate solutions (Klein, Rosage, & Shaw, 1999).

The rigid and variable interpretation of standards can also result in a lack of both creativity and flexibility when negotiating a design solution that meets the needs of both the code and the householder (Pynoos, Liebig, Alley, & Nishita, 2004). When access standards are used in residential settings, features are inflexible and noticeable, and their appearance can be clinical, oversized, and inelegant (Lund & Nygard, 2004). Dimensional standards are said to be based on dated lifestyle assumptions and not on a sophisticated understanding of interactions between people and their home environments (Imrie, 2006b).

How Therapists Can Use Access Standards

In most countries, it is not a mandatory requirement for existing domestic premises to incorporate public access provisions for people with disabilities into domestic designs or modifications. However, in countries such as the United States and Australia, some local building regulations can require compliance to aspects of the access standard in the construction of new dwellings or major modification work on an existing dwelling.

In occupational therapy practice, the application of access standards to home modifications is best understood in terms of where in the home modification process the standards are referred. If not required by local building regulations, access standards should not be the starting point of the home modification process, nor should they drive the design of the modification. However, they can be a useful reference when exploring physical changes to the environment and striving for accessibility. Specifications detailed in public access standards, such as circulation spaces, door clearances, changes in level between floor surfaces, width of corridors and paths, vertical height clearance of features, and other criteria, could be of use when developing options for individuals with characteristics like those in the population on whom the standards have been based. For example, the specifications in the standards for a roll-in shower can assist in designing a bathroom for a young adult who mobilizes independently in a wheelchair. The standards are also a useful guide for ensuring the safety and long-term viability of home modifications. For example, if a person has a degenerative health condition and is likely to become a wheelchair user in the future, the standards can assist in anticipating the minimum design requirements when redesigning areas of the home.

Occupational therapists might use public access standards to do the following:

+ Audit the built environment to identify features that are inaccessible

+ Identify key landmarks for measuring and drawing the environment

+ Assess the suitability of the access specifications, including the performance criteria for individuals using simulated spaces, layout, and measurements to provide information to clients on accessible features and their specifications

+ Act as a reference to inform the redesign of structures, spaces, fixtures, and fittings to stimulate ideas and develop alternative solutions

+ Alert designers and contractors to the specific design and construction criteria required for design and modification work

+ Guide the development of specifications, drawings, and wording for home modification reports

The access standards provide detail on specific design features for accessibility, such as circulation spaces, door widths or clearances, and heights of fittings and fixtures. The measurements in the standards can be used to identify changes required in the environment to accommodate a wheelchair user. The drawings in the standards illustrate the built environment landmarks that identify the points between which the measurement should be taken. For example, door clearance is measured between the door stop (the door stop is the part the door hits against when it closes) and the face of the door on the hinge side. Therapists then compare these measures against the dimensions of the person and his or her equipment and his or her ability to maneuver in a simulated environment. For example, as detailed in Chapter 8, recommended circulation spaces can be marked out on the floor using masking tape to test the client's ability to maneuver in the proposed area. Therapists refer to the specifications and drawings in the standard to explain to clients the characteristics of the proposed changes (e.g., ramp slope and hand rail design). Alternative options, such as bathroom layouts, detailed in the standards can be used to guide discussions and decision making about the best option, given the proposed use of the area and the existing space and structures in the built environment.

Therapists can direct contractors and designers to the specific design, construction, and installation criteria related to their recommendations. It is important that therapists ensure designers and contractors are aware of the defined scope and parameters of the access standards; that is, that these have been developed to address the access and mobility requirements of adult wheelchair users in public buildings and are generally minimum measurements that can be exceeded to meet the needs of the person, his or her equipment, and his or her carer.

Therapists should also confirm that designers and contractors understand that occupational therapy recommendations are based on a thorough assessment of the individual and the activities he or she undertakes within his or her particular home environment. Therapists can draw on the wording and diagrams used in the standards to document their recommendations. The use of industry language in the standards assists in the description of performance criteria in the occupational therapy report, minimizes misunderstandings, and ensures that the desired outcome is achieved.

The relevance of the specifications in the access standards to each situation depends greatly on the following:

+ Whether the person and his or her equipment fits the profile on which the standards have been based

+ The activities to be undertaken in the area

+ Characteristics of the existing built environment and the household

Before therapists consider using aspects of the access standards in developing home modification recommendations, it is important to determine whether the client fits the profile on which the standards are based, including his or her age, body dimensions, the nature of the disability, level of independence and mobility, and equipment type and size. The standards do not necessarily address the design requirements of older people, people outside the average range for weight and height, people with severe and multiple disabilities, or people who require caregiver assistance. In addition, equipment such as mobile shower commodes, common to many people requiring home modifications, is not a consideration in access standards because such devices normally would not be used in a public toilet. Homes may also accommodate floor-based or ceiling track hoists to enable people to move within or between rooms, whereas hoists are unlikely to be used in public facilities.

The standards provide detailed specifications for areas where functional tasks such as toileting are performed, but they provide limited guidance on the overall layout of the internal and external areas of the home or other domestic areas, such as the kitchen, bedroom, laundry, and car park, where many home-based activities are undertaken. Further, specific areas have been designed with only limited activities in mind. For example, in public buildings, the vanity has been designed for independent hand washing; however, in the home environment, people use the vanity for a range of activities, including shaving or brushing teeth.

Being primarily for new public buildings, the standards are not designed to apply to the design or modification of residential environments. Existing domestic premises have physical constraints; that is, they do not have the footprint or floor area to accommodate the public access standards design and layout requirements. For example, many bathrooms in existing older dwellings will have insufficient space to incorporate a fully accessible bathroom. Further, a range of people use areas of the home in a variety of ways, which is not a consideration of public access standards.

When tailoring modifications to the specific requirements of individuals, the activities they perform, and their home environment, therapists first determine the functional requirements of the individuals and then ensure that the designs and products recommended are safe and reliable. Occupational therapists use their expertise to tailor interventions to suit the individual (i.e., body dimensions, abilities, limitations, goals, preferences, and equipment used) to enable the person to undertake the task safely and independently, using his or her preferred method given the opportunities offered by the environment. Consequently, therapists might determine that the specifications in the standards do not adequately address the design requirement of the individual. For example, when recommending a grab bar to assist an older person in getting on and off a low toilet, the therapist would determine the best height, configuration, and location of grab bars for this situation. The relevance of public access standards to this modification is extremely limited because the height and position of grab bars in public toilet facilities is designed primarily to assist wheelchair users to transfer on and off a higher accessible toilet. These grab bars may not suit older people with different movement patterns (Dekker, Buznik, Molenbroek, & de Bruin, 2007; Kennedy et al, 2015; Sanford, 2002; Sanford, Arch, & Megrew, 1995). Another example of the limited relevance of the public access standards is in recommending a ramp for someone using a powered wheelchair. The length and turning space requirements of the equipment might necessitate a greater landing dimension compared with the recommendations in the standards.

Once the functional elements have been determined, therapists then consider the safety and reliability of interventions. The standards contain specifications related to the safety and reliability of several design features that are based on technical expertise and population anthropometric studies. These can assist therapists in selecting safe and reliable products and designs and ensuring that these can be installed appropriately. For example, several specifications contained in the access standards relate to the safety characteristics of grab bars, such as the amount of vertical and horizontal force a grab bar, fastener mounting device, or supporting structure should support and the horizontal space between the wall and grab bar to allow for safe hand placement and movement. Therapists should comply with these specifications unless the client's requirements are outside of the scope of the standards. For example, people who have bariatric requirements will require grab bars that are installed to withstand greater forces. Therapists do not have the technical expertise to determine the vertical and horizontal force requirements in this situation and should seek appropriate advice. Further, therapists are advised to comply with the stipulated ramp gradient in the standards unless they can produce supporting evidence to justify a steeper ramp installation. This may be achieved through providing research evidence to support the recommendation for the person, producing specification details on gradient capabilities of the powered mobility device, or testing the client's ability to mobilize on a steeper gradient under various conditions. Technical advice or evidence should be documented in the client's report to support recommendations that vary from technical specifications in the standards, where legislative compliance is not required.

Conclusion

This chapter has introduced the concept of standards and provided an overview of how these documents are developed by expert committees in various countries and supported by governments. A review of access standards and their development and applicability to the home modification process has also been discussed. Access standards for public buildings can be a useful resource for occupational therapists when determining the design of a home modification in certain instances, particularly if the individual home dweller is of similar profile to the population on which the standards were originally based. Caution needs to be taken in the indiscriminate use of access standards to inform home modification design, particularly if there is no local legislative requirement to use these documents. Therapists need to ensure that the starting point of all home modification interventions is a good understanding of the needs, desires, and goals of the individual home dweller and that, in most instances, it is this, and not the access standards, that drives the home modification design process. While there are benefits associated with the use of standards as a reference or guide, therapists need to be mindful of their limitations. This will ensure that occupational therapy practice in this field is not constrained by a poor understanding of the intent and application of standards to home modification scenarios, which can result in poor designs and poor outcomes for people with specific needs.

References

American National Standards Institute. (2009). *ICC/ANSI A117.1-2009: Accessible and usable buildings and facilities.* New York, NY: Author.

American National Standards Institute. (2017). Overview of the US standardization system. Retrieved from https://www.ansi.org/about_ansi/introduction/introduction

Balandin, S., & Chapman, R. (2001). Aging with a developmental disability at home: An Australian perspective. In W. F. E. Preiser & E. Ostroff (Eds.), *Universal design handbook* (pp. 38.1-38.15). New York, NY: McGraw Hill Handbooks.

Breitenberg, M. A. (1987). The ABC's of standards-related activities in the United States. Retrieved from https://ia800407.us.archive.org/2/items/abcsofstandardsr8735brei/abcsofstandardsr8735brei.pdf

Breitenberg, M. A. (2009). *The ABCs of standards activities.* Gaithersburg, MD: National Institute of Standards and Technology. Retrieved from https://www.nist.gov/sites/default/files/nistir_7614.pdf

Bridge, K., & Kendig, H. (2005). Housing and older people: Environments, professionals and positive ageing. In V. Minichiello & I. Coulson (Eds.), *Contemporary issues in gerontology: Promoting positive aging* (pp. 144-166). New York, NY: Allen & Unwin.

British Standards Institution. (2012). Pocket guide to standards development. Retrieved from https://www.bsigroup.com/Documents/about-bsi/NSB/BSI-pocket-guide-to-standards-development-UK-EN.pdf

British Standards Institution. (2017). Standards. Retrieved from https://www.bsigroup.com/en-GB/standards/

Centre for Inclusive Design and Environmental Access. (2009–2013). Visitability: An inclusive design approach for housing. Retrieved from http://udeworld.com/visbooklet/visitibility-booklet.pdf

Czaja, S. (1984). Hand anthropometrics. Technical paper prepared for the U.S. Architectural and Transportation Barriers Compliance Board, Washington, DC.

Danford, G. S., & Steinfeld, E. (1999). Measuring the influences of physical environments on the behaviors of people with impairments. In E. Steinfeld & G. S. Danford (Eds.), *Enabling environments: Measuring the impact of environment on disability and rehabilitation* (pp. 111-137). New York, NY: Plenum Publishers.

Dekker, D., Buzink, S. N., Molenbroek, J. F., & de Bruin, R. (2007). Hand supports to assist toilet use among the elderly. *Applied Ergonomics, 38*, 109-118.

Fair Housing Amendment Act of 1988, 42 U.S.C. §§ 3601 et seq. (1988).

Faletti, M. V. (1984). Human factors research and functional environments for the aged. In I. Altman, M. P. Lawton, & J. F. Wohlwill (Eds.), *Elderly people and the environment* (pp. 191-237). New York, NY: Plenum Press.

Harrison, M. (2004). Defining quality and environment: Disability standards and social factors. *Housing Studies, 19*(5), 691-708.

Imrie, R. (2006a). *Accessible housing: Quality, disability and design.* London, UK: Routledge Taylor and Francis Group.

Imrie, R. (2006b). Independent lives and the relevance of Lifetime Homes. *Disability and Society, 21*(4), 359-374.

Imrie, R., & Hall, P. (2001). *Inclusive design: Designing and developing accessible environments.* London, UK: Spon Press.

Imrie, R., & Kumar, M. (1998). Focusing on disability and access in the built environment. *Disability and Society, 13*(3), 357-374.

International Code Council & American National Standards Institute. (2003). *ICC/ANSI A117.1-2003. American National Standard—Accessible and usable buildings and facilities*. New York, NY: Author.

Jones, A., de Jonge, D., & Phillips, R. (2008). *The impact of home maintenance and modification services on health, community care and housing outcomes in later life*. Melbourne, Australia: Australian Housing and Urban Research Institute.

Kennedy, M.J., Arcelus, A., Guitard, P., Goubran, R.A., Eng, P., & Sveistrup, H. (2015) Toilet grab-bar preference and center of pressure deviation during toilet transfers in healthy seniors, seniors with hip replacements, and seniors having suffered a stroke. *Assistive Technology, 27*(2), 78-87, doi: 10.1080/10400435.2014.976799

Klein, S.K., Rosage, L., & Shaw, G. (1999). The role of occupational therapists in home modification programs at an area agency on aging. In E. D. Taira & J. L. Carlson (Eds.), *Aging in place: Designing, adapting, and enhancing the home environment* (pp. 19-38). Binghampton, NY: The Haworth Press.

Lawlor, D., & Thomas, M. A. (2008). *Residential design for aging in place*. Hoboken, NJ: John Wiley & Sons.

Lifetime Homes. (2017). For professionals: Policy and regulation. Retrieved from http://www.lifetimehomes.org.uk/pages/policy-and-regulation.html

Lund, M. L., & Nygard, L. (2004). Occupational life in the home environment: The experiences of people with disabilities. *Canadian Journal of Occupational Therapy, 71*(41), 243-251.

Pynoos, J., Liebig, P., Alley, D., & Nishita, C. M. (2004). Homes of choice: Towards more effective linkages between housing and services. *Journal of Housing for the Elderly, 18*(3/4), 5-49.

Pynoos, J., & Regnier, V. (1997). Design directives in home adaptation. In S. Lanspery & J. Hyde (Eds.), *Staying put: Adapting the places instead of the people* (pp. 41-54). Amityville, NY: Baywood Publishing Company Inc.

Pynoos, J., Sanford, J. A., & Rosenfelt, T. (2002). A team approach to home modifications. *OT Practice, 8*, 15-19.

Rapoport, A., & Watson, N. (1972). Cultural variability in physical standards. In R. Gutman (Ed.), *People and buildings* (pp. 33-53). New York, NY: Basic Books.

Rooney, C., Hadjri, K., & Craig, C. (2013). Assessing Lifetime Homes Standards and Part M building regulations for housing design in the UK. *The Design Journal, 16*(1), 29-50.

Sanford, J. A. (2001). Best practices in the design of toileting and bathing facilities for assisted transfers. Final report US Access Board. Retrieved from http://www.access-board.gov/research/Toilet-Bath/report.htm

Sanford, J. A. (2002). Time to get rid of those old gray grab bars and get yourself a shiny new pair. *Alzheimer's Care Quarterly, 3*(1), 26-31.

Sanford, J. A., Arch, M., & Megrew, M. B. (1995). An evaluation of grab bars to meet the needs of elderly people. *Assistive Technology, 7*, 36-47.

Sanford, J. A., & Bosch, S. J. (2013), An investigation of non-compliant toilet room designs for assisted toileting. *Health Environments Research and Design, 6*(2), 43-57.

Sanford, J. A., Echt, K., & Malassigné, P. (1999). An E for ADAAG: The case for accessibility guidelines for the elderly based on three studies of toilet transfer. *Journal of Physical and Occupational Therapy in Geriatrics, 16*(3,4), 39-58.

Standards Australia. (2009). *Design for access and mobility. Part 1: General requirement for access—New building work (AS 1428.1)*. Sydney, Australia: Author.

Standards Australia. (2017a). Benefits of standards. Retrieved from http://www.standards.org.au/StandardsDevelopment/What_is_a_Standard/Pages/Benefits-of-Standards.aspx

Standards Australia. (2017b). Red tape: Standards and the regulatory reform agenda. Retrieved from https://www.standards.org.au/StandardAU/Media/SA-Archive/OurOrganisation/Documents/SA-Red-Tape-Regulatory-Reform-Agenda.pdf

Steinfeld, E., Lenker, J., & Paquet, V. (2002). The anthropometrics of disability. Report prepared for the U.S. Access Board. Retrieved from http://www.ap.buffalo.edu/idea/Anthro/The%20Anthropometrics%20of%20Disability.html

Steinfeld, E., & Levine, D. (1998). *Technical report: CABO/ANSI A117.1 Standard*. Buffalo, NY: IDEA, University of Buffalo. Retrieved from http://www.ap.buffalo.edu/idea/Publications/technical%20reports.htm#CABO

Steinfeld, E., Levine, D., & Shea, S. (1998). Home modifications and the Fair Housing Law. *Technology and Disability, 8*, 15-35.

Steinfeld, E., Maisel, J., & Feathers, D. (2005). *Standards and anthropometry for wheeled mobility*. Buffalo, NY: Centre for Inclusive Design and Environmental Access, School of Architecture and Planning, University of Buffalo. Retrieved from http://idea.ap.buffalo.edu/Anthro/FinalAccessReport.pdf

Steinfeld, E., Maisel, J., Feathers, D., & D'Souza. (2010). Anthropometry and standards for wheeled mobility: An international comparison. *Assistive Technology, 22*, 51-67.

Steinfeld, E., Paquet, V., D'Souza, C., Joseph, C., & Maisel, J. (2010). Final report: Anthropometry of wheeled mobility project. Retrieved from http://www.udeworld.com/documents/anthropometry/pdfs/AnthropometryofWheeledMobilityProject_FinalReport.pdf

Steinfeld, E., Schroeder, S., & Bishop, M. (1979). *Accessible buildings for people with walking and reaching limitations*. Washington D.C.: US Department of Housing and Urban Development.

Steinfeld, E., Schroeder, & Shea, S. (1993). Enabling home environments: Identifying barriers to independence. *Technology and Disability, 2*(4), 69-79.

Tanner, B., Tilse, C., & de Jonge, D. (2008). Restoring and sustaining home: The impact of home modifications on the meaning of home for older people. *Journal of Housing for the Elderly, 22*(3), 195-215.

United Nations. (1975). Declaration on the rights of disabled persons. Retrieved from http://www1.umn.edu/humanrts/instree/t3drdp.htm

Ward, M., Franz, J., & Adkins, B. (2014). Livable housing design: The voluntary provision of inclusive housing in Australia. *Journal of Social Inclusion, 5*(1), 43-60.

Ethical, Legal, and Reporting Variables
Pathways to Best Practice

12

Elizabeth Ainsworth, MOccThy, Grad Cert Health Sci and
Barbara Kornblau, JD, OTR/L, FAOTA, FNAP, DASPE, CDMS, CCM, CPE

This chapter provides an overview of the potential ethical and legal issues that can arise in home modification practice, which occupational therapists should carefully consider when carrying out home visits and providing home modification recommendations to clients and services. Practitioners require an understanding of legal, ethical, and reporting issues to ensure effective working relationships with recipients of their services and to achieve best practice. This includes knowledge of frameworks and tools to analyze ethical issues and to evaluate decision making, and an awareness of their subsequent obligations and responsibilities as competent service providers (Doherty, 2014).

The chapter discusses the potential liability issues of occupational therapists who provide home modification services. It reviews basic principles and provides details on actions that clinicians can take to prevent litigation to lead them down the pathway to best practice. Further, there is advice on best practice with respect to good documentation, particularly in instances where the client, family member, guardian and/or conservator, or funding body might not accept the home modification recommendations.

Also examined in this chapter is the role of the occupational therapist as an expert witness in court, where judges make decisions about damage awards to clients for future home modification and care services. The chapter provides information on how the occupational therapy report becomes evidence and a source of information for the court on the person's future needs and contributes to the decision-making process the court uses to make its final judgement on the case.

CHAPTER OBJECTIVES

By the end of this chapter, the reader will be able to:

✦ Recognize and discuss some of the basic ethical and legal concepts, issues, and approaches relevant to home modification practice

✦ Identify sources of information relating to ethics and legal issues to guide professional practice

✦ Describe and apply a basic problem-solving framework for ethical issues in occupational therapy home modification practice

✦ Acknowledge the importance of good report writing by incorporating specific techniques to ensure protection from litigation, to aid court decisions, and to facilitate excellent clinical competence

✦ Explain the role of the occupational therapist as an expert witness and the process in preparing and presenting in court

Ainsworth, E., & de Jonge, D. *An Occupational Therapist's Guide to Home Modification Practice, Second Edition (pp. 259-282).*
© 2019 SLACK Incorporated.

ETHICAL AND LEGAL OBLIGATIONS

Contemporary professional life presents challenges that require occupational therapists to consider their actions and decisions in terms of their ethical and legal obligations (Cheyney Brandt & Yarett Slater, 2011). Occupational therapy assistants must also consider ethical and legal obligations in practice. However, because assistants carry out their work under the supervision of occupational therapists, and because the practice of home modifications is an advanced area, this chapter addresses the responsibilities of occupational therapists.

Occupational therapists must work within the context of ethics and law—two related fields but differing in terms of goals and sanctions (Doherty, 2014). Therefore, they must understand basic legal principles that constrict or empower them and ethical reasoning and decision making that affect competent practice (Dimond, 2010; Doherty, 2014). Ethical and legal obligations are rules of conduct grounded in moral theory. Ignorance of these rules neither abrogates therapists of these responsibilities, nor excuses them for non-compliance (Scott, 1997, 2009).

Ethical Issues

Ethical rules govern the conduct of professionals. They delineate the proprietary of official conduct, especially in relation to business dealings with people (Scott, 1997, 2009). Those areas of conduct regulated by codes of ethics include the nature of the professional-person relationship and the scope of business relationships.

Occupational therapists, as a group, have professional organizations such as the American Occupational Therapy Association (AOTA) that guide and maintain the ethics and values of the profession through standard setting and resources that explain the standards (Van Denend & Finlayson, 2007). The AOTA Ethics Commission reviews the Occupational Therapy Code of Ethics (AOTA, 2015a) that set the ethical standards of the profession (Doherty, 2014). The Code is a public statement tailored to address ethical concerns of the profession and the standards members of the public can expect from members of the occupational therapy profession (AOTA, 2015a). It serves as a guide for practitioners to determine appropriate moral and professional conduct toward clients and others that abides by laws and regulations. It also acts as a contract with the society that occupational therapists serve (Mosey, 1981). To ensure compliance with this ethical standard, AOTA established Enforcement Procedures for the Occupational Therapy Code of Ethics and Ethics Standards (2014), with oversight and enforcement provided by AOTA's Ethics Commission.

A professional code of ethics sets out the rules or principles intended to express the values of the profession (Kornblau & Burkhardt, 2012; Kornblau & Starling, 2000). The professional code of ethics provides the minimum standard for the occupational therapy profession (Kornblau & Burkhardt, 2012; Kornblau & Starling, 2000). A person's membership in a professional association means the occupational therapist accepts the responsibility to abide by the association's code of ethics (Kornblau & Burkhardt, 2012; Kornblau & Starling, 2000). Licensing or registration boards may embrace, adopt, or incorporate the code of ethics into their licensure or registration rules or regulations, requiring occupational therapists who are not members of the association to abide by the code of ethics pursuant to those rules or regulations (Kornblau & Burkhardt, 2012; Kornblau & Starling, 2000).

Like other codes of ethics for the profession around the world, the AOTA Code of Ethics is a public statement of principles used to promote high standards of professional conduct. Occupational therapists are required to promote inclusion, diversity, independence, and safety for all people at all stages of their lives, health, and illness, and to empower those who benefit from occupational therapy services (AOTA, 2015a).

The AOTA Code is an aspirational guide to professional conduct when ethical issues emerge in day-to-day practice with recipients of services as well as with other members of society (AOTA, 2015a). The code is based on ethical reasoning surrounding practice and professional issues and empathic reflection regarding practice situations (AOTA, 2015a).

Its purposes are to provide aspirational core values to guide members who are occupational therapy personnel such as students in occupational therapy programs, clinicians, educators, entrepreneurs, business owners, people elected or appointed, or other professional volunteer service, toward ethical courses of action in professional and volunteer roles (AOTA, 2015a). It also delineates principles and standards of conduct that apply to members of the association (AOTA, 2015a).

The AOTA Code:

✦ Helps guide and define ethical decision making

✦ Is a commitment to benefit others through good behaviors and "noble acts of courage"

✦ Explains to members that ethical practice goes beyond rote compliance with the ethical principles outlined

✦ Assists members in recognizing the complexities of ethical decision making and the specific steps involved in the process of resolving ethical dilemmas.

✦ Orients all occupational therapy personnel, including students of the Principles and Standards of Conduct in the Code, which they must follow

✦ Educates the public and members about the personnel roles played by members of the occupational therapy profession (AOTA, 2015a)

The various principles and standards of conducted described in the AOTA Code of Ethics (2015) that are enforceable for professional behavior include beneficence, nonmaleficence, autonomy, confidentiality, social justice, procedural justice, veracity, and fidelity.

Ethical Principles and Approaches

Various ethical approaches and theories support clinical decision making and aid in solving ethical dilemmas, such as adopting a principle-based approach (Shannon, 1993). The principle-based approach relates to the following fundamental ethical principles:

✦ Autonomy

✦ Nonmaleficence

✦ Beneficence

✦ Justice (Beauchamp & Childress, 2013)

Autonomy

Autonomy means different things in different contexts in relationship to privacy, individual choice, freedom of will, decisions about one's own behavior, and being one's own person (Beauchamp & Childress, 2013; Shannon, 1993). Autonomy refers to one's moral right to make choices and decisions about one's own life plan and course of action (Jonsen, Siegler, & Winslade, 2010; Kornblau & Burkhardt, 2012; Shannon, 1993). It involves freedom from controlling interference of others and limitations, such as inadequate cognitive functioning, which limits personal choice.

To exercise one's autonomy, an individual must have the ability to analyze alternatives, make responsible choices, and undertake intentional actions (Beauchamp & Childress, 2013). In contrast, others can limit the autonomy of people incapable of deliberating or acting because of their desires and plans (Beauchamp & Childress, 2013). In home modification practice, occupational therapists should provide clients with a choice to participate in the assessment process to respect their autonomy and should give clients choices of interventions where feasible. Therapists might have to constrain a person's freely chosen actions when that person's preferences and actions infringe on the rights and welfare of others (Jonsen et al., 2010).

Nonmaleficence

The principle of nonmaleficence asserts the obligation not to inflict harm on others (Beauchamp & Childress, 2013; Shannon, 1993). In medical ethics, it is associated with the Hippocratic Oath, which states, "I will use treatment to help the sick according to my ability and judgment but will never use it to injure or wrong them" (Beauchamp & Childress, 2013, p. 113). This means occupational therapists may not intentionally cause harm to individuals they serve (AOTA, 2015a; Bailey & Schwartzberg, 2003; Cheyney Brandt & Yarett Slater, 2011; Costa, 2007; Doherty, 2014). This includes ensuring they do not cause injuries extending beyond physical or psychological harm, such as harm to one's property, liberty, or reputation (Kornblau & Burkhardt, 2012). For example, to prevent falls during the home visit, the principle of nonmaleficence requires that therapists lock wheelchair wheels before clients attempt to transfer.

Beneficence

Some philosophers combine nonmaleficence with beneficence into a single principle (Beauchamp & Childress, 2013). Beneficence assures that a professional will treat individuals autonomously and refrain from harming them, but also will contribute to their welfare (Beauchamp & Childress, 2013; Jonsen et al., 2010; Shannon, 1993). It relates not only to refraining from doing harm but to taking positive steps to ensure the well-being of others (Beauchamp & Childress, 2013; Shannon, 1993). This ensures that people receive quality occupational therapy services in accordance with best practice (AOTA, 2015a; Bailey & Schwartzberg, 2003; Cheyney Brandt & Yarett Slater, 2011; Costa, 2007; Doherty, 2014). For example, an occupational therapist who does a home visit must evaluate the potential benefits of any proposed intervention in relation to its risks, make recommendations to the client, and solicit the client's preferences about whether to proceed with the intervention (Jonsen et al., 2010). Beneficence would also require therapists to recommend interventions, such as a home modification or assistive devices, should they see a client with a disability experience difficulty moving into sitting and rising from the toilet.

Justice

Justice relates to fairness, entitlement, and what one deserves (Doherty, 2014). It is viewed as fair, equitable, and appropriate treatment considering what is due or owed to the individual (Beauchamp & Childress, 2013; Shannon, 1993). Injustice relates to wrongful acts or omissions that deny individuals the benefits to which they have a right and/or distribute burdens unfairly (Beauchamp & Childress, 2013).

Ethicists identify various forms of justice:

- ✦ Distributive justice relates to fair, equitable, and appropriate distribution of benefits of society determined by justified norms that structure terms of social cooperation (e.g., a societal benefit can be the provision of health care).

- ✦ Criminal justice relates to the just infliction of punishment.

- ✦ Rectificatory justice relates to just compensation for transactional problems, such as malpractice (Beauchamp & Childress, 2013; Doherty, 2014).

During tough economic times involving budget constraints and debates over the appropriate allocation of funds to programs for older people and people with disabilities, distributive justice can be a significant issue in home modification practice.

Occupational therapy professional societies universally embrace the principles contained in the AOTA Code. For example, the World Federation of Occupational Therapists' (WFOT) Code of Ethics (2016), which sets standards for general categories of appropriate professional conduct, states that occupational therapists should exhibit personal attributes, such as personal integrity, reliability, open-mindedness, and loyalty, in all aspects of their professional role. On appropriate conduct, the WFOT Code of Ethics states that occupational therapists shall work responsibly with individuals and show respect and regard for their individual situations. It also stipulates that therapists not discriminate against individuals and that they take into consideration a person's values, preferences, and abilities when providing services. This includes ensuring the confidentiality of information. According to the code, therapists can provide information to others only with that person's consent. The WFOT Code of Ethics also states that occupational therapists participate in lifelong learning and seek knowledge based on best available evidence. Further, it prescribes that when therapists participate in research activities, they respect the ethical implications of this work. The code advocates that therapists aim to improve, develop, and promote the profession in an ethical manner (WFOT, 2016).

Codes of ethics rarely provide professionals with an absolute guide to behavior or decision making in any given circumstance. However, according to Kornblau and Burkhardt (2012), they do provide a starting point to seek guidance on professional practice and decisions. The occupational therapy profession itself imposes three major responsibilities with respect to ethics. Occupational therapists must:

1. Keep faith with the tenets and principles of the discipline by ensuring services continue to embrace client-centered, occupation-based practice

2. Preserve the integrity of the professional community through clearly established guidance on the competencies and professional development required for practitioners

3. Ensure the integrity of individual practitioners by encouraging ethical contemplation, reflection, and clinical reasoning based on perception, understanding, accountability, and sensitivity (Cheyney Brandt & Yarett Slater, 2011; Doherty, 2014)

Problem-Solving Frameworks for Ethical Issues

An ethical problem occurs when one believes a situation might question cherished moral values and duties and might involve difficult choices to determine a course of action (Doherty, 2014). An ethical dilemma occurs when the occupational therapist's response or actions can cause negative consequences or nullify the benefits of good consequences (Kornblau & Burkhardt, 2012). A true dilemma occurs when therapists face a strong persuasive argument both for and against a course of action, posing a moral conflict (Doherty, 2014; Kornblau & Burkhardt, 2012).

Ethical dilemmas can be viewed from personal, organizational, and societal perspectives, all of which should be given consideration (Kornblau & Burkhardt, 2012). A personal dilemma might relate to concern for the good of the individual. For example, a therapist might experience conflict when the client declines his or her recommendations. An organizational dilemma might relate to issues affecting institutions, such as businesses, professional associations, health care services or agencies, or the family. For example, the home modification service might experience conflict when deciding whether to provide limited services to many clients or a more comprehensive service to a limited number of clients. Societal dilemmas consider the well-being of the community or society (Kornblau &

Burkhardt, 2012). An example is when a government experiences conflict over priorities for allocation of resources in health services. The ethical dilemmas that occupational therapists might encounter in the home modification field include the following:

+ Confidentiality and disclosure of the person's private information

+ Resource allocation and priorities in home modification practice

+ Client's decision-making capacity

+ Personal and professional boundaries

+ Use of power

+ Cultural, religious, or family considerations

Confidentiality and Disclosure of Private Information

After a home modification visit, do occupational therapists respect the client's right to privacy or do they report that he or she is living in a state of neglect? Does it make a difference whether paid caregivers or family members provide the care in the home? Does the law require such a disclosure?

Resource Allocation and Priorities

Should home modification programs finance all types of modifications or only those alterations that improve the person's health and safety in the home? During tough economic times, should publicly or grant-funded programs still fund adaptations to enhance the individual's independence, community participation, and quality of life? How can occupational therapists provide services if they are working in settings with limited resources, while at the same time ethics and regulatory bodies require they provide quality care (Kinsella, Ji-Sun Park, Appiagyei, Chang, & Chow, 2008)?

Client's Decision-Making Capacity

Should occupational therapists rely solely on the self-report of people whom they believe are in the early stages of dementia or should they contact others to assist with decision making?

Personal and Professional Boundaries

How can occupational therapists deliver home modification services in a diagnostically driven health care system that conflicts with occupational therapists' values that are rooted in client-centered practice, social justice, enabling occupation, and, in some places, social models of care (Kinsella et al., 2008)?

Use of Power

Should occupational therapists place their clients and their families in situations that compel them to agree with professional recommendations, even in those instances where clients and their families do not feel comfortable with the proposed changes, or should they acquiesce to the views of clients and their families?

Cultural, Religious, or Family Considerations

Should occupational therapists alter their modification recommendations to suit another family member who also has a disability, or should they provide modifications only to benefit the client? Should occupational therapists consider the needs of caregivers in developing modification recommendations in addition to the needs of the client?

Ethical Terminology

Ethical terminology of relevance to occupational therapists includes the following:

+ Informed consent

+ Veracity

+ Confidentiality

+ Fidelity

+ Duty

+ Rights

+ Paternalism

Informed Consent

Informed consent obligates occupational therapists to provide clients with truthful, comprehensive information on all assessment and intervention strategies to ensure they can make willing, informed decisions (Kornblau & Burkhardt, 2012; Shannon, 1993).

Informed consent is defined as a client's willing acceptance of an intervention after adequate disclosure of the nature of the intervention and its risks and benefits and the alternatives and their risks and benefits (Jonsen et al., 2010; Shannon, 1993). One can determine the adequacy of disclosure by exploring what a reasonably prudent therapist would tell a client under similar circumstances (health professional-centered approach) or which information reasonable clients need to know to make rational decisions (client-centered approach; Jonsen et al., 2010).

Codes of ethics and licensure laws and federal and state laws and regulations require occupational therapists to seek informed consent (Kornblau & Starling, 2000).

The requirements of informed consent as described by Biano and Hirsh (1995; cited in Kornblau & Burkhardt, 2012, p. 37) include the following:

+ Occupational therapists must ensure the client understands the procedure or treatment and its risks, potential benefits, and any available alternatives.

+ Clients must freely give consent, willingly and without duress.

+ Clients must possess the capacity to give consent.

If clients have impaired decision-making capacity, the therapist must seek consent from a parent, guardian, or conservator. Further, clients who do not wish to participate in the occupational therapy process might refuse to give informed consent (Kornblau & Burkhardt, 2012).

Veracity

Veracity in occupational therapy practice involves the comprehensive, accurate, and objective transmission of information to individuals and the way the occupational therapist fosters their understanding (Beauchamp & Childress, 2008). It stems from respect for others; the obligations of fidelity, truth, and promise keeping; and trust (Beauchamp & Childress, 2008).

Occupational therapists must speak and act truthfully in all communication with clients. If the therapist fails to speak truthfully, it may interfere with the client's ability to make an informed decision (Kornblau & Burkhardt, 2012). When occupational therapists seek informed consent for assessment, treatment, or intervention, they must provide clients with comprehensive, accurate, and objective information as part of this process. For example, veracity can include providing clients and their caregivers accurate and complete information about the use of the home modifications and assistive devices in the home. Veracity also includes accurately representing one's occupational therapy qualifications to students seeking a home modification fieldwork experience (Costa, 2007) or when seeking employment with a service, company, or agency that requires personnel have experience performing major modification work.

Confidentiality

Privacy entails respecting a person's right to limit access to his or her personal sphere. In contrast, confidentiality focuses on informational privacy. It prevents disclosure of information previously disclosed within a confidential relationship (Beauchamp & Childress, 2001; Cheyney Brandt & Yarett Slater, 2011; Jonsen et al., 2010; Stallard, 2005). Occupational therapists need to ensure they familiarize themselves with practice requirements relevant to privacy and confidentiality. For example, in the United States, the Health Insurance Portability and Accountability Act (HIPAA, 1996) is a federal law that establishes the standards for the privacy and security of health information, as well as the standards for electronic data interchange of health information Health Insurance Portability and Accountability Act of 1996, Pub. L. No. 104-191 It creates a comprehensive system that defines the value, scope, and limits of confidentiality (Jonsen et al., 2010). Regulatory bodies, codes of ethics, and standards of practice usually require that occupational therapists, including those who practice home modifications, keep records of their interventions. They must maintain these records according to HIPAA's confidentiality requirements. The Summary of the HIPAA Privacy Rule (U.S. Department of Health and Human Services, 2015) provides particularly useful information regarding HIPAA's application to occupational therapy practice.

A breach in confidentiality occurs when professionals fail to protect information about people who have shared that information in confidence, or they share it without permission (Beauchamp & Childress, 2008; Stallard, 2005). Breaches in confidentiality can result in various actions, such as:

+ Employer disciplinary proceedings

+ Termination of contract of employment

+ Referral to the professional body for ethics violations

+ Legal proceedings for compensation

+ Criminal proceedings if the breach is prohibited by law (Stallard, 2005)

Occupational therapists might justify breaches in confidentiality if there is specific concern for the safety of others, such as instances of child or elder abuse, where a person is mortally threatened, or where there is concern for public welfare (Jonsen et al., 2010; Kornblau & Burkhardt, 2012). Occupational therapists may disclose information where clients agree to the disclosure and provide a HIPAA release or consent. Disclosure may be in the best interest of people with disabilities to ensure their health, safety, and independence in the home. In such instances, statutes or court orders might require the disclosure (Dimond, 2010; Stallard, 2005). For example, in the United States, state laws often require that occupational therapists and other health professionals report suspected elder abuse. Therapists who practice home modifications might find circumstances in the home that lead them to suspect possible elder abuse. Reporting this suspected elder abuse falls under an exception to HIPAA's confidentiality requirements and may be mandated by state law (e.g., Fla. Stat. §415.1034(1)(A) [2013]).

Where someone has impaired decision-making capacity, therapists might need to obtain consent for release of information from a guardian, conservator, or health care surrogate. Clients or substitute decision makers must sign written documentation as evidence of their agreement to release the information (Stallard, 2005). In the United States, the client or substitute decision maker must sign a HIPAA release. Further, the HIPAA release form must stipulate contents of the information and to whom it is being released. If therapists are in doubt about the process of sharing information with other parties, they should check with their employers or relevant others and review the HIPAA requirements.

Fidelity

Fidelity refers to faithfulness of one human being to another, in implicit or explicit promises and commitments (AOTA, 2015a; Bailey & Schwartzberg, 2003; Beauchamp & Childress, 2008; Cheyney Brandt & Yarett Slater, 2011; Costa, 2007; Doherty, 2014). This principle justifies the obligation to act in good faith to keep vows and promises, fulfill agreements, maintain relationships, and discharge fiduciary responsibilities (Beauchamp & Childress, 2008). In occupational therapy, fidelity means upholding responsibilities to clients. This might include, for example, a program or department following through with its commitment to perform scheduled home modification evaluations or to keep shared information confidential (Kornblau & Burkhardt, 2012).

Duty

A duty is a responsibility that therapists have to their patients or clients. It refers to obligations required of professionals by society, codes of ethics, standards of practice, laws, and regulations, or self-imposed actions. For example, occupational therapists have a duty to their patients and clients to maintain their level of competence in their area of practice through lifelong learning, so they can deliver quality care (Costa, 2007; WFOT, 2016).

Rights

Rights refer to a justified claim or entitlement warranted by moral principles and rules (Beauchamp & Childress, 2008). Rights relate to the moral entitlement to protect life, liberty, expression, and property. When respected, rights can provide a basis to protect against oppression, unequal treatment, intolerance, and invasion of privacy, among others (Beauchamp & Childress, 2008; Shannon, 1993).

For example, during their interactions in home modification practice, occupational therapists must ensure clients' rights to autonomy, privacy, and confidentiality.

Paternalism

Historically, decision making in the medical field has been "paternalistic." Physicians made diagnoses, prescribed treatments, and gave "orders," providing the patient with limited information (Jonsen et al., 2010). In occupational therapy practice, paternalism occurs when occupational therapists fail to respect clients' autonomy and act without regard of the person's individual rights (Kornblau & Burkhardt, 2012).

Paternalism may emerge when there is conflict between beneficence and autonomy. It can involve interference with, or refusal to conform to, individual clients' preferences regarding their own good (Beauchamp & Childress, 2008; Shannon, 1993). Paternalistic acts can involve force, coercion, deception, lying, manipulation, or nondisclosure of information; overriding one's known preferences; or restricting a person's autonomous choice (Beauchamp & Childress, 2008). For example, paternalism would occur in home modification practice if therapists coerced clients into accepting home modification recommendations the client may not want, insisting that they knew best as an "expert."

In the middle of the 20th century, this pattern of paternalism shifted, in theory, to patient autonomy in which the patient or client was the authoritative decision maker (Jonsen et al., 2010). The current view sees shared decision making between the health professional and the client as the preferred relationship (Jonsen et al., 2010).

Problem-Solving Tools for Ethical Issues

Although the study of ethical theory provides the basis for formulating solutions, it might not readily solve the problem identified. Instead of easy answers, it can raise a variety of questions and issues. Occupational therapists require knowledge of a range of resources and tools that help translate their judgments into specific action steps to solve ethical dilemmas (Kornblau & Burkhardt, 2012). Resources and tools help analyze the situation in a structured and systematic way, including, for example, referring to the profession's codes of ethics, such as the AOTA's code (AOTA, 2015a), which incorporates ethical principles. It might also include referring to textbooks in the field that provide guidance and information to assist in the analysis of ethical issues (Van Denend & Finlayson, 2007).

Analysis of ethical dilemmas is a multistep process guided by various sets of values and principles (Kornblau & Burkhardt, 2012). Though there are various methods or processing tools available to analyze ethical dilemmas, the CELIBATE Method (Clinical Ethics and Legal Issues Bait All Therapists Equally) for Analyzing Ethical Dilemmas provides occupational therapists in home modification practice with a workable tool for addressing problems they might come across. This method, developed by Kornblau and Starling (2000), provides therapists with a clear framework that considers both legal and ethical issues (Table 12-1). The title of the method is an acronym where each letter provides a cue for the user of the framework:

+ C—Clinical situation
+ E—Ethical issues
+ L—Legal issues
+ I—Information
+ B—Brainstorming actions
+ A—Analyzing actions
+ T—Taking action
+ E—Evaluating the results

Occupational therapists need not use the CELIBATE method alone. In fact, working with other members of the team, therapists can ensure a range of insights into ethical problem solving. Kornblau and Burkhardt (2012) provide further information on the application of this approach.

Tymchuck (1982) developed another model for resolving dilemmas, whereby it provides steps on how to describe the ethical issues and assess this information. The process for making ethical decisions is a seven-step procedure.

1. Describe the parameters of the situation.
2. Describe the potential issues involved.
3. Describe the guidelines already available that might affect each issue (e.g., values, laws, codes, practice, and research).
4. Enumerate the alternative decisions for each issue.
5. Enumerate the short-term, ongoing, and long-term consequences for each alternative.
6. Present evidence (or the lack thereof) for those consequences as well as the probability of their occurrence.
7. Rank, order, and vote on the decisions (Tymchuck, 1982).

It may be necessary for occupational therapy personnel to seek out additional resources to assist in resolving complex ethical issues including ethics committees, ethics officers, the AOTA Ethics Commission or Ethics Program Manager, or an ethics consultant (AOTA, 2014).

Ethical Breaches and Consequences

Unethical practice is practice that fails to conform to established professional standards (Kornblau & Burkhardt, 2012). This can include unreasonable, unjustified, ineffective, immoral, questionable, and knowingly harmful or wrong practice (Kornblau & Burkhardt, 2012). Clients, colleagues, employers, family members, and others can raise breaches of the code of ethics with the various registration or certification bodies that monitor professional conduct.

Employers can also have codes of conduct that impose professional and/or contractual duties on occupational therapists as workplace requirements. Employers might respond to ethics complaints with disciplinary proceedings, which could result in demotion or dismissal. Therapists who are self-employed or working on a contractual basis might find their contract terminated.

Numerous rules and regulations govern the basic ethical and legal requirements of professional conduct. These include the following:

+ The profession's code of ethics
+ State licensure laws
+ Malpractice standards
+ State and federal criminal or civil statutes
+ Case law (Bailey & Schwartzberg, 2003)

Ethical and legal matters differ in the types of penalties professionals can face because of their behaviors (Table 12-2). The AOTA Code's Enforcement Procedures (AOTA, 2014) describe the process used to address ethical violations by association members (and associated members, where applicable; AOTA, 2014). AOTA's Code is intended to as a freestanding document, guiding ethical dimensions of professional behavior, responsibility, practice, and decision making, but it can also be used in combination with licensure board regulations and laws (AOTA, 2014).

Therapists who violate the professional code of ethics may also violate a criminal law and find themselves subject to legal action (Costa, 2007; Scott, 1997). While ethics and law are not synonymous, occupational therapists need to be aware of

Table 12-1. CELIBATE Method for Analyzing Ethical Dilemmas

1. What is the problem?
2. What are the facts of the situation?
3. Who are the interested parties? Facility, patient, other therapists, observers, payers, etc.
4. What is the nature of the interest? Why is this a problem? Professional Personal Business Economic Intellectual Societal
5. Ethical? Does it violate a professional code of ethics? Which section(s)?
6. Legal? Is there a legal issue? Practice act/licensure law & regulations? Other laws: Check the CELIBATE Checklist
7. Do I need more information? What information do I need? Is there a treatment, policy, procedure, law, regulation, or document that I do not know about? Can I obtain a copy of the treatment, policy, procedure, law, regulation, or document in writing? Do I need to research the issue further? Do I need to consult with a mentor, an expert in this area, and/or a lawyer?
8. Brainstorm possible action steps.
9. Analyze action steps. Eliminate obvious wrong or impossible choices. How will each alternative affect my patients, other interest parties, and me? Do your choices abide by the Code of Ethics? Do your choices abide by the practice act and regulations? Are my choices consistent with my moral, religious, and social beliefs?
10. Choose your course of action. The Rotary Four-Way Test Is it the truth? Is it fair to all concerned? Will it build goodwill and better friendships? Will it be beneficial to all concerned? Is it win-win? How do you feel about your course of action?
Reprinted with permission from Kornblau, B. L., & Burkhardt, A. (2012). *Ethics in rehabilitation: A clinical perspective* (2nd ed.). Thorofare, NJ: SLACK Incorporated.

Table 12-2. Possible Ethical and Legal Penalties in the United States

FEATURE	ETHICS	LAW
Comprised of:	Standards of practice	Federal statutes
	Codes of Ethics	State statutes
	Social values	State regulations
	Religious values	Federal regulations
	Cultural values	Case law
	Moral value	Licensure laws
Penalties	Fines	Fines
	Loss of provisional privilege, license, or certification	Monetary damages (punitive, compensatory, or restitution)
	Relinquishment of membership in professional organization	Imprisonment
	Reprimand—public or private	Injunctions
	Censure—usually public	Revocation or suspension of license
	Publication of the ethical violation and penalty imposed	Publication of revocation or suspension of license
	Report to licensure or certification board	License placed in probationary status
	Termination	Termination

Adapted with permission from Kornblau, B. L., & Burkhardt, A. (2012). *Ethics in rehabilitation: A clinical perspective* (2nd ed.). Thorofare, NJ: SLACK Incorporated.

the effect of law on decisions they make in practice because not all legal actions are ethical and not all ethical actions are legal (Cheyney Brandt & Yarett Slater, 2011). At times, therapists might consider a law wrong or contrary to their ethical principles (Dimond, 2010). Under these circumstances, they need to determine what personal action to take, in full awareness that they subject themselves to penalties (Dimond, 2010). For example, a therapist receives a request for a home modification intervention and, during the initial visit, discovers that the client has a guardian/conservator who must approve the visit. The therapist calls the guardian to explain the need and seek consent. However, the guardian refuses to allow the visit to proceed and tells the therapist "to stay out of family business." According to the law, without the consent of the guardian, the therapist cannot visit the client and provide the service. However, the therapist may feel an ethical and moral obligation to not abandon the client and to provide the services. At the same time, the law and ethical obligations require the therapist not to see the client without informed consent. The therapist needs to decide what action to take, which may include petitioning the court for permission to see the client.

When ethical conflicts occur in practice, legal requirements might sometimes set limits to ethical options or can even create ethical conflicts (Jonsen et al., 2010). For example, therapists might feel conflicted between their ethical duty to protect confidential information and their legal duty to report required information to protect a person or community's health and safety (Jonsen et al., 2010). In another example, an occupational therapist visiting a client to undertake a home modification assessment may find that he or she is living in a state of abuse and neglect despite residing with family. The occupational therapist may feel conflicted between his or her ethical duty to respect the confidentiality of the client's circumstances as per the family's wishes and his or her legal duty to report the client's suspected state of abuse and neglect.

Occupational therapists in home modification practice can face situations that raise both ethical and legal concerns. It is important that therapists' problem solve ethical issues using ethical concepts and reasoning because the law, though relevant to various cases, rarely settles ethical problems (Jonsen et al., 2010).

LEGAL ISSUES

The law has been described as "a collection of rules and regulations by which society is governed" (Bailey & Schwartzberg, 2003). They are generally manmade and involve the blending of court decisions (also called case law, common law or judge-made law), state and federal statutes, regulations, and procedures to ensure people's rights are protected (Bailey & Schwartzberg, 2003). Laws commonly reflect society's needs, attitudes, and mores and serve to regulate social conduct in a formal and binding manner.

The two legal issues commonly raised in relation to the negligence of occupational therapists include professional standard of care and professional negligence.

Professional Standard of Care

A health professional must practice according to a specific standard of care, which is the standard that a reasonably prudent person in the same profession would demonstrate under similar circumstances (Ekelman Ranke & Moriarty, 1995). Under the law, occupational therapists who possess average skill and competence in the exercise of their profession, establish the standard of care (Jarvis, 1983).

Standard of care comes from the person who testifies to what the standard is (the expert witness), the profession's standards of practice and codes of ethics, professional literature, standard textbooks, licensure laws and regulations, and how 51% of occupational therapists would act under similar circumstances (Simon, 2005). Failure to perform to these standards constitutes negligence or malpractice (Ekelman Ranke & Moriarty, 1995). For example, during a home modification evaluation, an occupational therapist must review a client's occupational performance in a range of areas in the home if he or she believes the client may have requirements extending beyond those indicated in the initial referral.

The law, codes of ethics, and standards of practice require that occupational therapists competently provide assessments and interventions (Neeman, 1979). The concept of competence in professional practice is important because it relates to employee expectations in the workplace and involves more than the accomplishment of several discrete or separate tasks (Occupational Therapy Australia, 2010).

Competence is described as "a complex interaction and integration of knowledge, judgment, higher order reasoning, personal qualities, skills, values and beliefs" (Occupational Therapy Australia, 2010). Competent professionals recall and apply facts and skills, evaluate evidence, create explanations from available facts, develop hypotheses, and synthesize information from their own knowledge base (Occupational Therapy Australia, 2010). Competence also involves the capacity to generalize or transfer skills and knowledge from one situation to another (Occupational Therapy Australia, 2010). Consequently, it is "a construction that is both abstract and tangible" (Occupational Therapy Australia, 2010) The occupational therapy profession accepts responsibility for the competence of its members. It sets standards for their preparation and practice, provides a means of achieving competence, identifies those qualified as competent, and implements measures to oversee occupational therapy practice (Neeman, 1979). The Occupational Therapy Code of Ethics (AOTA, 2015a) clearly imposes requirements for individual occupational therapists to engage in competent practice and recommends continuing competence plans (Moyers & Hinojosa, 2011). Continuing competence requires one to participate in a process to examine of one's current skills and competence, while developing one's capacity for the future (AOTA, 2015b).

All occupational therapists must ensure their own competence in the area in which they practice by keeping abreast of current developments in the field through the professional literature. At a minimum, they must know what other reasonable and competent occupational therapists in the same specialty know or should know (Jarvis, 1983; Neeman, 1979). Employers have a duty to hire people with appropriate qualifications, and supervisors have a duty to delegate tasks within the individual's sphere of competence (Neeman, 1979).

The consequences of incompetent performance could include occupational therapists' self-dissatisfaction with respect to their own performance, as well as clients' and employers' dissatisfaction with their work practices (Moyers & Hinojosa, 2011). Incompetent practice can result in a decline in business, a reduction in revenue for the business, limited opportunities for promotion, job loss, and difficulty obtaining new employment (Moyers & Hinojosa, 2011). Incompetent occupational therapists could face actions for malpractice or loss of their state licenses, certifications, and/or professional association memberships (Moyers & Hinojosa, 2011).

Because home modification is a specialized area, various occupational therapy professional organizations around the world, such as AOTA, have developed home modification training and specialty certification programs. While students can acquire some training through education and fieldwork, they are likely to need further education and training to establish skills and knowledge in home modification practice, particularly after they receive a license (Yarett Slater & AOTA, 2016). Occupational therapists should document their competence in home modification practice and update it regularly to ensure consistency of skill and knowledge (Yarett Slater & AOTA, 2016). This is particularly important if specific countries do not have their own set of documented competencies for this area (Yarett Slater & AOTA, 2016). If a patient or client is harmed, occupational therapists who perform home modification work beyond their professional knowledge, skill, and expertise might open themselves to allegations of professional incompetence or malpractice (Bull, 1998).

Legal frameworks in state practice acts, such as those in effect in the United States, establish the scope of practice of occupational therapy (Yarett Slater & AOTA, 2016). State licensure laws in the United States, also called *practice acts*, legally define the profession's scope of practice to protect consumers of occupational therapy services (Yarett Slater & AOTA, 2016). Other countries or inter-country councils might have other frameworks that establish the domain of practice of occupational therapy. Additionally, occupational therapy professional bodies might also have specific practice guidelines for home modification practice that can assist individuals who work in this area. Therapists can acquire information about home modification practice from professional literature, standard textbooks, licensure laws and regulations, and other occupational therapists with expertise in this area.

Professional Negligence

To appreciate the risks involved in home modification practice and to implement strategies to reduce these risks, occupational therapists will find it useful to understand the laws of negligence and professional malpractice (Ekelman Ranke & Moriarty, 1995).

In the United States, two sets of laws govern behavior toward one another: criminal and civil (Ekelman Ranke & Moriarty, 1995). Under civil law, everyone in society has a duty to exercise due care or reasonable care for his or her own safety and the safety of others (Ekelman Ranke & Moriarty, 1995). Failure to ensure this safety of self or others is considered negligent, which can result in a civil lawsuit (Ekelman Ranke & Moriarty, 1995).

Negligence is a common civil action where the defendant, the occupational therapist, owed a duty of care to the client; the defendant breached that duty; and the breach of the duty caused reasonably foreseeable harm to person or property (Dimond, 2010; Jarvis, 1983). The harm to the person or property results from an action that a "reasonable person" would not take or the failure to take an action that a reasonable person would take under similar circumstances (Jarvis, 1983). If an action or failure to act occurs without damage or harm, there is no negligence. At the same time, if damage or harm occurs but the action taken meets the "reasonable person" test, then it does not constitute negligence (Jarvis, 1983).

Negligence is not synonymous with malpractice (Jarvis, 1983). Malpractice, a broader concept, applies to all wrongful acts against a person, such as treating without valid consent, as well as negligence (Costa, 2007; Jarvis, 1983; Stallard, 2005). Malpractice occurs when professionals participate in professional misconduct, lack reasonable skills, and fail to deliver appropriate professional services with the degree of skill and learning expected of members of the profession, which results in injury, loss, or damage to service recipients or those entitled to services (Costa, 2007; Jarvis, 1983; Stallard, 2005). Malpractice includes malicious practice or illegal and immoral conduct (Costa, 2007; Jarvis, 1983; Stallard, 2005).

The fundamental guiding principle in professional practice is the "reasonable occupational therapist standard," and the courts decide what is reasonable under the law (Jarvis, 1983). Courts have the fundamental obligation to apply the same standards to similar cases. They might look to the standard of care of a similarly situated professional, or the court may look to the profession's own standards to determine potential liability (Hertfelder & Crispen, 1990).

The "reasonable person standard" applies to all members of the public. However, a higher standard applies to health professionals, such as occupational therapists (Jarvis, 1983). There are various reasons why the law holds professionals to a higher standard than nonprofessionals. First, the law sees the skills of professionals coming from validated, theoretical bodies of knowledge, which laypeople do not bring to the equation (Jarvis, 1983). Second, professional practice is based on research and the ongoing development of new theories compared with laypeople, who base what they do on general knowledge (Jarvis, 1983). Finally, the law views professionals as those who can provide the best solution to meet the clients' need based on their own knowledge as professionals and the needs of the client. The client is not usually in a position to question the judgment of the professional, compared with the judgment of a layperson, who may provide customer service or other nonskilled tasks (Jarvis, 1983).

The Four Elements of Negligence-Based Malpractice

Most malpractice claims are based on negligence. The courts consider four elements when determining whether a professional's action or lack of action constitutes negligence (Jarvis, 1983). They include duty of care, breach of duty, harm, and causation.

Duty of Care

By the nature of the relationship, occupational therapists always owe a duty of care to the clients with whom they establish relationships. This relationship starts when the therapist first establishes contact with the client (Dimond, 2010; Jarvis, 1983; Kornblau & Burkhardt, 2012). A duty of care arises when a person can reasonably foresee that his or her actions or omissions (the failure to do something one should do) could cause reasonably foreseeable harm to another person (Dimond, 2010; Mu, Lohman, & Scheirton, 2005).

Occupational therapists may find themselves liable for damages caused by actions they took, acts of commission, as well as the actions they failed to take, acts of omissions (Kornblau & Burkhardt, 2012). To achieve success in a negligence action, the person claiming the harm, the plaintiff, must show that the person he or she claims harmed him or her, the defendant, owed the plaintiff a duty of care (Dobbs, 2000). Occupational therapists' duties compel them to exercise the reasonable care and skills expected of a reasonably prudent occupational therapist. In fact, the courts will inquire as to whether a reasonably prudent occupational therapist would act in a similar manner under similar circumstances (Kornblau & Burkhardt, 2012).

Breach of Duty

After presenting evidence that the defendant had a duty of care, the plaintiff must show the defendant had to practice according to a minimum standard of practice (Dobbs, 2000). Occupational therapists breach the duty of care if they fail to meet the standard of practice required by law (Jarvis, 1983). This can be established through first determining the most appropriate standard of practice, including care and proficiency (Dimond, 2010; Wright, 1985). This involves examining the following:

+ The reasonableness of the practice
+ The degree of risk of an incident or accident occurring
+ The consequences of not providing a service (Dimond, 2010)

The expert witness' role in court is to help prove breach of duty or providing care that falls below the standards of a reasonably prudent occupational therapist (Kornblau & Burkhardt, 2012). Expert witnesses are usually practitioners in the same field who testify to provide their opinion on the standard of care to which occupational therapists must practice situations (Kornblau & Burkhardt, 2012). Standards of practice, codes of ethics, licensure laws, professional literature, and standard texts provide evidence to the court as to the standard of care.

The type of relationship an occupational therapist has with an employer, hospital, or agency affects the determination of liability for therapists' acts of negligence (Ekelman Ranke & Moriarty, 1995). The two most common relationships involving occupational therapists include the employer/employee relationship and the relationship between occupational therapy independent contractors and the contracting entities, such as hospitals, agencies, and individual clients (Ekelman Ranke & Moriarty, 1995). In the United States, under the doctrine of "respondent superior" ("let the master answer"), occupational therapists can find themselves liable for the action of subordinates unless they are independent contractors (Ekelman Ranke & Moriarty, 1995; Kornblau & Burkhardt, 2012). Under this doctrine, the law can impute liability to occupational therapists or employers who direct and supervise employees if they delegate therapy services to staff who are not qualified or who fail to perform these services properly (Kornblau & Burkhardt, 2012).

If occupational therapists work in a private capacity under an independent contractor agreement and their actions result in damage to the person receiving the services, the contracting agency or entity would generally not be held liable for the independent contractor's negligence (Ekelman Ranke & Moriarty, 1995). Under these circumstances, occupational therapists are liable for their own actions. Independent contractors should consider professional liability insurance to protect themselves from malpractice actions (Ekelman Ranke & Moriarty, 1995). In the United States, however, attorneys are more likely to sue occupational therapists with malpractice insurance than those without.

Harm

In a negligence case, breach of duty must result in some sort of harm (Dobbs, 2000). The person to whom the duty of care was owed must prove the harm. Harm is established when the person experiences some loss or injury (Jarvis, 1983). Examples of recognizable harm include personal injury, death, lost wages, and property damage (Dimond, 2010).

This harm or loss is referred to as damages and forms the basis for the claim (Dimond, 2010).

Occupational therapists might act in a manner that falls below the standard of care without causing any harm. Should no harm occur, one cannot make a case for malpractice (Kornblau & Burkhardt, 2012). Additionally, therapists might act reasonably and provide effective services, but the person's condition does not improve. This also fails to rise to the level of malpractice (Kornblau & Burkhardt, 2012).

Causation

The plaintiff must show that the occupational therapist's negligent conduct was responsible for the reasonably foreseeable harm to the client (Dimond, 2010). The standard is the "but for" test: But for the occupational therapist's negligence, the client's injury would not have occurred (Kornblau & Burkhardt, 2012).

Example: Suppose Mrs. Smith hired an occupational therapist to evaluate her 85-year-old mother's home to determine modifications necessary for her mother to age in place. The occupational therapist provides Mrs. Smith with a report with diagrams of the bathroom and kitchen and a list of equipment. The occupational therapist forgets to report the need for a grab bar near the bathtub. Mrs. Smith's mother falls and breaks her hip 1 month later while stepping into the bathtub. If Mrs. Smith sued the occupational therapist, the court would find that the treating therapist owed a duty of due care to Mrs. Smith's mother. An occupational therapy expert would testify that any competent occupational therapist would have recommended a grab bar near the bathtub to get in and out of the tub safely. The court would probably find that Mrs. Smith's mother was harmed by the failure of the occupational therapist to recommend the grab bar near the bathtub, something even a new occupational therapy graduate would recommend.

OTHER LEGAL-RELATED PRACTICAL ISSUES

Assault and Battery

During home visits, occupational therapists might provide physical assistance to clients as they complete various activities to demonstrate how they manage in the home. This involves the client cooperating and giving informed consent before undertaking any activities in the home (Kornblau & Burkhardt, 2012). Occupational therapists need to know that if they place someone in a position where he or she is apprehensive of being touched in an offensive manner without consent, this is considered assault. Intentionally touching someone without consent defines battery to the person (Dimond, 2010; Kornblau & Burkhardt, 2012).

Occupational therapists must take reasonable care in their interactions with clients (Dimond, 2010). A chaperone could prove useful should therapists later find themselves accused of harming a client (Dimond, 2010). It is also essential that the occupational therapist clearly document any incidents that might have occurred at the time of the interaction with the client to ensure that he or she has a clear record of the event for future reference.

Breach of Fiduciary Duty

Another type of action is breach of fiduciary duty, which can apply to professionals in specific situations. Under the law, occupational therapists owe a fiduciary duty to their clients (Jonsen et al., 2010). As defined in the law, a fiduciary owes undivided loyalty to clients and must work for their benefit (Jonsen et al., 2010). Fiduciaries have specialized expertise; are held to high standards of honesty, confidentiality, and loyalty; and must avoid all conflicts of interest that could prejudice their client's interests (Jonsen et al., 2010).

Where professionals use their relationships to procure a benefit for themselves without disclosing the private interest to clients, the law requires that they account for those benefits to the client. For example, the law does not look kindly on therapists who recommend products and fittings for a home that come from a company in which they have a personal financial interest and fail to disclose this to the client. Additionally, the law prohibits therapists from obtaining any financial benefit from a client's acquisition of products and finishes. This creates a conflict between occupational therapists' private interest and their duty to their client. If they are receiving "kickbacks" or commissions from the company that provides the products and fittings, they could face ethical charges, criminal charges, and disciplinary action from the licensure or certification boards, that could include permanent loss of their license or exclusion from certain government health programs.

DEFENSES TO AN ACTION

Even when the plaintiff can prove all the specific elements of negligence, the court might accept some defenses against allegations of negligence (Dobbs,

2000). This means that defendants might justify some actions, even though they were negligent and individuals suffered losses from those actions (Dobbs, 2000). If negligent actions are defensible, individuals harmed might find that they cannot pursue claims for compensation from the people who caused their harm (Dobbs, 2000).

The plaintiff must prove facts corresponding to the various acceptable legal defenses, which can include the following:

+ Contributory negligence: Where the claimant is partly responsible for the harm

+ Exemption from liability for loss or damage to property or person: Where, for example, individuals might waive their right to sue via a contract or fail to follow proper procedures; or the government limits the right to sue, such as the doctrine of sovereign immunity; or where a statute prevents suing a government employee, such as the Federal Tort Claim Act 28 U.S.C. §§ 1346(b), 2671-2680 (1948)

+ Statute of limitation: Where the claimant fails to initiate a lawsuit within the time allowed by law

+ Assumption of risk: Where injured parties knowingly and willingly place themselves at risk of harm (Dimond, 2010; Dobbs, 2000)

IMPLICATIONS FOR OCCUPATIONAL THERAPY PRACTICE

Occupational therapists must use diligence, care, knowledge, skill, and caution in their interactions with clients during home visits (Wright, 1985). To guard against negligence and malpractice, occupational therapists need to follow safe and acceptable work practices and procedures.

They must ensure their knowledge is up-to-date and commensurate with peers who practice in the home modification field. Therapists must use reasoned judgment in all situations (Jarvis, 1983). This can be accomplished by following the recommendations of Costa (2007), Kornblau and Burkhardt (2012), Moyers and Hinojosa (2011), and Wright (1985). Occupational therapists are to:

+ Maintain professional standards: Maintain professional membership and keep abreast of ethical and legal practice requirements; comply with the profession's standards of practice and quality assurance programs; and attend conferences and workshops, read the professional literature, and participate in lifelong learning and regular professional development.

+ Manage day-to-day practice effectively: Request policies and instructions in writing from employers and those with whom therapists contract; provide close supervision to students on placements; establish a relationship with a mentor or professional supervisor; take time out to think through issues and seek advice; recognize when to hand over clients to another occupational therapist with more expertise.

+ Communicate clearly and comprehensively: Establish sound communication with individuals in their homes and provide an explanation of occupational therapy's role and the purpose of any activities undertaken in the home for the housing-needs assessment process; complete contemporaneous, complete, and comprehensive documentation accurately and truthfully, and save these documents for future reference; ensure written documentation demonstrates sound clinical reasoning, rationale, and consultation throughout the housing-needs assessment process.

+ Deal with ethical and legal issues appropriately: Report ethical and legal violations to ethics and licensure boards; seek counsel, support, and assistance from other experts or a legal representative if issues arise.

Preventing Occupational Therapy Errors

In the United States in 1999, the Institute of Medicine (IOM) produced a report entitled *To Err is Human: Building a Safer Health System* (Kohn, Corrigan, & Donaldson, 2000). Kohn et al. (2000) reported that errors in health care professional practice cause significant harm to the population. This report defined safety as freedom from accidental injury and error as the failure to take planned action to be completed as intended or the use of a wrong plan to achieve an aim (Jonsen et al., 2010). The report highlighted personal and financial costs of errors. It noted some errors occurred because of incompetence, mistaken judgment, and unrecognized and uncorrected system failures, which resulted in a breach of the health care professional's responsibility (Jonsen et al., 2010). After the publication of this report, the IOM publications *Crossing the Quality Chasm: A New Health System for the 21st Century* (IOM, 2001) and *Patient Safety: Achieving a New Standard for Care* (IOM, 2004) have provided more information to guide practice.

Given the complexities of issues that occupational therapists deal with, there is a risk of errors occurring in practice (Clark, Gray, & Mooney, 2013). Research shows that errors occur in occupational therapy practice (Lohman, Mu, & Scheirton, 2003; Mu, Lohman, & Scheirton, 2005, 2006; Scheirton, Mu, & Lohman, 2003). Much of occupational therapy research in practice errors relates to personnel working in geriatric and physical rehabilitation settings (Clark et al., 2013) with a paucity of studies in home modification practice. Mu et al. (2011) indicates that errors can be classified as technical errors (methods, skills, or approaches that lead to physical harm to clients) or moral errors (relating to behaviors that undermine the practitioner-client relationship or are ethically inconsistent). Findings from various studies have shown that practice errors have occurred in the intervention phase, and often have a moral or ethical dimension (Mu et al., 2006; Scheirton, Mu, Lohman, & Cochran, 2007).

Practice errors may also include near-misses and mistakes, issues that are largely underinvestigated in research (Mu et al., 2011). Near-misses are defined as an event that could have caused an accident, injury or illness that was averted because of chance or intervention (Wagner, Capezuti, & Ouslander, 2006). Mistakes are defined as untoward, undesirable and unanticipated events that cause harm to a person or the mission of an organization (Ebright, Urden, Patterson, & Chalko, 2004). Such mistakes may result in harm or death (Wagner et al., 2006). Near-misses and mistakes are considered practice errors or adverse events (Clark et al., 2013).

Lohman et al. (2013) highlighted other common occupational therapy practice errors, their causes, prevention, and other implications. For example, practice errors can be physical or psychosocial in nature (Lohman et al., 2003) and can occur because of something the therapist does or fails to do (Lohman et al., 2003; Mu et al., 2005). Examples of practice errors in home modification practice include causing a client unnecessary fatigue and falls during a transfer; errors in communication about the home modification; incorrect use of the home modification; poor documentation (Clark et al., 2013). Mistakes that put the occupational therapist themselves or their colleagues at risk include not taking precautions with a client known to be aggressive, making a mistake during manual handling, poor communication, and providing insufficient documentation (Clark et al., 2013).

Research indicates a range of causes of errors, including human factors, equipment factors, controllable and uncontrollable environmental factors, and poorly structured organizations and systems (Mu et al., 2005). In occupational therapy, major causes of errors included misjudgment of situations, poor preparation and consideration of precautions, lack of experience, inadequate training and knowledge, miscommunication, poor attention, heavy workload, and inadequate supervision, or a combination of these factors (Clark et al., 2013; Lohman et al., 2003). Fewer years of occupational therapy work experience were associated with the types and frequency of errors made, and inexperience or lack of knowledge were more often linked to error commission (Mu et al., 2011). Further, the culture of organizations in which therapists' work and responses to practice errors by others affect how therapists develop and implement strategies for addressing the errors (Mu et al., 2011).

Practice errors may be prevented when occupational therapists do the following as part of their professional socialization and lifelong learning routines:

+ Undertake cultural and systematic change within the workplace: Provide error information to administrators and insurance agencies to enable them to formulate more reasonable productivity expectations; participate in assertiveness training during professional education.

+ Create a supportive work environment: Create a nonpunitive work culture to encourage reporting of errors and learning from these experiences; create policies and procedures and require staff to follow them; re-examine existing policies and procedures to improve them; conduct orientation and training of all new staff and students and highlight potential areas for errors during training; strengthen existing orientation and mentoring programs; maintain appropriate staffing levels; and facilitate collaborative teamwork.

+ Enhance existing or establish new safety policies and procedures: Contribute to the work of safety committees and quality assurance officers that provide safety orientation, in service training for occupational therapists, educate clients and collect error data.

+ Develop structures for monitoring, reporting, and analyzing errors: Develop monitoring and reporting structures; encourage staff to become more vigilant, pay attention to all circumstances, and do not rush decisions; encourage staff honesty and error disclosure; encourage staff to seek assistance from colleagues with more expertise.

+ Provide training: Provide client safety and error reduction education; establish programs for areas of concern; provide in-services for different intervention approaches; provide staff assertiveness training

✦ Mentor and complete performance competency checks: Undertake regular performance-based competency checks parallel to continuing education and in-service opportunities (Lohman et al., 2003; Mu et al., 2005, 2006, 2011).

Managers can help create a culture of safety by developing mechanisms for optimizing teamwork and strengthening communication, developing safety related policies, standardizing processes, building in redundancies, conducting competency checks to key error issues in practice, and systemizing reporting and learning from errors (Mu et al., 2011, p. 74).

Research shows that occupational therapists need to disclose practice errors to enable them to learn from their experiences and to develop preventative strategies to reduce errors and improve client safety rather than feeling pressured to attain 100% perfection (Clark et al., 2013; Mu et al., 2006). The Occupational Therapy Code of Ethics and Good Practices (AOTA, 2015a) Principle 6D on "Veracity," indicates that a therapist should identify and fully disclose to all appropriate persons, errors that compromise recipients' safety.

It is inevitable that occupational therapists will make practice errors and this includes novice therapists as well as the most highly trained, skilled, and experienced occupational therapists who deal with clients whose needs and their environments are quite complex (Mu et al., 2011). Disclosure of these errors and subsequent learning best occurs in nonpunitive, supportive environments that have processes established for reporting of practice errors and supporting staff through this process, and to investigate, analyze, and plan improvements to occupational therapy practice (Mu et al., 2006). Competent clinical practice requires sound clinical reasoning informed by consumer need, principles of best practice, and research.

Occupational therapists can minimize or prevent practice errors by careful analysis and management of potentially injurious situations. Therapists must understand adverse events and risks and learn how to reduce them. This promotes effective service delivery and helps prevent incidents, accidents, adverse events, or death, and all harm to clients that can result in litigation. Chapter 7 contains further information on risk assessment and risk management.

Therapists working in home modifications practice are frequently exposed to situations that place their clients at risk. For example, when evaluating a person's ability to perform activities in their own environment, a therapist needs first to determine the potential risk involved in this assessment and how it can be managed. The therapist needs to determine the probability of an incident occurring and the likely consequences. He or she would then need to reduce the likelihood of an event occurring and minimize an injury by avoiding the task altogether or putting strategies in place to reduce the risk. Further, therapists should constantly monitor the clients, tasks, and environment during home visits to avoid potentially hazardous situations, and thoroughly document all issues that arise during interactions with clients.

DOCUMENTATION

Documentation is an essential aspect of occupational therapy practice and is critical to ensuring best practice and minimizing harm. Occupational therapists must determine the most appropriate type of documentation within their scope of practice and provide it in accordance with the requirements of their practice settings, government agencies, licensure, external accreditation programs, payers, and occupational therapy association documents (AOTA, 2008).

Documentation serves many purposes. First, it provides information on the rationale behind the provision of occupational therapy services and the relationship of this service to the client outcomes. Second, documentation reflects the occupational therapist's clinical reasoning and professional judgment. Third, it communicates information about the client from an occupational therapy perspective. Fourth, it provides a chronological record of the client's status, the occupational therapy services provided, and the outcome of the interventions (AOTA, 2010, 2013; Stallard, 2005). Finally, adequate documentation reduces risk and legal liability (Ekelman Ranke, 1998).

AOTA's *Guidelines for Documentation of Occupational Therapy* (2013) explain different types of documentation provided by occupational therapists, the required contents of reports, and the fundamental elements of reports. According to the guidelines, therapists must be thorough in documentation of home modification assessments and must ensure information is accurate. Inadequate or incomplete documentation can lead to misunderstandings, duplication of effort, and errors that can ultimately result in harm. It is generally difficult, if not impossible, to defend poor documentation in court where the attorney's view of a medical record is adversarial (Ekelman Ranke, 1998). The plaintiff's attorney might argue that poor documentation is proof of careless judgment or poor practice. If therapists fail to document proceedings, there is no evidence to prove that it ever happened. For example, if the therapist fails to document a recommendation for grab bars and the patient falls, there is no proof that the therapist made the recommendation (Ekelman Ranke, 1998).

Occupational therapists seeking to demonstrate best practice in documenting client information can use the following list as a guideline. Reports are to contain the following:

+ All relevant demographic information about the client including his or her contact details and phone number

+ The date of the home visit and a summary of all people present at that time

+ A summary of the client's health background or disability, functional implications, prognosis, and level of risk of accident or injury and his or her past and present health history as it relates to housing needs

+ The source of the medical or disability information, including the name of the author of reports reviewed and the date of the report, information about the client's self-report, or the therapist's observation of the client

+ Information on the impact of the person's health or disability on his or her everyday roles and activities and how the person presents functionally

+ A statement about the client's anticipated future function

+ Information on the person's mobility, including how he or she manages transfers, use of equipment, and how he or she accesses community facilities

+ Detail about the person's level of independence with respect to completing his or her self-care and household tasks (and any other relevant activities around the home)

+ A summary of the type and level of support services, including current and future need for medical intervention, family or caregiver support, and location of services

+ Equipment dimensions and anthropometric measurements (static and dynamic) where appropriate (including information on future equipment needs where possible)

+ A record of the use of any standardized assessment tools and a statement of the goals set by the client

+ A description of the home and the environmental barriers identified

+ A description of the options considered when discussing the various interventions

+ A list of the client's preferred options

+ Information on the person's preferences, which might differ from the occupational therapist's recommendations

+ The occupational therapist's opinions, including a discussion of concerns where the occupational therapist's and the client's preferences differ

+ A detailed list of the final interventions selected and the reasons as to why they were chosen (e.g., to enhance the client's health, safety, independence, and home and community participation)

+ A statement of possible risks associated with not proceeding with list of final interventions recommended for implementation

+ An indication of whether the client agrees with the recommended options

+ References to relevant peer-reviewed literature that supports the modifications or specific assistive devices recommended

+ A summary list of the home modification requirements and detailed diagrams and photos in a separate section of the report, to be used by the builder for quoting purposes

+ Information about the author of the report, including name, job title, qualifications, hours of work and contact number; the author's signature; and the date of the report (DeMaio-Feldman, 1987; Dimond, 2010)

Detailed reports are essential where there has been a compromise because of a conflict with client wishes, environmental constraints, service policy, or financial limitations. The occupational therapist must report and document to the employer, insurance company, or service that has engaged him or her any difficulties in negotiating options with the client. Good practice recommends the occupational therapist, client, and a witness, who need not be independent, sign documentation to indicate the client has declined the occupational therapist's recommendations. Readers may find an example home visit checklist for collection of information in the field, a report template, and an example client report in Appendices G, H, and I.

Documentation must not contain the following:

+ Inconsistencies, mistakes, and omissions that might support the claim of malpractice or raise a question of veracity

+ Inappropriate alterations or extraneous hand-written notes

+ Veiled criticisms of another service provider

+ Alterations or criticisms that may raise concerns about the care provided or the competency of the provider

+ Contradictory or inconsistent sequence of events

+ Documentation of staff shortages that could support a claim of corporate negligence (Ekelman Ranke, 1998)

The nature and type of documentation occupational therapists keep is likely to depend on who requested the home modifications and the type of documentation they want. For example, in the United States, an attorney might not want the therapist to prepare a written report as part of a trial strategy; instead, he or she might hire a therapist to complete an assessment only, without any documentation or intervention.

Errors in documentation may result in duplication of effort, poor decision making, inaccurate assessments, and loss of court cases (Dimond, 2010). Inaccurate information will not help the occupational therapist's defense. In serious cases, it can lead to civil or criminal proceedings (Stallard, 2005). All documentation, including notes and reports, must be clear, factual, contemporaneous, comprehensive, relevant, and objective in style (Dimond, 2010; Ekelman Ranke, 1998; Stallard, 2005). This includes documenting the following:

+ Facts, rather than assumptions, about the situation

+ The time and date of calls therapists made to others, to whom they spoke, and the content of the discussions

+ Evidence of client compliance or non-compliance with instructions

+ Date and time of follow-up visits (Ekelman Ranke, 1998)

Further, occupational therapists should prepare documentation to suit the reporting requirements of the audience or readers (Sames, 2014). Each audience reads documentation with a different focus, depending on their practice setting, education level, understanding of medical terminology, and/or cultural background (Sames, 2014).

Occupational therapists should ensure that their documentation:

+ Is jargon-free and written at the appropriate literacy level for the reader

+ Is devoid of spelling and grammatical errors

+ Uses accepted abbreviations for the practice area

+ Is legible and written in black or blue ink or typed

+ Is dated and signed and accompanied by the legible name and position of the professional (Ekelman Ranke, 1998; Stallard, 2005)

Illegible or messy handwriting makes deciphering records difficult. It also prevents the reader from discerning information that might lead to provider liability or support him or her in accusations of liability. It may cause mistakes to be made by other providers. Plaintiff's counsel or regulatory agencies can interpret illegible documentation as a deliberate attempt to disguise incorrect decisions or oversight in client care (Ekelman Ranke, 1998). However, as electronic medical records become the norm, this might not present itself as an issue any longer.

An intentional destruction or change to another person's documentation is called spoliation. The destruction or alteration of documentation destroys its value as evidence in a legal proceeding. Occupational therapists can face discipline if they change records after the fact. For example, once an attorney or a client requests copies of reports or records, the therapist cannot change them. Once therapists submit records to the service or court, including the occupational therapy report and the architect or building contractor's drawings or specifications, they cannot alter them. If changes are required, therapists should send them back to the source to request changes before submitting them for use by the service or in court.

Occupational therapists must advise clients when they cease the provision of services and document this information to ensure comprehensive records of occupational therapy services (Stallard, 2005). Finally, therapists must remember their records are legal documents subject to subpoena and entry as evidence in any type of legal proceeding involving malpractice, fraud, negligence, or incompetence. Documentation includes e-mail, rough notes on paper, and all references to the patient. Attorneys may present any type of documentation as evidence in a proceeding, without the occupational therapist present to provide further explanation (Sames, 2014).

Recommendations Rejected by Referral Source

Occupational therapists might receive referrals for home modification evaluations where the referral source might not agree with the final proposals.

Therapists should document their recommendations based on their professional assessments, client preferences, and consequences to the client if the modifications are not provided. Referral sources make the final decision if they are paying for the modifications and consequently hold the responsibility for choosing an alternative option. Therapists should not alter their recommendations or reports considering fiscal constraints, but rather identify the best option to optimize the person's occupational performance and discuss relative benefits and limitations of the alternatives. Decisions regarding the affordability of the option should remain the responsibility of the person providing the funding approval.

APPEARING IN COURT AS AN EXPERT WITNESS

Occupational therapists might need to appear in court because of problems arising from their home modification practice or to provide information as an expert witness. Legal systems generally recognize two types of witnesses: fact witnesses and expert witnesses. Fact witnesses testify as to something they saw, heard, or otherwise experienced first-hand (Carson, 1990). Expert witnesses, as well as testifying as to facts, provide opinions (Carson, 1990). The courts decide who may testify as an expert (Carson, 1990). For example, occupational therapists with expertise in home modification could testify as to design and modification requirements of the individual (Forrester & Griffiths, 2015).

The right expert witnesses can make or break a case (Friedman & Klee, 2001). However, not anyone can be an expert witness. Courts use specific criteria to determine whether the person qualifies as an expert (DeMaio-Feldman, 1987). The person must possess specialized qualifications or experience, which might include relevant qualifications, such as board certifications, knowledge, experience, and specialized training. An examination of curriculum vitae will provide the court with an overview of the prospective expert witness's training, professional interests, research, and teaching experience (DeMaio-Feldman, 1987; Friedman & Klee, 2001).

Some courts in the United States follow the Supreme Court's decision in the case of Daubert v. Merrell Dow Pharmaceuticals, 509 U.S. 579 (1993). The court limited expert witness testimony to what it considered scientific knowledge that would assist the judge in deciding. The court announced four factors to consider in determining whether to admit scientific expert witness testimony under the Federal Rules of Evidence:

1. Has the theory or technique been tested?
2. Has the theory or technique been subjected to peer review and publication?
3. In the case of a scientific technique, is there a known or potential rate of error and standards controlling the technique's operation?
4. Is the underlying technique generally accepted in the scientific community (Daubert, 509 U.S. 579, 1993)?

An occupational therapist who could not pass the four-factor test as an expert witness could only testify to first-hand knowledge and facts as a fact witness. In such instances, courts would probably exclude reports from nonexperts that contain opinions.

Experts must develop unbiased conclusions as opposed to acting as a "hired gun" to advocate for one specific position (Friedman & Klee, 2001). Experts can provide opinions based on what they know and what other witnesses have told them. This includes their professional opinion about matters related to the case, such as a description of the client's needs for assistive technology in the home and how often specific devices might need replacement. An expert may be defined as someone associated with characteristics or criteria of professional engagement and critical self-reflection, and who is informed by evidence, and several years' experience.

For the expert witness role, the occupational therapist should prepare a comprehensive resumé or curriculum vitae summarizing all relevant experience. If requested by the attorney, occupational therapists should prepare thorough reports supported by relevant peer-reviewed literature. Sometimes, because of trial strategy, attorneys might not want experts to prepare anything in writing, including notes.

Occupational therapists have a range of skills to offer the legal system. In civil cases, they can testify about the impact an injury might have on an individual's life, how he or she might manage on a day-to-day basis, and the kinds of home modifications needed to maximize independence (DeMaio-Feldman, 1987). Courts value this holistic approach to evaluating individuals, and an objective expert opinion helps relate judgments to awards of monetary damages for future housing options. Additionally, they can also contribute to, and testify about, design/modifications for future housing needs.

The entry into the expert witness role begins when an attorney (solicitor), who represents the plaintiff or claimant, or the defendant contacts the occupational therapist to seek assistance with a person's compensation claim. The therapist must evaluate the case to determine whether it is appropriate for his or her area and level of expertise. Potential experts must decide whether they can be fair and impartial or if they have ethical or other reasons not to take the case. Occupational therapists may decline cases if, after reviewing the files, they find ethical or other reasons to turn down a case. They must provide clear verbal feedback to the attorney (solicitor) who requested their services so alternative assistance can be sought (DeMaio-Feldman, 1987).

Occupational therapists prepare various types of reports for use in court proceedings. For example, in claims where individuals seek compensation for injuries or losses suffered and to prevail they need to prove negligence and damages, either party's attorneys (solicitors) can request reports that outline needs (Stallard, 2005). In home modification practice, this requires therapists to make a home visit to complete a full housing needs assessment of the home. Various laws and rules exist in different countries, states, and provinces that govern how therapists proceed with their roles as expert. This includes an overriding duty to the court rather than to the person requesting the report (Stallard, 2005). Various rules might also dictate the contents of reports and the scope and duties of the expert. Experts might be subpoenaed and questioned about their expert opinions before administrative bodies, courts, tribunals, or at depositions (Allen, Carlson, Ownsworth, & Strong, 2006).

Insurance companies and employers might request reports where individuals file insurance claims for a work-related or non-work-related accident or injury. Individuals might experience difficulty carrying out their job duties. A housing-needs assessment, as part of the process, will recommend modifications to assist people with managing their work and lifestyle. For example, a person with a disability might need bathroom modifications and a ramp to enable him or her to manage his or her self-care and entrance and exit from home to the workplace.

Preparation and Information Gathering

If requested, the occupational therapist must prepare thorough documentation to help establish the facts and/or assess the person's needs. This includes a comprehensive review of all reports and records provided by the attorney or agency that requested the housing-needs assessment for either new construction or home modification solutions.

To gather information not available in reports and records, the therapist should interview and observe individuals in their homes and complete standardized assessments where possible. Before interviews, the therapist must review available documentation to ensure that he or she is familiar with the individual's situation to date. Conversation with the referral source can provide other unwritten information about the case.

If requested, the therapist must independently prepare an unbiased report. This report should detail specific, factual information that can assist organizations, agencies, or courts to establish the scope of the person's disability, medical condition resulting in disability, and the impact on function and roles. Information is also provided on the outcome of the assessment process and references to supporting research literature. This helps to provide evidence of a clear process for clinical reasoning and justification of recommendations. Therapists may complete the report in consultation with contractors or architects experienced in home modification work. They address the housing-needs assessment report to the court or the party that requested their home modification services, which might include an attorney, case manager, rehabilitation counselor, or insurance adjustor, among others.

Therapists should not imply responsibility for the actual physical modifications in their recommendations. Rather, their report should clearly indicate the needed changes to the contractor or licensed tradesman. The final report should include a description of the home and photographs of areas around the home, with an emphasis on the areas to be modified. Diagrams of the existing area and proposed changes also provide the reader with the necessary details of the changes.

Throughout this process, if requested, not only must therapists complete a housing-needs assessment report, but they must also keep other notes on conversations with various parties and the outcomes of any standardized assessments, research, or other activities. This ensures clear information in the record as the work progresses. For court purposes, therapists need to work with attorneys. Attorneys might not want a report or other notes because any written documents are discoverable and can be subpoenaed by the opposing party.

Based on the review of documentation, the attorney might prepare a diary of events, conduct a review of policies and procedures, perform background checks of personnel, and/or review available incident reports (Ekelman Ranke, 1998).

Appearing in Court or at a Deposition

Various authors provide guidelines for professionals who appear in court or at sworn depositions. Some examples include the following:

+ Prepare materials for the testimony carefully to ensure an orderly sequence of materials. Do not bring material to court or depositions unless specifically requested.

+ Speak slowly, loudly, and clearly to ensure the judge and jury can follow the testimony.

+ Answer only the question asked, and avoid unnecessary comments to the judge or opposing counsel.

+ Remain courteous, firm, and even-tempered.

+ State qualifications fully.

+ Explain the methods used to reach conclusions and reference the literature that supports opinions presented.

+ Present the testimony convincingly, concisely, and with relevant detail to resolve any doubts in the mind of the judge.

+ Avoid unimportant details and keep to the essentials of the testimony.

+ Indicate when a question requires additional information for a response or whether the question is based on erroneous assumptions (DeMaio-Feldman, 1987).

Some helpful points for therapists to follow to prepare for the role of expert witness include the following:

+ Consult with established experts in the field.

+ Visit courts and watch a trial.

+ Attend criminal and civil trials to observe other health professionals testifying.

+ Visualize oneself giving a high-level performance in the courtroom.

+ Visit an empty courtroom to prepare psychologically.

+ Prepare, especially reference materials.

+ Research and review the relevant peer-reviewed literature.

+ Develop good knowledge through reading medico-legal material.

+ Study academic literature to seek out evidence to support practice.

+ Develop sound public speaking skills (Allen et al., 2006).

Occupational therapists, who provide expert witness testimony, form their opinions based on the facts and act independent of the pressures of litigation. Occupational therapist expert witnesses should assist the court by providing objective, unbiased opinions on matters within their own expertise. They must remember when they serve the court as independent experts that they do not serve in as an advocate for either party (Dimond, 2010; Ministry of Justice, 2015; Winistorfer & Yarett Slater, 2016).

OTHER OCCUPATIONAL THERAPY ROLES

Occupational therapists working in home modifications can act as advocates for individuals. As an advocate, therapists speak on behalf of individuals with disabilities to promote the provision of supports or services (Tannous, 2000). In the United States, therapists might have to advocate on behalf of clients who need home modifications installed in rental units. The Fair Housing Amendments Act (1989) requires property owners to allow home modifications under certain circumstances. Therapists might have to inform property owners of their obligation to allow tenants to make modifications at their own cost. Further, should the owner refuse to allow the modifications, the therapist might advise the client to file an administrative complaint with the Department of Housing and Urban Development. Chapter 4 provides details about the role of the occupational therapist in relation to this legislation.

CONCLUSION

A range of issues contribute to the complexities of ethical, legal, and reporting practices. Occupational therapists need to familiarize themselves with these issues as described in this chapter and the resources they can use to guide them to make sound ethical and legal decisions. Through increased awareness of legal issues and measures to prevent medical errors, therapists can reduce their risk of exposure to malpractice liability (Ekelman Ranke & Moriarty, 1995). Best practice requires that therapists understand legal processes, such as court proceedings and investigation of malpractice cases, and use clear and concise documentation that comports with legal, ethical, and/or organizational requirements (Ekelman Ranke, 1998) as described in this chapter.

REFERENCES

Allen, S., Carlson, G., Ownsworth, T., & Strong, J. (2006). A framework for systematically improving occupational therapy expert options on work capacity. *Australian Journal of Occupational Therapy, 53*, 293-301.

American Occupational Therapy Association. (2010). Occupational therapy code of ethics and ethics standards. Retrieved from http://www.aota.org/Consumers/Ethics/39880.aspx

American Occupational Therapy Association. (2013). Guidelines for documentation of occupational therapy. *American Journal of Occupational Therapy, 67*(6), S32-S38. doi:10.5014/ajot.2013.67S32

American Occupational Therapy Association. (2014). Enforcement procedures for the occupational therapy code of ethics and ethics standards. *American Journal of Occupational Therapy, 68*(Suppl. 3), S3-S15. http://dx.doi.org/10.5014/ajot.2014.686S02

American Occupational Therapy Association. (2015a). Occupational therapy code of ethics (2015). Retrieved from https://www.aota.org/~/media/Corporate/Files/Practice/Ethics/Code-of-Ethics.pdf

American Occupational Therapy Association. (2015b). Standards for continuing competence. *American Journal of Occupational Therapy, 69*(Suppl. 3), 6913410055. http://dx.doi.org/10.5014/ajot.2015.696S16

Bailey, D. M., & Schwartzberg, S. L. (2003). *Ethical and legal dilemmas in occupational therapy* (2nd ed.). Philadelphia, PA: FA Davis.

Beauchamp, T. L., & Childress, J. F. (2001). *Principles of biomedical ethics* (5th ed.). New York, NY: Oxford University Press.

Beauchamp, T. L., & Childress, J. F. (2008). *Principles of biomedical ethics* (6th ed.). New York, NY: Oxford University Press.

Beauchamp, T. L., & Childress, J. F. (2013). *Principles of biomedical ethics* (7th ed.). New York, NY: Oxford University Press.

Bull, R. (1998). Making the most of an occupational therapist's skills in housing for people with disabilities. In R. Bull (Ed.), *Housing options for disabled people* (pp. 40-77). London, UK: Jessica Kingsley Publishers Incorporated.

Carson, D. (1990). Reports to court: A role in preventing decision error. *Journal of Social Welfare Law, 12*(3), 151-163.

Cheyney Brandt, L., & Yarett Slater, D. (2011). Ethical dimensions in occupational therapy. In K. Jacobs, & G. L. McCormack, (Eds.), *The occupational therapy manager* (5th ed., pp. 469-484). Bethesda, MD: AOTA Press.

Clark, M., Gray, M., & Mooney, J. (2013). New graduate occupational therapists' perceptions of near-misses and mistakes in the workplace. *International Journal of Health Care Quality Assurance, 26*(6), 564-576.

Costa, D. (2007). *Clinical supervision in occupational therapy: A guide for fieldwork and practice*. Bethesda, MD: AOTA Press.

Daubert v. Merrell Dow Pharmaceuticals, 509 U.S. 579 (1993).

DeMaio-Feldman, D. (1987). The occupational therapist as an expert witness. *American Journal of Occupational Therapy, 41*(9), 590-594.

Dimond, B.C. (2010). *Legal aspects of occupational therapy* (3rd ed.). Oxford, UK; Blackwell Publishing.

Dobbs, D. B. (2000). *The law of torts*. St. Paul, MN: West Group.

Doherty, R. F. (2014). Ethical practice. In B. A. Boyt Schell, G. Gillen, & M.E. Scaffa (Eds.), *Willard & Spackman's occupational therapy* (12th ed., pp. 413-424). Philadelphia, PA: Lippincott, Williams & Wilkins.

Ebright, P., Urden, L., Patterson, E., & Chalko, B. (2004). Themes surrounding novice near-miss and adverse-event situations. *Journal of Nursing Administration, 34*(11), 531-538.

Ekelman Ranke, B. A. (1998). Documentation in the age of litigation. *OT Practice*, 20-24.

Ekelman Ranke, B. A., & Moriarty, M. P. (1995). An overview of professional liability in occupational therapy. *American Journal of Occupational Therapy, 51*(8), 671-680.

Fair Housing Amendment Act, 24 C.F.R. § 100.204 (1989).

Federal Tort Claims Act. 28 U.S.C. §§ 1346(b),1402(b), 2401(b), 2671-2680 (1948).

Forrester, K., & Griffiths, D. (2015). *Essentials of law for health professionals* (4th ed.). Sydney, Australia: Harcourt.

Friedman, H. J., & Klee, C. H. (2001). The roles of experts and litigation support consultants in medical-legal claims. *Neurorehabilitation, 16*, 123-130.

Galt, K. A., & Paschal, K. A. (2011). *Foundations in patient safety for health professionals*. Sudbury, MA: Jones and Bartlette Publishers.

Hertfelder, S. D., & Crispen, C. (1990). *Private practice: Strategies for success*. Rockville, MD: AOTA Press.

Health Insurance Portability and Accountability Act (HIPAA) of 1996. P.L.104-191.

Institute of Medicine Committee on Quality of Health Care in America. (2001). *Crossing the quality chasm: A new health system for the 21st century*. Washington, DC: National Academies Press (US). (2001). Retrieved from https://www.ncbi.nlm.nih.gov/books/NBK222274/

Institute of Medicine. (2004). *Patient safety: Achieving a new standard for care*. Washington, DC: The National Academies Press.

Jarvis, H. (1983). Professional negligence and the occupational therapist. *Canadian Journal of Occupational Therapy, 50*(2), 45-48.

Jonsen, A. R., Siegler, M., & Winslade, W. J. (2010). *Clinical ethics: A practical approach to ethical decisions in clinical medicine* (7th ed.). Stamford, CT: Appleton & Lange.

Kinsella, E. A., Ji-Sun Park, A., Appiagyei, J., Chang, E., & Chow, D. (2008). Through the eyes of students: Ethical tensions in occupational therapy practice. *Canadian Journal of Occupational Therapy, 75*(3), 176-183.

Kohn, L., Corrigan, J., Donaldson, M., (Eds.). (2000). *To err Is human: Building a safer health system*. Washington, DC: Committee on Quality of Health Care in America, Institute of Medicine. National Academies Press.

Kornblau, B. L., & Burkhardt, A. (2012). *Ethics in rehabilitation: A clinical perspective* (2nd ed.). Thorofare, NJ: SLACK Incorporated.

Kornblau, B. L., & Starling, S. P. (2000). *Ethics in rehabilitation: A clinical perspective*. Thorofare, NJ: SLACK Incorporated.

Lohman, H., Mu, K., & Scheirton, L. (2003). Occupational therapists' perspectives on practice errors in geriatric practice settings. *Physical and Occupational Therapy in Geriatrics, 21*(4), 21-39.

Ministry of Justice. (2015). Practice direction 35—Experts and assessors. Retrieved from http://www.justice.gov.uk/courts/procedure-rules/civil/rules/part35/pd_part35

Mosey, A. C. (1981). *Occupational therapy: Configuration of a profession*. New York, NY: Raven Press.

Moyers, P. A., & Hinojosa, J. (2011). Continuing competency. In K. Jacobs & G. L. McCormack, (Eds.), *The occupational therapy manager* (pp. 485-502). Bethesda, MD: AOTA Press.

Mu, K., Lohman, H., & Scheirton, L. S. (2005). To err is human! Common practice errors and preventative strategies in occupational therapy. *OT Practice*, September 19, 13-17.

Mu, K., Lohman, H., & Scheirton, L. S. (2006). Occupational therapy practice errors in physical rehabilitation and geriatric settings: A national survey study. *American Journal of Occupational Therapy, 60*(3), 288-297.

Mu, K., Lohman, H., Scheirton, L. S., Cochran, T.M., Coppard, B.M., & Kokesh, S. R. (2011). Improving client safety: Strategies to prevent and reduce practice errors in occupational therapy. *American Journal of Occupational Therapy, 65*, e69-e76.

Neeman, R. L. (1979). Specialization: Legal and administrative implications. *American Journal of Occupational Therapy, 33*(2), 118-119.

Occupational Therapy Australia Limited. (2010). *Australian minimum competency standards for new graduate occupational therapists.* Melbourne, Australia: Author. Retrieved from https://www.otaus.com.au/sitebuilder/onlinestore/files/37/australiancompetencystandardsentryleveleleccopy.pdf

Sames, K. S. (2014). Documentation in practice. In E. Blesedell Crepeau, E. S. Cohn, & B. A. Boyt Schell (Eds.), *Willard & Spackman's occupational therapy* (12th ed., pp. 466-475). Philadelphia, PA: Lippincott, Williams & Wilkins.

Scheirton, L., Mu, K., & Lohman, H. (2003). Occupational therapists' responses to practice errors in physical rehabilitation settings. *American Journal of Occupational Therapy, 57*(3), 307-314.

Scheirton, L. S., Mu, K., Lohman, H., & Cochran, T. M. (2007). Error and patient safety: Ethical analysis of cases in occupational and physical therapy practice. *Medicine, Health Care, and Philosophy, 10*(3), 301-311.

Scott, R. W. (1997). *Promoting legal awareness in physical and occupational therapy.* St Louis, MO: Mosby.

Scott, R. W. (2009). *Promoting legal and ethical awareness: A primer for health professionals and patients.* St Louis, MO: Mosby.

Shannon, T. A. (Ed.). (1993). *Bioethics: Basic writings on the key ethical questions that surround the major modern biological possibilities and problems* (4th ed.). Mahwah, NJ: Paulist Press.

Simon, R. E. (2005). Standard-of-care testimony: Best practices or reasonable care? *Journal of the American Academy of Psychiatry and Law, 33*, 8-11.

Stallard, E. (2005). Legal influences on practice. In T. J. Clouston, L. Westcott, A. Turner, & N. Palastagna (Eds.), *Working in health and social care* (pp. 161-181). New York: Elsevier/Churchill Livingstone.

Tannous, C. (2000). Therapists as advocates for their clients with disabilities: A conflict of roles? *Australian Occupational Therapy Journal, 47*, 41-46.

Tymchuck, A. J. (1982). Strategies for resolving value dilemmas. *The American Behavioural Scientist, 26*, 159-175.

United States Department of Health and Human Services. (2015). Summary of the HIPAA Privacy Rule. Retrieved from https://www.hhs.gov/hipaa/for-professionals/privacy/laws-regulations/index.html

Van Denend, T., & Finlayson, M. (2007). Ethical decision making in clinical research: Application of CELIBATE. *American Journal of Occupational Therapy, 61*(1), 92-95.

Wagner, L. M., Capezuti, E., & Ouslander, J. G. (2006). Health care policy: Reporting near-miss events in nursing homes. *Nursing Outlook, 54*(2), 85.

Winistorfer, W. L. & Yarett Slater, D. (2016). The role of an occupational therapist as an expert Witness. American Occupational Therapy Association Advisory Opinion for the Ethics Commission. Retrieved from https://www.aota.org/-/media/corporate/files/practice/ethics/advisory/expert-witness.pdf

World Federation of Occupational Therapists. (2016). Code of ethics. Retrieved from http://www.wfot.org/ResourceCentre.aspx

Wright, M. (1985). Legal liability for occupational therapists. *Canadian Journal of Occupational Therapy, 52*(1), 16-19.

Yarett Slater, D., & American Occupational Therapy Association. (2016). *Reference guide to the occupational therapy code of ethics 2015.* Bethesda, MD: AOTA Press.

13

Evaluating Outcomes

Desleigh de Jonge, MPhil (OccThy), Grad Cert Soc Sci and
Melanie Hoyle, BSc (Psych), MOccThySt, Grad Dip Health Sci, Post Grad Dip Psych

Outcomes are the result of the occupational therapy process and describe what an intervention achieves (American Occupational Therapy Association [AOTA], 2014). Evaluating the outcomes of home modifications is an essential aspect of service delivery. At a basic level, a review of a modification immediately following installation allows evaluation of the quality and consistency of service delivery and an opportunity to determine the client's level of satisfaction with the nature and quality of service provided. An evaluation of outcomes can also confirm that the modifications fulfilled the service, client, and household goals and have not resulted in any unexpected negative outcomes. Over time, this accumulated information can inform practice and develop evidence of the efficacy of various environmental interventions. Further, specifically designed evaluations can establish the effectiveness of modification interventions for a client population. Systematic and consistent use of outcome measures allows the benefits and cost of environmental interventions to be established and compared with other interventions.

There is a range of measures used to evaluate the effectiveness of interventions, each with a focus and purpose. Some document the specific benefits of an intervention to an individual or group of clients, whereas others are designed to capture the outcomes of a service or the impact of an intervention on a sector of society. The purpose of the evaluation generally determines the type of outcome measures selected and used.

This chapter examines why it is important to evaluate environmental interventions and discusses some of the difficulties in undertaking an evaluation of outcomes and selecting suitable outcome measures. It describes the types and levels of evaluation used to establish the quality, effectiveness, value, and impact of home modifications and the implications for the measures used. This chapter also outlines the range of tools available and their contribution to evaluating home modifications and discusses the value of using tools with sound psychometric properties.

CHAPTER OBJECTIVES

By the end of this chapter, the reader will be able to:

✦ Discuss the importance of undertaking outcome evaluations

✦ Outline the issues in evaluating outcomes

✦ Describe the different purposes of outcome evaluations

✦ Identify a range of outcomes measures and distinguish their focus and purpose

Ainsworth, E., & de Jonge, D. *An Occupational Therapist's Guide to Home Modification Practice, Second Edition (pp. 283-311).*
© 2019 SLACK Incorporated.

+ Describe outcomes measures used in evaluating the outcomes of home modification interventions

+ Explain the psychometric properties to be considered when selecting outcome measures

IMPORTANCE OF EVALUATING OUTCOMES OF HOME MODIFICATION INTERVENTIONS

It has become increasingly important to evaluate the outcomes of interventions provided in health and social services, including home modification interventions. Concerns about rising costs of health and social care services, the aging population, inequities and inefficiencies in service delivery, practice errors, and inconsistencies in the quality of services has resulted in many governments establishing accreditation systems to monitor service provision. These systems require services to develop quality assurance frameworks to review, evaluate, and improve the quality and consistency of service delivery and outcomes (Arah, Westert, Hurst, & Klazinga, 2006). Further, a shift to a market-oriented approach to health and social care service delivery that places an emphasis on value for money demands interventions that are both clinically and cost-effective (Laver Fawcett, 2007). These and other developments require therapists to make a meaningful contribution to the review and documentation of processes and outcomes within the health and social care services in which they work. This necessitates that therapists develop measurement strategies to evaluate the effectiveness and impact of the interventions they provide.

Professionals also have an ethical responsibility to evaluate the outcomes of their interventions. All health professionals are bound by a code of ethics, which compels them to make a positive contribution to people's lives, beneficence, and ensures that they do not cause harm, nonmaleficence. Historically, professionals are always assumed to have behaved in an ethical manner. They were rarely questioned about their practice. However, practitioners are increasingly being required to account for decisions and to defend their actions. Occupational therapists are particularly vulnerable to complaints in home modification practice because they are working in a complex environment, and the consequences of an incident or accident resulting from a modification can be significant. Modifications have been found to be unacceptable, ineffective, and, in some cases,

harmful (Heywood, 2004a; Heywood & Turner, 2007). Evaluating outcomes enables therapists to confirm that they have improved the client's situation, thereby meeting their ethical responsibilities and reducing the likelihood of legal action. Outcome evaluation also provides individual therapists and services with feedback that can be used to improve service delivery and increase effectiveness. This information is essential for informing home modification practice and refining the design of future environmental interventions.

Client-centered practice also highlights the importance of outcome evaluation. A client-centered approach requires therapists to provide clients with sufficient information about interventions to make informed decisions. Clients are increasingly becoming well informed and frequently request information on the effectiveness of interventions (DeRuyter, 2001). Consequently, they are less likely to rely solely on professional expertise and anecdotal evidence when making decisions involving expensive changes to their homes. Documenting outcomes assists therapists to clearly communicate the effectiveness of various interventions to clients. Client-centered practice also requires therapists to address clients' priorities and goals. Outcome evaluation affords therapists an opportunity to confirm that interventions have met clients' goals and have not resulted in any unexpected issues.

The demand for evidence-based practice has also heightened the need for outcome evaluation (Dunn, 2017; Laver Fawcett, 2007). Though occupational therapists currently base their modification recommendations on strong theoretical knowledge and experience (Luebben & Royeen, 2005), the profession has yet to establish a body of research to inform and refine home modification practice. In an increasingly competitive funding environment, the profession needs to establish evidence on the efficacy of home modifications and build a body of knowledge on the relative effectiveness of various interventions to understand how, what, when, where, and why particular interventions are most effective.

Funding for health and social care services has become increasingly dependent on establishing the cost-effectiveness of interventions. Services are likely to receive funding only if they can demonstrate that their interventions are cost-effective. To date, the effectiveness of home modification has been determined using global measures, such as morbidity, mortality, and quality of life. While these benefits are important, there has been little attention paid to the benefits gained from investing in people's well-being, safety, activity engagement, and participation in the home and community. Information gathered by therapists on the broad benefits of home modifications will assist in identifying the value of these interventions to clients and to the society and will promote environmental interventions as an investment rather than a discretionary cost (Frisch, 2000; Hurstfield, Parashar, & Schofield, 2007).

ISSUES IN EVALUATING OUTCOMES

Evaluating the outcomes of home modifications presents several challenges. Combining to increase the complicated nature of this task are complexities in the way home modification services are delivered, the unique approach and experience of each therapist providing advice, the diversity of people and households undertaking home modifications, and the variety of housing forms being modified.

Home modifications are generally provided in conjunction with a number of other interventions, such as assistive technologies, education and training, and personal care. Consequently, it might be difficult to ascertain the degree to which the modifications are responsible for the outcomes achieved. Service delivery is diverse and fragmented, with modifications being provided within several systems with very different briefs (e.g., health, home, and social care, housing, and not-for-profit organizations; Jones, de Jonge, & Phillips, 2008). There is immense variation across services in terms of the nature of information collected and solutions provided. This makes it difficult to collate and meaningfully analyze any information that might be collected. Change is best measured by using consistent and standardized measures before and after an intervention. Currently, there are few standardized tools that adequately measure changes resulting from modifications, and these are not routinely used.

To date, therapists have been reluctant to engage in outcome measurement in home modification practice. This is largely because service managers and funders have not deemed it necessary and have not allocated time and payment for follow-up and evaluation. Consequently, little is known about the usefulness of modifications once installed. Home modifications, as with assistive devices, are regarded as a practical intervention. It is assumed that once the problem has been appropriately identified and a solution put in place, the problem has been solved and there is no need to evaluate the impact or effectiveness of the intervention. Further, therapists experience difficulties in evaluating outcomes. They often have limited time and find it easier and more informative to use non-standardized measures, such as observation and informal client feedback

(Bowman, 2006). Therapists have also reported difficulty in identifying what and how to measure the outcomes of occupational therapy interventions (Bowman, 2006). Limited knowledge of outcomes measures and skill in the use of standardized measures also hampers the evaluation of outcomes (Bowman, 2006).

Outcome evaluation is further complicated by the heterogeneity of the clients receiving home modifications, the nature and extent of their impairments, the range of individualized goals, and the variety of interventions used. This variation makes it difficult to identify measures capable of addressing the breadth and diversity in outcomes sought. The complexity of the person-environment-occupation transaction and the home environment also makes it difficult to define the expected outcomes. Further, people's needs and expectations change over time, and these might shift during the process of exploring needs and options. Expectations also influence perceptions of outcomes. The goals people begin with might not be the same as the goals they have at the end of the process, after they have learned what is possible. When developing environmental interventions, people often must make compromises as a result of the availability of products, the suitability of the design to the existing dwelling, as well as the costs involved. Given their original expectations, these concessions can result in clients having limited appreciation of the effectiveness of the modification.

Poor outcomes can result from any number of reasons other than the suitability of the recommendation, namely, changes in the person's health or social situation since the modification, disruptions experienced during the modification process, or unexpected expenses resulting from the work or quality of the workmanship or quality of the product installed. There are also variables, such as a past negative experience or an unsupportive household, that might also contribute to the perceived failure of an intervention (Gelderblom & De Witte, 2002). Perception of effectiveness can sometimes differ from actual performance and separating these and other issues can be a challenge when evaluating outcomes.

PURPOSES OF OUTCOME EVALUATION

Despite the complexities inherent in assessing outcomes, it is essential to evaluate the impact and consequences of modifications. Traditionally, occupational therapists have thought about evaluation predominantly in terms of determining an individual's needs. As noted in Chapter 6, therapists use a range of formal and informal evaluation strategies to understand clients' abilities and occupational performance difficulties, and they use information gained from these evaluations to develop interventions. However, evaluating and recording the consequences of occupational therapy interventions is critical to the ongoing improvement of service delivery, ensuring good outcomes for clients, "building a body of evidence to support practice" (Sells, 2005), and establishing the value or cost-effectiveness of home modifications. To be successfully undertaken, it is important to first understand the purpose of the evaluation (Barak & Duncan, 2006) because this determines its aim and focus.

An outcome evaluation can be focused on the following:

+ Monitoring the quality and consistency of service provision

+ Determining whether service, client, or therapist goals have been met

+ Building a body of knowledge or evidence

+ Demonstrating the efficiency and value of interventions

Monitoring Service Provision

Many services have some form of quality assurance process in place to ensure the ongoing quality and consistency of service delivery. This level of evaluation is generally concerned with establishing whether the service is responding to and meeting the expectations of the client group in terms of what the service delivers and how it is delivered.

Organizations generally want to confirm that the service has been delivered in an efficient and effective manner and that all clients are satisfied with the timing, level and quality of service. Service managers generally monitor the ongoing responsiveness and quality of service provision using a quality assurance framework. This framework can involve the routine collection of information about the timing of service events or periodic survey of service recipients. Undertaking post modification evaluations can assess the quality of the completed works with a view to evaluating the workmanship of the contractor and confirming that the work was carried out according to the recommendations and the appropriate building legislation, codes and standards.

The main indicators of a quality home modification service are:

+ A timely response

+ Clients feel that they are treated respectfully and are consulted throughout the home modification process

+ Clients have a clear understanding of the process and the responsibilities of the stakeholders involved

+ Clients are satisfied with the service and outcome

+ Clients are satisfied with the quality of the modification

+ Work has been completed successfully and in accordance with recommendations and relevant legislation, codes and standards

+ The modification meets performance expectations in terms of reliability, maintenance, and durability (Rossi, Lipsey, & Freeman, 2004)

Generally, therapists can monitor these outcomes through the following:

+ Reviews of documentation and databases—Tracking service events from date of referral and date of completion

+ Telephone surveys and questionnaires—Seeking clients' feedback on their satisfaction with the service and the modification, and information about the impact of the modification on their day to day lives

+ Auditing the modification work—Designed to evaluate the workmanship of the installation and its compliance with the recommendations and relevant legislation, codes and standards

Therapists can assist in tracking the timing of activities associated with the home modification and developing survey questions to capture the service and outcome quality indicators that reflect the priorities of occupational therapists and their clients. For example, therapists might be interested in knowing the time taken to complete modification work so they can advise clients of the likely timing of service events. They might also wish to know whether the work resulted in any disruptions to daily routines in the household, so that they can assist clients to prepare for modification work. Therapists would be particularly interested in finding out whether the work was completed according to their recommendations and reasons for any incongruence. This feedback will assist them to understand how well their scope of works and concept drawings were interpreted and the factors that prevented recommendations from being implemented.

By evaluating the accessibility, adequacy, appropriateness, and sustainability of the program, occupational therapists can also assist service managers with a broader view of the effectiveness and efficiency of services. For example, therapists can contribute to the ongoing development of the service by examining whether the program is:

+ Reaching everyone with a home modification need and meeting their need/s

+ Efficient in the delivery of services

+ Providing all the environmental interventions that are required

+ Supplying the most effective modifications to address identified barriers and issues

+ Building adequate structures, resources, and capacity to support the program, and the knowledge and skills of its employees' long term

By reviewing the demographic data of the population in the area, waiting lists for home modifications services, and hospital admissions and discharge data, therapists can identify people at risk who may benefit from an environmental intervention. A review of the service database will also provide information about the timeliness of response times to those requests. By analyzing referral rates and the range of modifications provided, therapists can understand the nature of services provided and where resources need to be invested. This information can also be compared with service events in a similar service in another region so that differences can be identified and analyzed. Information gathered on the return rate of clients and the nature of return requests provides an indication of the effectiveness of previous service events. Finally, information gathered in this type of evaluation can be used to identify where the system requires improvement. These data provide a sound foundation for justifying the development of service structures and resources and building capacity within the system by improving staff knowledge and skills.

Determining Whether Goals Have Been Met

While it is important to ensure that the quality of home modification services is consistent, it is equally important to establish that services are making a positive contribution to the client's and family's ability to carry out activities in the home, and that the environmental interventions have not resulted in any unexpected or undesirable outcomes.

This type of evaluation ensures that interventions are targeted appropriately. Most home modification services have broad goals of promoting the health, safety, independence, quality of life, home and community participation, and well-being of their clients. Services are generally interested in determining whether the modifications have addressed health and safety issues and improved the person's independence and quality of life. It is also important at this time to affirm that the environmental interventions have not created any additional safety risks for the client or other householders or any challenges to their independence and well-being.

Occupational therapists and their clients are generally focused on reducing occupational performance difficulties and concerns in everyday activities and increasing participation in the home and community. Clients usually have issues they want addressed, and a post modification evaluation provides the therapist with an opportunity to confirm that the client's specific concerns and other occupational performance difficulties have been adequately resolved. At this point, the therapist might also want to confirm that the client is using the modification successfully and that the home environment (i.e., the physical, personal, social temporal, occupational, and societal dimension of the home) has not been unduly disrupted by the environmental changes.

Routine evaluation of home modification outcomes allows services and therapists to monitor the effectiveness of environmental interventions for individuals and groups of clients as well as their impact on other householders, and care givers. The main indicators that the interventions have been effective in meeting the goals of the client, and significant others, are that they:

+ Feel their goals and priorities were adequately addressed

+ Are using the solution as intended without adverse effects

+ Have maintained or improved with respect to their health and safety, and have reduced the risk of incident, accident, or injury

+ Are not experiencing any additional risk or difficulties resulting from the modification

+ Have maintained or increased their independence

+ Experience less difficulty in performing activities in the home and community

+ Are satisfied with their performance of activities in the home and community

+ Have maintained or increased engagement in activities in the home and community

+ Do not feel that the home environment, and the activities of the household, have been adversely affected by the modification

If the therapist can follow up with clients, these outcomes are generally monitored through informal evaluation strategies, such as informal interview or observation. Routine follow-up is essential to allow therapists to confirm that their recommendations have been useful in meeting the service, therapist, and client goals. Follow-up can also include the use of structured and standardized measures to assist in determining the extent to which the intended outcomes have been achieved. For example:

+ Telephone surveys/questionnaires seeking clients' feedback on their level of satisfaction with the service and modification and how well it has maintained or improved their health, safety, independence, and quality of life in the home and community

+ Structured observation of the client's occupational performance and of obstacles and risks in the environment

+ Standardized outcome measures related to goal attainment, occupational performance and participation, or the accessibility, safety, and quality of the home and community environment. Global measures of quality of life and well-being may be of interest to the service

Building a Body of Evidence

There is a growing requirement for therapists to use evidence-based interventions. Evidence has been derived from a combination of clinical expertise and knowledge and relevant published research (Cohen & Kearney, 2005; Sackett, Rosenberg, Gray, Haynes, & Richardson, 1996). Traditionally, therapists accumulated expertise and knowledge through clinical experience; however, this is not a very effective way for a profession to build a body of knowledge. Further, when a profession does not have a well-established body of evidence, clients can be repeatedly subjected to uninformed advice from novice therapists. Because there is limited research to support practice in this area, it is essential that therapists establish a mechanism for gathering evidence on the effectiveness of home medication interventions.

Therapists generate volumes of detailed data in clinical practice, which can be used as evidence if therapists are systematic in collecting and organizing evaluation data (Cohen & Kearney, 2005). For easy retrieval of this valuable information, individual data can be stored in databases with fields for client demographics (i.e., age, gender, health condition, medications), specific goals and occupational performance issues, modifications provided, outcomes achieved, and unexpected or unintended events and consequences (Cohen & Kearney, 2005). With the accumulation of client information and judicious use of outcome measures, occupational therapists can build a body of evidence to support their home modification practice.

To establish evidence, therapists need information on the following:

+ The number and demographics of people requiring home modifications, the nature of issues they encounter in the home, and the type of modifications undertaken

+ The outcomes of modifications and the extent to which they met client goals and addressed difficulties identified in the home and community

+ The outcomes of specific home modifications in various situations

+ Whether there were any unexpected or unintended consequences of environmental interventions

By systematically evaluating the outcomes of various environmental interventions with a range of clients, therapists can gather information on where and when various interventions are most effective. They can then make comparisons between alternative options, so they can generate a body of knowledge about the relative effectiveness of various modifications in a range of situations.

Evidence-based practice also requires therapists to review the literature for research on environmental interventions and their effectiveness. To date, research on home modifications has been patchy, unsystematic, and variable in quality (Heywood & Awang, 2011; Jones et al., 2008). In addition, many research questions critical to informing home modification practice remain unanswered (Gitlin, 2003). There have been some studies detailing the need and demand for modifications; environmental difficulties experienced by various client groups in the home; the effectiveness of environmental interventions in terms of health, safety, and independence; and their impact on the client's well-being and the home environment. Specific evaluations of the effectiveness of modifications, especially in relation to alternative options, are less prevalent. More detailed data collection by therapists regarding the outcomes of home modification interventions and more focused, systematic research on the effectiveness of specific interventions would greatly assist in informing practice in this area (Heywood & Awang, 2011).

The Efficacy and Value of Environmental Interventions

Therapists employ a wide variety of interventions, such as home modifications, assistive devices, and in-home care services, to address a range of difficulties experienced by older people and people with disabilities in the home. While these multifactorial interventions have been found to produce savings to health and social care (Heywood & Turner, 2007), little is known about the specific cost-benefits of home modifications (Fänge & Iwarsson, 2007; Heywood & Turner, 2007). Home modifications, in combination with interventions previously mentioned, have been found to reduce the cost of care and improve the outcomes for clients (Heywood & Turner, 2007), but more information is required on the cost-effectiveness of modifications specifically and whether some environmental interventions are more cost-effective than others and in which circumstances (Pynoos, Rose, Rubenstein, Choi, & Sabata, 2006).

Cost-effectiveness analysis (CEA) and cost-benefit analysis (CBA) are formal methods for comparing the costs and consequences of an intervention to determine whether the intervention is worth doing (Rossi et al., 2004). CEA measures benefit in terms of an outcome (e.g., health outcomes, quality-adjusted life years), whereas CBA calculates benefit in terms of money (e.g., dollar outlays averted [value of reductions in re-admissions to hospitals] and value of life years saved).

CEA and CBA need to:

+ Define the intervention under investigation
+ Identify relevant costs
+ Identify relevant effects and benefits
+ Measure costs (direct and indirect)
+ Measure effects and calculate benefits for individuals and the community at large (Rossi et al., 2004)

Once again, therapists can provide input into identifying the direct and indirect costs of environmental interventions and identifying and measuring the relevant effects or benefits of home modifications. Cost considerations include the cost of the investment, maintenance, and services (Andrich & Caracciolo, 2007). For home modifications, these costs are likely to be:

+ The cost of purchasing the products
+ The cost of installation

+ Ongoing maintenance, repair, servicing, running costs, and replacement costs over a specified period
+ Additional expenses incurred during the work (e.g., replacing electrical wiring to bring it up to the standard expected by legislation)
+ Personal support required to use the modification effectively

The benefits of interventions are generally discussed in terms of the benefits to society. For example, the benefit of home modifications is often conceptualized in terms of savings made from reduction of care costs or life years saved. It is in the interests of occupational therapists to contribute to identifying the cost-benefits to society; however, therapists are most likely to be able to identify the cost-benefits to the client and/or caregivers in terms of maintenance of, or increase in, health, safety, independence, and participation in home and community activities. The benefits of home modification interventions could be identified as:

+ Reduced risk of incident or accident resulting in injury
+ Reduced reliance on formal and informal supports
+ Maintenance of, or increase in, health and independence
+ Reduced difficulty in performing activities in the home and community
+ Maintenance of, or increase in, engagement in activities in the home and community
+ Maintenance of, or improvement in, satisfaction with performance of activities in the home and community
+ Maintenance of, or improvement in, quality of life

By routinely collecting information on the outcomes of home modifications for each client, therapists can ensure that the benefits for clients (and their caregivers) can be used in CEA and CBA analyses. These outcomes are preferable to the global measures commonly used in these analyses because they acknowledge the impact of these interventions for the clients rather than their general benefit to society. This data will assist in-home modifications being reconceptualized as an investment rather than a discretionary cost or as a substitute for care (Frisch, 2000; Hurstfield et al., 2007).

TRADITIONAL APPROACHES TO MEASURING HOME MODIFICATION OUTCOMES

As discussed earlier in this chapter, there are a number of clear reasons why home modification outcomes need to be evaluated. The question now remains: What are the best ways for this evaluation to happen? To date, most of the evaluations of home modifications have focused on the impact and cost-benefits of environmental interventions, which have been measured in terms of reduced injuries, morbidity and mortality, and the cost of ongoing care. For example, one randomized controlled trial involving 90 frail, elderly, home-based people found that members of the intervention group, who were systematically provided with assistive technologies and environmental interventions, were found to decline at a slower rate, experiencing reduced morbidity, than the control group and had reduced institutional and in-home personal care costs (Mann, Ottenbacher, Fraas, Tomita, & Granger, 1999). Another study found that home modifications reduced the hours of unpaid help for wheelchair users who live alone (Allen, Resnik, & Roy, 2006). Other studies have found that home modifications, in combination with other interventions, reduce falls (Gillespie et al., 2003; Nikolaus & Bach, 2003) and other injuries (Plautz, Beck, Selmar, & Radetsky, 1996). A retrospective study on the costs of home modifications and assistive technologies, using seven detailed case studies, found substantial savings resulting from the interventions (Andrich, Ferrario, & Moi, 1998). This information is useful to funders and policymakers when justifying funding for environmental interventions, however, it provides only indirect evidence of the efficacy of these interventions and does not inform day-to-day clinical practice.

Whilst the outcomes of health conditions and interventions have traditionally relied on morbidity and mortality data, new understandings of health have resulted in a shift in focus to evaluating the impact on the individual's day-to-day functioning (World Health Organization [WHO], 2002). The introduction of the *International Classification of Functioning, Disability and Health* (ICF; WHO, 2001) saw the concept of health expand from an absence of illness to physical, mental, and social well-being (AOTA, 2014). The focus of health, education and community care systems has extended beyond remediating impairments to being interested in function, well-being, and quality of life (Law, Baum, & Dunn, 2017). Disability is no longer viewed as simply a personal problem, directly caused by disease, trauma, or health conditions, but also as resulting from barriers in the environment (WHO, 2002). The ICF has extended the concept of function to encompass engagement in activities and involvement in life (participation), which are important determinants of health (WHO, 2002). This framework recognizes the dynamic interaction between the person and contextual factors (Jette & Haley, 2005). Over the last decade, it has informed outcomes evaluation practices, and has resulted in the growth in number of measures focused on activity engagement, participation, and the environment.

This shift in the focus aligns well with the broad and overarching outcome of occupational therapy services, identified by the Occupational Therapy Practice Framework as "achieving health, well-being, and participation in life through engagement in occupation" (AOTA, 2014). Occupation or the daily activities that people engage in are described as "personal activities that individuals choose or need to engage in and the ways in which each individual actually experiences them" (Crepeau, Schell, Gillen, & Scaffa, 2014). Occupational therapy models, such as the person-environment-occupation transactional models, also recognize the role of the environment in occupational performance; however, few outcome measures that capture the person-environment-occupation transaction and are responsive to changes, are available for use.

With the scope of occupational therapy practice in mind, a review of research into home modification interventions for adults and older people was undertaken to determine its efficacy in supporting home and community participation. This systematic review of 36 studies found strong evidence for home modification interventions, both single and multicomponent interventions, to improve function for people with a variety of health conditions and the risk of falls for older adults and moderate evidence for reducing caregiver demand for people with dementia (Stark, Keglovits, Arbesman, & Lieberman, 2017). A wide range of outcome measures was used across the studies (Table 13-1), with most studies examining the impact of modifications on function and independence in personal and instrumental activities of daily living (IADL).

Existing Measures

An extensive range of outcome measures has been developed, each with a focus (see Table 6-2 for complete list). They come in a variety of formats: self-administered questionnaires and interviewer-administered telephone interviews, face-to-face interviews, or computerized/web-based interviews with the client or a proxy, such as a family member (Barak & Duncan, 2006). In addition, several observational assessments have been developed to be undertaken by a trained assessor.

Table 13-1. Outcomes Measures Used in Home Modification Research

TYPE OF OUTCOME	MEASURE/TOOL
Health status	Hospital admission and injury rates
	Mortality
Injuries and falls	Abbreviated Injury Scale
	Self-report
Pain	Functional Status Index
Self-efficacy	Fear of falling
	Self-efficacy and Upset Likert scales
	Sense of Competence Questionnaire
Function	Craig Handicap Assessment
	Multnomah Community Ability Scale
	Occupational Therapy Functional Assessment Compilation
	Self-report
	Sickness Impact Profile: Mobility
	Social and Occupational Functioning Scale
ADL and IADL	Barberger Gateau et al. IADL
	Barthel Index, Klein-Bell, ADL Staircase—Revised
	Deterioration of Daily Activities in Dementia
	Disability Rating Index (ADL/IADL Performance)
	Frenchay Activities Index
	Functional Independence Measure (FIM)
	Groningen Activity Restriction Scale
	Katz Index of Independence in Activities of Daily Living
	Lawton-Brody Questionnaire
	Older Americans Resources and Services
	Self-report and caregiver report
Occupational performance	Assessment of Motor and Process Skills (AMPS)
	Canadian Occupational Performance Measure (COPM)
	Client Clinical Assessment Protocol (C-CAP): Part I Self-Report
Participation	Social Participation
Quality of Life	EuroQual
	WHO Quality of Life Instrument—BREF
Caregiver burden	Caregiver Mastery Index, Task Management Strategy Index
	Caregiver (reaction/upset) scales
	Caregiver-reported information including scores on the affect and activity
	Limitation-Alzheimer's Disease Assessment
	Zarit Burden Interview Memory and Behavior Problem Checklist
Environmental assessments	Dedicated environmental hazards checklist
	Environmental FIM
	Home Safety Assessment
	Westmead Home Safety Assessment, Self-Report of Hazards
	Usability in my Home Instrument (UIMH)

Adapted from Stark, S., Keglovits, M., Arbesman, M., & Lieberman, D. (2017). Effect of home modification interventions on the participation of community-dwelling adults with health conditions: A systematic review. *American Journal of Occupational Therapy, 71*(2), 7102290010p1-11A.

Whilst measurement has traditionally focused on evaluating body structure and functions; with the introduction of the ICF, there has been an increased number of tools developed to examine activity performance and participation and aspects of the environment. In home modification practice, therapists are most interested in measuring the impact of the intervention on:

+ The person's, or caregiver's, physical and mental health and well-being

+ Occupational performance and participation

+ Aspects of the home environment and the person's experience of home

Measures of Physical and Mental Health

Modifications are designed to reduce the environmental "press" placed on people within and around the home. Environmental interventions can reduce dependence as well as physical and mental stress by decreasing physical or cognitive effort or the pain and difficulty when completing or supporting someone to complete activities. For some people, especially those who spend a lot of time at home or have mental health vulnerabilities, the general ambiance of the home can also affect their mood or mental health. In addition, modifications can increase an individual's sense of safety and security, self-efficacy, general well-being, and quality of life (Jones et al., 2008).

Dependence, or independence, in personal ADL and IADL can be assessed using a range of tools such as the Modified Barthel Index (MBI; Shah, Vanclay, & Cooper, 1989), FIM (Uniform Data System for Medical Rehabilitation [UDSMR], 1997, 2009), FIM for Children (Msall et al., 1994), Katz Index of Activities of Daily Living (Katz, Ford, Moskowitz, Jackson, & Jaffe, 1963), ADL Staircase (Sonn & Hulter-Åsberg, 1991) and the ADL Staircase—Revised (Iwarsson & Isacsson, 1997). These assessments focus on determining the level of dependence/independence across a range of daily activities for the purposes of screening or measuring outcomes. However, these global measures can have ceiling effects and are not sensitive to changes to the quality of performance such as the effort involved, or difficulties experienced (Gitlin, 2003) that result from environmental interventions. The ADL Staircase is designed as a hierarchical scale and has been used in combination with self-rated difficulty to evaluate the effectiveness of home modifications (Ekström, Schmidt, & Iwarsson, 2016; Fänge & Iwarsson, 2005a; Iwarsson, Horstmann, & Sonn, 2009). It has been found to have an acceptable construct validity and reliability (in terms of internal consistency) for most age groups

however, seems to be most valid and reliable for people aged 18 to 29 and 75 to 89 years (Jakobsson, 2008).

Traditional measures of functional independence, such as the FIM (UDSMR, 1997, 2009), have become benchmarks in outcome measurement in hospital settings, because they allow comparisons across client groups and care settings. Many independence measures developed in the context of rehabilitation in the 1960s and 1970s have been useful in informing and evaluating care by providing information on people's ability to perform the basic ADL independently (Jette & Haley, 2005). However, the modest goals of inpatient rehabilitation at that time do not reflect current professional, client, and societal expectations of community-based services and interventions (Jette & Haley, 2005). Though the values, beliefs, and principles underlying the development of these tools are not always stated explicitly, they are generally embedded in the measure's conceptual foundation, item inclusion, standardization, and scale design (Klein, Barlow, & Hollis, 2008). The purpose of these tools is not well suited to a home modification evaluation. Independence has not been found to be an effective measure of an individual's ability in daily life or of the impact of modifications (Johansson, Lilja, Petersson, & Borell, 2007; Petersson, Lilja, Hammel, & Kottorp, 2008). In addition, generic scales, such as the FIM, are not very responsive to the impact of environmental adaptations (Klein et al., 2008). Though ADL assessment has historically been a key aspect of occupational therapy practice, the scores on many of these tools are negatively affected by the use of a modification or device and are not sufficiently sensitive to measure changes in performance, such as reduced effort or difficulty. Outcome measures developed within a traditional medical framework are not designed to capture the complexities of the person-environment interaction (Gitlin, 2003) and do not reflect a contemporary understanding of health and well-being.

There are also several standardized self-report measures that evaluate perceived efficacy and pain. Self-efficacy questionnaires have been found to be useful in examining people's confidence in various activities. The Falls Efficacy Scale (Tinetti, Richman, & Powell, 1990) was modified by Sanford and colleagues (2006) to evaluate people's confidence in performing 10 household activities on a scale of 1 (not confident at all) to 10 (completely confident). Questions in the Falls Efficacy Scale, such as, "How confident are you in performing the following activities without falling?" were adapted by removing the words "without falling" from the end of each question. Activities included in the measure were getting dressed and undressed, cleaning the house, preparing simple meals, bathing, shopping, going up and down stairs, reaching into cabinets or cupboards, getting in and out of a chair, walking around the neighborhood, and hurrying to answer the phone.

Pain experienced during activities can be evaluated using the dedicated pain questionnaires and various verbal, visual, and picture pain-rating scales (Patterson, Jensen, & Engel-Knowles, 2002). Common pain measures include the McGill Pain Questionnaire (Melzack, 1975) and the Faces Pain Scale (Bieri, Reeve, Champion, Addicoat, & Ziegler, 1990). Tools have also been developed to evaluate the level of burden or stress on caregivers in terms of their physical and mental health, disruption to family life, and financial difficulties (Gupta, 2008). The Caregiver Strain Index (Robinson, 1983) is brief and easily administered and is one of the most commonly used scales for caregiver burden (Post, Festen, van de Port, & Visser-Meily, 2007). This tool contains 13 statements related to strain experienced by caregivers. If the caregiver agrees with seven or more statements, he or she is experiencing a high level of burden (Robinson, 1983). The Perceived Change Index has also been used to examine the impact of home modification and related interventions on caregiver well-being (Gitlin, Hauck, Winter, Dennis, & Schulz, 2006). This is a 13-item scale, including, for example, change in affect, ability to manage difficult behaviors, and somatic feelings (fatigue). The caregiver rates how often in the past month things have become worse or improved, using a 5-point Likert scale (Gitlin et al., 2006). Measures of mood states, such as the Beck Depression Inventory II (Beck, Ward, Mendelson, Mock, & Erbaugh, 1961), might also be useful in measuring changes in mood following modifications to the home. It is important, however, when using these generic measures to assess mental well-being, to be aware of the many other factors that can contribute to fluctuations in mood.

As discussed previously, global measures of quality of life and well-being have become increasingly popular in health and social settings when measuring and comparing the impact of various interventions. There are several quality-of-life measures available. One of the most popular is the Short Form 36 (Ware, Snow, Kosinski, & Gandek, 1993), a self-report survey comprising 36 questions. The scale measures eight dimensions—namely, vitality, physical functioning, bodily pain, general health perceptions, physical role functioning, emotional role functioning, social role functioning, and mental health. It provides functional health and well-being scores as well as psychometrically based physical and mental health summary measures and a preference-based health utility index (Ware & Sherbourne, 1992). However, it is important to be aware that quality-of-life measures are not without criticism. Some consider quality of life to be a dynamic construct, the reference value of which might not remain constant (Allison, Locker, & Feine, 1997; Carr, Gibson, & Robinson, 2001). People's expectations can have an impact on their perceptions of quality of life. Those with high expectations find changes in the environment to have less of an impact than those with low expectations. In addition, this construct has been linked to personality (DeNeve, 1999) and core affects (Davern, Cummins, & Stokes, 2007), thus making measures of quality of life vulnerable to individual interpretations of life events.

Quality of life has also been used to evaluate the impact of interventions, with modifications or adaptations being found to have a positive impact on people's quality of life (Andrich et al., 1998; Heywood, 2001). As a global measure, quality-of-life measures are relatively inexpensive to administer and are therefore popular in public health and social care settings to evaluation the impact of services generally. Quality-of-life outcomes are also used in the research community (Douglas, Swanson, Gee, & Bellamy, 2005; Haigh et al., 2001) and in economic analyses to review the impact of interventions and compare the cost-effectiveness of various interventions. This information is then used to inform policy, which in turn influences the allocation of funding. Although there are numerous quality-of-life measures available, they are not routinely used in clinical settings to evaluate client outcomes (Douglas et al., 2005). These measures provide a mechanism for reviewing the indirect benefits of home modifications and associated interventions; however, they do little to confirm that the client, therapist, and service goals have been addressed. Further, they do not inform therapists about the effectiveness of specific modifications for clients.

Measures of Occupational Performance and Participation

Occupational therapists need to use valid and reliable measures of occupational performance and participation if they are to establish the efficacy of their interventions (Law et al., 2017). It is believed that modifications enable people to be more independent in daily activities and to increase their participation in the home and the community. There are an ever-growing number of tools available that measure occupational performance and participation.

Some tools, such as the COPM (Law et al., 1998, 2014), are used to gain an understanding of the client's current occupational performance goals and perceptions of performance. This individualized evaluation tool uses a semi-structured interview to identify specific problems in occupational performance areas, such as self-care, work, and leisure. It allows clients to rate the importance of each problem on a scale of 1 (not important) to 10 (very important) and their perceptions of their current level of performance and satisfaction with their performance are rated on scales of 1 (unable to perform, not satisfied) to 10 (able to perform, extremely satisfied). This tool can then be used to assess changes in their perceptions following an environmental intervention. The COPM has been translated into 30 languages and is used with a variety of client groups in practice and in outcomes research over the last decade (Carswell et al., 2004; McColl, & Pollock, 2017). It has been used in over 45 studies and demonstrated excellent psychometric properties (McColl, & Pollock, 2017) More specifically, several studies have used it to determine the impact of rehabilitation (Donnelly et al., 2004), equipment and adaptation service (Davis & Rodd, 2014), and in-home modifications (Stark, 2004). The COPM has been found to be sensitive to changes that result from home modifications and to provide information that cannot be obtained from less individualized measures (Dedding, Cardol, Eyssen, Dekker, & Beelen, 2004; McColl, & Pollock, 2017). When compared with other instruments, the COPM is identified as an accurate measure of perceived changes in occupational performance (Eyssen et al., 2011; Schultz-Krohn, 2014). Test-retest reliability at 1- to 2-week intervals ranges from 0.63 to 0.89 for performance and 0.76 to 0.88 for satisfaction (Schultz-Krohn, 2014). A systematic review of the COPM undertaken by Parker and Sykes (2006) demonstrates the value of the COPM in promoting client-centered practice and evaluating occupational performance outcomes.

Though self-report measures provide a perception of ability, they do not provide therapists with objective or detailed information on the quality of performance. An objective measure of the effort involved in completing activities might be determined by taking the person's pulse rate or recording the time taken to perform tasks. The quality of performance can be identified and recorded using some ADL and IADL assessments. For example, tools, such as the AMPS (Fisher, 1995; Fisher & Jones, 2011a, 2011b), and the Performance Assessment of Self-Care Skills (PASS; Chisholm, Toto, Raina, Holm, & Rogers, 2014; Rogers & Holm, 1994) allow therapists to standardize their observations of occupational performance with people undertaking relevant tasks in the usual way in their own environment. These tools might also

be useful in identifying changes in the safety and quality of performance of everyday activities once the environment has been modified. Changes in performance might be noted if environmental barriers are removed or facilitators introduced. For example, reduced physical demands might be observed in the showering task when a step into the shower is removed and a grab rail is installed; and decreased cognitive demands might be observed during a coffee-making task when the required items are moved and stored within the person's field of vision.

The AMPS is a performance based assessment that allows trained therapists to rate 16 motor and 20 process skills when clients undertake activities selected from a menu of over 50 ADL and IADL tasks. The AMPS demonstrates high test-retest and intra-rater reliability and has established validity across age, culture, ethnic and diagnostic groups and between genders in multiple studies (Furphy & Stav, 2014). Although the AMPS requires specialist training and standardized setup, it has an established history of item response theory research studies and provides therapists with access to databases of reference groups for client comparisons (Holm & Rogers, 2017).

The home, and clinic, version of the PASS includes 26 core tasks, specifically: 5 functional mobility, 3 personal self-care, 18 IADL tasks (14 with cognitive emphasis and 4 with physical emphasis). As a standardized tool, it provides clear description of the required assessment conditions, practitioner directions, and hierarchy of assists as well as a scoring protocol. Each task stands alone, allowing therapists to select tasks relevant to the client's priorities or lifestyle or use a template to develop a criterion for a specific task of importance to the client. The tool allows therapists to identify the precise point of task breakdown and to record the independence, safety, adequacy of the process, and outcome of each task using a 4-point scale, where 0 = unable to complete/requires maximum assistance or unacceptable level of safety or quality, and 4 = independent, safe, and acceptable performance. Both versions of the PASS have demonstrated good test-retest reliability, internal consistency and inter-rater reliability. Each has also been found to demonstrate responsiveness with the PASS Home (PASS-H) being responsive of both short-term changes in stroke survivors ($P < .01$) for independence and adequacy; and long-term changes in older adults ($P < .001$) for independence and adequacy with safety remaining high in both instances, Content, construct and criterion validity has also been established. The PASS has been used in a variety of settings, including homes, and is appropriate for healthy populations as well as people with a range of health conditions and impairments (Holm & Rogers, 2017).

The C-CAP (Lilja, 2002; Petersson, Fisher, Hemmingsson, & Lilja, 2007) was also designed to assess an individual's performance in activities in terms of independence, difficulty, and safety. It uses both self-report and observation of an individual's performance in terms of independence, difficulty, and safety of activities, including mobility (14) and personal (10) and instrumental (12) ADL (Thomas Jefferson University, n.d.). It has four parts. Part I provides questions to build rapport and explore routines and support systems. Part II is a client self-report of perceived ability to perform daily life tasks and records assistive devices currently in use. Part III examines the clients' readiness to change while Part IV consists of occupational therapist observations and rating of the client's ability to perform daily life tasks and records assistive devices used (Petersson et al., 2007). One study provided some evidence of internal scale validity, person response validity, and person separation reliability, although the qualities of the three scales differed (Petersson et al., 2007). The tool has been used to demonstrate positive impact of home modifications on self-rated ability in everyday life, specifically on decreasing the level of difficulty and increasing safety (Petersson et al., 2008).

Measures of participation would also be useful in examining the full impact of home modifications. People have described modifications as a "godsend" (Jones et al., 2008) and as releasing them from being a prisoner in their own home (Heywood, 2004b). This suggests that modifications allow people to achieve much more than successfully completing nondiscretionary activities within the home. Access into, within, around, and out of the house can have a substantial impact on an individual's ability to participate actively. Increased independence, ease, and safety in undertaking daily activities within the home also afford people the time and energy to invest in family and community activities.

Measures such as the Activity Card Sort (ACS) (Baum & Edwards, 2001, 2008) allow therapists to compare the number of activities someone was able to participate in prior to the modification and following the intervention. The ACS is a client-centered, interview-based activity measure where clients sort 80 photographs of instrumental, low-demand and high-demand, and social leisure activities into groups of never done, not done as an older adult, do now, do less, or given up (Law et al., 2017). The activities and photographs have been tailored to specific groups and populations of interest including older adults, children and young adults with Israeli,

U.K., Australian, Puerto Rican, Hong Kong, Arabic and Dutch versions available. Although not used to date in research or practice related to the outcomes of home modifications, this tool has great potential for examining the broader impact of home modifications on the person's participation.

The ICF also provides a checklist of activities (WHO, 2005). These include learning and applying knowledge; general tasks and demands; communication; mobility; self-care; domestic life; interpersonal relationships; major life areas such as work; and community, social, and civic life, which can evaluate an individual's performance in activities and participation domains. The performance qualifier measures the difficulty an individual experiences when undertaking various activities using scores that range from 0 (no difficulty in performance) to 4 (complete difficulty); that is, there is a problem present more than 95% of the time with an intensity that totally disrupts the person's day-to-day life (WHO, 2005). This checklist is useful when comparing the person's level of activity engagement and participation pre- and post-modification.

A range of outcome tools has also been developed to measure the quality of activity engagement and level of participation in various aspects of community life. Global tools, such as OTFACT (Smith, 2002) and the Assessment of Life Habits (Noreau, Fougeyrollas, & Vincent, 2002), examine people's level of engagement in an extensive range of activities and participation across life areas. OTFACT (Smith, 2002) and the developing ICFFACT software-based data collection system enable therapists to record performance in a range of activities. It uses the Trichotomous Tailored Sub-Branching Scaling to customize the question set to the specific needs of the client (Smith, 2002). The Trichotomous Tailored Sub-branching Scaling system provides a mechanism for customizing scales to the needs of everyone. As issues are identified in an area, the software branches out, breaking the activity into subsections so that discrete aspects of the performance can be examined in detail (Smith, 2002). A percentage score is then calculated for activities, relevant to the individual where he or she is not able to fully participate. Therapists can then compare scores obtained prior to the modification with scores obtained post-modification.

Autonomy is another important aspect of participation and outcome of home modifications. The Impact of Participation and Autonomy Questionnaire (IPA) examines the extent of autonomy people experience in their day-to-day lives (Cardol, de Haan, de Jong, van den Bos, & de Groot, 2001; Sibley et al, 2006). The IPA is a 39-item questionnaire that examines an individual's perceived participation and perceived problems in a range of domains, such as autonomy indoors and outdoors, family role, social situations, and paid work and education. Perceived participation is rated on a 5-point scale, with 1 being very good and 5 being very poor (Cardol et al., 2001). Perceived problems are rated from being no problem (0) to a severe problem (2). Although, to date, the IPA has been used to examine participation and perceived problems of people with spinal cord injuries (Lund, Nordlund, Nygard, Lexell, & Bernspang, 2005), it has not been used to examine the impact of home modifications. Test-retest reliability has been confirmed for all subscales and construct validity was demonstrated through confirmatory factor analysis (Martin, 2014).

Measures of the Home Environment

Many standardized measures of the environment have been developed with the purpose of identifying safety hazards (e.g., the Home Falls and Accident Screening Tool [Mackenzie, Byles, & Higginbotham, 2000], the Home Environmental Assessment Protocol [HEAP; Gitlin et al., 2002], and the Westmead Home Safety Assessment [Clemson, 1997]). Other developed standardized measures determine the accessibility of the environment (e.g., the Americans with Disabilities Act [ADA] Checklist for Existing Facilities [Adaptive Environments, 1995]). These tools evaluate the environment based on a recognized set of risks or an established standard, such as the ADA. Other tools, such as the Safety Assessment of Function and the Environment for Rehabilitation (SAFER; Oliver, Blathwayt, Brackley, & Tamaki, 1993) and the Housing Enabler (Iwarsson & Slaug, 2001), have been designed to evaluate the person-environment fit.

Although these tools are useful in identifying needs and confirming that identified risks or barriers have been removed, they are not suited to assessing the suitability or effectiveness of an environmental intervention in supporting or promoting occupational performance in the home or its impact on various dimensions of the home environment. Furthermore, they are not sufficiently sensitive to detect changes resulting from modifications. In recognition of the limitations of existing measures, Chiu and Oliver (2006) revised the SAFER to evaluate the effectiveness of intervention in addressing home safety concerns.

SAFER-HOME v.3 (Chiu & Oliver, 2006; Chui et al., 2006) allows therapists to use a combination of interviews, observation, and task performance to rate the safety of 74 activities. It consists of 12 domains: living situation, mobility, kitchen, environmental hazards, household, eating, bathroom and toilet, medication, addiction and abuse, leisure, communication and scheduling, personal care and wandering. The binary scale in the original SAFER tool was expanded to a 4-point scale, where 1 = no identified concern and 4 = severe problem, high safety risk to client's function and/or environment with 67% to 100% chance of negative consequences (Chiu & Oliver, 2006). This tool is well grounded in theory and has been carefully developed (Cooper, Letts, Rigby, Stewart, & Strong, 2005). Its unique focus on the person-environment interaction provides a comprehensive evaluation of home safety (Rigby, Craciunoiu, Stier, & Letts, 2017). Further, it has been found to be clinically useful, practical to administer, and sensitive in detecting changes (Chiu & Oliver, 2006). Using a factor analysis of 1,173 observations, Chiu and Oliver found the tool had an internal consistency coefficient alpha value of 0.86. Though test-retest reliability was established for the total score, only moderate reliability was established for the subscales for SAFER-HOME v.2 (Gitlow, 2014). Weak correlation with another functional assessment supported the hypothesis that home safety was related, but not limited, to functioning (Chiu & Oliver, 2006).

Developed specifically for people living with dementia, HEAP is an objective evaluation of the hazards, adaptations, and level of clutter and comfort across eight areas of the home (Gitlin et al., 2002). The assessment uses caregiver interview, direct observation and caregiver clarification to rate 192 items in the living room, dining room, bedroom, bathroom, kitchen, hallway and stairs. Content validity was established through an expert panel of occupational therapists and convergent validity was demonstrated by correlations of lower cognitive ability and mental status of clients to more adaptations and less clutter on HEAP scores (Gitlow, 2014). Due to the large number of items, interrater agreement varied widely on dichotomous items ranging from slight (0.01) to almost perfect (0.95). This tool has recently been revised (Struckmeyer, 2016) to reduce the number of items. The HEAP-R reformatted items into a table to make it easier to navigate the tool and record data. Content validity was established using a literature review and expert panel with scores (0.86 to 0.1). Concurrent validity with the original HEAP ranged was strong for hazards, adaptations clutter and comfort. Test-retest reliability was examined using experts who scored 10 home environment videos and ranged from 0.487 for visual cues and 0.696 for clutter to 0.82 for hazards and 0.887 for adaptations (Struckmeyer, 2016). Interrater reliability was low (0.252 to 0.313; Struckmeyer, 2016).

In-Home Occupational Performance Evaluation (I-HOPE; Stark, Somerville, & Morris, 2010) was created to fill the gap in availability of assessments that reviewed function in relation to the environment by providing a performance-based measure focused on home-based activities for older adults (60+). Specifically, it examines the fit between the person and their environment, drawing attention to any "mis-fits" and the associated effects (Stark et al., 2010). In addition to acknowledging the influence of the environment on performance the I-HOPE also considers the client's perspective on both their performance in the environment and their associated satisfaction with this performance. The completion of the measure results in four subscales, which represent the client's participation in daily activities, ability to perform activities, satisfaction with their performance and the influence of environmental barriers on activity performance (Stark et al., 2010). These four subscales demonstrate good internal consistency ($a = 0.85$ [38 items], 0.78 [6 items], 0.77 [6 items], and 0.77 [8 items], respectively) and excellent strength of agreement between raters with intraclass correlations between 0.94 and 1.0 (Stark et al., 2010). Further the measure demonstrates convergent validity as all four subscales were found to be significantly correlated to the FIM. In addition to its sound psychometric properties, the I-HOPE supports the review of outcomes post modification and has been shown to demonstrate potential for measuring changes in performance, satisfaction and environmental barrier scores. Specifically, when implemented pre-and post-intervention the I-HOPE has demonstrated statistically significant differences between pre and posttest scores and has also been found to be sufficiently sensitive to detect changes in performance after reductions in environmental barriers (Stark et al., 2010). These features have contributed to the suggestion that the I-HOPE is a clinical useful tool that enables the measurement of the effectiveness of interventions, like modifications, that focus on the reduction of environmental barriers (Stark et al., 2010).

Measures have been developed to assess the perceived quality of housing. These measures have been used in cross-cultural research to examine the relationship between perceived housing and healthy aging outcomes in very old age and could be useful in evaluating the impact of modifications on householders' perceptions of usability, meaning, and housing-related control beliefs. Usability in this instance is defined as the extent to which an individual's housing needs and preferences can be fulfilled with respect to activity performance in the home (Fänge & Iwarsson, 2005a). The UIMH (Fänge, 2002; Fänge & Iwarsson, 1999) is a self-administered questionnaire that asks clients to rate the usability of various aspects of the environment using a 7-point scale, with 7 indicating the most positive response alternative. Its 16 items target physical, activity, and personal/social aspects of the home environment. The authors of the UIMH have carefully developed this tool, establishing usability as a valid construct with three independent aspects (Fänge & Iwarsson, 2003, 2005b) and using an expert panel to establish content validity. The tool was also determined to have moderate to very good test-retest reliability with agreement for each item achieving correlation scores between 0.57 and 0.88 (Fänge & Iwarsson, 1999).

The dimensions of home as outlined in Chapters 1 and 6 provide a framework for understanding clients' experience of home. An outcome measure evaluating these dimensions was developed based on the outcomes and experiences of home modification clients (Aplin, 2013). The tool named the Dimensions of Home Measure (DOHM) was specifically designed for home modification practice and is a self-administered questionnaire examining the personal, social, occupational, temporal, physical and societal dimensions of home. The tool uses a 4-point Likert scale of strongly disagree, disagree, agree and strongly agree (Aplin, de Jonge & Gustafsson, 2014). Items for the personal dimension for example include, "I have the privacy I want from others in my home" and "my home reflects who I am." For the social dimension example questions include "all the areas of my home are easy for others to use" and "I would like to do more social activities at home" (Aplin et al., 2014). The DOHM has initial evidence of reliability and construct validity based on the Rasch Rating Scale Model although further psychometric evaluation is required as additional items were added to enhance the targeting of the tool (Aplin, 2013; Aplin, Chien, & Gustafsson, 2016).

Another tool evaluating the experience home is the Meaning of Home Questionnaire (Oswald et al., 2006). The meaning of the home concept incorporates subjective evaluations, values, goals, cognitions, and emotions of an individual in relation to his or her home (Marcus, 1995; Moore, 2000; Nygren et al., 2007; Oswald & Wahl, 2005). The Meaning of Home Questionnaire is a self-administered questionnaire that examines four different aspects of the meaning of home: physical (7 items), such as "being at home means for me living in a place that is well designed and geared to my needs"; activity (6 items), such as "being able to do whatever I please"; cognitive/emotional (10 items), such as "feeling comfortable and cozy"; and social (5 items), such as "being able to receive visitors" (Iwarsson, Horstmann, & Slaug, 2007; Nygren et al., 2007). Factor analysis and structural equation modeling techniques have been used to confirm four component models of perceived housing, which has held up in cross-cultural analysis of the same (Oswald et al., 2006).

A tool that has proved useful in examining perceptions of control in the home environment is the Housing-Related Control Beliefs Questionnaire (Oswald, Wahl, Martin, & Mollenkopf, 2003). This 24-item questionnaire uses a 5-point scale to measure agreement with statements based on the psychological dimensions of internal control (8 items); external control powerful others (8 items); and external control: chance (8 items; Iwarsson et al., 2007). The Internal Control subscale examines housing events related to a person's own behavior, such as "I have been able to set up my home in accordance with my own personal ideas," "Everything in my home will stay the way it is; no one is going to tell me what to do," or "I myself decide whose help to accept within or outside my home" (Oswald, Wahl, Schilling, & Iwarsson, 2007). The two external control subscales examine events related to another person and chance, such as "Other people have told me how to arrange the furnishings in my home," "Whether I can stay in my home depends on luck and circumstance," or "Where and how I live has happened more by chance" (Oswald et al., 2007). To date, only internal consistency has been established for the external control dimensions of this tool (Iwarsson et al., 2007).

SELECTING OUTCOME MEASURES

To date, home modification therapists have mostly used informal and qualitative strategies to determine needs and evaluate the effectiveness of interventions. While these methods allow therapists to deal with the complexity and uniqueness of each person-environment-occupation transaction, they do not allow them to determine the extent of the need or improvement afforded by the modification for each individual or to compare the effectiveness of modifications in different situations. Reliance on informal evaluation strategies makes it difficult to communicate the impact of modifications and accumulated knowledge of the effectiveness of various modifications to colleagues, service managers, and funding bodies. An outcomes-oriented approach to delivering home modification services allows occupational therapists to monitor the impact and effectiveness of specific recommendations and inform

practice by building a body of knowledge about the effectiveness of a range of modifications.

The use of standardized outcomes measures would greatly improve practice in this area and would allow data relating to the needs and outcomes of individual clients to be systematically recorded and accumulated to document the needs of the population of which the clients are a part (Sells, 2005). This information could also be used to record the outcomes of the interventions provided by the service for the population being served, which in turn could contribute to a broader understanding of the impact of modifications. A change in the way therapists understand evaluation requires them to not only think carefully about what outcomes to evaluate but to also consider how these are best evaluated.

Sometimes measures are selected because they are easy to use and are readily available, and insufficient consideration is given to their purpose and limitations (Backman, 2005). Because the tools used, and the variables measured often become the operational definition for the outcome, occupational therapists need to select outcome measures carefully. For example, the FIM has become the gold standard for measuring independence in ADL in some settings. Though the FIM might be considered to define people's levels of independence, in reality, independence is much more complex. While people who perform well on this assessment might be able to perform the defined activities independently in the hospital environment, this does not ensure that they will be independent at home. First, environmental challenges that are not present in the hospital environment might compromise their performance. Second, being independent assumes that the person can perform tasks safely, confidently, and with ease; however, the FIM does not explicitly evaluate these parameters. Finally, independence in basic self-care tasks is often not a good indication of an individual's ability to cope at home on his or her own because there are many other critical tasks required to ensure health and safety in the home environment, such as cooking, mopping up spills, and taking out the trash.

Outcome evaluations need to be undertaken carefully, ensuring that the outcome tools are:

+ Congruent with the needs, desires and goals of clients

+ Valid, reliable and appropriately sensitive to desired changes

+ Based on their actual and purported ability to predict future outcomes (AOTA, 2014)

Client-Centered Outcomes Evaluation

Outcome evaluations have conventionally focused on the person's clinical status as defined and evaluated by the therapist (Law, 1998). However, research on the acceptance and outcomes of home modifications highlight the importance of understanding the complexity of the home environment and the person-occupation-environment transaction and routinely reviewing the effectiveness of the recommended modifications for the client and other householders (Gitlin, 2003).

Many therapists have encountered clients who decline a modification suggestion or refuse the contractor entry to the property once the recommendation has been made. There are many reasons why a client might find a therapist's recommendations unacceptable. First, the client and therapist might have different priorities or concerns. For example, a client might be more concerned about the threat of a home invasion and might therefore not be as concerned with their safety and difficulty in the bathroom. Second, the client might have a specific concern that might not have been fully captured in the therapist's recommendations. Consequently, what the therapist believes to be appropriate might not be acceptable to the client (Gitlin, Luborsky, & Schemm, 1998). Third, clients might also reject a modification if they perceive that it will impact negatively on their sense of independence and autonomy (Messecar, Archbold, Stewart, & Kirschling, 2002). Overemphasis on safety and performance problems can detract attention from other important issues, such as independence, injury prevention, caregiver health, and social integration (Duncan, 1998; Pynoos, 2004). Finally, home modifications have been found to impact negatively on people's self-image and connection with the home (Heywood, 2005), as well as on their routines and sense of heritage when the needs of the person were not fully understood or considered (Heywood, 2005). Adaptations to the home can result in people being labeled as different and, more importantly, making them vulnerable to ridicule or violence (Fisher, 1998). It is therefore important that the client's priorities, goals, and preferences are not only considered in designing the modification, but that these are also incorporated into an evaluation of the intervention.

As noted in Chapter 6, evaluation methods, including outcome evaluation, should allow clients to identify their specific concerns about valued occupations, record their unique occupational performance requirements, and document the impact of interventions on their lives (Law et al., 2017). This requires that outcome evaluation strategies also:

+ Allow occupational performance issues or problems to be identified by the client and household members and not solely by the therapist and team

+ Permit the unique nature of each person's participation in occupations to be recognized

+ Provide opportunities for both the subjective experience and the observable qualities of occupational performance to be recorded

+ Afford the client (and relevant others) to have a say in evaluating the outcomes of the interventions

+ Recognize the unique qualities of the home environment

+ Assist clients and household members to develop a mutual understanding of therapists' safety, prevention, or health-maintenance concerns (Law & Baum, 2017)

Using a client-centered approach encourages clients to identify goals and outcomes that are meaningful to them (Law, 1998). It also ensures that the factors that affect the client and the way they operate in, and relate to, the home environment are acknowledged (de Jonge, Scherer, & Rodger, 2007). The personal meaningfulness of occupations is also an important consideration when evaluating outcomes (Klein et al., 2008). Because everyone is unique, this challenges therapists to choose outcome measures that reflect an individualized perspective (Donnelly & Carswell, 2002).

Conceptual Framework for Outcome Evaluation

As noted earlier, there are numerous outcome tools, each founded on a theory or understanding and with a specific purpose in mind. The challenge for occupational therapists is to choose outcome measures that are in harmony with the health and social care system in which they work but also reflect the scope and focus of occupational therapy interventions (in this case, environmental interventions). Increasingly, the ICF is used to define and organize outcomes and measures around the constructs of body structures and function, activity and participation, environmental conditions, and personal characteristics (Backman, 2005). The ICF aims to provide an interprofessional and international framework for studying and understanding health outcomes, having a means of collecting and comparing data across countries for research, and for developing health and social policy (Hemmingsson & Jonsson, 2005). Its recognition of the relationship between people's daily activities and health and the role of the environment in promoting health make the ICF, and tools developed using this framework, useful to occupational therapists, allowing them to communicate their understandings to others. Although there are a number of commonalities between the ICF and occupational therapy models, it is also important not to underestimate the differences (Kjeken & Lillemo, 2006).

Occupational therapists have a unique and thorough understanding of occupation and its role in promoting health. Further, they appreciate the dynamic interaction between the person, occupation, and the environment. Consequently, they need their own language, frameworks, and tools to develop and evaluate occupational therapy interventions. Several conceptual models (see Chapter 3) have been developed in occupational therapy to understand and explain the complex reality that therapists encounter in daily practice (Stamm, Cieza, Machold, Smolen, & Stucki, 2006). Whether therapists use these models consciously or unconsciously, they direct clinical decisions and shape choice of evaluation measures and interventions. It is therefore important, when choosing outcome measures, that therapists review the theoretical foundation of the tools and ensure that they are compatible with occupational therapy's conceptual frameworks and goals (Miller Polgar, 2009). Measures that reflect the aims and principles of occupational therapy practice allow therapists to demonstrate their unique contributions to health and social care (Klein et al., 2008). If the expected outcome of occupational therapy, namely occupational performance, is improved, then "measuring the presence, absence, or magnitude of change in occupational performance should be a primary outcome measure for occupational therapy" (AOTA, 2014; Backman, 2005, p. 259).

Occupational performance is variously defined as the experience of being engaged in, or the act of doing and accomplishing, everyday life activities that hold value and meaning to the individual, referred to as occupations. It is described as having a subjective experiential element or meaning to the person as well as an objective observable component (McColl & Pollock, 2001). Measurement of occupational performance must therefore capture both the subjective and objective aspects of occupational performance (McColl & Pollock, 2001). Occupational therapy's understanding of occupational performance is also guided by several pervasive values and beliefs, such as holism, client-centeredness, and the uniqueness of each individual and his or her life situation (Klein et al., 2008). These values and beliefs are reflected in transactional models that recognize the dynamic relationship between the person, the environment,

and the occupations in which he or she chooses to engage (Klein et al., 2008). Occupational therapists also see occupational performance in the home environment as an orchestration of valued activities that allow the person to fulfill meaningful roles in the home and community (Crepeau et al., 2014; Larson, 2000) rather than a series of disconnected routine tasks. When selecting home modification outcome measures, therapists need to evaluate the capacity of each tool to capture these important occupational therapy constructs.

Klein et al. (2008) developed a construct rating review form (Figure 13-1) for reviewing the cohesion between evaluation measures and the value and principles of occupational therapy practice.

This review form alerts therapists to the elements essential to an occupational therapy evaluation of occupational performance. It enables them to select measures that are better aligned with the profession's aims and understanding of people as occupational beings; the dynamic relationship between the person, his or her occupations, and the environment; and the extent to which occupational performance or engagement is afforded by changes in the environment. In their review of existing ADL measures, Klein et al. (2008) identified six tools that adequately reflected the values and beliefs of occupational therapy. The review of these tools explains the dissatisfaction occupational therapists have with existing measures and alert the profession to a need for measures based on conceptual foundations that are better aligned with occupational therapy practice. The profession needs to be actively involved in developing tools that fit well with occupational theory and practice rather than relying on tools developed within other frameworks.

Psychometric Properties of Outcome Measures

All selected outcome measures should have sound psychometric properties, including validity, reliability, responsiveness (Barak & Duncan, 2006; Jerosch-Herold, 2005; Magasi, Gohil, Burghart, & Wallisch, 2017), and clinical utility (Corr & Siddons, 2005). These properties are important because the quality of the measure impacts on the quality of the data obtained (Gelderblom & De Witte, 2002). When a tool has established validity, you can be certain that it is measuring what it purports to measure and that there is general agreement about what is being measured (Dunn, 2017). A reliable tool ensures that the measures are consistent across time and assessors (Dunn, 2017). Tools also need to be responsive to changes in the parameter being measured. Using

This form is intended to be used for reviewing established ADL measures for constructs identified as important for the assessment of ADL in occupational therapy practice. Please keep in mind the following:

- Each question has some examples that were raised to help illustrate this construct. This is not meant to be exhaustive, just to help recall the construct.
- Many of these measures will not have the construct you are looking for outlined clearly in the supporting documentation (that would be too easy!).

You will need to examine the measure, the way it has the tester examine ADL, and how the tester scores it to see if that particular construct is "implied" or "inherent" by the way it is structured. For example, the measure may not overtly state that they consider the environment, but it may have a place on the score sheet to describe the test environment. For this reason, we are asking you to comment on what drew you to that conclusion about that particular question. This will be very important for our review.

Score measure based on the following scale:
(0) Construct not present
(1) Some elements of construct present
(2) Construct present

	0	1	2
1. Is the measure client-centred? 1.1 Does the measure allow the tester to identify tasks important to the client? For example: • does the test have a total score or can it be done in components valued by the client? • is the measure comprised of a scoring format that allows the client to prioritize tasks where he or she wants to invest his or her energy? • does the measure acknowledge role expectations of self and others (gender, culture, age, how acceptable it is to get assistance from other family members, how the culture values independent occupational performance)? 1.2 Does the measure identify if the client is motivated to learn new ways to be independent? 1.3 Does the measure identify when the client is willing to persist with the task to complete it?			
2. Does the client have a general knowledge of task demands? 2.1 Does the measure identify the client's knowledge of the task demands? • does he or she know the steps of the task? 2.2　Does the measure recognize the client's awareness of strengths, challenges, and ability to prioritize tasks, e.g. decide what he or she wants to invest their energy in doing)? 2.3 Does the measure allow for making informed decisions about taking risks? • is the client aware that going down to the bottom of the tub may increase the risk of a fall, but that is the way he or she wants to do it.			

Figure 13-1. ADL Construct Rating Review Form. (Reprinted with permission from Klein, S., Barlow, I., & Hollis, V. [2008]. Evaluating ADL measures from an occupational perspective. *Canadian Journal of Occupational Therapy, 75*[2], 69-81.) *(continued)*

3. Is the client's performance competent?

3.1   Is task competence identified/defined* by the client?

3.1.1 Does the measure allow for the task success to be defined by the client?
- the client has identified getting clean while bathing as a task that requires submersion in a tub bath, not showering.

3.1.2 Does the measure allow for different ways or processes for completing the task?
- task success vs. doing it "correctly"
- task process is only important if the client has identified that as a concern—such as speed of dressing.
- allows for how the culture affects the way an ADL task is done (China bowl for eating, rather than with plate, knife, fork).

3.2   Where is the performance breaking down?

3.2.1 Does the measure recognize or acknowledge interaction between the person, environment, and task?

3.2.2 Does the measure allow for qualitative observation?

3.3   Does the client have the ability (performance components)?

3.3.1 Does the measure identify or allow observation of underlying performance components (e.g., sensation, motor control, and perception)?

3.4 Are the demands/supports of the task appropriate for the person's ability and environmental situation (i.e., task modification)?

3.4.1 Does the measure recognize/identify modifications needed for success?
- does the measure identify issues related to time restraints – dressing for work/school vs. less pressured time restrictions?
- a client is unable to dress independently due to limited ROM, but would be able to if long-handled aids were available, or a different dressing technique.

3.5 Are the demands/supports of the environment appropriate for the person's ability and task difficulty?

3.5.1 Does the measure identify the "assessment" environment and the demands of the "discharge" or "typical" environment?
- hospital vs. home
- when role requires changing environments for task

3.5.2 Does the measure acknowledge the social support environment?
- does it identify who lives with the client and how much they are able to assist?
- does it identify the client's role expectations of self and others related to how acceptable it is to get assistance from another family member?

3.5.3 Does the measure identify whether financial resources/supports are available?
- does the client have the ability to pay for equipment or environmental modification that may be needed to be independent?

Total Score   **/60**

© CAOT PUBLICATIONS ACE

Figure 13-1 (continued). ADL Construct Rating Review Form. (Reprinted with permission from Klein, S., Barlow, I., & Hollis, V. [2008]. Evaluating ADL measures from an occupational perspective. *Canadian Journal of Occupational Therapy, 75*[2], 69-81.).

Table 13-2. Checklist for Reviewing the Validity, Reliability, and Sensitivity of Outcomes Measures

RESULTS: VALIDITY YES NO RESULTS
1. Does the measure make intrinsic sense—face validity (expert opinion/consensus)?
2. Does the measure sample the content/domain adequately?
3. Is there evidence of the test's construct validity?
(i) Does the test discriminate between healthy and diseased groups (known-groups method)?
(ii) Do the test values agree with the values of a similar test or gold standard (concurrent or convergent validity) or with a future outcome (predictive validity)?
If yes, then:
(a) What is the strength of the correlation?
(b) What are the confidence limits, if given?
(iii) What is the internal consistency (relevant where scales have multiple items that sum up to a total score)?
RESULTS: RELIABILITY YES NO RESULTS
4. What is the test-retest reliability?
(i) Have appropriate statistical measures been used to assess agreement between two or more occasions using the same observer?
(ii) What is the level of agreement (for example, kappa or ICC)?
(iii) What are the confidence limits, if given?
5. What is the inter-tester reliability?
(i) Have appropriate statistical measures been used to assess agreement between two or more observers?
(ii) What is the level of agreement (for example, kappa or ICC)?
(iii) What are the confidence limits, if given?
RESULTS: RESPONSIVENESS YES NO RESULTS
6. Does the instrument capture clinical change?
(i) What is the magnitude of the responsiveness of the instrument (for example, effect size or standard response mean)?
(ii) Is there evidence of floor or ceiling effects?
Reprinted with permission from the College of Occupational Therapists Ltd and Christina Jerosch-Herold from Jerosch-Herold, C. (2005). An evidence-based approach to choosing outcome measures: A checklist for the critical appraisal of validity, reliability and responsiveness studies. *British Journal of Occupational Therapy, 68*(8), 347-353.

tools with sound psychometric properties ensures that any improvements detected by the measure are the result of real change and not random error.

The psychometric properties of outcome measures and the quality of data they obtain is not just a concern for researchers. Therapists and their clients also need to be confident in the outcomes measures used. When selecting them, therapists need to consider whether the tool is:

✦ Appropriate for the purpose and population for which it is being used (valid for the purpose and application)

✦ Able to produce accurate information repeatedly (reliable)

✦ Sensitive to small but clinically important changes (responsive)

✦ Useful and easy to use (has clinical utility; Jerosch-Herold, 2005)

Jerosch-Herold (2005) provides a useful checklist for reviewing the validity, reliability, and sensitivity of outcomes measures (Table 13-2).

It is important to remember that the validity, reliability, and responsiveness of tools are not fixed properties; but rather, they are influenced by where and how the tool is used (Jerosch-Herold, 2005). For example, a tool designed to assess falls risk in a clinical setting will not be a valid measure of falls risk in a home environment unless validated for that context. A tool designed solely for use with the frail aged is no longer valid if used with young adults. Tools designed to measure changes in quality of life following surgery are not always responsive to subtle changes that occur over time with regular therapy. Measures of independence that penalize the use of assistive technologies will respond negatively to the introduction of aids and equipment. It is therefore important that therapists select tools that are appropriate to the purpose and the population to which they will be applied. The tools also need to be used in accordance with the instructions and scored in the correct manner to retain their validity and reliability (Corr & Siddons, 2005; Sells, 2005). A "pick and mix" approach, where only sections of standardized measures are used, is also not appropriate when using standardized tools because this "invalidates the tool and renders the results meaningless" (Corr & Siddons, 2005).

To evaluate the psychometric quality of tools, it is useful to understand each of the properties and how these are established.

Validity

As noted previously, validity refers to "the degree to which a test measures the phenomenon that it purports to measure" (Jerosch-Herold, 2005, p. 349). There are several kinds of validity. The types of concern to therapists are face, content, construct, and ecological validity. As the lowest form of validity, face validity is assessed subjectively in terms of whether the items make sense to the assessor and the client (Jerosch-Herold, 2005). This ensures that therapists and clients understand what the test is assessing, which is usually established by several practicing therapists reviewing the test items.

Content validity refers to the extent to which the items in the assessment fully represent the attribute being examined (Magasi et al., 2017). The comprehensiveness of a measure is generally established through consultation with experts and consensus (Jerosch-Herold, 2005).

Construct validity is the extent to which an assessment supports the theory on which it is founded (Crist, 2005). This is generally established by demonstrating that the measure:

+ Correlates with an established test that measures a similar construct (convergent validity)

+ Can differentiate between someone known to experience difficulties and those without concerns (discriminant validity; Crist, 2005)

Convergent and discriminant validity are usually established using a "gold standard," or established tool, as a basis for comparison, with correlations of 0.6 and above being considered excellent (Salter, Jutai, Teasell, Foley, & Bitensky, 2005).

When a test has established content and construct validity, therapists can be assured that the test has adequate theoretical foundation and that experts have confirmed all of the relevant elements.

Occupational therapists using tests developed in other conceptual frameworks may, however, feel that a test does not adequately measure the attribute as they understand it or that it does not assess it appropriately. Therefore, although a test may have established validity from one perspective, it might not be adequate within an occupational therapy context. Similarly, validity of an older tool might no longer be considered adequate because understandings of the attribute being examined might have changed. For example, ADL assessments have traditionally focused on determining whether someone requires assistance, independence, in basic self-care activities. Increasingly, however, therapists are concerned with measuring the quality of performance and outcomes of a broad range of daily activities, paying attention to the safety and ease of performance.

In home modification practice, less structured measures are considered more suitable because they allow therapists to evaluate the uniqueness of performance within the dynamic person-environment-occupation interaction (Klein et al., 2008). The ecological validity of a measure (i.e., the extent to which the assessment reflects performance in the real world [Bottari, Dutil, Dassa, & Rainville, 2006; Sbordone & Guilmette, 1999]) is very important when evaluating a person's performance in the home environment. However, even within the home environment, the use of simulated tasks can limit the ecological validity of measures, such as ADL assessments (Bottari et al., 2006). These tasks are selected and structured by the therapist where environmental elements differ from actual performance (e.g., time of day, lighting conditions, time pressures, occupational context of the tasks, and the presence of the therapist).

There have been attempts to improve several ADL tools by increasing their ecological validity and the accuracy of inferences based on these assessments. A less structured approach in the natural environment has been used, considering environmental demands and incorporating a larger sample of more complex tasks (Bottari et al., 2006). Criterion-referenced assessments, such as the Activities of Daily Living Profile (Dutil, Bottari, Vanier, & Gaudreault, 2005; Dutil, Forget, Vanier, & Gaudreault, 1990), AMPS (Fisher, 1995; Fisher & Jones, 2011a, 2011b), and the PASS Home (Rogers & Holm, 1994; Rogers, Holm, & Chisholm, 2016), allow therapists to observe and record performance difficulties experienced by clients when undertaking activities in the usual way and in their natural environment. Occupational performance, therefore, can be measured more accurately than using traditional standardized independence measures (Bottari et al., 2006).

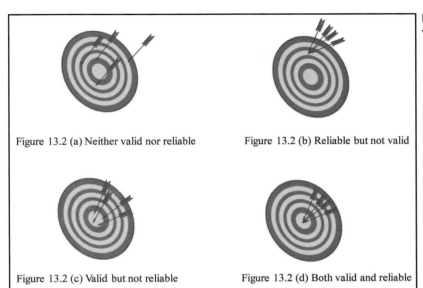

Figure 13-2. Target analogy for reliability and validity.

Figure 13.2 (a) Neither valid nor reliable

Figure 13.2 (b) Reliable but not valid

Figure 13.2 (c) Valid but not reliable

Figure 13.2 (d) Both valid and reliable

Reliability

While ecological validity requires that measures allow for variability in task performance so that they more accurately reflect real situations, reliability is strengthened by standardization and repeatability of test items (Klein et al., 2008). As noted earlier, reliability reduces the likelihood of measurement error and ensures that the measure is used correctly (intra-rater reliability) and that measurement remains stable over time (test-retest reliability) and across different testers (inter-rater reliability; Jerosch-Herold, 2005). Intra-rater reliability (i.e., consistency in test administration and scoring) requires each therapist to undertake training in using the tool and to calibrate its use regularly (Crist, 2005). Test-retest reliability is particularly important when measuring changes resulting from an intervention because it ensures that the change in score reflects the true change and is not a result of the instability of the measure (Crist, 2005). Inter-rater reliability is reliant on all therapists learning to use the test appropriately, adhering to published administration and scoring procedures (Crist, 2005). The reliability of tools is generally reported in terms of correlation coefficients. The closer the correlation between testing events or testers is to 1.0, the more reliable the test is considered (Laver Fawcett, 2007). Correlation scores of 0.7 or more are considered to have high reliability (Corr & Siddons, 2005; Magasi et al., 2017).

A good outcome measure must have good reliability and validity if it is to measure outcomes accurately (Laver Fawcett, 2007). A target analogy, first presented by Pynsent, Fairbank, and Carr (2004), provides a useful illustration of the impact of having neither, both, or only one of these properties present on the accuracy of the outcome. In this analogy, the bulls-eye stands for the true outcome being measured and each arrow stands for a single application of the outcome tool (Laver Fawcett, 2007). When a measure is neither valid nor reliable, the arrows are scattered across the target (Figure 13-2A), indicating that the tool is not capturing the true purpose consistently. A measure that is reliable but not valid will have the arrows clustered together closely but not near the bulls-eye (Figure 13-2B), signifying that the tool is reliably measuring something but not necessarily what needs to be measured. A measure that is valid but not reliable will have the arrows near the bulls-eye, but they will be dispersed widely (Figure 13-2C), demonstrating that the tool is appropriately focused but not consistent. Finally, a measure that is both valid and reliable will have the arrows clustered closely together within the bulls-eye area (Figure 13-2D), establishing that the tool is both appropriately focused and accurate in capturing what it needs to measure.

Responsiveness

Outcome measures need to be able to detect small changes over time (Corr & Siddons, 2005; Salter et al., 2005). Some standardized tools are not responsive to changes that result from environmental interventions. For example, measures of independence such as the FIM (UDSMR, 1997, 2009) typically penalize reliance on assistive devices or modifications and do not register subtle changes in performance, such as reduced completion time and improved safety (Corr & Siddons, 2005). Consequently, they are not considered responsive or sensitive enough for this purpose. Responsiveness is evaluated using a variety of statistical measures, such as standardized effects size that quantify the magnitude of change (Jerosch-Herold, 2005). These calculations involve correlations where values of more than 0.8 are considered a large effect (Jerosch-Herold, 2005; Salter et al., 2005).

Another important consideration in terms of a tool's sensitivity is its capacity to detect changes at the upper and lower ends of the scale (Jerosch-Herold, 2005). If a test is too difficult, scores will cluster at the lower end of the scale and exhibit "floor" effects (Jerosch-Herold, 2005; Salter et al., 2005). Alternatively, if a test is too easy, and scores cluster at the upper end, it is considered to show "ceiling" effects (Jerosch-Herold, 2005; Salter et al., 2005). Consequently, tests that have floor or ceiling effects will not be sufficiently sensitive to detect changes in people at the upper and lower ends of the range. The size of the ceiling effect is examined by determining the percentage of people obtaining maximum or minimum scores (Laver Fawcett, 2007). If more than 20% of the test population score minimum or maximum scores, the test is considered to have ceiling effects (Salter et al., 2005). It is important that the outcome measures used by therapists can detect changes across a broad range of people. Many existing ADL measures fail to determine the full extent of the difficulties people experience in daily activities or the tasks people need to complete safely to live a full life. In other words, people are considered capable of performing tasks even when they find them effortful or challenging, or they are assumed independent when there are activities they cannot do.

Clinical Utility

The overall utility of a tool is reflected in its usefulness in a clinical situation (Laver Fawcett, 2007). Therapists are interested in the availability, ease of use, acceptability, portability, cost, administrative burden, and training requirements of a measure (Laver Fawcett, 2007; Law, 2005; Miller Polgar, 2009) as well as the meaning and clinical relevance of the information it provides (Miller Polgar, 2009). Many valid and reliable tools remain unused if therapists find them too cumbersome, complicated, or time-consuming to administer (Laver Fawcett, 2007). Equally, the measure must provide information that is useful in informing clinical practice or determining the impact of the intervention. As discussed earlier, global measures, such as measures of independence, provide little information on the specific difficulties someone is experiencing in carrying out a task and cannot establish whether an intervention addresses these specific difficulties.

CONCLUSION

This chapter has discussed the importance of evaluating the outcomes of home modifications. The rising costs of health and social care services, the aging population, inequities and inefficiencies in service delivery, practice errors, and inconsistencies in the quality of services have resulted in governments establishing accreditation systems to monitor service provision. The profession's ethical responsibilities and client-centered approach also require therapists to continually monitor their clients' outcomes and establish evidence to support their recommendations. Without adequate proof of the effectiveness of home modification interventions, occupational therapists and the services they provide are at risk of losing funding. Several challenges to evaluating the outcomes of home modifications have been presented (namely, the complexities in the way home modification services are delivered, the unique approach and experience of each therapist providing advice, the diversity of people and households undertaking home modifications, and the variety of housing forms being modified), all of which combine to increase the difficulty associated with this task.

The chapter reviewed four different purposes of outcome evaluation, each with a focus. Outcome evaluations can focus on monitoring the quality and consistency of service provision; determining whether service, client, or therapist goals have been met; building a body of knowledge/evidence; or demonstrating the efficiency and value of interventions. In doing so, it outlined the indicators of quality or effectiveness for each of these approaches and detailed how therapists can gather information to contribute to these evaluations in a way that informs day-to-day home modification practice.

This chapter reported on the outcome measures used in research on the effectiveness of home modifications. A review of outcome measures well suited to gathering information on the impact of home modification on the physical and mental health of clients, their occupational performance and participation, as well as their perceptions and experience of the home environment was also provided.

A shift in the definition of health has resulted in traditional approaches to measurement being less appropriate in this community context. This chapter discussed the importance of choosing evaluation tools that are client centered and in line with occupational therapy's values, principles, and conceptual frameworks. In particular, it has highlighted the value of choosing tools that reflect an individualized perspective, focus on occupational performance, and recognize the dynamic interaction between person, occupation, and environment. Finally, the chapter also emphasized the value of using tools with sound psychometric properties. It described validity, reliability, responsiveness, and clinical utility and the role of each in ensuring the quality of the data gathered.

REFERENCES

Adaptive Environments. (1995). *Checklist for existing facilities.* Boston, MA: Author.

Allen, S., Resnik, L., & Roy, J. (2006). Promoting independence for wheelchair users: The role of home accommodations. *Gerontologist, 46*(1), 115-123.

Allison, P., Locker, D., & Feine, J. (1997). Quality of life: A dynamic concept. *Social Science Medicine, 45*(2), 221-230.

American Occupational Therapy Association. (2014). Occupational therapy practice framework: Domain and process (3rd ed.). *American Journal of Occupational Therapy, 68,* S1-S48.

Andrich, R., & Caracciolo, A. (2007). Analysing the cost of individual assistive technology programs. *Disability and Rehabilitation: Assistive Technology, 2*(4), 207-234.

Andrich, R., Ferrario, M., & Moi, M. (1998). A model of cost-outcome analysis for assistive technology. *Disability and Rehabilitation, 20*(1), 1-24.

Aplin, T. (2013). Development and psychometric analysis of the Dimensions of Home Measure (DOHM): A measure of the home environment for home modification practice (Doctoral dissertation, The University of Queensland, Australia). Retrieved from http://espace.library.uq.edu.au/

Aplin, T., Chien, C. W., & Gustafsson, L. (2016). Initial validation of the Dimensions of Home Measure (DOHM). *Australian Occupational Therapy Journal, 63*(1), 47-56.

Aplin, T., de Jonge, D., & Gustafsson, L. (2014). *The dimensions of home measure.* St Lucia, Australia The University of Queensland.

Arah, O. A., Westert, G. P., Hurst, J., & Klazinga, N. S. (2006). A conceptual framework for the OECD health care quality indicators project international. *Journal for Quality in Health Care, 18*(Suppl. 1), 5-13.

Backman, C. L. (2005). Outcomes and outcome measures: Measuring what matters is in the eye of the beholder. *Canadian Journal of Occupational Therapy, 72*(5), 259-261.

Barak, S., & Duncan, P. W. (2006). Issues in selecting outcome measures to assess functional recovery after stroke. *NeuroRx: The Journal of the American Society for Experimental NeuroTherapeutics, 3,* 505-524.

Baum, C., & Edwards, D. (2001). *Activity card sort.* St. Louis, MO: Washington University at St. Louis.

Baum, C., & Edwards, D. (2008). *Activity card sort* (2nd ed.). Bethesda, MD; AOTA Press.

Beck, A. T., Ward C. H., Mendelson, M., Mock, J., & Erbaugh, J. (1961). An inventory for measuring depression. *Archives of General Psychiatry, 4,* 561-571.

Bieri, D., Reeve, R. A., Champion, G. D., Addicoat, L., & Ziegler, J. B. (1990). The Faces Pain Scale for the self-assessment of the severity of pain experienced by children: Development, validation and preliminary investigation for ratio scale properties. *Pain, 41,* 139-150.

Bottari, C., Dutil, E., Dassa, C., & Rainville, C. (2006). Choosing the most appropriate environment to evaluate independence in everyday activities: Home or clinic? *Australian Occupational Therapy Journal, 53*(2), 98-106.

Bowman, J. (2006). Challenges to measuring outcomes in occupational therapy: A qualitative focus group study. *British Journal of Occupational Therapy, 69*(10), 464-472.

Cardol, M., de Haan, R. J., de Jong, B. A., van den Bos, G. A., & de Groot, I. J. (2001). Psychometric properties of the questionnaire Impact on Participation and Autonomy Questionnaire. *Archives of Physical Medicine and Rehabilitation, 82,* 210-216.

Carr, A. J., Gibson, B. A., & Robinson, P. G. (2001). Is quality of life determined by expectations or experience? *British Medical Journal, 322,* 1240-1243.

Carswell, A., McColl, M. A., Baptiste, S., Law, M., Polatajko, H., & Pollock, N. (2004). The Canadian Occupational Performance Measure: A research and clinical literature review. *Canadian Journal of Occupational Therapy, 71*(4), 210-222.

Chisholm, D., Toto, P., Raina, K., Holm, M., & Rogers, J. (2014). Evaluating capacity to live independently and safely in the community: Performance Assessment of Self-care Skills. *British Journal of Occupational Therapy, 77*(2), 59-63.

Chiu, T., & Oliver, R. (2006). Factor analysis and construct validity of the SAFER-HOME. *Occupational Therapy Journal of Research: Occupation, Participation and Health, 26*(4), 132-142.

Chiu, T., Oliver, R., Ascott, P., Choo, L., Davis, T., Gaya, A., . . . Letts, L. (2006). *Safety assessment of function and the environment for rehabilitation: Health outcome measurement and evaluation (SAFER-HOME) Version 3 Manual.* Toronto, ON: COTA Health.

Clemson, L. (1997). *Home fall hazards: A guide to identifying fall hazards in the homes of elderly people and an accompaniment to the assessment tool the Westmead Home Safety Assessment.* Victoria, Australia: Co-ordinates Publications.

Cohen, M. E., & Kearney, P. J. (2005). Use of evaluation data to support evidence-based practice. In J. Hinojosa, P. Kramer, & P. Crist (Eds.), *Evaluation: Obtaining and interpreting data* (2nd ed., pp. 263-282). Bethesda, MD: AOTA Press.

Cooper, B., Letts, L., Rigby, P., Stewart D., & Strong, S. (2005). Measuring environmental factors. In M. Law, C. Baum, & W. Dunn (Eds.), *Measuring occupation performance: Supporting best practice in occupational therapy* (2nd ed., pp. 316-344). Thorofare, NJ: SLACK Incorporated.

Corr, S., & Siddons, L. (2005). An introduction to the selection of outcome measures. *British Journal of Occupational Therapy, 68*(5), 202-206.

Crepeau, E. B., Schell, B. A. B., Gillen, G., & Scaffa, M. E. (2014). Analyzing occupations and activity. In B. A. B. Schell, G. Gillen, & M. E. Scaffa (Eds.), *Willard & Spackman's occupational therapy* (12th ed., pp. 234-248). Philadelphia, PA: Wolters Kluwer Health/Lippincott Williams & Wilkins.

Crist, P. (2005). Reliability and validity: The psychometric properties of standardized assessments. In J. Hinojosa, P. Kramer, & P. Crist (Eds.), *Evaluation: Obtaining and interpreting data* (2nd ed., pp. 175-194). Bethesda, MD: AOTA Press.

Davern, M. T., Cummins, R. A., & Stokes, M. A. (2007). Subjective well-being as an affective-cognitive construct. *Journal of Happiness Studies, 8*(4), 429-499.

Davis, R., & Rodd, R. (2014). Proving the effectiveness of community occupational therapy in the equipment and adaptation setting using the Canadian Occupational Performance Measure. *The British Journal of Occupational Therapy, 77*(2), 91-95.

de Jonge, D., Scherer, M. J., & Rodger, S. (2007). *Assistive technologies in the workplace.* St. Louis, MO: Mosby.

Dedding, C., Cardol, M., Eyssen, I. C., Dekker, J., & Beelen, A. (2004). Validity of the Canadian Occupational Performance Measure: A client-centred outcome measurement. *Clinical Rehabilitation, 18*(6), 660-667.

DeNeve, K. M. (1999). Happy as an extroverted clam? The role of personality for subjective well-being. *Current Directions in Psychological Science, 8*(5), 141-144.

DeRuyter, F. (2001). Outcomes and performance monitoring. In D. A. Olson & F. DeRuyter (Eds.), *Clinician's guide to assistive technology* (pp. 67-74). St. Louis, MO: Mosby.

Donnelly, C., & Carswell, A. (2002). Individualized outcome measures: A review of the literature. *Canadian Journal of Occupational Therapy, 69*(2), 84-94.

Donnelly, C., Eng, J. J., Hall, J., Alford, L., Giachino, R., Norton, K., & Kerr, D. S. (2004). Client-centered assessment and the identification of meaningful treatment goals for individuals with a spinal cord injury. *Spinal Cord, 42*(5), 302-307.

Douglas, H., Swanson, C., Gee, T., & Bellamy, N. (2005). Outcome measurement in Australian rehabilitation environments. *Journal of Rehabilitation Medicine, 37*(5), 325-329.

Duncan, R. (1998). Blueprint for action: The National Home Modifications Action Coalition. *Technology and Disability, 8*(1-2), 85-89.

Dunn, W. (2017). Measurement concepts and practices. In M. Law, C. Baum, & W. Dunn (Eds.), *Measuring occupational performance: Supporting best practice in occupational therapy* (3rd ed., pp. 17-28). Thorofare, NJ: SLACK Incorporated.

Dutil, E., Bottari, C., Vanier, M., & Gaudreault, C. (2005). *ADL Profile: Performance-based assessment user's guide* (Version 5). Montreal, Quebec: Emersion.

Dutil, E., Forget, A., Vanier, M., & Gaudreault, C. (1990). Development of the ADL Profile: An evaluation for adults with severe head injury. *Occupational Therapy in Health Care, 7*, 7-22.

Ekström, H., Schmidt, S. M., & Iwarsson, S. (2016). Home and health among different sub-groups of the ageing population: a comparison of two cohorts living in ordinary housing in Sweden. *BMC Geriatrics, 16*(1), 90.

Eyssen, I. C., Steultjens, M. P., Oud, T. A., Bolt, E. M., Maasdam, A., & Dekker, J. (2011). Responsiveness of the Canadian occupational performance measure. *Journal of Rehabilitation Research and Development, 48*(5), 517-528.

Fänge, A. (2002). *Usability in my home*. Lund, Sweden: Lund University, Division of Occupational Therapy.

Fänge, A., & Iwarsson, S. (1999). Physical housing environment: Development of a self-assessment instrument. *Canadian Journal of Occupational Therapy, 66*, 250-260.

Fänge, A., & Iwarsson, S. (2003). Accessibility and usability in housing: Construct validity and implications for research and practice. *Disability and Rehabilitation, 25*, 315-326.

Fänge, A., & Iwarsson, S. (2005a). Changes in ADL dependence and aspects of usability following housing adaptation—A longitudinal perspective. *American Journal of Occupational Therapy, 59*, 296-304.

Fänge, A., & Iwarsson, S. (2005b). Changes in accessibility and usability in housing: An exploration of the housing adaptation process. *Occupational Therapy International, 12*, 44-59.

Fänge, A., & Iwarsson, S. (2007). Challenges in the development of strategies for housing adaptation evaluations. *Scandinavian Journal of Occupational Therapy, 14*(3), 140-149.

Fisher, A. (1995). *Assessment of motor and process skills*. Fort Collins, CO: Three Star Press.

Fisher, A. G. (1998). Uniting practice and theory in an occupational framework. *American Journal of Occupational Therapy, 52*(7), 509-520.

Fisher, A. G., & Jones, K. B. (2011a). *Assessment of Motor and Process Skills: Development, standardization, and administration manual* (7th ed. Rev.). Fort Collins, CO: Three Star Press.

Fisher, A. G., & Jones, K. B. (2011b). *Assessment of Motor and Process Skills: User manual* (7th ed. Rev.). Fort Collins, CO: Three Star Press.

Frisch, J. (2000). Some notes on the economics of disability. Paper presented at Disability and Law Conference in Canberra, Australia, December 4, 2000. Retrieved from http://www.members.optushome.com.au/jackfrisch/EcsOfDisbltyNotes.pdf

Furphy, K. A., & Stav, W. B. (2014). Occupational performance assessments. In I. E. Asher (Ed.), *Asher's occupational therapy assessment tools: An annotated index* (4th ed., pp. 29-64). Bethesda, MD: American Occupational Therapy Association, Inc.

Gelderblom, G. J., & De Witte, L. (2002). The assessment of assistive technology outcomes, effects and cost. *Technology and Disability, 14*, 91-94.

Gillespie, L., Gillespie, W., Robertson, M., Lamb, S., Cumming, R., & Rowe, B. (2003). Interventions for preventing falls in elderly people (Cochrane Review). *The Cochrane Database of Systematic Reviews, 4*, CD000340.

Gitlin, L. N. (2003). Next steps in home modifications and assistive technology research. In N. Charness & K. W. Schaie (Eds.), *Impact of technology on successful aging* (pp. 188-202). New York, NY: Springer.

Gitlin, L. N., Hauck, W. W., Winter, L., Dennis, M. P., & Schulz, R. (2006). Effect of an in-home occupational and physical therapy intervention on reducing mortality in functionally vulnerable older people: Preliminary findings. *Journal of American Geriatric Society, 54*, 950-955.

Gitlin, L. N., Luborsky, M. R., & Schemm, R. L. (1998). Emerging concerns of older stroke patients about assistive devices. *The Gerontologist, 38*(2), 169-180.

Gitlin, L. N., Schinfeld, S., Winter, L., Corcoran, M., Boyce, A., & Hauck, W. (2002). Evaluating home environments of persons with dementia: Inter-rater reliability and validity of the Home Environmental Assessment Protocol (HEAP). *Disability and Rehabilitation, 24*(1), 59-71.

Gitlow, L. (2014). Assessments of Context: Physical Environment. In I. E. Asher (Ed.), *Asher's occupational therapy assessment tools: An annotated index* (4th ed., pp. 335-360). Bethesda, MD: American Occupational Therapy Association, Inc.

Gupta, A. (2008). *Measurement scales used in elderly care*. Oxford, UK: Radcliffe Publishing.

Haigh, R., Tennant, A., Biering-Sorenson, F., Grimby, G., MarinCek, C., Phillips, S., . . . Thonnard, J-L. (2001). The use of outcome measures in physical medicine and rehabilitation within Europe. *Journal of Rehabilitation Medicine, 33*(6), 273-278.

Hemmingsson, H., & Jonsson, H. (2005). An occupational perspective on the concept of participation in the International Classification of Functioning, Disability and Health: Some critical remarks. *American Journal Occupational Therapy, 59*(5), 569-576.

Heywood, F. (2001). *Money well spent: The effectiveness and value of housing adaptations*. Bristol, UK: Policy Press.

Heywood, F. (2004a). The health outcomes of housing adaptations. *Disability and Society, 19*(2), 129-143.

Heywood, F. (2004b). Understanding needs: A starting point for quality. *Housing Studies, 19*(5), 709-726.

Heywood, F. (2005). Adaptation: Altering the house to restore the home. *Housing Studies, 20*(4), 531-547.

Heywood, F., & Awang, D. (2011). Developing a housing adaptation genome project. *British Journal of Occupational Therapy, 74*(4), 200-203.

Heywood, F., & Turner, L. (2007). *Better outcomes, lower costs: Implications for health and social care budgets of investment in housing adaptations, improvements and equipment: A review of the evidence.* Leeds, UK: Department for Works and Pensions under license from the controller of Her Majesty's Stationery Office by Corporate Document Services.

Holm, M. B. & Rogers, J. C. (2017). Measuring performance in instrumental activities of daily living. In M. Law, C. Baum, & W. Dunn (Eds.), *Measuring occupational performance: Supporting best practice in occupational therapy* (3rd ed., pp. 305-332). Thorofare, NJ: SLACK Incorporated.

Hurstfield, J., Parashar, U., & Schofield, K. (2007). *The costs and benefits of independent living.* Norwich, UK: Office of Disability Issues, Department for Work and Pensions.

Iwarsson, S., Horstmann, V., & Slaug, B. (2007). Housing matters in very old age—Yet differently due to ADL dependence level differences. *Scandinavian Journal of Occupational Therapy, 14*, 3-15.

Iwarsson, S., Horstmann, V., & Sonn, U. (2009). Assessment of dependence in daily activities combined with a self-rating of difficulty. *Journal of Rehabilitation Medicine, 41*(3), 150-156.

Iwarsson, S., & Isacsson, Å., (1997). On scaling methodology and environmental influences in disability assessments: The cumulative structure of personal and instrumental ADL among older adults in a Swedish rural district. *Canadian Journal of Occupational Therapy, 64*, 240-251.

Iwarsson, S., & Slaug, B. (2001). *The Housing Enabler: An instrument for assessing and analyzing accessibility problems in housing.* Navlinge och Staffanstorp, Sweden: Veten & Stapen HB & Slaug Data Management. Retrieved from http://www.enabler.nu

Jerosch-Herold, C. (2005). An evidence-based approach to choosing outcome measures: A checklist for the critical appraisal of validity, reliability and responsiveness studies. *British Journal of Occupational Therapy, 68*(8), 347-353.

Jette, A. M., & Haley, S. M. (2005). Contemporary measurement techniques for rehabilitation outcomes assessment. *Journal of Rehabilitation Medicine, 37*, 339-345.

Jakobsson, U. (2008). The ADL-staircase: further validation. *International Journal of Rehabilitation Research, 31*(1), 85-88.

Johansson, K., Lilja, M., Petersson, I. A., & Borell, L. (2007). Performance of activities of daily living in a sample of applicants for home modification services. *Scandinavian Journal of Occupational Therapy, 14*, 44-53.

Jones, A., de Jonge, D., & Phillips, R. (2008). *The role of home maintenance and modification services in achieving health, community care and housing outcomes in later life: Research report.* Melbourne, Australia: Australian Housing and Urban Research Institute. Retrieved from https://www.ahuri.edu.au/__data/assets/pdf_file/0003/2100/AHURI_Final_Report_No123_The-role-of-home-maintenance-and-modification-services-in-achieving-health-community-care.pdf

Katz, S., Ford, A. B., Moskowitz, R. W., Jackson, B. A., & Jaffe, M. W. (1963). Studies of illness in the aged. The index of ADL, a standardized measure of biological and psychological function. *Journal of the American Medical Association, 185*(12), 914-919.

Kjeken, I., & Lillemo, S. (2006). Exploration of the link between conceptual occupational therapy models and the International Classification of Functioning, Disability and Health: A response from colleagues in Norway. A*ustralian Occupational Therapy Journal, 54*, 142-143.

Klein, S., Barlow, I., & Hollis, V. (2008). Evaluating ADL measures from an occupational perspective. *Canadian Journal of Occupational Therapy, 75*(2), 69-81.

Larson, E. A. (2000). The orchestration of occupation: The dance of mothers. *American Journal of Occupational Therapy, 54*, 269-280.

Laver Fawcett, A. (2007). The importance of accurate assessment and outcomes measurement. In A. Laver Fawcett (Ed.), *Principles of assessment and outcome measurements for occupational therapists and physiotherapists: Theory, skills and application* (pp. 15-44). West Sussex, UK: John Wiley & Sons Ltd.

Law, M. (1998). *Client-centered occupational therapy.* Thorofare, NJ: SLACK Incorporated.

Law, M. (2005). Outcome measures rating form guidelines. In M. Law, C. Baum, & W. Dunn (Eds.), *Measuring occupational performance: Supporting best practice in occupational therapy* (2nd ed., pp. 396-409). Thorofare, NJ: SLACK Incorporated.

Law, M., Baptiste, S., Carswell, A., McColl, M., Polatajko, H., & Pollock, N. (1998). *Canadian occupational performance measure* (3rd ed.). Toronto, ON: CAOT Publications ACE.

Law, M., Baptiste, S., Carswell, A., McColl, M., Polatajko, H., & Pollock, N. (2014). *Canadian occupational performance measure* (5th ed.). Ottawa, ON: CAOT Publications ACE.

Law, M. C., & Baum, C. M. (2017). Measurement in occupational therapy. In M. Law, C. Baum, & W. Dunn (Eds.), *Measuring occupational performance: Supporting best practice in occupational therapy* (3rd ed., pp. 1-16). Thorofare, NJ: SLACK Incorporated.

Law, M., Baum, C., & Dunn, W. (2017). *Measuring occupational performance: Supporting best practice in occupational therapy* (3rd ed.). Thorofare, NJ: SLACK Incorporated.

Lilja, M. (2002). *Riktlinjer för användning av Client-Clinician Assessment Protocol (C-CAP). [Guidelines for Using the Client-Clinician Assessment Protocol (C-CAP)].* Karolinska Institutet, Stockholm.

Luebben, A. J., & Royeen, C. B. (2005). Non-standardized testing. In J. Hinojosa, P. Kramer, & P. Crist (Eds.), *Evaluation: Obtaining and interpreting data* (2nd ed., pp. 125-146). Bethesda, MD: AOTA Press.

Lund, M. L., Nordlund, A., Nygard, L., Lexell, J., & Bernspang, B. (2005). Perceptions of participation and predictors of perceived problems with participation in persons with spinal cord injury. *Journal of Rehabilitation Medicine, 37*(1), 3-8.

Mackenzie, L., Byles, J., & Higginbotham, N. (2000). Designing the Home Falls and Accidents Screening Tool (HOME FAST): Selecting the items. *British Journal of Occupational Therapy, 63*(6), 260-269.

Magasi, S., Gohil, A., Burghart, M., & Wallisch, A. (2017). Understanding measurement properties. In M. Law, C. Baum, & W. Dunn (Eds.), *Measuring occupational performance: Supporting best practice in occupational therapy* (3rd ed., pp. 29-41). Thorofare, NJ: SLACK Incorporated.

Mann, W. C., Ottenbacher, K. J., Fraas, L., Tomita, M., & Granger, C. V. (1999). Effectiveness of assistive technology and environmental interventions in reducing home care costs for the frail elderly: A randomized control trial. *Archives of Family Medicine, 8*(May/June), 210-217.

Marcus, C. (1995). *House as a mirror of self.* Berkeley, CA: Conrai Press.

Martin, L. (2014). Social Participation Assessments. In I. E. Asher (Ed.), *Asher's occupational therapy assessment tools: an annotated index* (4th ed., pp. 335-360). Bethesda, MD: American Occupational Therapy Association, Inc.

McColl, M. A., & Pollock, N. (2001). Measuring occupational performance using a client-centered perspective. In M. Law, C. Baum, & W. Dunn (Eds.), *Measuring occupational performance* (pp. 81-91). Thorofare, NJ: SLACK Incorporated.

McColl, M. A., & Pollock, N. (2017). Measuring occupational performance using a client-centered perspective. In M. Law, C. Baum, & W. Dunn (Eds.), *Measuring occupational performance: Supporting best practice in occupational therapy* (3rd ed., pp. 83-94). Thorofare, NJ: SLACK Incorporated.

Melzack, R. (1975). The McGill Pain Questionnaire: Major properties and scoring methods. *Pain, 1,* 277-299.

Messecar, D. C., Archbold, P. G., Stewart, B. J., & Kirschling, J. (2002). Home environmental modification strategies used by caregivers of elders. *Research in Nursing and Health, 25,* 357-370.

Miller Polgar, J. (2009). Critiquing assessments. In E. Crepeau, E. Cohn, & B. Schell (Eds.), *Willard & Spackman's occupational therapy* (11th ed., pp. 519-536). Philadelphia, PA: Wolters, Kluwer, Lippincott, Williams, & Wilkins.

Moore, J. (2000). Placing home in context. *Journal of Environmental Psychology, 20,* 207-217.

Msall, M. E., DiGaudio, K., Rogers, B. T., LaForest, S., Catanzaro, N. L., Campbell, J., . . . Duffy, L. C. (1994). The Functional Independence Measure for Children (WeeFIM): Conceptual basis and pilot use in children with developmental disabilities. *Clinical Pediatrics, 33*(7), 421-430.

Nikolaus, T., & Bach, M. (2003). Preventing falls in community-dwelling frail older people using a home intervention team. *Journal of the American Geriatric Society, 51,* 300-305.

Noreau, L., Fougeyrollas, P., & Vincent, C. (2002). The LIFE-H: Assessment of the quality of social participation. *Technology and Disability, 14,* 113-118.

Nygren, C., Oswald, F., Iwarsson, S., Fänge, J., Sixsmith, J., Schilling, O., . . . Wahl, H-W. (2007). Relationships between objective and perceived housing in very old age. *The Gerontologist, 47,* 85-95.

Oliver, R., Blathwayt, J., Brackley, C., & Tamaki, T. (1993). Development of the Safety Assessment of Function and the Environment for Rehabilitation (SAFER) tool. *Canadian Journal of Occupational Therapy, 60*(2), 78-82.

Oswald, F., Schilling, O., Wahl, H. W., Fänge, A., Sixsmith, J., & Iwarsson, S. (2006). Homeward bound: Introducing a four-domain model of perceived housing in very old age. *Journal of Environmental Psychology, 26,* 187-201.

Oswald, F., & Wahl, H. W. (2005). Dimensions of the meaning of home in later life. In G. D. Rowles & H. Chaudhury (Eds.), *Home and identity in later life: International perspectives* (pp. 21-46). New York, NY: Springer.

Oswald, F., Wahl, H. W., Martin, M., & Mollenkopf, H. (2003). Toward measuring proactivity in person-environment transactions in late adulthood: The Housing-Related Control Beliefs Questionnaire. *Journal of Housing for the Elderly, 17,* 135-152.

Oswald, F., Wahl, H. W., Schilling, O., & Iwarsson, S. (2007). Housing-related control beliefs and independence in activities of daily living in very old age. *Scandinavian Journal of Occupational Therapy, 14,* 33-43.

Parker, D. M., & Sykes, C. H. (2006). A systematic review of the Canadian Occupational Performance Measure: A clinical practice perspective. *British Journal of Occupational Therapy, 69*(4), 150-160.

Patterson, D. R., Jensen, M., & Engel-Knowles, J. (2002). Pain and its influence on assistive technology use. In M. J. Scherer (Ed.), *Assistive technology: Matching device and consumer for successful rehabilitation* (pp. 59-76). Washington, DC: American Psychological Association.

Petersson, I., Fisher, A. G., Hemmingsson, H., & Lilja, M. (2007). The client-clinician assessment protocol (C-CAP): Evaluation of its psychometric properties for use with people aging with disabilities in need of home modifications. *Occupational Therapy Journal of Research: Occupation, Participation and Health, 27*(4), 140-148.

Petersson, I., Lilja, M., Hammel, J., & Kottorp, A. (2008). Impact of home modification services on ability in everyday life for people ageing with disabilities. *Journal of Rehabilitation Medicine, 40*(4), 253-260.

Plautz, B., Beck, D., Selmar, C., & Radetsky, M. (1996). Modifying the environment: A community-based injury-reduction programme for elderly residents. *American Journal of Preventative Medicine, 12*(4), 33-38.

Post, M. W. M., Festen, H., van de Port, I. G., & Visser-Meily, J. M. A. (2007). Reproducibility of the Caregiver Strain Index and the Caregiver Reaction Assessment in partners of stroke patients living in the Dutch community. *Clinical Rehabilitation, 21,* 1050-1055.

Pynoos, J. (2004). On the forefront of the ever-changing field of home modification. *Rehabilitation Management, 17*(3), 34-35, 50.

Pynoos, J., Rose, D., Rubenstein, L., Choi, H., & Sabata, D. (2006). Evidence-based interventions in fall prevention. *Home Health Care Services Quarterly: The Journal of Community Care, 25*(1/2), 55-72.

Pynsent, P., Fairbank, J., & Carr, A. (2004). *Outcome measures in orthopaedics and trauma* (2nd ed.). London, UK: A Hodder Arnold Publication.

Rigby, P., Craciunoiu, O., Stier, J. & Letts, L. (2017). Measuring environmental factors. In M. Law, C. Baum, & W. Dunn (Eds.), *Measuring occupational performance: Supporting best practice in occupational therapy* (3rd ed., pp. 351-390). Thorofare, NJ: SLACK Incorporated.

Robinson, B. C. (1983). Validation of a Caregiver Strain Index. *Journal of Gerontology, 38,* 344-348.

Rogers, J. C., & Holm, M. B. (1994). *The performance assessment of self-care skills (PASS)—Version 3.1.* Pittsburgh, PA: University of Pittsburgh.

Rogers, J. C., Holm, M. B., & Chisholm, D. (2016). The Performance Assessment of Self-Care Skills (PASS)—Version 4.1. Pittsburgh, PA: University of Pittsburgh. In M. Law, C. Baum, & W. Dunn (Eds.), *Measuring occupational performance: Supporting best practice in occupational therapy* (3rd ed., pp. 351-390). Thorofare, NJ: SLACK Incorporated.

Rossi, P. H., Lipsey, M. W., & Freeman, H. E. (2004). *Evaluation: A systematic approach* (7th ed.). Thousand Oaks, CA: Sage Publications.

Sackett, D. L., Rosenberg, W. M. C., Gray, J. A. M., Haynes, R. B., & Richardson, W. S. (1996). Evidence-based medicine: What it is and what it isn't. *British Journal of Medicine, 312,* 71-72.

Salter, K., Jutai, J. W., Teasell, R., Foley, N. C., & Bitensky, J. (2005). Issues for selection of outcome measures in stroke rehabilitation: ICF body functions. *Disability and Rehabilitation, 27*(4), 191-207.

Sanford, J. A., Patricia C., Griffiths, P. C., Richardson, P. N., Hargraves, K., Butterfield, T., & Hoenig, H. (2006). The effects of in-home rehabilitation on task self-efficacy in mobility-impaired adults: A randomized clinical trial. *Journal of the American Geriatrics Society, 54*(11), 1641-1648.

Sbordone, R. J., & Guilmette, T. J. (1999). Ecological validity: Prediction of everyday and vocational functioning from neuropsychological test data. In J. J. Sweet (Ed.), *Forensic neuropsychology: Fundamentals and practice* (pp. 227-254). Exton, PA: Taylor & Francis.

Schultz-Krohn, W. (2014). Occupational Performance Assessments. In I. E. Asher (Ed.), *Asher's occupational therapy assessment tools: an annotated index* (4th ed., pp. 29-64). Bethesda, MD: American Occupational Therapy Association, Inc.

Sells, C. H. (2005). Additional uses of evaluation data. In J. Hinojosa, P. Kramer, & P. Crist (Eds.), *Evaluation: Obtaining and interpreting data* (2nd ed., pp. 283-305). Bethesda, MD: AOTA Press.

Shah, S., Vanclay, F., & Cooper, B. (1989). Improving the sensitivity of the Barthel Index for stroke rehabilitation. *Journal of Clinical Epidemiology, 42*, 703-709.

Sibley, A., Kersten, P., Ward, C. D., White, B., Mehta, R., & George, S. (2006). Measuring autonomy in disabled people: validation of a new scale in a UK population. *Clinical Rehabilitation, 20*(9), 793-803.

Smith, R. O. (2002). OTFACT: Multi-level performance-oriented software assistive technology outcomes protocol. *Technology and Disability, 14*, 133-139.

Sonn, U., & Hulter-Åsberg, K., (1991). Assessment of activities of daily living in the elderly. *Scandinavian Journal of Rehabilitation Medicine, 23*, 193-202.

Stamm, T. A., Cieza, A., Machold, K., Smolen, J. S., & Stucki, G. (2006). Exploration of the link between conceptual occupational therapy models and the International Classification of Functioning, Disability and Health. *Australian Occupational Therapy Journal, 53*, 9-17.

Stark, S. (2004). Removing environmental barriers in the homes of older adults with disabilities improves occupational performance. *Occupation, Participation and Health, 24*(1), 32-40.

Stark, S., Keglovits, M., Arbesman, M., & Lieberman, D. (2017). Effect of Home Modification Interventions on the Participation of Community-Dwelling Adults with Health Conditions: A Systematic Review. *American Journal of Occupational Therapy, 71*(2), 7102290010p1-11A.

Stark, S. L., Somerville, E. K., & Morris, J. C. (2010). In-Home Occupational Performance Evaluation (I-HOPE). *American Journal of Occupational Therapy, 64*(4), 580-589.

Struckmeyer, L. R. (2016, December). Reliability and Validity of the Home Environmental Assessment Protocol-Revised (Doctoral dissertation, Texas Woman's University, Denton, Texas). Retrieved from http://search.proquest.com.ezproxy.library.uq.edu.au/docview/1832952513/previewPDF/EF2FA89B22B04F72PQ/1?accountid=14723

Thomas Jefferson University. (n.d.). Center for Applied Research on Aging and Health. Retrieved from http://www.jefferson.edu/jchp/carah/researchers.cfm

Tinetti, M. E., Richman, D., & Powell, L. (1990). Falls efficacy as a measure of fear of falling. *Journal of Gerontology: Psychological Sciences, 45*, 239-243.

Uniform Data System for Medical Rehabilitation. (1997). *Functional Independence Measure (Version 5.1).* Buffalo, NY: Buffalo General Hospital, State University of New York.

Uniform Data System for Medical Rehabilitation. (2009). *The FIM System Clinical Guide—Version 5.2.* Buffalo, NY: UDSMR, State University of New York at Buffalo.

Ware, J., & Sherbourne, C. (1992). The MOS 36-Item Short Form Health Survey (SF36): Conceptual framework and item selection. *Medical Care, 30*(6), 473-481.

Ware, J. E., Snow, K. K., Kosinski, M., & Gandek, B. (1993). *SF-36 health survey manual and interpretation guide.* Boston, MA: New England Medical Center, The Health Institute.

World Health Organization. (2001). *The International Classification of Function, Activity and Participation.* Geneva, Switzerland: Author.

World Health Organization. (2002). *Towards a common language for functioning, disability and health.* Geneva, Switzerland: Author.

World Health Organization. (2005). ICF checklist. Retrieved from http://www.who.int/classifications/icf/training/icfchecklist.pdf

14

Literature Review
Home Modification Outcomes for
Older Adults and Adults With Disabilities

Elizabeth Ainsworth, MOccThy, Grad Cert Health Sci;
Tammy Aplin, PhD, BOccThy (Hons); Louise Gustafsson, PhD, BOccThy (Hons);
and Desleigh de Jonge, MPhil (OccThy), Grad Cert Soc Sci

This chapter presents a review of the research on the outcomes of home modification for adults. The intent is to detail the benefits and unintended consequences of home modifications and provide an evidence base for home modification practice. The review identified that modifications result in outcomes that are highly valued by service providers, such as health, safety, and independence. It also highlighted the potential for modifications to enrich the lives of clients, and others in the household, neighborhood, and community. However, home modifications were also found to have devastating impacts on the lives of older people and people with a disability when not completed well. A summary of the strength of evidence in each outcome area is provided, and areas for future research to enhance the evidence base for home modification practice is presented.

CHAPTER OBJECTIVES

By the end of the chapter, the reader will be able to:

✦ Describe the research reporting outcomes of home modifications

✦ Identify knowledge gaps and limitations in the current body of research

GENERAL OVERVIEW

A pragmatic synthesis approach was used to complete this narrative literature review (Green, Johnson, & Adams, 2006). The review was conducted by searching a range of databases including the Cumulative Index of Nursing and Allied Health Literature, Pub Med, OT Seeker, SCOPUS, PsycARTICLES, the Cochrane Library, and Web of Science. Research articles reviewed included those published from 1990 to 2017. Findings of the articles specific to the aim of this review were extracted and summarized into themes. A summary of the limitations associated with the findings, directions for future research, and implications for occupational therapy practice are described.

The literature describing home modification outcomes originates from Western countries such as America, Canada, Europe, the United Kingdom, and Australia with some more recent studies emerging from Asia. Predominantly this has been conducted in the health care sector with a smaller number emerging from the housing sector (Carnemolla & Bridge, 2015). The range of studies reviewed differ in their use of language and meaning in relation to home modifications (Iwarsson, 2015; Russell, 2016). For the purposes of this review, home

Ainsworth, E., & de Jonge, D. *An Occupational Therapist's*
Guide to Home Modification Practice, Second Edition (pp. 313-335).

modifications are defined as individually tailored interventions that eliminate barriers in the home environment (Granbom, Taei, & Ekstam, 2017). They include nonstructural and permanent structural modifications to the physical home environment. Nonstructural modifications, referred to as minor modifications, include the installation or alteration of fittings and fixtures (Jones, de Jonge, & Phillips, 2008). Permanent structural modifications, defined as major modifications, involve changes to the fabric, space, and layout of the home (Jones et al., 2008). The type of modification provided depends on the ability of the individual, the activities to be performed and the standard and design of the home (Pettersson, Löfqvist, & Fänge, 2012).

Alternative terminology for home modifications found in the international literature includes *housing adaptations* and *environmental adaptation*, resulting in debate about what constitutes a home modification (Russell, 2016). The term *home modifications* is often used interchangeably with *housing adaptations*. Iwarsson (2015) defines home modifications broadly to include interventions in the home such as housing adaptations, alterations to the physical structure of the home and the immediate outdoor environment, home hazard counselling, and provision of assistive technology (Iwarsson, 2015). In the United States, researchers also consider home modifications to include a wider range of strategies that compensate for impairments and improve performance of daily activities (Gitlin, Hauk, Winter, Dennis, & Schultz, 2006; Siebert, Smallfield, & Stark, 2014). These strategies include medical equipment, universally designed products, architectural modifications, major home renovations, or a learning strategy to use the environment a different way (Siebert et al., 2014). An additional overlap exists between the use of the term *home modifications* and *assistive technology* (Jones et al., 2008; Pynoos, Tabbarah, Angelelli, & Demiere, 1998). In some countries such as the United States, home modifications are classified as an assistive technology and are defined as "any device or system that allows an individual to perform a task that they would otherwise be unable to do or increases the ease and safety with which the task can be performed" (Cowan & Turner-Smith, 1999). In many countries, assistive devices are typically considered to be mobile and not attached to the structure of the house (Pynoos et al., 1998), whereas home modifications are more permanent, secure, and fixed in place (Jones et al., 2008). Despite the difference in viewpoints about what constitutes a home modification, there appears to be general agreement that the intent of home modifications is to alter the physical home environment, to reduce the physical barriers in the home, and enhance a person's activity and participation (Fänge & Iwarsson, 2005a; Russell, 2016; Sanford, 2012; Stark, 2004; Steinfeld & Maisel, 2012).

A large proportion of the studies examined home modification outcomes for older community-dwelling adults. However, these studies do not have a consistent definition for the age range of older adults. For example, researchers indicate the age range as 60 years and older (Stark, Landsbaum, Palmer, Somerville & Morris, 2009), 65 years and older (Close et al., 1999), 70 years and older (Palvanen et al., 2014; Tinetti, Mendes de Leon, Doucette, & Baker, 1994), or 73 years and older (Naik & Gill, 2005). Other research has focussed on the needs of children, people with low vision, people with schizophrenia, and people undergoing hip surgery (Stark, Keglovits, et al., 2017), but not to the same extent.

Research into home modification outcomes has largely been undertaken using quantitative methodology, investigating the delivery of minor home modifications in combination with other interventions. These studies have examined the outcome of home modifications in relation to hazard reduction and falls prevention; maintaining and improving functional ability, reducing morbidity and mortality; limiting the impact of care on caregivers; and achieving cost savings to services in relation to delivery of care (Stark, Keglovits, Arbesman, & Lieberman 2017; Stark, Somerville, et al., 2017; Wahl, Fänge, Oswald, Gitlin, & Iwarsson, 2009). The most common outcomes of home modifications investigated has been functional ability and falls (Fänge & Iwarsson, 2005a, 2005b; Gillespie et al., 2012; Haak, Fänge, Iwarsson, & Dahlin-Ivanoff, 2007; Keall et al., 2015; Petersson, Kottorp, Bergström, & Lilja, 2009; Petersson, Lilja, Hammel, & Kottorp, 2008; Petersson, Löfqvist, & Fänge, 2012; Wahl et al., 2009). Much of this quantitative research appears to be derived from a health service focus on function and safety.

Qualitative studies have reported greater diversity in subject age range, health conditions, and disabilities than those in quantitative studies. This research supports that home modifications reduce falls (Adams & Grisbrooke, 1998); improve function (Pettersson et al., 2012); improve health and well-being and caregiver outcomes (Andrich, Ferrario, & Moi, 1998; Calkins & Namazi, 1991; Heywood, 2005) and result in cost savings (Heywood & Turner, 2007). However, qualitative studies describe broader outcomes such as enabling people to remain in their own homes and participate in valued roles in the home and community. Home modifications have been found to foster freedom, autonomy, and control; restore self-image, privacy, and dignity (Haak,

Fänge, et al., 2007) and assist in restoring and fostering relationships (Heywood, 2005). They are also described as enhancing the experience of home as a place of significance and personal meaning (Aplin, de Jonge, & Gustafsson, 2015). This qualitative research, while less prolific, is likely representing the most meaningful outcomes to older people and people with a disability.

The following sections further summarize and describe the outcomes reported in literature under the themes of falls and injuries, mortality and morbidity, institutional and home care costs, impact on caregivers, activities of daily living and the experience of home. Table 14-1 provides an overview of the strength of the research evidence for each theme.

FALLS AND INJURIES

Most home modification research lies in falls prevention. Falls and the consequences thereof are common amongst older people, often resulting in injuries, morbidity, the need for care assistance and increased health care costs (Ekstam, Carlsson, Chiatti, Nilsson, & Fänge, 2014; Pynoos, Steinman, Nguyen, & Bressette, 2012). Injury and hospital admissions are a major expense for public and private organisations (Pynoos et al., 2012), and consequently there is a large body of research focused on falls, including home modifications as an intervention preventing falls. The strongest evidence for fall reduction is when home modification interventions are targeted at older people who are at high risk of falls, rather than people in a younger age groups with a range of health conditions or disabilities (Chase, Mann, Wasek, & Arbesman, 2012; Clemson, Mackenzie, Ballinger, Close, & Cumming, 2008; Costello & Edelstein, 2008; Lord, Menz, & Sherrington, 2006; Tse, 2005).

A range of systematic reviews have investigated the home environment's relationship to injury prevalence or falls prevention (Carnemolla & Bridge, 2015). Most studies included within these reviews measured the effect of home modifications in combination with other interventions such as caregiver training, assistive devices, and behavioral change strategies (Carnemolla & Bridge, 2015). It has been consistently demonstrated that these multicomponent prevention programs using an individualized approach, prevent falls (Pighills, Ballinger, Pickering, & Chari, 2016; Pynoos et al., 2012). However, it remains difficult to determine the specific influence of home modifications within these multicomponent interventions (Chase et al., 2012; Stark, Keglovits, et al., 2017).

Seven randomized controlled trials have examined the clinical effectiveness of home modifications and assessment in isolation from other interventions (Pighills et al., 2016) with three demonstrating statistically significant reductions in falls (Campbell et al., 2005; Nikolaus & Bach, 2003; Pighills, Torgerson, Sheldon, Drummond, & Bland, 2011), one indicated a borderline result (Cumming et al., 1999) and the remaining three were unable to demonstrate a statistically significant effect on falls (Day et al., 2002; Lin, Wolf, Hwang, Gong, & Chen, 2007; Stevens, Holman, & Bennett, 2001). Pighills et al. (2016) concluded that to be effective in reducing falls, the interventions should be of high intensity (involving comprehensive validated functional assessment of people in their home environment with follow-up), provided by an occupational therapist, and directed toward high-risk populations such as those aged over 65 years of age, with one or more risk factors. These risk factors included having a history of falls in the previous year, recent hospital admission, a chronic condition, or a vision impairment (Pighills et al., 2016). The most recent of the systematic reviews stated that interventions focussing on home safety assessment and modifications reduced falls by 19% (relative rate 0.81, 95% confidence interval (CI) 0.68-0.97; 6 trials with 4,208 total participants; Gillespie et al., 2012).

With respect to injury outcomes, a Cochrane review demonstrated that multifactorial injury prevention interventions have been shown to reduce injuries in the home (Turner, Arthur, & Lyons, 2011). However, few studies focused specifically on the impact of home modifications. Twenty-eight published and one unpublished study were included in the review and were categorized into three groups: children, older people, and the general population that included a mix of age groups. None of the studies focusing on children or older people demonstrated a reduction in injuries that were a direct result of home modifications. One study focusing on older people demonstrated a reduction in falls (Campbell et al., 2005) and another, a reduction in falls and injurious falls that may have been due to hazard reduction (Jensen, Lundin-Olsson, Nyberg, & Gustafson, 2002). A meta-analysis was performed which examined the effects on falls of multifactorial interventions consisting of home hazard assessment and modification, medication review, health and bone assessment and exercise, finding that multifactorial fall prevention programs designed for older people who had fallen in the previous twelve months did not reduce the risk of falling (risk ratio [RR] 1.09, 95% CI 0.97-1.23; Turner et al., 2011). Campbell et al.'s 2005 study was the only study to demonstrate a direct association between the home

Table 14-1. Strength of Current Evidence

OUTCOME	STRENGTH	CONTEXT
Falls	++++	Community-dwelling older adults with a history of falls (multifactorial interventions)
		Community-dwelling older adults with a history of falls (single interventions)
Injuries	++	Community-dwelling older adults
Mortality and morbidity	+++	Community-dwelling older adults and younger populations
		Multicomponent approach
Institutional and in-home care costs	+	Community-dwelling older adults
Caregiver's role, personal health and well-being	+++	Multicomponent approach
		Caregivers of people with dementia or related disorders; people with spinal injury; family caregivers
Activities of daily living (Personal and Instrumental)	+++	Community-dwelling older adults and younger populations with a range of health conditions and disabilities; caregivers
Safety, security, and comfort	++++	Community-dwelling older adults and younger populations with a range of health conditions and disabilities; caregivers
Sense of permanency and continuity	++++	Community-dwelling older adults and younger populations with a range of health conditions and disabilities; caregivers
Privacy and dignity	++++	Community-dwelling older adults and younger populations with a range of health conditions and disabilities; caregivers
Freedom, choice, and control	++++	Community-dwelling older adults and younger populations with a range of health conditions and disabilities; caregivers
Identity and self esteem	++++	Community-dwelling older adults and younger populations with a range of health conditions and disabilities; caregivers
Appearance and ambience of the home	++++	Community-dwelling older adults and younger populations with a range of health conditions and disabilities; caregivers
Usability of the home	++++	Community-dwelling older adults and younger populations with a range of health conditions and disabilities; caregivers
Maintaining and enhancing valued roles and occupations	++++	Community-dwelling older adults and younger populations with a range of health conditions and disabilities; caregivers
Fostering relationships, social connections, and participation in social activities	++++	Community-dwelling older adults and younger populations with a range of health conditions and disabilities; caregivers
Perception of value and potential resale of the home	++++	Community-dwelling older adults and younger populations with a range of health conditions and disabilities

++++   High: Consistent findings; further research is unlikely to change our confidence in the finding

+++   Moderate: Further research is likely to have an impact on our confidence

++   Low: Further research is required to develop our confidence

+   Very low: Impact is uncertain

safety component of the intervention, that is, home modification, and a significant reduction in injuries in relation to falls. However, the authors reported that there was no significant difference between falls occurring inside and outside the home, where the home modification intervention could not have influenced the risk of falling. Overall, the Cochrane review concluded that there is insufficient evidence to determine if home modifications reduce injuries. Suggesting that the effect of modifications within the included multifactorial interventions was either inseparable or insignificant.

In summary, most studies relating to falls prevention have focused on the impact of home modifications on falls for older people (Cumming et al., 1999; Day et al., 2002; Lannin et al., 2007; Pardessus et al., 2002; Stevens et al., 2001) and consider home modifications to be effective in reducing falls for the older population at falls risk (Gillespie et al., 2012). The effects of home modifications on falls and fall-related injuries are difficult to isolate in multicomponent approaches (Robinovitch, Scott, & Feldman, 2014). Consequently, there is a need for more adequately designed randomized controlled trials with large populations to provide more conclusive evidence of injury outcomes and a need consider using factorial designs to allow the evaluation of individual components of multifactorial interventions (Turner et al., 2011).

HEALTH, MORTALITY, AND MORBIDITY

A decline in health and associated accidental injuries are a significant cause of morbidity and mortality among older populations (Plautz, Beck, Selmar, & Radetsky, 1996). As per the previous section, a multicomponent approach is adopted, and home modifications are often combined with other interventions to reduce the likelihood of mortality and morbidity. Studies have identified that home modifications combined with assistive technologies may slow the progression of frailty, and prevent and postpone morbidity and mortality (Mann, Ottenbacher, Fraas, Tomita, & Granger, 1999). For example, a prospective cohort study found that the progression of frailty and mortality in 574 older adults 65 years and older who required a low or moderate level of care in their home was slowed due to the provision of home modifications with assistive technology (Mitoku & Shimanouchi, 2014). The mortality of participants who had home modifications was significantly lower than those without home modifications at 2 years

(adjusted hazard ratio [HR] = 0.52; 95% CI [0.32, 0.87]), 3 years (HR = 0.57, 95% CI [0.54, 0.81]), and 4.7 years (HR = 0.65, 95% CI [0.65, 0.91]). Another study explored the effectiveness of a multicomponent intervention, including home modifications, behavioral and cognitive strategies, with a group of 319 urban community living older people aged 70 years and older (Gitlin, Winter, et al., 2006). This randomized controlled trial found that the intervention offset the functional consequences of chronic disease and reduced mortality risk, with intervention participants exhibiting a 1% rate of mortality, compared with a 10% rate for the no-treatment control participants (P = 0.003, 95% CI [52.4-15.04]). These studies contribute to the evidence base for multicomponent interventions, but further research would assist in determining the specific impact of home modifications on morbidity and mortality.

Focusing on morbidity, home modifications have been found to positively influence pain and breathlessness. For example, the provision of grab bars for 144 people, including older people and people with a disability, resulted in people performing tasks within the home with less pain (Clemson & Martin, 1996). Reduction in pain levels has similarly been reported for people receiving major modifications (Heywood, 2004b), and for people with physical disabilities receiving level access showers (Adams & Grisbrooke, 1998). The introduction of level access showers was also found to decrease breathlessness in participants (Adams & Grisbrooke, 1998), a finding similarly reported in a quasi-experimental study with 14 people with asthma aged between 15 to 49 years of age (Frisk et al., 2006). Pre- and postmodification outcome measurement also identified that the removal of carpet resulted in the improvement of lung function, respiratory symptoms, and indoor air quality (Frisk et al., 2006). A more recent randomized controlled study reinforced this finding, showing that home modifications (including removal of carpets) contribute to reduction in the onset of asthma and resultant hospitalizations in people aged 18 to 64 years of age in an asthma management program (Shelledy, Legrand, Gardner, & Peters, 2009). At 6 months post modifications, people had significantly fewer (P < 0.05) hospitalizations, inpatient days, lower hospitalizations, and greater health related quality of life physical component summary scores, and patient satisfaction scores, than those patients receiving usual care (Shelledy et al., 2009).

The findings above suggest that home modifications may have a role in limiting morbidity and mortality, particularly when delivered within the home as part of a multicomponent intervention program. Further investigation is required into whether home modifications that are not delivered as part of a multicomponent intervention program, impact morbidity and mortality.

INSTITUTIONAL AND IN-HOME CARE COSTS

Home modifications have also been found to contribute to cost savings in relation to institutional and in-home care costs. A literature review completed in 2007 found that when modifications removed the need for a daily home care visit, or reduced the number of such visits, they paid for themselves in a time-span ranging from a few months to 3 years and then produced annual savings (Heywood & Turner, 2007). These positive impacts on institutional and home care costs occur when the provision of home modifications enables discharge from hospitals more quickly or avoids residential care, saving money, sometimes on a considerable scale (Heywood & Turner, 2007; Mann et al., 1999; Mathieson, Kronenfeld, & Keith, 2002; Newman, Struyk, Wright & Rice, 1990; Oswald & Rowles, 2007). For example, increased expenditure on nurse visits and case manager visits for home based frail older persons was avoided with the purchase of assistive technology and environmental interventions (Mann et al., 1999). Other researchers have demonstrated the cost savings of home modifications using a series of constructed case studies, whereby environmental interventions were shown to cost significantly less than providing ongoing residential care, except in cases where people have severe impairments (Lansley, McCreadie, & Tinker, 2004). Predictive costs associated with the installation of home modifications have also been shown to reduce ongoing costs using vignette-like descriptions of fictional cases to evaluate hypothetical interventions for the same individual case (Chiatti & Iwarsson, 2014).

The first known cost-effective analysis of a home modification program was undertaken by Jutkowitz and colleagues (2012). This analysis was based on a randomized control trial (Gitlin, Winter, et al., 2006) where the intervention group was provided with occupational and physical therapy sessions and a home modification intervention. Using data from the National Death Index records, the length of time of survivorship was compared between the intervention and control group to calculate the cost of enabling one additional year of life. The authors concluded that the additional cost to bring about one additional year of life to older adults living at home with functional difficulties was low using

the multifactorial intervention described in Gitlin, Winter, et al.'s (2006) study compared with the high cost of medical and drug therapies. With the intent of generating some economic evidence for home modifications to progress research in this area, Slaug and colleagues conducted a secondary analysis of data from 266 older people who were at risk of developing dependence in instrumental activities of daily living. The analysis simulated a policy change to remove the five most severe environmental barriers in their homes and found that the need for home services would be reduced, thereby saving costs (Slaug, Chiatti, Oswald, Kaspar, & Schmidt, 2017).

Whilst this literature suggests the potential cost savings of home modifications, few studies have undertaken economic appraisals (Chiatti & Iwarsson, 2014; Fänge & Iwarsson, 2007; Heywood & Turner, 2007; Mann et al., 1999; Newman et al., 1990). Two factors contribute to this. Firstly, there is limited access to data in countries whose public policy does not support home modifications (Slaug et al., 2017). Secondly, when public policy supports home modifications, such as in Sweden, the provision of home modification as a legal right for all prevents controlled trials that can evaluate cost effectiveness (Slaug et al., 2017).

The above-mentioned research, while limited, indicates that home modifications contribute to cost savings for organisations and individuals but there is scope for further research to explore home modifications applying health economic models. Although there are challenges associated with comprehending and isolating the effects of home modification interventions, researchers have identified that new experimental data regarding costs and outcomes of home modification interventions will be needed to assist policy and practice (Chiatti & Iwarsson, 2014).

IMPACT ON CAREGIVERS' ROLE, PERSONAL HEALTH, AND WELL-BEING

Home modifications can reduce or even eliminate care needs in the home (Allen, Resnik, & Roy, 2006; Granbom et al., 2017; Jones et al., 2008; Liu & Lapane, 2009; U.K. Home Adaptations Consortium, 2017). Most research relating to caregiver outcomes involve home modifications as part of multicomponent approaches and focus on caregivers of people with dementia. A recent systematic review supported that home modifications combined with other interventions improved the ability of carers to provide care for people with dementia or related disorders (Stark, Keglovits, et al., 2017). Specifically, it was reported that the multicomponent intervention resulted in less caregiver upset, enhanced self-efficacy in managing complex behavioral problems (Gitlin, Corcoran, Winter, Boyce, & Hauck, 2001), a reduction in feelings of caregiver burden (Dooley & Hinojosa, 2004; Gitlin, 2003), and less service assistance for caregivers of people who were aging in their own home (Gitlin, 2003). The impact on paid and unpaid care hours is less clear. While Allen and colleagues (2006) survey of 899 wheelchair users found that the odds of receiving unpaid help were decreased by 14% with the presence of each additional home modification, this was not the case for paid help. Further, a randomized controlled study with 91 participants with a range of disabilities found that home modifications did not necessarily reduce caregiver hours which was attributed to peoples' general functional changes and decline over time (Wilson, Mitchell, Kemp, Adkins, & Mann, 2009).

The health and well-being benefits of home modifications to caregivers has been demonstrated strongly in qualitative research (Aplin et al., 2015; Granbom et al., 2017; Heywood, 2002, 2003, 2004a, 2004b, 2005; Jones et al., 2008; Tanner, Tilse, & de Jonge, 2008). Home modifications have been found to improve well-being (Gitlin et al., 2001; Heywood, 2004a, 2005; Tanner et al., 2008), alleviate or reduce mental stress and physical strain, improve personal relations and happiness, and allow caregivers to continue caring (Heywood, 2002, 2005, 2007). For example, in one qualitative study the health and safety of 48% of family caregivers improved after the installation of major modifications, which reduced the stress of caring and positively impacted their mental health (Heywood, 2005). In another qualitative study, the role of the caregiver and the activities of caregivers were made easier through the installation of home modifications, with caregivers reporting less physical demand and strain, and a decreased risk of injuries (Aplin et al., 2015). This is particularly important for caregivers who are aging and at risk of serious injury from prolonged stresses on their body (Jones et al., 2008).

Home modifications may also provide caregivers capacity to participate in activities outside the home, enhancing their mental and physical health (Tanner et al., 2008). For example, spouses or family members who were caregivers, were less tied to the home and more able to engage in other activities without needing to provide as much care to the client (Tanner et al., 2008). Further, home modifications resulted in people no longer relying on others to assist in personal care or to provide meals, with

an alteration in the relationship with their caregiver (often a spouse of family member; Tanner et al., 2008). Findings from a recent qualitative study found that the home modifications improved the everyday life of the caregiver by allowing opportunity for the caregiver to undertake activities without the need to continually check on the person they were caring for (Granbom et al., 2017).

The abovementioned findings indicate that home modifications reduce or even eliminate care needs in the home, reduce negative health consequences for carers, and allow them to participate in other life roles. Further research is required to examine the needs and perceptions of home modifications by caregivers, particularly those people who have health conditions or disabilities themselves (Australian Bureau of Statistics, 2015; Velkoff & Lawson, 1998).

ACTIVITIES OF DAILY LIVING (PERSONAL AND INSTRUMENTAL)

The impact of home modifications on activities of daily living is a well-researched outcome area. The ability of individuals to complete personal and instrumental activities of daily living (including household activities) is an important outcome as it enables people to remain living in their own homes (Stark, Keglovits, et al., 2017). Research studies indicate that home modifications may reduce dependence in personal and instrumental activities of daily living (Fänge & Iwarsson, 2005b; Gill et al., 2002; Gitlin et al., 2001; Johansson, Lilja, Petersson, & Borell, 2007; Petersson et al., 2008, 2009; Pighills et al., 2011; Stark, 2004). Notably, three systematic reviews have concluded that home modifications reduce difficulty with activities of daily living (Chase et al., 2012; Stark, Keglovits, et al., 2017; Wahl et al., 2009).

Once again, much of the research in this area includes home modifications as part of a multicomponent intervention. Four randomized controlled trials report positive results of multicomponent interventions on improving function including independence and self-care (Gitlin et al., 2001; Mann et al., 1999; Szanton et al., 2011; Wilson et al., 2009). Mann et al. (1999) found that although older adults experienced functional decline over time, the rate of decline was slowed through a systematic approach of providing assistive technology and environmental interventions. Older adults with Alzheimer's disease have been found to experience less difficulty with both instrumental and personal tasks of everyday life up to 1 year after the implementation of a multi-component program (Gitlin et al., 2001). In addition, this approach positively impacts on both the caregiver and the person with dementia by slowing the rate of functional decline particularly in bathing and toileting (Gitlin et al., 2001).

Home modifications provided in isolation have also been found to reduce dependence in personal and instrumental activities of daily living (Allen et al., 2006; Fänge & Iwarsson, 2005b; Fox, 1995; Gill et al., 2002; Gitlin et al., 2001; Johanssen et al., 2007; Liu & Lapane, 2009; Petersson et al., 2008; Pighills et al., 2011; Stark, 2004). A few studies have found that older community-dwelling adults experience lower levels of difficulty with getting in and out of the home, managing mobility indoors, and undertaking self-care activities in the bathroom after provision of home modifications (Hagsten, Svensson & Gardulf, 2004; Petersson et al., 2008, 2009). A single group prospective study that evaluated a client-centered home modification program for 67 older adults reported a significant improvement in daily activity performance immediately after individualized home modifications and training (Stark et al., 2009). People's perception of their performance and satisfaction with daily activities were also maintained at a 2-year period after the intervention (Stark et al., 2009).

A strong finding in qualitative research is the positive effect of home modifications on the completion of self-care and household routines. For example, a study of 12 older people aged 65 years and over living in social housing (Tanner et al., 2008) found that home modifications increased independence, allowing the maintenance of habitual personal routines with some participants no longer relying on others to assist in personal care or household routines. Home modifications made everyday life easier for participants in a qualitative study of 42 households, describing that they could live in their home without effort (Aplin et al., 2015). This and a range of other studies with people of a range of ages and living circumstances highlighted that it was easier to move around and access the home, to do everyday activities like showering, toileting, laundry and to care for children and family members (Aplin et al., 2015; Boniface & Morgan, 2017; Felix, de Haan, Vaandrager, & Koelen, 2015; Granbom et al., 2017; Mackenzie, Curryer, & Byles, 2015).

The above-mentioned findings support that home modifications have a positive impact on people's capacity to manage their self-care and household tasks and routines. Because the home is considered a complex environment for a range of people of different backgrounds and ages, further investigation is required into the impact of home modifications on activities of daily living for a diverse range of people, aside from older community living adults (Gitlin, 2003).

EXPERIENCE OF HOME

The literature to date has prioritized the assessment of quantitative research and empirical research outcomes, with comparatively little consideration of valuable qualitative outcomes (Annear et al., 2014). As noted earlier, qualitative studies have been undertaken with diverse populations differing in age ranges, and health conditions and disabilities. The intent of a home modification is to transform the home, eliminating the barriers that confine the person and restoring their home to them (Heywood, 2005). Qualitative research reports on the experience of home beyond completing tasks and being able to function in the environment (Tanner et al., 2008). This experience of home includes the subjective feelings and resulting meaning that people assign to their home and the usability of the environment (Aplin et al., 2015). To date, the literature demonstrates that this experience of home for older people and people with a disability is complex, multifaceted, and individually experienced (Aplin, Thornton, & Gustafsson, 2017). Table 14-2 outlines the breadth of qualitative research that has been considered in this review that considers the complexity of the experience of home. It has been included to provide a succinct summary of the range and background of the studies and to illustrate the breadth of research emerging in this area. The strength of this qualitative research is that it examines the impact of home modifications from the perspective of people who receive home modifications and therefore, provides a valuable perspective on the benefits and the intended and unintended consequences of this intervention. This understanding is critical in ensuring quality home modification service provision.

The qualitative literature indicates that home modifications impact on people's experience of home in a range of ways, altering the person's identity, the comfort and ease of living in the home, and changing relationships within the home. The qualitative research also demonstrates the personal and individual experience of home modifications, the complexity of this experience, and the diversity of outcomes. For example, one qualitative study found that people preferred not to modify their home, as overcoming the everyday challenges posed by one's own frailties, such as stairs, afforded feelings of achievement (Sixsmith et al., 2014). Some people

Table 14-2. Summary of Qualitative Research

AUTHOR (DATE)	PARTICIPANTS (NUMBER AND NATURE OF COHORT)	DATA COLLECTION METHOD	TYPE OF MODIFICATIONS (MAJOR/MINOR)
Ahn & Ledge (2011)	N = 3175, aged 60 to 94 years, living at home	Questionnaires	Both
Aplin, de Jonge, & Gustafsson (2013)	N = 55, aged 25 to 87 years, living at home	Interviews	Major
Aplin et al. (2015)	N = 55, aged 25 to 87 years, living at home	Interviews	Major
Aplin et al. (2017)	N = 9, aged 3.5 to 74 years	Interviews	Major
Bailey, Foran, Scanaill, & Dromey (2011)	N = 5, 70 to 87 years	Life-space diary study	Major
Boniface & Morgan (2017)	N = 64 families	Online questionnaires, interviews	Both
Danziger & Chaudrey (2009)	N = 26, aged 50 to 86 years, living at home	Interviews	Minor
de Jonge, Jones, Phillips, & Chung (2011)	N = 49 cases and 48 controls aged 15 to 49 years	Interviews	Both
Frisk et al. (2006)	N = 49 cases and 48 controls aged 15 to 49 years	Surveys	Minor
Granbom et al. (2017)	N = 9, aged 52 to 90 years	Interviews	Both
Haak, Dahlin-Ivanoff, Fänge, Sixsmith, & Iwarsson (2007)	N = 8, aged 80 to 89 years	Interviews	Both
Haak, Fänge, et al. (2007)	N = 40, aged 80 to 89	Interviews	Both
Heywood (2001)	Children to adults (oldest 98 years)	Interviews	Both
Heywood (2002)	Children to adults (oldest 98 years)	Interviews	Both
Heywood (2003)	N = 69, aged 0 to 65+ years	Interviews	Both
Heywood (2004a)	N = 69, aged 0 to 65+ years	Interviews	Both
Heywood (2004b)	N = 69, aged 0 to 65+ years	Interviews	Major
Heywood (2005)	N = 69, aged 0 to 65+ years	Interviews	Major
Johannson, Borrel, & Lilja (2009)	N = 4, aged 40+ years	Interviews, field notes	Both
Jones et al. (2008)	N = 31, aged 56 to 90 years	Interviews	Both
Mackenzie et al. (2015)	N = 202, aged 75 to 79 years	Interviews	Both
Morgan, Boniface, & Reagon (2016)	N = 39 staff, 48 families with children with disabilities	Interviews, on-line surveys	Both
Niva & Skar (2006)	N = 5, aged 70 to 84 years	Case study	Both
Nocon & Pleace (1997)	N = 24 people with disabilities, 26 professional staff, 210 postal questionnaire	Focus groups, postal questionnaires	Both

(continued)

Table 14-2. Summary of Qualitative Research (continued)

AUTHOR (DATE)	PARTICIPANTS (NUMBER AND NATURE OF COHORT	DATA COLLECTION METHOD	TYPE OF MODIFICATIONS (MAJOR/MINOR)
Nord, Eakin, Astley, & Atkinson (2009)	N=6 clients, 4 OTs, 6 grant surveyors, 3 builders	Interviews	Major
Pettersson et al. (2012)	N=4, aged 39 to 75 years	Interviews, survey assessments	Both
Randström, Asplund, & Svedlund (2012)	N=10, aged 68 to 93 years	Interviews	Not started
Roy, Rousseau, Allard, Feldman, & Majnemer (2008)	N=11 parents of children with disabilities	Interviews, focus groups	Major
Sixsmith et al. (2014)	N=190, aged 75 to 89 years, living alone in urban setting	Interviews	Not started
Tanner et al. (2008)	N=12, aged 60 to 90 years; residing in public housing	Interviews	Both
Vik, Lilja, & Nygard (2007)	N=14, aged 68 to 81 years	Interviews	Not started

also preferred to maintain a living environment that was familiar and reflective of self rather than one that was modified (Sixsmith et al., 2014). However, a modified environment can reduce people's concerns about a home's capability to meet their future needs, their satisfaction with their home, and their perception of safety in the home (Ahn & Ledge, 2011; Granbom et al., 2017). Another strong finding from the qualitative literature is that the home modifications done without regard for the entire experience of home can impact negatively on people's self-image, their connection with the home and their routines and sense of heritage (Heywood, 2005). The seminal qualitative study by Tanner et al. (2008) indicates that home modifications can impact negatively on the meaning of home or homeliness of the dwelling. Such variable qualitative findings demonstrate the unique and complex individual experiences of modifications and indicate the need for modification recommendations to be carefully considered by therapists as they work with people in their home (Felix et al., 2015).

The review of the research identified 10 key impacts of home modifications. These are listed below, and each will be introduced and discussed in turn. While the focus is on qualitative literature, quantitative studies have also, on occasion, been included in these topics below where relevant and not reported above:

1. Usability of the home
2. Safety, security, and comfort

3. Sense of permanency and continuity
4. Privacy and dignity
5. Freedom, choice, and control within the home
6. Maintaining and enhancing valued roles and occupations
7. Identity and self-esteem
8. Appearance and ambience of the home
9. Fostering relationships, social connections, and participation in social activities
10. Perception of value and the potential resale of the home

USABILITY OF THE HOME

A strong research finding from both qualitative and quantitative literature is that home modifications enhance the usability of the home, that is, the experience of performing daily activities within the home (Fänge & Iwarsson, 2003). Usability is a perceived aspect of home that includes the extent to which the environment supports occupational performance, which involves a transaction between a person, the environment, and the activity (Fänge & Iwarsson, 2005a; Granbom, Iwarsson, Kylberg, Pettersson, & Slaug, 2016). It is based on the person's subjective evaluation of the constraining or supportive impact of the environment on activities and is a separate concept to accessibility (Fänge & Iwarsson,

2003). Other studies have described the outcome of home modifications on usability of the home whereby people described home modifications as having the greatest impact on making everyday life easier, enabling them to live in their own home with ease and without effort or thought (Aplin et al., 2015). This includes being able to move around the home and access all areas to manage activities such as showering, toileting, laundry activities (Aplin et al., 2015). Others reported that home modifications enabled them undertake activities they had become unable to engage in and restored access to areas of the home (Heywood, 2005).

In one longitudinal study, home modifications resulted in improved activity performance and usability in housing (Fänge & Iwarsson, 2005a). Specifically, home modifications resulted in a decrease in dependence in bathing but not necessarily overall activities of daily living dependence (Fänge & Iwarsson, 2005a). The changes also demonstrated that the highly individualized home modifications facilitated caregiving and enabled participants to perform activities with less effort (Fänge & Iwarsson, 2005a). A finding of this study was the need for research into home modification processes as they may differ considerably amongst clients, impacting on the outcomes of home modifications. The research also highlighted that there is a lack of systematic approaches to interventions, whereby most aspects of home modifications represent a "black box," challenging traditional approaches to evaluation. This highlights the need to undertake research to examine the value of systematizing intervention procedures and completing long-term follow-up of clients.

SAFETY, SECURITY, AND COMFORT

A commonly reported outcome of home modifications in the qualitative literature is the enhanced sense of safety, security, and comfort in the home (Aplin et al., 2015; Tanner et al., 2008). Tanner et al. (2008) found that home modifications positively affected the experience of home as a place of security, safety, and comfort by decreasing the demands of the environment. Participants valued being able to decorate their home to achieve pleasing aesthetics or regulate the temperature in their environment to achieve comfort (Tanner et al., 2008). In one qualitative study the houses of several families had been so cold that they were at risk of both pain and illness. They described the change once heating was installed as restoring a sense of home (Heywood, 2005). Additionally, people confined to their home

have reported that windows, which allow light into the home and provide contact with the outside world, as being vital to their well-being (Heywood, 2004b). Another qualitative study reported that minor modifications had a range of lasting positive consequences including "improved safety and reduced risk of accidents" with major modifications such as bathroom conversions, extensions and lifts were perceived as having a greater impact, having "transformed people's lives" (Heywood, 2001). The transformative and restorative effect of modifications was also reported in Heywood's 2005 study when participants reported the ability to take a bath or shower, and use the toilet and stairs was a relief due to experiencing a reduction in pain, and restoration of autonomy and access to areas around the home (Heywood, 2005).

Home modifications, which removed danger and suffering, were not only preventing accidents or alleviating conditions but were restoring the dwelling's power to be a home that provided a place of security (Heywood, 2005). In contrast, some home modifications have been found to create unsafe situations due to the use of substandard materials or features being missed in the home modification (Aplin et al., 2015). For example, dangerous materials used on step ramps were found to be slippery or to deteriorate with the weather (Aplin et al., 2015). Similarly, features missing such as handrails or kerbing on paths could result in a wheelchair slipping off the edge of a pathway (Aplin et al., 2015). This information highlights that further research is required to determine home modifications that undermine a person's and household's experience of safety, security and comfort, and to further examine modifications that have a preventative, restorative and transformative effect on people's lives.

SENSE OF PERMANENCY AND CONTINUITY

Another frequently reported and important outcome from participants in qualitative studies is that home modifications contribute to a sense of permanency and continuity in the home when they consider the recipient's current and future needs (Aplin et al., 2015; Tanner et al., 2008). Several studies have reported that people wish to remain in their own home as they age, preferring to make changes to the home rather than relocate (Aplin et al., 2015; Jones et al., 2008; Tanner et al., 2008). Home modifications enable people to "stay put" rather than being forced to relocate (Heywood, 2005). In one study, the capacity to age in place was enhanced for 70% of participants who had made home modifications to their home in the previous 5 years (Mackenzie et al., 2015). This demonstrates that home modifications provide possibilities for people to stay at home and be part of their home and community rather than move into an institution (Hwang, Cummings, Sixsmith, & Sixsmith, 2011).

A recent study found that the installation of a home modification that removes environmental barriers can change the person's mind about wanting to move (Granbom et al., 2017). Highlighting the life changing impact that modifications can make, another study reported that home modifications supported a participant to leave residential care and move in with family in the community (Heywood, 2002). In contrast, home modifications may also trigger a desire to move to alternative accommodation as discussions or initial modifications can result in people questioning the long-term suitability of the current residence (Granbom et al., 2017). Further research is required to explore the range of home modifications that are required at different points in time in a person's life that allow them to remain in their home as their needs change. There is also a need to examine those modifications that can address people's needs if they want to move from institutions back into a home environment (Callaway, Tregloan, Williams, & Clark, 2016) and how to best support people to relocate if their home is no longer meeting their needs (Jones et al., 2008).

PRIVACY AND DIGNITY

Home modifications can restore and maintain privacy and dignity in the home (Fänge & Iwarsson, 2005b; Heywood, 2002, 2004a, 2004b, 2005). A strong finding from Heywood's work was the ability of modifications to restore and offer people privacy and dignity (Heywood, 2002) and provide a positive image of self (Heywood, 2004b). Privacy and dignity in Heywood's later 2005 study was also found to be restored within the home, through the provision of home modifications that provided independence in self-care activities (Heywood, 2005). There was a joy of restored dignity and sense of self when people could toilet or bathe themselves with space, time, and privacy. People experienced privacy when they could have time away from others, which was valued by them and others in the home (Heywood, 2005). When these factors were not restored, a lack of privacy and dignity that was described as "degrading" was felt by people (Heywood, 2004b, 2005). When people were unable to shower, maintain

their hygiene, or left to use commodes in communal areas, people's sense of self was deeply impacted (Heywood, 2004a, 2004b, 2005). For some people, when home modifications were provided, they were viewed as a threat as the home now reflected them in a not so "perfect and self-sufficient light" (Heywood, 2004b).

In one study examining the perception of parents who were the carers of their children with health conditions or disabilities, families acknowledged the need to maintain privacy and dignity for their children as they were growing up (Aplin et al., 2017). Parents have also reported being disappointed by home modifications that made the child's health condition or disability "visible for all to see" (Roy et al., 2008. p. 365). Heywood (2005) describes a loss of privacy at home as a betrayal or assault on its meaning (p. 540). Heywood (2004b) found that the need to retain or restore dignity, to have values recognized, to be afforded choice and to take an active part in society are important aspects of the home environment for home modification recipients, more than material needs such as access and safety. This is particularly important where people have a need to see their home as a positive reflection of themselves (Heywood, 2004b).

Research is required to examine the specific types of home modifications that can be introduced into a home to restore the sense of privacy and dignity to individuals, and a positive reflection of themselves. Additionally, it would be valuable to examine the perceptions of clients, parents, carers, and others living in households about the privacy and dignity provided by modification. This information may provide good insight into important features to consider over time as a person's experience of their home may change as they mature (Aplin et al., 2017) or as there are changes to their health condition or disability.

FREEDOM, CHOICE, AND CONTROL

Commonly reported in both qualitative and quantitative literature is the finding that home modifications enhance the sense of independence and autonomy in the home by providing freedom of movement, choice, and control (Aplin et al., 2015; de Jonge et al., 2011; Fänge & Iwarsson, 2005a; Haak, Fänge, et al., 2007; Heywood, 2004b, 2005; Tanner et al., 2008). Home modifications provide opportunity and choice to participate in day-to-day routines and activities (Heywood, 2004b). People long for freedom to go where they want and to do what they want, such as being able to do things for one self, to choose activities freely, to move from room to room, to use stairs to access different areas of the home, and to undertake independent routines and spontaneous activities (Aplin et al., 2015; Heywood, 2004b, 2005). Home modifications enable people the opportunity to master the environment and exercise control over many of their day-to-day activities including their own private habitual routines (Lansley et al., 2004; Oswald et al., 2007; Tanner et al., 2008). In one study, people enjoyed having a shower when they chose, without having to ensure their spouse or family member was present (Aplin et al., 2015). In another study, where people could not undertake all activities themselves, people still valued the opportunity to be able to maximize their sense of freedom through being able to participate in tasks with assistance (Heywood, 2004b). This included for example, the person sitting in the shower rather than a strip wash with a bowl or using a vanity basin during a self-care routine (Heywood, 2004b).

Other studies highlighted that if home modifications are done well, they afford people the freedom to remain in the home, a factor that was central to their feeling of autonomy and independence (de Jonge et al., 2011; Heywood, 2005). Home modifications were described as critical to enabling people to do what they wanted (Jones et al., 2008). Homes were transformed from a place of imprisonment to one of autonomy and control (Tanner et al., 2008). Home modifications enabled the home to become a base to return to, rather than be a place of confinement providing no opportunity for people to go out at all (Heywood, 2005). Specific home modifications such as lifts, and ramps were reported as restoring freedom of movement (Heywood, 2004b).

The freedom and independence provided by home modifications have been described by some as a "godsend" and fundamental to their capacity to manage in the home (Jones et al., 2008). For others, home modifications resulted in disappointment when they restricted their freedom to act in ways they desired, such as being able to access all areas of the home (Heywood, 2005). In one study, one participant's autonomy was not improved as she wasn't provided with modifications that enabled her to access her garden and outdoor area (Aplin et al., 2015).

Older people and people with a disability value being listened to and having their needs and wishes respected. A failure to consult with the person during the home modification process can result in a loss of autonomy and control (Aplin et al., 2015; Heywood 2004b, 2015; Nord et al., 2009; Pettersson et al., 2012; Picking & Pain, 2003). Further, loss of autonomy and control occurs when the service restricts the type, location, and features of the home

modifications (Aplin et al., 2015; Heywood, 2005). A group of older adults described difficulties with the home modification system, where standards, a lack of consultation and limited information provision from service providers resulted in unsatisfactory outcomes (Johansson et al., 2009). Families experienced issues where there were delays to processes, uncertainty around the nature and funding of home modifications, and the need for the family to fight for what the family felt was required (Boniface & Morgan, 2017; Morgan, Boniface, & Reagon, 2016). This reflects a provider-led rather than a user-led approach to service provision (Morgan et al., 2016). This lack of control and choice can result in home modifications that are not wanted and rarely used (Heywood 2005; Morgan et al., 2016). For example, Heywood (2005) describes one mother, who chose to continue to carry her child even though a through-ceiling lift had been installed, because she wanted an extension and could not accept the alternative solution offered.

The above information highlights that there is a need to ensure individuals are respectfully involved in the entire home modification process from concept development to the implementation of the home modifications to achieve positive home modification outcomes (Burns, Pickens, & Smith, 2017; Heywood, 2004b, 2005; Renaut, Ogg, Petite, & Chamahian, 2015). More research is needed to examine the full impact of modifications that don't recognize the complex and unique nature of the home environment (de Jonge et al., 2011); are restricted by service guidelines or do not involve the residents in all stages of the consultation process. Further, information about the short- and long-term impact of these outcomes for a range of client groups such as children, families, and people aging into disability would also be valuable.

MAINTAINING AND ENHANCING VALUED ROLES AND MEANINGFUL OCCUPATIONS

Studies have reported that home modifications enable people to maintain, enhance, or restore participation in valued roles such as being a parent, worker, caregiver; and in meaningful occupations such as gardening, cooking, social activities, and work (Aplin et al., 2015; de Jonge et al., 2011; Mann et al., 1999; Pettersson et al., 2012; Stark, 2004). They support people as they age and spend increasing amounts of time in the home by enabling occupational engagement and performance (Gitlin, 2003). For example, in the Tanner et al. (2008) study, one participant, a resident of social housing was offered relocation to a location with better accessibility, but this was not considered a priority by the participant as despite the environmental barriers in the current home, she felt she had a role in monitoring the safety of others' children at her local bus stop which contributed to her sense of identity (Tanner et al., 2008). In another example, people aged between 80 and 89 years of age reported that homes supported engagement in valued roles, routines and everyday activities following the installation of home modifications (Dahlin-Ivanoff, Haak, Fänge, & Iwarsson, 2007). Conversely, a poorly designed environment can create disability and limit people's capacity to maintain or enhance their valued roles and occupations (Aplin et al., 2015).

Service models that have a preoccupation with providing home modifications to prioritize independence in self-care activities over other valued activities have been reported to devalue the home as a place of meaningful occupation (Heywood, 2005). This was highlighted in one study where participants spoke of financing their own modifications to incorporate broader occupations and roles which were outside of the recommended changes from their service provider (Aplin et al., 2013). Client-centered goal setting has been proposed as a means by people's occupational performance (roles and occupations) can be promoted (Stark, 2004; Stark et al., 2009). Further research is needed to describe the value of home modifications for fostering people's engagement in valued roles and meaningful occupations over time, in the home and community (Aplin et al., 2013; Stark, 2004).

IDENTITY AND SELF-ESTEEM

The impact of modifications on people's identity and self-esteem is commonly reported in the qualitative literature with many people describing the experiences as being life altering. A home's appearance is linked to the occupant's identity, reflecting who they are (Aplin et al., 2015). The appearance and the connection to identity have been reported to be both positively and negatively impacted by home modifications (Aplin et al., 2015; Heywood, 2004b; Jones et al., 2008).

Home modifications have been reported to enhance a person's self-esteem through enabling greater independence (Aplin et al., 2015; Roy et al., 2008; Tanner et al., 2008). Home modifications also support the continuation of habitual personal routines or rituals that connected older people to their home (Tanner et al., 2008). In one study, the appearance of a bathroom area was enjoyed by participants who felt they could welcome people into their home (Heywood, 2005). In another study, a new ramp provided a sense of enjoyment as it improved the look of the home (Aplin, et al., 2015). When modifications reinforced the control, individuals could have of their routines, daily activities, and privacy from others, people felt that home was a place of personal control, mastery and self-efficacy - giving meaning and influencing their sense of self and identity (Tanner et al., 2008).

Alternatively, the appearance of home modifications can make a home feel like a hospital or look disabled (Aplin et al., 2015). People were dissatisfied with home modifications that had a clinical appearance, did not match the look of their home, reflected disability, and did not represent their own view or sense of self (Heywood, 2005; Jones et al., 2008). For some people, home modifications have resulted in them labelled as different, making them vulnerable to ridicule or violence (Fisher, 1998).

Heywood (2004b) identified that people were grateful and satisfied with their home modification whenever their values were considered in the home modification process and discussed their distress when these values were ignored. For example, problems arose when a lack of thought was given to the cleaning and maintenance of home modifications, resulting in people feeling a loss of control and harm to their self-respect (Heywood, 2004b). Further, when unwelcome home modifications were installed, some participants felt that the installation reflected their sense of helplessness, reminded them of their disability, and contributed to depression (Heywood, 2004a). These studies highlight that when the physical aspects of accessibility and functionality are emphasized, and the personal and social meanings of home such as the impact on identity and self-esteem are neglected, the experience of home for people diminishes (Aplin et al., 2015; Tanner et al., 2008). Further research is required to examine those home modifications that are have an influence on a person's sense of self, identity, and self-esteem, that may be considered life altering.

APPEARANCE AND AMBIENCE

The conflict between the function of the home modification and the aesthetics and design has often been reported in qualitative studies (Hawkins & Stewart, 2002; Pettersson et al., 2012; Winfield, 2003). The physical appearance of modifications is an important contributor to a person's satisfaction with their modification (Heywood, 2001; Jones et al., 2008; Morgan et al., 2016; Nord et al., 2009; Pettersson et al., 2012). Peoples' satisfaction with home modifications was found to be substantially derived from the aesthetic components (Heywood, 2001) not just its practical use. Some modifications are reported as enhancing the person's pride in their own home and providing self-affirming meaning that contributes to their sense of status and well-being (Heywood, 2005). Home modification recipients have also reported modifications as improving the appearance of the home and making spaces more enjoyable (Aplin et al., 2015; Jones et al., 2008).

Some studies, however, have reported that people have not been concerned with the impact of the home modifications on the look of their home, preferring to focus on function or comfort over aesthetics (Aplin et al, 2015, 2017; Granbom et al., 2017; Jones et al., 2008; Pettersson et al., 2012). For example, Granbom et al.'s (2017) and Ahn and Ledge's (2011) studies report that a modified home environment does not necessarily impact on how the older person perceives the home environment. In Granbom et al.'s (2017) research even if some cohabitants raised concerns that a ramp could disrupt the aesthetics of the exterior and maybe reduce the property value at a future sale, over time, once the home modification was installed, this was no longer a concern. When the home modification was installed, and if there was an improvement in the person's health status, carers and their partners did not give much consideration to the effect of the home modification on appearance (Granbom et al., 2017). Aplin et al.'s (2015, 2017) studies also found that the functionality and practicality of the home, as well as the modifications were considered priorities by some participants over appearance.

In contrast, stories of negative consequences are somewhat more common with modifications making "ugly intrusions into what had once been a well-loved home" and people experiencing a great deal of distress (Heywood, 2004b, p. 718) and disappointment (Jones et al., 2008). People have felt that their homes have been medicalized (Morgan et al., 2016; Roy, et al., 2008). Others have described modifications as embarrassing or stigmatizing, a signifier of old age or disability (Auriemma, Faust, Sibrian, & Jimenez, 2000; de Jonge et al., 2011; Hawkins & Stewart, 2002; Heywood, 2004b, 2005; Montreuil, Després, & Beauregard, 2011; Orrell et al., 2013; Tanner et al., 2008). In a range of qualitative studies, modifications that have been described as appearing "disabled", "like a hospital", "clinical", and not in the style or décor of the home, and those that

were left unfinished, resulted in dissatisfaction and disappointment (Aplin et al., 2013, 2015; Heywood, 2004b, 2005; Jones et al., 2008; Morgan et al., 2016). Such modifications have the potential to impact on the identity of the person and family using the home and result in nonacceptance or nonuse (Hawkins & Stewart, 2002; Heywood, 2005; Nocon & Pleace, 1997). People concerned about the look of the home modifications, at times have opted to make the modifications more acceptable by paying for additional changes, or they may pay for the changes themselves rather than accept a home modification provided free of charge by a service (Jones et al., 2008; Pettersson et al., 2012). One study reports that when people were able to modify the aesthetic aspects of home modifications, some were able to do this in a way that did not compromise the functionality of the feature (Aplin et al., 2017). This included, for example, using color and smaller panels to enable the exterior of a lift to blend in with the look of the external area of the home.

The ambience of the home may include the lighting, airflow, shade and weather, or the impact of the climate on the temperature and comfort of the home (Sanford & Bruce, 2010). The amount of daylight a home receives, the level of thermal and sound insulation, the quality of technical installations (Oswald & Wahl, 2005; Sixsmith, 1986), the use of sustainable materials, and the ease of maintenance (Percival, 2002), are valued in relation to their connection to deeper feelings of privacy, safety, freedom, and independence (Oswald, Wahl, Naumann, Mollenkopf, & Hieber, 2006; Rowles, 2006; Smith, 1994). People concerned about home modifications affecting the ambience of the home reported negative impacts such as the installation or removal of features that may affect the lighting, view, or "feel" of a room (Aplin et al., 2013). For example, in some instances the installation of home modifications such as lifts, landings and stairs, resulted in people being exposed to the weather and needing protection from the rain, wind, and sun (Aplin et al., 2015). Some home modifications may also affect the temperature of the environment, impacting on the thermal comfort of residents (Aplin et al., 2015). For example, the design of a modified bathroom made it difficult for some people to keep warm. People in in another study reported several examples where inadequate heating either made people ill, made their conditions worse or prevented them from using the space they needed, including a newly adapted shower-room (Heywood, 2004a).

Further investigation is required in this area as manufacturers of home modification products continue to introduce new products into the market to address people's requests for more aesthetically pleasing and functional environments. For example, the baby boomer generation as they age, are likely to expect more choice of product and finishes (de Jonge, Aplin, Larkin, & Ainsworth, 2016). In addition, the impact of home modifications on the ambience of the home requires further examination to identify those that enable people to feel "in place" or "at home," comfortable or "at one" with their environment (de Jonge et al., 2011).

FOSTERING RELATIONSHIPS, SOCIAL CONNECTIONS, AND PARTICIPATION IN SOCIAL ACTIVITIES

Home modifications have also been found to enhance relationships, social connections, and participation in social activities in the home and community (Boniface & Morgan, 2017; de Jonge et al., 2011; Heywood, 2001, 2005; Niva & Skar, 2006; Pettersson et al., 2012; Tanner et al., 2008). While there are limited studies that report on the social outcomes of modifications, the importance of the social nature of home cannot be underestimated. Home has multiple meanings for families; it is a space in which family life is enacted and it is also a social space (Morgan et al., 2016). Tanner et al.'s (2008) study of people living in social housing reported that home was a place to strengthen and secure important relationships. Participants reported that their relationships were of greater importance and value than other aspects of the home including comfort, ease of access and functionality (Tanner et al., 2008).

Home modifications can either preserve/restore relationships or have a negative impact on social connections and relationships within and outside the home (Heywood, 2005; Tanner et al., 2008). Relationships can be preserved or restored by reducing people's dependency on others thus alleviating feelings of being a burden and the threat that this poses to family relationships (Heywood, 2005; Tanner, et al., 2008). For example, children having the opportunity to play together has improved family relationships (Heywood, 2005). Home modifications have also been found to reduce the stress on relationships, foster family interaction, and enable easier monitoring of household members (Heywood, 2005). For example, in one study families commented that a good home modification was life-changing, enabling them to function and live as a family and function as a family unit (Boniface & Morgan, 2017).

Several studies have reported that home modifications enable people to access the neighborhood and community to develop social connections and participate in social activities (Aplin et al., 2015; Haak, Dahlin-Ivanoff, et al., 2007; Niva & Skar, 2006; O'Day & Corcoran, 1994; Ostensjö, Carlberg, & Völlestad, 2005; Pettersson et al., 2008, 2012; Randström et al., 2012; Tanner et al., 2008; Vik et al., 2007). For older adults, this included activities such as visiting friends, going for a walk, and going to town (Niva & Skar, 2006). Home modifications also allowed people to have friends visit fostering social connections (Aplin et al., 2015). For many people, particularly those who are in the older age group, the ability to remain in their own home is important for maintaining social contact with people within their neighborhood and community (Bailey et al., 2011; de Jonge et al., 2011; Mackenzie et al., 2015; Pettersson et al., 2012; Tanner et al., 2008). By enabling people to continue to live in their own homes, home modifications allow social connections to continue and can also enhance these connections. For example, home modifications could be used by visiting family and guests such as someone using a wheelchair (Aplin et al., 2015). The home modifications enabled one participant to wheel into his garden, to interact with people walking past rather than being confined to a patio (Aplin et al., 2015).

Conversely, research demonstrates that if home modifications create further barriers such as lost space, they can strain relationships within the household and with neighbors (Heywood, 2005). Further, when home modifications focus on the person with the disability and disregarded the consequences for others in the home, they result in distorted relationships with family and neighbors (Heywood, 2005) and threaten the meanings attributed to home (Morgan et al., 2016). For example, the lack of access to specific areas in the home and space within the home had a negative impact on families' capacity to maintain social networks (Heywood, 2003; Morgan et al., 2016).

There is less research on the impact of home modifications on people's relationships with others and social activities which occur within and outside the home, particularly the negative outcomes. This is an area that requires further investigation as existing social networks are reported to contribute strongly to the essence of what a home means and are reported to reinforce other outcomes of home modifications such as providing individuals with a sense of identity (Tanner et al., 2008).

PERCEPTION OF THE VALUE AND RESALE VALUE OF THE HOME

A small amount of research exists that highlights that people perceive that home modifications may limit the market appeal of a home, impacting the value and potential resale of the home (Jones et al., 2008). However, some people feel that home modifications do not make a big difference to the value of their home, reasoning that the home modifications could be removed by the next owner or before sale (Jones et al., 2008) or stating that there may be a specific market for homes with accessibility features that may appeal to the aging population (Jones et al., 2008). One study found that the major modifications may be in use for many years, by other people in the household with a disability and subsequent occupiers of the property, demonstrating that this one-off capital investment may provide a service for years (Heywood, 2002). Further research is required to determine the specific home modifications that influence the positive and negative perceptions of the value and potential resale of the home; and how they provide value as a capital investment to save costs relating to accident and injury prevention, and the relocation of people into residential care.

SUMMARY OF ISSUES ARISING FROM THE REVIEW

To conclude, home modifications are valuable interventions that have a mixed impact on the lives of older people and people with a disability, and result in a range of outcomes in the short and longer term. Home modification outcomes may be perceived as either positive or negative. This review highlights that there is a need to complete more research in areas that have received limited attention to date to ensure outcomes of interest to the recipients of home modifications are duly recognized. It would also be of value to study the outcome of home modifications over a longer period in people's lives to have a longitudinal perspective on these outcomes (Pettersson et al., 2008). Research in this area is essential as there continues to be massive growth anticipated for older people wanting to remain in the community rather than move to care facilities (Kendig, Clemson, & Mackenzie, 2012). Further investigation is also required to examine those home modifications that result in poor outcomes to ensure this information can be used to inform solutions are tailored to the needs of individuals (Fänge & Iwarsson, 2005a) and improve occupational therapy practice.

This review highlights that qualitative reports of the outcomes as perceived by the people experiencing them are just as important as the quantitative findings relating to home modifications reducing falls and injuries; mortality and morbidity; institutional and in-home care costs; the impact on caregiver's roles, personal health and well-being; and activities of daily living. This qualitative research provides insights into how occupational therapy practice can contribute to achieving positive outcomes. This includes therapists taking a client-centered approach that includes individualized goal setting, and considering home modifications that promote health, safety, security, and comfort; valued roles and occupational performance; foster relationships, social connection, and participation; and afford people freedom, choice, and control. It also highlights the importance of working with residents to ensure the modifications are acceptable, aesthetically pleasing, fit with the ambience of the home, and are perceived to add value for the value and resale of the property to contribute to positive client perception.

Despite the range of themes relating to home modification outcomes, research in this area remains under developed and limited to a restricted range of users (Gitlin, 2003; Nagib & Williams, 2016). There is a need to examine wider age groups, beyond older adults, for example the baby boomer population is a large group who have expectations about their lifestyle and will place significant demand on services within the community as they seek to remain in their own homes as they age (Judd, Liu, Easthope, Davy, & Bridge, 2014). There is also a need for more research from the perspective of younger adults, caregivers and other householders using home modifications (Pettersson et al., 2008). There is a range of studies focusing on home modifications for older people living in urban areas, yet more research is needed with people of varying ages living in rural and remote areas, and with those who may be renting or who have less stable housing histories (Mackenzie et al., 2015).

Finally, the current range of studies have been criticized as fragmented and limiting progress toward a strong body of evidence, possessing poor research quality and inconsistencies between measures of outcomes (Awang, 2004; de Jonge et al., 2011; Gitlin, 2003; Heywood & Awang, 2011; Mackenzie et al., 2015; Wahl et al., 2009). Methods of recruitment, small samples, limited age ranges, specific geographical locations of study samples, and high participant homogeneity impact the depth of information able to be sourced, and limit potential for generalisation (Danziger & Chaudhury, 2009; de Jonge et al., 2011; Mackenzie et al., 2015). There is a need for clear and consistent definition of home modifications to ensure that the evidence base under review is measuring a consistently applied intervention (Carnemolla & Bridge, 2015). Some researchers have also commented on the individual nature of home modifications requiring more individualized methodologies to identify home modification outcomes (Fänge & Iwarsson, 2005a; Felix et al., 2015; Golant, 2003; Pettersson et al., 2008). There is also more research required on home modifications as a single intervention as current studies have combined home modifications with other interventions such as assistive technologies (Heywood & Awang, 2011; Pettersson et al., 2008).

IMPLICATIONS FOR OCCUPATIONAL THERAPISTS

The knowledge and insights gained from this review of research provide new understanding of best practices that could enhance home modification outcomes. The broad range of outcomes that have been reported in this literature review demonstrate that home modifications are complex, multi-faceted and individually experienced by older people and people with a disability, and their caregivers. Occupational therapists need to seriously consider this information in relation to their home modification process and interventions proposed, to determine how to best support older people and people with a disability, and their caregivers, and ensure services are provided in a manner which achieves positive outcomes, that value and enhance their experience of home (Aplin et al., 2017). The number of positive and negative outcomes reported also illustrate that occupational therapists need to understand what clients value about their home and intended modifications in relation to their personal needs and preferences. They also need to ensure they involve the client in all stages of the home modification process and undertake a process of evaluation once home modifications are installed (Aplin et al., 2015; Oswald et al., 2007).

REFERENCES

Adams, J., & Grisbrooke, J. (1998). The use of level access showers 12 months after installation. *British Journal of Therapy and Rehabilitation, 5*(10), 504-510. doi:10.12968%2Fbjtr.1998.5.10.14041

Ahn, M. & Ledge, A. L. (2011) Perceived aspects of home environment and home modifications by older people living in rural areas. *Journal of Housing for the Elderly, 25*(1), 18-30. doi:10.1080/02763893.2011.545735

Allen, S., Resnik, L., & Roy, J. (2006). Promoting independence for wheelchair users: The role of home accommodations. *The Gerontologist, 46*(1), 115-123. doi: https://doi.org/10.1093/geront/46.1.115

Andrich, R., Ferrario, M., & Moi, M. (1998). A model of cost-outcome analysis for assistive technology. *Disability and Rehabilitation, 20*(1), 1-24. doi:10.3109/09638289809166850

Annear, M., Keeling, S., Wilkinson, T., Cushman, G., Gidlow, B., & Hopkins, H. (2014). Environmental influences on healthy and active aging: A systematic review. *Ageing & Society, 34*, 590-622. doi: 10.1017/S0144686X1200116X

Aplin, T., de Jonge, D., & Gustafsson, L. (2013). Understanding the dimensions of home that impact on home modification decision making. *Australian Occupational Therapy Journal, 60*(2), 101-109. doi:10.1111/1440-1630.12022

Aplin, T., de Jonge, D., & Gustafsson, L. (2015). Understanding home modifications impact on clients and their family's experience of home: A qualitative study. *Australian Occupational Therapy Journal, 62*(2), 123-131. doi:10.1111/1440-1630.12156

Aplin, T., Thornton, H., & Gustafsson, L. (2017). The unique experience of home for parents and carers of children with disabilities. *Scandinavian Journal of Occupational Therapy*, 1-10. doi: 10.1080/11038128.2017.1280079. [Epub ahead of print]

Auriemma, D., Faust, S., Sibrian, K., & Jimenez, J. (2000). Home modifications for the elderly: Implications for the occupational therapist. *Physical & Occupational Therapy in Geriatrics, 16*(3-4), 135-144. doi:10.1080/J148v16n03_08

Australian Bureau of Statistics. (2015). Survey of disability, ageing, and carers. Retrieved from http://www.abs.gov.au/ausstats/abs@.nsf/mf/4430.0

Awang, D. (2004). *Building in evidence: Reviewing housing and occupational therapy*. London, England: College of Occupational Therapists.

Bailey, C., Foran, T., Scanaill, C., & Dromey, B. (2011). Older adults, falls and technologies for independent living: A life space approach. *Ageing & Society, 31*(5), 829-848. doi:https://doi.org/10.1017/S0144686X10001170

Boniface, G., & Morgan, D. (2017). The central role of the occupational therapist in facilitating housing adaptations/home modifications for disabled children. *British Journal of Occupational Therapy, 80*(6), 375-383.

Burns, S. P., Pickens, N. D., & Smith, R. O. (2017). Interprofessional client-centred reasoning processes in home modification practice. *Journal of Housing for the Elderly, 31*(3), 213-228. doi:10.1080/02763893.2017.1280579

Calkins, M. P., & Namazi, K. H. (1991). Caregivers' perceptions of the effectiveness of home modifications for community living adults with dementia. *American Journal of Alzheimer's Disease and Other Dementias, 6*(1), 25-29.

Callaway, L., Tregloan, K., Williams, G., Clark, R. (2016). Evaluating access and mobility within a new model of supported housing for people with neurotrauma: A pilot study. *Physical Activity in Neurological Populations, 71*(1), 64-76. doi: https://doiorg.ezproxy.library.uq.edu.au/10.1017/BrImp.2016.7

Campbell, A. J., Robertson, M. C., La Grow, S. J., Kerse, N. M., Sanderson, G. F., Jacobs, R. J., . . . Hale, L. A. (2005). Randomised controlled trial of prevention of falls in people aged ≥75 with severe visual impairment: The VIP trial. *British Medical Journal, 331*, 817. doi: https://doi.org/10.1136/bmj.38601.47731.55

Carnemolla, P., & Bridge, C. (2015). *Systematic review: Evidence on home modifications.* Sydney, Australia: Enabling Built Environment Program, University of New South Wales.

Chase, C. A., Mann, K., Wasek, S., & Arbesman, M. (2012). Systematic review of the effect of home modification and fall prevention programs on falls and the performance of community-dwelling older adults. *American Journal of Occupational Therapy, 66*, 284-291. doi: 10.5014/ajot.2012.005017

Chiatti, C., & Iwarsson, S. (2014). Evaluation of housing adaptation interventions: Integrating the economic perspective into occupational therapy practice. *Scandinavian Journal of Occupational Therapy, 1*(5), 323-333. doi:http://dx.doi.org/10.3109/11038128.2014.900109

Clemson, L., Mackenzie, L., Ballinger, C., Close, J. C., & Cumming, R. G. (2008). Environmental interventions to prevent falls in community-dwelling older people: A meta-analysis of randomized trials. *Journal of Aging and Health, 20*(8), 954-971. doi: http://dx.doi.org/10.1177/0898264308324672

Clemson, L., & Martin, R. (1996). Usage and effectiveness of rail, bathing, and toileting aids. *Occupational Therapy in Health Care, 10*(1), 41-58. doi: http://dx.doi.org/10.1080/J003v10n01_04

Close, J., Ellis, M., Hooper, R., Glucksman, E., Jackson, S., & Swift, C. (1999). Prevention of Falls in the Elderly Trial (PROFET): A randomised controlled trial. *The Lancet, 353*(9147), 93-97. doi: http://dx.doi.org/10.1016/S0140-6736(98)06119-4

Costello, E., & Edelstein, J. E. (2008). Update on falls prevention for community-dwelling older adults: Review of single and multifactorial intervention programs. *Journal of Rehabilitation Research and Development, 45*(8) 1135-1152. doi: https://doi.org/10.1682/JRRD.2007.10.0169

Cowan, D., & Turner-Smith, A. (1999). The role of assistive technology in alternative models of care for older people. In *Royal commission on long-term care* (Volume 2, Appendix 4, pp. 325-346). London, England: Stationery Office. Retrieved from http://citeseerx.ist.psu.edu/viewdoc/download?doi=10.1.1.123.1879&rep=rep1&type=pdf

Cumming, R. G., Thomas, M., Szonyi, G., Salkeld, G., O'Neill, E., Westbury, C., & Frampton, G. (1999). Home visits by an occupational therapist for assessment and modification of environmental hazards: A randomized trial of falls prevention. *Journal of the American Geriatrics Society, 47*(12), 1397-1402. doi:10.1111/j.1532-5415.1999.tb01556.x

Dahlin-Ivanoff, S., Haak, M., Fänge, A., & Iwarsson, S. (2007). The multiple meaning of home as experienced by very old Swedish people. *Scandinavian Journal of Occupational Therapy, 14*(1), 25-32. doi: 10.1080/11038120601151714

Danziger, S., & Chaudhury, H. (2009). Older adults' use of adaptable design features in housing units: An exploratory study. *Journal of Housing for the Elderly, 23*(3), 134-148. doi: http://dx.doi.org/10.1080/02763890903035498

Day, L., Fildes, B., Gordon, I., Fitzharris, M., Flamer, H., & Lord, S. (2002). Randomised factorial trial of falls prevention among older people living in their own homes. *British Medical Journal, 325*, 128. doi: https://doi.org/10.1136/bmj.325.7356.128

de Jonge, D., Aplin, T., Larkin, S., & Ainsworth, E. (2016). The aesthetic appeal of assistive technology and the economic value baby boomers place on it: A pilot study. *Australian Occupational Therapy Journal, 63*(6), 415-423. doi: 10.1111/1440-1630.12286

de Jonge, D., Jones, A., Phillips, R., & Chung, M. (2011). Understanding the essence of home: Older people's experiences of home in Australia. *Occupational Therapy International, 18*(1), 39-47. doi: 10.1002/oti.312

Dooley, N. R., & Hinojosa, J. (2004). Improving quality of life for persons with Alzheimer's disease and their family caregivers: Brief occupational therapy intervention. *American Journal of Occupational Therapy, 58*, 561-569. doi: 10.5014/ajot.58.5.561

Ekstam, L., Carlsson, G., Chiatti, C., Nilsson, M. H., & Fänge, A. M. (2014). A research-based strategy for managing housing adaptations: Study protocol for a quasi-experimental trial. *BMC Health Services Research, 14*, 602. doi:10.1186/s12913-014-0602-5

Fänge, A., & Iwarsson, S. (2003). Accessibility and usability in housing: Construct validity and implications for research and practice. *Disability and Rehabilitation, 25*(23), 1316-1325. doi: 10.1080/09638280310001616286

Fänge, A., & Iwarsson, S. (2005a). Changes in accessibility and usability in housing: An exploration of the housing adaptation process. *Occupational Therapy International, 12*(1), 44-59. doi:10.1002/oti.14

Fänge, A., & Iwarsson, S. (2005b). Changes in ADL dependence and aspects of usability following housing adaptation: A longitudinal perspective. *American Journal of Occupational Therapy, 59*, 296-304. doi:10.5014/ajot.59.3.296

Fänge, A., & Iwarsson, S. (2007). Challenges in the development of strategies for housing adaptation evaluations. *Scandinavian Journal of Occupational Therapy, 14*(3), 140-149. doi:10.1080/11038120600840150

Felix, E., de Haan, H., Vaandrager, L., & Koelen, M. (2015). Beyond thresholds: The everyday lived experience of the house by older people. *Journal of Housing for the Elderly, 29*(4), 329-347. doi:10.1080/02763893.2015.1055027

Fisher, A.G. (1998). Uniting practice and theory in an occupational framework. *The American Journal of Occupational Therapy, 52*(7), 509-520.

Fox, P. L. (1995). Rehabilitation in practice: Environmental modifications in the homes of elderly Canadians with disabilities. *Disability and Rehabilitation, 17*(1), 43-49. doi:10.3109/09638289509166626

Frisk, E., Arvidsson, H., Kiviloog, J., Ivarsson, A. B., Kamwendo, K., & Stridh, G. (2006). An investigation of the housing environment for persons with asthma and persons without asthma. *Scandinavian Journal of Occupational Therapy, 13*(1), 4-12. doi: 10.1080/11038120510031824

Gill, T. M., Baker, D. I., Gottschalk, M., Peduzzi, P., Allore, H., & Byers, A. (2002). A program to prevent functional decline in physically frail, elderly persons who live at home. *New England Journal of Medicine, 347*(14), 1069-1074. doi: 10.1056/NEJMoa020423

Gillespie, L. D., Robertson, M. C., Gillespie, W. J., Sherrington, C., Gates, S., Clemson, L. M., & Lamb, S. E. (2012). Interventions for preventing falls in older people living in the community. *Cochrane Database of Systematic Reviews*, (9), CD007146. doi: 10.1002/14651858.CD007146.pub3

Gitlin, L. N. (2003). Conducting research on home environments: Lessons learned and new directions. *The Gerontologist, 43*(5), 628-637. doi: 10.1093/geront/43.5.628

Gitlin, L. N., Corcoran, M., Winter, L., Boyce, A., & Hauck, W. W. (2001). A randomized, controlled trial of a home environmental intervention: Effect on efficacy and upset in caregivers and on daily function of persons with dementia. *The Gerontologist, 41*(1), 4-14. doi: http://dx.doi.org/10.1093/geront/41.1.4

Gitlin, L. N., Hauck, W. W., Winter, L., Dennis, M. P., & Schulz, (2006). Effect of an in-home occupational and physical therapy intervention on reducing mortality in functionally vulnerable older people: Preliminary findings. *Journal of the American Geriatrics Society, 54*(6), 950-955. doi: 10.1111/j.1532-5415.2006.00733.x

Gitlin, L. N., Winter, L., Dennis, M. P., Corcoran, M., Schinfeld, S., & Hauck, W. W. (2006). A randomised trial of a multicomponent home intervention to reduce functional difficulties in older adults. *Journal of the American Geriatrics Society, 54*(5), 809-816. doi:10.1111/j.1532-5415.2006.00703.x

Golant, S. M. (2003). Conceptualizing time and behavior in environmental gerontology: A pair of old issues deserving new thought. *The Gerontologist, 43*(5), 638-648. doi: https://doi.org/10.1093/geront/43.5.638

Granbom, M., Iwarsson, S., Kylberg, M., Pettersson, C., & Slaug, B. (2016). A public health perspective to environmental barriers and accessibility problems for senior citizens living in ordinary housing. *BMC Public Health, 16*, 772. DOI: 10.1186/s12889-016-3369-2

Granbom, M., Taei, A., & Ekstam, L. (2017). Cohabitants' perspective on housing adaptations: A piece of the puzzle. *Scandinavian Journal of Caring Studies, 31*(4), 805-813.

Green, B. N., Johnson, C. D., & Adams, A. (2006). Writing narrative literature reviews for peer-reviewed journals: Secrets of the trade. *Journal of Sports Chiropractic Rehabilitation, 15*(3), 5-19. doi: 10.1016/S0899-3467(07)60142-6e

Haak, M., Dahlin-Ivanoff, S., Fänge, A., Sixsmith, J., & Iwarsson, S. (2007a). Home as the locus and origin of participation: Experiences among very old Swedish people. *Occupational Therapy Journal of Research: Occupation, Participation, and Health, 27*(3), 95-103. doi: 10.1177/153944920702700303

Haak, M., Fänge A., Iwarsson, S., & Dahlin-Ivanoff, S. (2007b). Home as a signification of independence and autonomy: Experiences among very old Swedish people. *Scandinavian Journal of Occupational Therapy, 14*(1), 16-24. doi: 10.1080/11038120601024929

Hagsten, B., Svensson, O., & Gardulf, A. (2004). Early individualized postoperative occupational therapy training in 100 patients improves ADL after hip fracture: A randomized trial. *Acta Orthopaedica Scandinavica, 75*(2), 177-183. doi: http://dx.doi.org/10.1080/00016470412331294435

Hawkins, R., & Stewart, S. (2002). Changing rooms: The impact of adaptations on the meaning of home for a disabled person and the role of occupational therapists in the process. *British Journal of Occupational Therapy, 65*(2), 81-87. doi: 10.1177/030802260206500206

Heywood, F. (2001). *Money well spent: The effectiveness and value of housing adaptations.* Bristol, England: Policy Press.

Heywood, F. (2002). Adaptations: Key evidence for managers. *Journal of Integrated Care, 10*(5), 13-17. doi: http://dx.doi.org/10.1108/14769018200200042

Heywood, F. (2003). Adaptation policies especially for children: Key factors in effective outcomes. *Journal of Integrated Care, 11*(1), 22-27. doi:http://dx.doi.org/10.1108/14769018200300006

Heywood, F. (2004a). The health outcomes of housing adaptations. *Disability & Society, 19*(2), 129-143. doi: http://dx.doi.org/10.1080/0968759042000181767

Heywood, F. (2004b). Understanding needs: A starting point for quality. *Housing Studies, 19*(5), 709-726. doi: http://dx.doi.org/10.1080/0267303042000249161

Heywood, F. (2005). Adaptation: Altering the house to restore the home. *Housing Studies, 20*(4), 531-547. doi: http://dx.doi.org/10.1080/02673030500114409

Heywood, F., & Awang, D. (2011). Developing a housing adaptation genome project. *British Journal of Occupational Therapy, 74*(4), 200-203. doi: 10.4276/030802211X13021048723372

Heywood, F., & Turner, L. (2007). Better outcomes, lower costs: Implications for health and social care budgets of investment in housing adaptations, improvements, and equipment: A review of the evidence. Retrieved from http://www.wohnenimalter.ch/img/pdf/better_outcomes_report.pdf

Hwang, E., Cummings, L., Sixsmith, A., & Sixsmith, J. (2011). Impacts of home modifications on aging-in-place. *Journal of Housing for the Elderly, 25*(3), 246-257. doi: 10.1080/02763893.2011.595611

Iwarsson, S. (2015). Housing adaptations and home modifications. in I. Soderback (Ed.). *International handbook of occupational therapy interventions* (pp. 177-187). Switzerland: Springer International Publishing.

Jensen, J., Lundin-Olsson, L., Nyberg, L., & Gustafson, Y. (2002). Fall and injury prevention in older people living in residential care facilities: A cluster randomized trial. *Annals of Internal Medicine, 136*(10), 733-41. doi: 10.7326/0003-4819-136-10-200205210-00008

Johansson, K., Borrell, L., & Lilja, M. (2009) Older persons' navigation through the service system towards home modification resources, *Scandinavian Journal of Occupational Therapy, 16*(4), 227-237, doi: 10.3109/11038120802684307

Johansson, K., Lilja, M., Petersson, I., & Borell, L. (2007). Performance of activities of daily living in a sample of applicants for home modification services. *Scandinavian Journal of Occupational Therapy, 14*(1), 44-53. doi: 10.1080/11038120601094997

Jones, A., de Jonge, D., & Phillips, R. (2008). *The impact of home maintenance and modification services on health, community care and housing outcomes in later life (Positioning paper).* Melbourne, Australia: Australian Housing and Urban Research Institute. Retrieved from https://www.ahuri.edu.au/__data/assets/pdf_file/0022/2893/AHURI_Positioning_Paper_No103-The-impact-of-home-maintenance-and-modification-services-on-health.pdf

Judd, B., Liu, E., Easthope, H., Davy, L., & Bridge, C. (2014). *Downsizing amongst older Australians (AHURI Final Report No. 214).* Melbourne, Australia: Australian Housing and Urban Research Institute. Retrieved from http://www.ahuri.edu.au/research/final-reports/214

Jutkowitz, E., Gitlin, L. N., Pizzi, L. T., Lee, E., & Dennis, M. P. (2012). Cost effectiveness of a home-based intervention that helps functionally vulnerable older adults age in place at home. *Journal of Aging Research, 2012*, 680265. doi: 10.1155/2012/680265. Epub 2011 Aug 16.

Keall, M. D., Pierse, N., Howden-Chapman, P., Cunningham, C., Cunningham, M., Guria, J., & Baker, M. G. (2015). Home modifications to reduce injuries from falls in the Home Injury Prevention Intervention (HIPI) study: A cluster-randomised controlled trial. *The Lancet, 385*(9964), 231-238. doi: 10.1016/S0140-6736(14)61006-0

Kendig, H., Clemson, L., & Mackenzie, L. (2012). Older people: well-being, housing, and neighbourhoods. In S. Smith, M. Elsinga, O. S. Eng, L. O'Mahony, & S. Wachter (Eds.), *International encyclopedia of housing and home* (pp. 150-155). Oxford, England: Elsevier.

Lannin, N. A., Clemson, L., McCluskey, A., Lin, C-W. C., Cameron, I. D., & Barras, S. (2007). Feasibility and results of a randomised pilot-study of pre-discharge occupational therapy home visits. *BMC Health Services Research, 7*(42), 1-8. doi: 10.1186/1472-6963-7-42

Lansley, P., McCreadie, C., & Tinker, A. (2004). Can adapting the homes of older people and providing assistive technology pay its way? *Age and Ageing, 33*(6), 571-576. doi-org.ezproxy.library.uq.edu.au/10.1093/ageing/afh190

Lin, M-R., Wolf, S.L., Hwang, H-F., Gong, S-Y., & Chen, C-Y. (2007). A randomized, controlled trial of fall prevention programs and quality of life in older fallers. *Journal of the American Geriatrics Society, 55*(4), 499-506.

Liu, S. Y., & Lapane, K. L. (2009). Residential modifications and decline in physical function among community-dwelling older adults. *The Gerontologist, 49*(3), 344-354. doi: 10.1093/geront/gnp033

Lord, S., Menz, H., & Sherrington, C. (2006). Home environment risk factors for falls in older people and the efficacy of home modifications. *Age and Ageing, 35*(Suppl. 2), ii55-ii59.

Mackenzie, L., Curryer, C., & Byles, J. E. (2015). Narratives of home and place: Findings from the Housing and Independent Living Study. *Ageing & Society, 35*, 1684-1712. doi: 10.1017/S0144686X140000476

Mann, W. C., Ottenbacher, K. J., Fraas, L., Tomita, M., & Granger, C. V. (1999). Effectiveness of assistive technology and environmental interventions in maintaining independence and reducing home care costs for the frail elderly: A randomized controlled trial. *Archives of Family Medicine, 8*, 210-217. doi: http://dx.doi.org/10.1001/archfami.8.3.210

Mathieson, K. M., Kronenfeld, J. J., & Keith, V. M. (2002). Maintaining functional independence in elderly adults: The roles of health status and financial resources in predicting home modifications and use of mobility equipment. *The Gerontologist, 42*(1), 24-31. doi: https://doi.org/10.1093/geront/42.1.24

Mitoku, K., & Shimanouchi, S. (2014). Home modification and prevention of frailty progression in older adults: A Japanese prospective cohort study. *Journal of Gerontological Nursing, 40*(8), 40-47. doi: 10.3928/00989134-20140311-02

Montreuil, C., Després, C., & Beauregard, L. (2011). Impact of housing modifications on the meaning of home for people with disabilities. Paper presented at the International Conference on Best Practices in Universal Design, Toronto, Canada. Retrieved from https://udeworld.com/presentations/powerpoints/FICCDAT2011_impactofhousingmodificationsonthemeaningofhomeforpeoplewithdisabilities_Montreuil,C..pdf

Morgan, D. J., Boniface, G. E., & Reagon, C. (2016). The effects of adapting their home on the meaning of home for families with a disabled child. *Disability & Society, 31*(4), 481-496. doi: 10.1080/09687599.2016.1183475

Nagib, W., & Williams, A. (2016). Toward an autism friendly home environment. *Housing Studies, 32*(2), 140-167. doi:http://dx.doi.org/10.1080/02673037.2016.1181719

Naik, A. D. & Gill, T. M. (2005). Underutilization of environmental adaptations for bathing in community-living older persons. *Journal of the American Geriatrics Society, 53*(9), 1497-1503. doi: 10.1111/j.1532-5415.2005.53458.x

Newman, S. J., Struyk, R., Wright, P., & Rice, M. (1990). Overwhelming odds: Caregiving and the risk of institutionalization. *Journal of Gerontology, 45*(5), S173-183.

Nikolaus, T., & Bach, M. (2003). Preventing falls in community-dwelling frail older people using a home intervention team (HIT): Results from the randomized Falls-HIT trial. *Journal of the American Geriatrics Society, 51*(3), 300-305. doi: http://dx.doi.org/10.1046/j.1532-5415.2003.51102.x

Niva, B., & Skar, L. (2006). A pilot study of the activity patterns of five elderly persons after a housing adaptation. *Occupational Therapy International, 13*(1), 21-34. doi: 10.1002/oti.21

Nocon, A., & Pleace, N. (1997). Until disabled people get consulted: The role of occupational therapy in meeting housing needs. *British Journal of Occupational Therapy, 60*(3), 115-122. doi: 10.1177/030802269706000305

Nord, C., Eakin, P., Astley, P., & Atkinson, A. R. (2009). An exploration of communication between clients and professionals in the design of home adaptations. *British Journal of Occupational Therapy, 72*(5), 197-204. doi: 10.1177/030802260907200504

O'Day, B. L., & Corcoran, P. J. (1994). Assistive technology: Problems and policy alternatives. *Archives of Physical Medicine and Rehabilitation, 75*(10), 1165-1169.

Orrell, A., McKee, K., Torrington, J., Barnes, S., Darton, R., Netten, A., & Lewis, A. (2013). The relationship between building design and residents' quality of life in extra care housing schemes. *Health & Place, 21*, 52-64. doi: https://doi.org/10.1016/j.healthplace.2012.12.004

Ostensjö, S., Carlberg, E. B., & Völlestad, N. K. (2005). The use and impact of assistive devices and other environmental modifications on everyday activities and care in young children with cerebral palsy. *Disability and Rehabilitation, 27*(14), 849-861. doi: 10.1080/09638280400018619

Oswald, F., & Rowles, G.D. (2007). Beyond the relocation trauma in old age: New trends in elders' residential decisions. In H.-W. Wahl, C. Tesh-Romer, & A. Hoff (Eds.), *New dynamics in old age: Individual, environmental, and societal perspectives* (pp. 127-152). Amityville, New York: Baywood Publishing Company Inc.

Oswald, F., & Wahl, H. W. (2005). Dimensions of the meaning of home in later life. In G. D. Rowles & H. Chaudhury (Eds.), *Home and identity in late life: International perspectives* (pp. 21-45). New York, NY: Springer.

Oswald, F., Wahl, H. W., Naumann, D., Mollenkopf, H., & Hieber, A. (2006). The role of the home environment in middle and late adulthood. In H. W. Wahl, H. Brenner, H. Mollenkopf, D. Rothenbacher, & C. Rott (Eds.), *The many faces of health, competence and well-being in old age* (pp. 7-24). Dordrecht, The Netherlands: Springer.

Oswald, F., Wahl, H.-W., Schilling, O., Nygren, C., Fänge, A., Sixsmith, A., . . . Iwarsson, S. (2007). Relationships between housing and healthy aging in very old age. *The Gerontologist, 47*(1), 96-107. doi: https://doi.org/10.1093/geront/47.1.96

Palvanen, M., Kannus, P., Piirtola, M., Niemi, S., Parkkari. J., & Jarvinen, M. (2014). Effectiveness of the Chaos Falls Clinic in preventing falls and injuries of home dwelling older adults: A randomised controlled trial. *International Journal of Care of the Injured, 45*, 265-271. doi: http://dx.doi.org/10.1016/j.injury.2013.03.010

Pardessus, V., Puisieux, E., Di Pompeo, C., Gaudefroy, C., Thevenon, A., & Dewailly, P. (2002). Benefits of home visits for falls and autonomy in the elderly: A randomized trial study. *American Journal of Physical Medicine and Rehabilitation, 81*, 247-252. doi: http://dx.doi.org/10.1097/00002060-200204000-00002

Percival, J. (2002). Domestic spaces: Uses and meanings in the daily lives of older people. *Aging and Society, 22*, 729-749. doi:doi.org/10.1017/S0144686X02008917

Petersson, I., Kottorp, A., Bergström, J., & Lilja, M. (2009). Longitudinal changes in everyday life after home modifications for people aging with disabilities. *Scandinavian Journal of Occupational Therapy, 16*(2), 78-87. doi: 10.1080/11038120802409747

Petersson, I., Lilja, M., Hammel, J., & Kottorp, A. (2008). Impact of home modification services on ability in everyday life for people ageing with disabilities. *Journal of Rehabilitation Medicine, 40*(4), 253-260. doi: 10.2340/16501977-0160

Pettersson, C., Löfqvist, C., & Fänge, A. M. (2012b). Clients' experiences of housing adaptations: A longitudinal mixed-methods study. *Disability and Rehabilitation, 34*(20), 1706-1715. doi: http://dx.doi.org/10.3109/09638288.2012.660596

Picking, C., & Pain, H. (2003). Home adaptations: User perspectives on the role of professionals. *British Journal of Occupational Therapy, 66*(1), 2-8.

Pighills, A., Ballinger, C., Pickering, R., & Chari, S. (2016). A critical review of the effectiveness of environmental assessment and modification in the prevention of falls amongst community-dwelling older people. *British Journal of Occupational Therapy, 79*(3), 133-143. doi: 10.1177/0308022615600181

Pighills, A. C., Torgerson, D. J., Sheldon, T. A., Drummond, A. E., & Bland, J. M. (2011). Environmental assessment and modification to prevent falls in older people. *Journal of the American Geriatrics Society, 59*(4), 26-33. doi: http://dx.doi.org/10.1111/j.1532-5415.2010.03221.x

Plautz, B., Beck, D. E., Selmar, C., & Radetsky, M. (1996). Modifying the environment: A community-based injury-reduction program for elderly residents. *American Journal of Preventive Medicine, 12*(Suppl.), 33-38.

Pynoos, J., Steinman, B. A., Nguyen, A., Bressette, M. (2012). Assessing and adapting the home environment to reduce falls and meet the changing capacity of older adults. *Journal of Housing for the Elderly, 26*(1-3), 137-155. doi:10.1080/02763893.2012.673382

Pynoos, J., Tabbarah, M., Angelelli, J., & Demiere, M. (1998). Improving the delivery of home modifications. *Technology and Disability, 8*(1), 3-14. doi: 10.1016/S1055-4181(98)00004-1

Randström, K. B., Asplund, K., & Svedlund, M. (2012). Impact of environmental factors in home rehabilitation: A qualitative study from the perspective of older persons using the International Classification of Functioning, Disability, and Health to describe facilitators and barriers. *Disability and Rehabilitation, 34*(9), 779-787. doi:10.3109/09638288.2011.619621

Renaut, S., Ogg, J., Petite, S., & Chamahian, A. (2015). Home environments and adaptations in the context of ageing. *Ageing and Society, 35*(6), 1278-1303.

Robinovitch, S. N., Scott, V., & Feldman, F. (2014). Home-safety modifications to reduce injuries from falls. *The Lancet, 385*(9964), 205-206. doi: http://dx.doi.org/10.1016/S0140-6736(14)61188-0

Rowles, G. D. (2006). Commentary: A house is not a home, but can it become one? In H. W. Wahl, H. Brenner, H. Mollenkopf, D. Rothenbacher, & C. Rott(Eds.), *Many faces of health, competence and well-being in old age* (pp. 25-32). Dordrecht, The Netherlands: Springer.

Roy, L., Rousseau, J., Allard, H., Feldman, D., & Majnemer, A. (2008). Parental experience of home adaptation for children with motor disabilities. *Physical and Occupational Therapy in Pediatrics, 28*(4), 353-368. doi: doi.org/10.1080/01942630802307101

Russell, R. (2016). The development of a design and construction process protocol to support occupational therapists in delivering effective home modifications (Unpublished Doctoral Dissertation). University of Salford, UK.

Sanford, J. (2012). *Universal design as a rehabilitation strategy: Design for the ages.* New York, NY: Springer.

Sanford, J. & Bruce, C. (2010). Measuring the impact of the physical environment. In: E. Mpofu & T. Oakland (Eds.), *Rehabilitation and health assessment* (pp. 207-228). New York: Springer.

Shelledy, D. C., Legrand, T. S., Gardner, D. D., & Peters, J. I. (2009). A randomized, controlled study to evaluate the role of an in-home asthma disease management program provided by respiratory therapists in improving outcomes and reducing the cost of care. *Journal of Asthma, 46*(2), 194-201. doi: http://dx.doi.org/10.1080/02770900802610068

Siebert, C., Smallfield, S., & Stark, S. (2014). *Occupational therapy practice guidelines for home modifications.* Bethesda, MD: American Occupational Therapy Association.

Sixsmith, A. (1986). Independence and home in later life. In C. Phillipson, M. Bernard, & P. Strang (Eds.), *Dependency and interdependency in old age: Theoretical perspectives and policy alternatives* (pp. 338-347). London, England: Croom Helm.

Sixsmith, J., Sixsmith, A., Fänge, A.M., Naumann, D., Kucsera, C., Tomsone, S., . . . Woolrych, R. (2014). Healthy ageing and home: The perspectives of very old people in five European countries. *Social Science & Medicine, 106*, 1-9. http://dx.doi.org/10.1016/j.socscimed.2014.01.006

Slaug, B., Chiatti, C., Oswald, F., Kaspar, R., & Schmidt, S.M. (2017). Improved housing accessibility for older people in Sweden and Germany: Sort term costs and long-term gains. *International Journal of Environmental Research and Public Health, 14*(964), 1-13. doi: 10.3390/ijerph14090964

Smith, S. G. (1994). The essential qualities of a home. *Journal of Environmental Psychology, 14*, 31-46. doi.org/10.1016/S0272-4944(05)80196-3

Stark, S. (2004). Removing environmental barriers in the homes of older adults with disabilities improves occupational performance. *OTJR: Occupation, Participation, and Health, 24*(1), 32-39. doi:10.1177/153944920402400105

Stark, S., Keglovits, M., Arbesman, M., & Lieberman, D. (2017). Effect of home modification interventions on the participation of community-dwelling adults with health conditions: A systematic review. *American Journal of Occupational Therapy, 71*, 7102290010p1-p11. doi:10.5014/ajot.2017.018887

Stark, S., Landsbaum, A., Palmer, J., Somerville, E.K., & Morris, J.C. (2009). Client-centred home modifications improve daily activity performance of older adults. *Canadian Journal of Occupational Therapy, 76*(1 Suppl.), 235-245. doi:10.1177/000841740907600s09

Stark, S., Somerville, E., Keglovits, M., Conte, J., Li, M., Hu, Y-L., & Yan, Y. (2017). Protocol for the home hazards removal program (HARP) study: A pragmatic, randomized clinical trial, and implementation study. *BMC Geriatrics, 17*, 90. doi:10.1186/s12877-017-0478-4

Steinfeld, E., & Maisel, J. (2012). *Universal design: Creating inclusive environments.* Hoboken, NJ: John Wiley & Sons.

Stevens, M., Holman, C. D., & Bennett, N. (2001). Preventing falls in older people: Impact of an intervention to reduce environmental hazards in the home. *Journal of the American Geriatric Society, 49*(11), 1442-1447. doi:10.1046/j.1532-5415.2001.4911235.x

Szanton, S. L., Thorpe, R. J., Boyd, C., Tanner, E. K., Leff, B., Agree, E., . . . Gitlin, L. N. (2011). Community aging in place, advancing better living for elders: A bio-behavioral environmental intervention to improve function and health related quality of life in disabled older adults. *Journal of the American Geriatrics Society, 59*, 2314-2320. https://doi.org/10.1111/j.1532-5415.2011.03698.x

Tanner, B., Tilse, C., & de Jonge, D. (2008). Restoring and sustaining home: The impact of home modifications on the meaning of home for older people. *Journal of Housing for the Elderly, 22*(3), 195-215. doi: http://dx.doi.org/10.1080/02763890802232048

Tinetti, M. E., Mendes de Leon, C. F., Doucette, J. T., & Baker, D. I. (1994). Fear of falling and fall-related efficacy in relationship to functioning among community-living elders. *Journal of Gerontology: Medical Sciences, 49*(3), M140-M147.

Tse, T. (2005). The environment and falls prevention: Do environmental modifications make a difference? *Australian Occupational Therapy Journal, 52*(4), 271-281. doi:10.1111/j.1440-1630.2005.00525.x

Turner, S., Arthur, G., & Lyons, R. A. (2011). Modification of the home environment for the reduction of injuries. *Cochrane Database of Systematic Reviews*, (2), CD003600. doi:10.1002/14651858.CD003600.pub3

U.K. Home Adaptations Consortium. (2017). Data and evidence. Retrieved from https://homeadaptationsconsortium.wordpress.com/data-and-evidence/

Velkoff, V., & Lawson, V. A. (1998). US Department of Commerce, Economics, and Statistics Administration Bureau of the Census international brief: Gender and ageing. Retrieved from https://www.census.gov/population/international/files/ib-9803.pdf

Vik, D., Lilja, M., & Nygard, L. (2007). The influence of the environment on participation subsequent to rehabilitation as experienced by elderly people in Norway. *Scandinavian Journal of Occupational Therapy, 14*(2), 86-95. doi: http://dx.doi.org/10.1080/11038120600971047

Wahl, H-W., Fänge, A., Oswald, F., Gitlin, L. N., & Iwarsson, S. (2009). The home environment and disability-related outcomes in aging individuals: What is the empirical evidence? *The Gerontologist, 49*(3), 355-367. doi:10.1093/geront/gnp056

Wilson, D. J., Mitchell, J. M., Kemp, B. J., Adkins, R. H., & Mann, W. (2009). Effects of assistive technology on functional decline in people aging with a disability. *Assistive Technology, 21*, 208-217. doi: http://dx.doi.org/10.1080/10400430903246068

Winfield, J. (2003). Best adaptation redeeming people's homes: Enlightened occupational therapy. *British Journal of Occupational Therapy, 66*(8), 376-377. doi.org/10.1177/030802260306600807

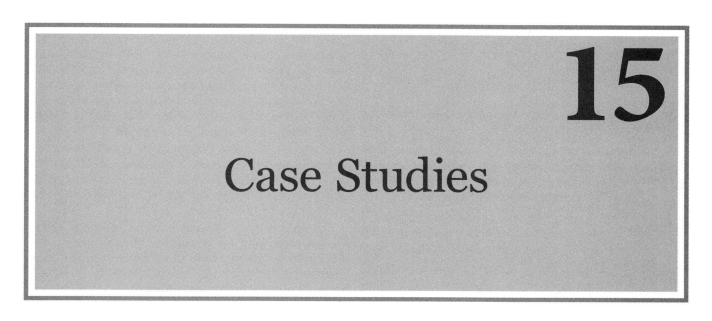

Case Studies

Elizabeth Ainsworth, MOccThy, Grad Cert Health Sci;
Kathleen Baigent, Dip COT, Dip Health Prom; Ruth Cordiner, Dip COT, Grad Cert Occ Thy;
Shirley Darlison, BOccThy; and May Eade, BOccThy

This chapter synthesizes the information from previous chapters by providing the reader with a range of case studies relating to older people and people with disabilities across the lifespan. Each case study highlights the home modification process. This chapter includes detail on the clinical reasoning process used to determine the range of environmental interventions selected to enhance the health, safety, independence, and home and community participation of a range of clients. Additionally, it provides evidence of the value of post modification evaluation to review client outcomes and to contribute to the occupational therapist's practice knowledge.

The first case study relates to a young man with spina bifida who lives with his aging parents in a newly acquired home built in the late 1800s. Home modifications were recommended to provide access to and within the home, and would meet his short term and long-term needs.

The second case study provides information about a young woman with a spinal injury who has recently purchased a house that has needed extensive home modifications. She has received finance for her modifications through an insurance claim. The completed home modifications had to meet the requirements of "reasonable and necessary" as indicated in legislation.

The third case study describes an elderly gentleman who is experiencing a deterioration in his physical and functional status. Modifications are provided to enable him to remain at home or as long as possible, in the care of his wife, who also has health conditions.

The fourth case study describes the home modification needs of two men residing together and sharing 24-hour caregiver support. These two men have intellectual and physical disabilities and tend to damage property. This section discusses the home modifications required to improve the usability of the environment and to prevent ongoing damage.

The fifth case study provides information to the reader on a range of home modifications that have been considered for a person with a visual impairment living alone in her own home.

The sixth case study showcases the effect of housing types and home modifications on a young man with a psychiatric disability who has made the transition from an institution into the community. Changes discussed include home modifications that aim to prevent neighborhood disputes and improve the client's sense of safety and security in his own home.

The final case study describes the home modification requirements of an elderly couple where one partner is caring for a spouse who has dementia.

Ainsworth, E., & de Jonge, D. *An Occupational Therapist's*
Guide to Home Modification Practice, Second Edition (pp. 337-380).
© 2019 SLACK Incorporated.

Chapter Objectives

By the end of this chapter, the reader will be able to:

+ Explain the role of the occupational therapist in the home modification process

+ Recognize and discuss the application of the transactive approach to examining the person, his or her home environment, and occupations during the home modification process

+ Describe and apply the processes for home modification practice, including using clinical reasoning, for a range of people with varying health conditions and disabilities

+ Identify a range of products, designs, and solutions that could be considered when developing intervention options for individuals with specific housing requirements

Clinical Reasoning, Evaluation, and Justification for Recommendations

The following case studies provide examples of minor and major modification recommendations provided by occupational therapists that include the process of clinical reasoning. This has included the therapists using a combination of narrative, scientific, pragmatic, ethical, and interactive reasoning approaches in examining each client's access to, and performance in, the different areas in and around the home. The therapists have used the information gathered at the time of the visit, the advice of a builder who attended the interview either part way through the occupational therapy assessment or at the time of a second visit, and the views of client and other people who may be involved in their day-to-day lives, to formulate options for discussion.

At times, builders attended the home visits with the therapists to provide advice on the proposed structural modifications and compliance and building approval considerations associated with any such work. The therapists recorded equipment dimensions and the clients' anthropometric and reach range measurements, and client eye height, to use in developing the modifications where there was an emphasis on modifying for physical access. Photos were also taken, and measurements of the built environment were recorded by the builders and therapists.

Factors considered during the process of formulating options included the cost of the work, ensuring the home modifications were designed in keeping with the look of the home without creating an institutional appearance; and the needs of other household members and visitors including children, grandchildren, friends, and caregivers.

Clinical reasoning began once information was provided by the referrers at the time of initial contact, documentation from the health services were received, and through discussion and observing the clients in their own homes.

Scientific reasoning was used to interpret information regarding each person's health condition. Where some clients may deteriorate, acquire new equipment, and experience change in function because of their health condition, it was anticipated that in some circumstances, they will continue to encounter changing environmental demands and barriers. Scientific reasoning was used to collect cues throughout the assessment process as to how each person's skills and deficits were likely to affect his or her performance and when evaluating the effectiveness of the solution in addressing his or her occupational performance needs.

Narrative reasoning assisted occupational therapists to understand and interpret information relating to past and present life and each person's goals for the future. The therapists became aware, for example, that some clients wanted to set up the home so that they would not be a burden to their partners as they deteriorated. Some clients had a strong desire to stay in their home for as long as possible. It was determined that such preferences and lifestyle choices would continue to impact on people's future goals.

Pragmatic reasoning was used to consider contextual factors, choice of materials and relevant measurements for modifications, as well as funding issues. For example, the age of homes and people's plans for the staying in the home or selling the home when people no longer wanted to reside in their properties were considered in recommending the extent of the home modifications in various areas of each homes. Funding options such as whether there was a government contribution available, were considered within a framework for determining the most reasonable and necessary home modification solutions.

Pragmatically, the choice of materials was considered. For example, basic quality fittings and fixtures were selected for a range of clients because they were considered a reasonable cost, matched the look of the home, and did not appear out of place in the design of the property. Anthropometric and equipment measurements were considered in planning clearances and circulation space and for positioning fittings and fixtures in all areas of the home.

Ethical reasoning was used in considering alternative decisions for each issue identified by clients, including those that were not addressed and the consequences of recommendations made. Ethical reasoning was also considered in relation to the appropriate use of funding for a short- to medium-term planning of home modification solutions. For example, despite some clients receiving funding from the government through non-government organizations, the therapists did not make home modification recommendations that might have been considered extravagant or wasteful of resources. The therapists kept this information in mind while they considered client's preferences for changes in their home.

The builders provided samples of products and finishes that were discussed with clients and their families and other householders. After concluding the home visits, the therapists, and the builders, over a period of several weeks, developed concept drawings with layouts for the clients and their families and carers to consider. The therapists visited the home for a second time to show clients their concept drawings. The chosen options were finalized, and the final therapy reports, including the builder's specifications, were forwarded to clients and the relevant organizations providing funding for approval.

CASE STUDY 1: A YOUNG ADULT WITH A PHYSICAL CONDITION

Client Interests and Daily Activities

Dave is a 32-year-old who lives with his parents in a beautifully restored detached house in a quiet suburban area. Dave works full time in the city and enjoys driving himself to work in his new car. He has an active social life, playing sports on the weekends and has a keen interest in gaming on the internet. His parents are retired and enjoy community activities and travel. He has no other siblings.

Health Condition and Functional Performance

Dave has myelomeningocele, also known as open spina bifida, a condition where there was incomplete closure of the backbone and membranes around the spinal cord. His lesion is at the L2-L3 level of the spine which results in loss of sensation below the lumbar level affected in the spine resulting in paraplegia, with some inner thigh feeling; some incontinence of the bowels and bladder; reduced fine motor skills in the upper limbs, with associated tremor at times. Dave has good upper limb strength and balance and full reach range in the seated position. He has a history of having a range of operations but none in over 10 years. He has not had any significant illnesses or diseases in the last few years, and reported being in good health. He has had the same equipment, a manual wheelchair and mobile shower commode, for general use, for several years. Over the long term, Dave may have a change in his equipment needs and as he ages further into disability.

Location and Description of the House

The occupational therapist visited the home on the outskirts of a major metropolitan city. The home, a detached house, was built in the late 1800s, has been renovated over time, and was recently relocated from a small town to its current location. The family have just purchased the high set house situated on land that slopes away at the rear. The home is positioned at the end of a cul-de-sac and has a high fence (6-ft/1,800-mm high) at the front of the property. It is located high in a hilly area, and the family have a beautiful view of the city.

The house has six risers at the front entry with bilateral handrails, and four risers with no handrails at the side entry off the carport. There are other stairs located at the rear of the home. The front entry with the front and side stairs is the main entry used by the family and visitors.

The house has:

✦ Four bedrooms

✦ Large kitchen overlooking the rear yard

✦ Combined dining room and living room areas

✦ Laundry located downstairs

✦ A self-contained flat under the home

✦ Three bathrooms

✦ A double carport adjacent to the home

The house is of timber construction with polished floors in all areas except in the kitchen, laundry, and bathroom where there is tile on the floor. There is a small change in level between the hallway outside the toilet and laundry, and the bathroom area. There are level thresholds at the two doorways leading into the laundry area. There are timber thresholds at the doorways leading into the home.

Client Goals

A home visit referral requested an occupational therapist visit to make home modification recommendations to ensure that Dave would be able to live in the home without having to rely on his family to assist him accessing the front of the house from the carport, and the bathroom and its fittings and features.

The Canadian Occupational Performance Measure (COPM) was used with Dave. He indicated that his goals included the following:

+ Gaining access to the home from the carport without relying on his family to set up a temporary ramp to wheel him up and down the stairs near the carport

+ Gaining access to the bathroom and toilet close to his bedroom, to enable him to do his own self-care routine independently

Evaluating Occupational Performance and Identifying Needs

Prior to the home visit, the therapist reviewed the health information to gather information on Dave's current physical and functional status.

During the home visit, the therapist interviewed Dave to identify his goals and to ascertain Dave's capacity to function in the home that had not yet been modified to suit his needs. He was observed undertaking transfers, wheeling himself around in his manual wheelchair and mobile shower commode, and completing various activities in areas such as the bathroom, carport, and front yard area.

Mobility and Transfers

Dave reported that he used his manual wheelchair to propel himself short and long distances. He stated that he could negotiate curbs independently. He demonstrated his capacity to wheel up and down steep inclines during the time of the visit, including the steep driveway. He reported that although he could manage side-on transfers on and off the bed, toilet, a self-propelling mobile shower commode, and a chair, and a tub transfer bench with ease, he was struggling at home because of the inaccessible environment. Dave was observed to transfer on and off the bed independently and demonstrated that he could transfer from the bed and then into a mobile shower commode that he wheeled around the bedroom area. He was not able to wheel the mobile shower commode into the bathroom due to the narrow doorway and presence of the step at the

doorway. He was just able to fit his manual wheelchair through the bathroom doorway but scraped the timber door frames. His parents assisted him in the bathroom as he transferred from his wheelchair onto a tub transfer bench with difficulty. His parents wheeled him in his wheelchair up and down the four risers located at the front of the home near the carport but were struggling due to his size and weight in the wheelchair.

Self-Care and Household Activities

Dave showed the therapist where he undertook the various self-care tasks in the bathroom and bedroom. He stated that he could manage some of his self-care activities independently, including dressing, and basic grooming. He reported that he needed assistance to get in and out of the bath and on and off the toilet because of the lack of space for equipment and positioning of the wheelchair for transfers. He also stated that he could not access the bathroom sink fully and had to use a bowl. His mother and father aided with showering, drying, and managing his transfers due to the poor design of the bathroom.

Dave relied on his parents to do the cooking as the kitchen is not accessible. He did some light cleaning and shopping though his parents managed the heavier tasks such as completing the larger shopping and heavier cleaning tasks, lawn mowing, and gardening.

Anthropometric Measurements and Equipment

Dave's anthropometric measurements including his reach range and eye height were taken while seated in his wheelchair, and mobile shower commode.

Environmental Issues and Intervention Options

Various environmental issues and intervention options were discussed during the walk-through of the home with Dave and his parents.

Access to the Property

Wheelchair Access to the Home

Dave required assistance in his wheelchair to negotiate the stairs at the front of the home after transferring out his car under cover under the carport (Figure 15-1). Options considered included the installation of an elevator or a ramp at one set of stairs. The elevator was considered too costly compared with the installation of a ramp.

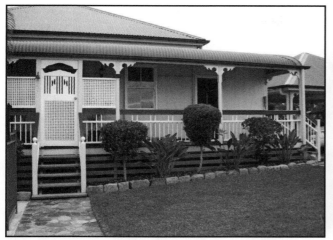

Figure 15-1. Before home modifications—front external access.

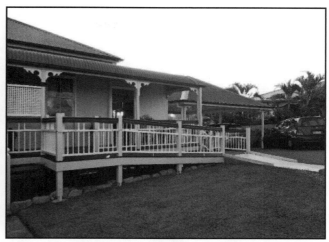

Figure 15-2. After home modifications—front external access.

The final recommendation included the installation of a ramp at the front of the property that led from the side of the driveway, along the front of the house, to adjoin the existing front verandah (Figure 15-2). This modification was designed to ensure the two sets of stairs leading onto the verandah could be retained, for people who did not suit or want to use the ramp. The lower landing would provide the client with close access to the driveway, so that he could wheel to his car under the carport. As well, the ramp was installed in such a way that it blended in with the look of the home. This was important to the family even though there was a high fence at the front of the home that blocked the view of the front entry from the street.

Internal Access

Adequate Door Widths

Dave had trouble wheeling through the narrow hallways and doorways leading into the bathroom, and his bedroom and was damaging his knuckles using the wheel rims to maneuver through these areas.

Options considered included limiting the client's access to specific areas of the home or completing some structural modifications to the timber frames in the home at the doorways.

The final recommendation included widening the doorways leading from the hallway into Dave's bedroom and the remodeled bathroom.

Access Within the Bathroom

Wheelchair and Mobile Shower Commode Access

Because of the presence of a low bath, inaccessible vanity, high mirror, narrow storage cupboard, and a step into the bathroom, Dave had trouble managing his routine in the bathroom (Figure 15-3). He had trouble getting into the bathroom and positioning himself to the side or in front of various features. He was over-reaching to access the sink, and there was no space to do a side-on transfer on and off the tub transfer bench. The mobile shower commode was not sitting over the toilet properly, resulting in his need for alternative ways to transfer on and off the toilet with help.

Solutions considered included leaving the features with their current location and design, resulting in Dave having limited use of the facilities, or redesigning the area to include an accessible vanity and shower, large storage area, and eliminating the step at the entry to the bathroom.

The final recommendation included the redesign and relation of the features to ensure that Dave had safe wheelchair and mobile shower commode access (Figure 15-4). This included the removal of all existing features, and the redesign to include the installation of a wheel-in shower, handheld shower, single lever mixer tap, and soap holder; a semi-recessed basin set into a vanity counter with a large mirror above the sink; a power point; a new "slip-resistant-when-wet" floor covering with no step at the doorway; and the relocation of the existing toilet suite.

Additional Factors Considered for Final Home Modification Solution

The age of the house and whether the client would continue to reside there in the short and long term were considered in recommending the extent of the home modifications in various areas of the home. Funding for the home modifications had become available through a government funded home modifications program and, though limited, was allocated

Figure 15-3. Before home modifications—bathroom. (A) Entry area. (B) Vanity. (C) Shower over bath. (D) Toilet.

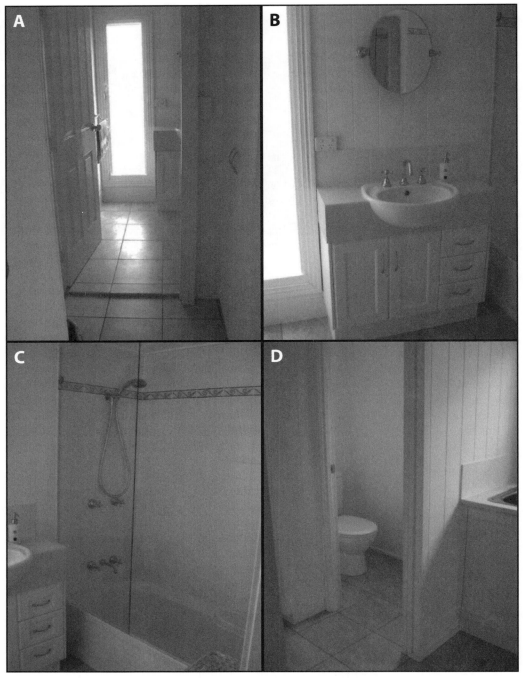

based on his home modification needs for at the next 5 years of his life. Dave was seriously considering his accommodation options for subsequent years and recognized that home modification funding would be required for an alternative solution to the family home if he chose to rent or purchase a unit in the area.

The choice of materials was considered. For example, an external timber ramp was selected because it was considered a reasonable cost compared with hiring a portable ramp for the short- to medium-term. The timber ramp also matched the look of the home and did not appear out of place in the design of the property. The bathroom was designed with the client's color preferences in mind for the wall tiles, to keep the modification looking aesthetically appealing in relation to the look of the rest of the home. Anthropometric, reach range, eye height, and equipment measurements were considered in planning clearances and circulation space and for positioning fittings and fixtures in all areas of the home.

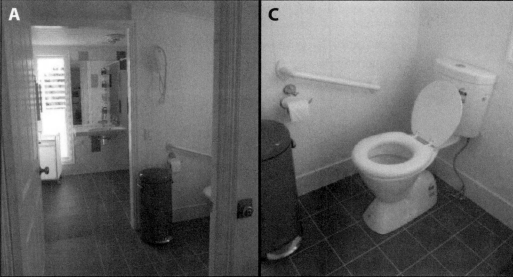

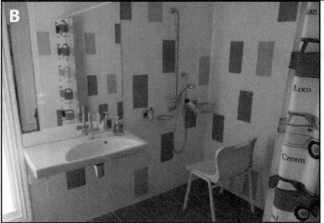

Figure 15-4. After home modifications—bathroom. (A) Entry area. (B) Vanity and shower area. (C) Toilet area.

The clients negotiated with the builder and provided extra funding at their own expense, for features such as additional tiling.

Outcomes

Quotes were obtained by staff at the government funded major modifications project. This included information from the builder who attended the visit and a second builder, for cost comparison. The original builder was selected to provide the home modifications. These were installed, and the therapist visited Dave in his home to complete a post modification evaluation. The therapist conducted an interview and structured observation of Dave in the various areas of the home. The interview included the review of the original occupational therapy report and the readministration of the COPM to determine whether there had been any improvement in the scores to demonstrate a change in Dave's capacity to

manage the various activities in the home and community (Table 15-1).

The scores indicated change in his performance and satisfaction with respect to his goals. The therapist observed that he had clearly improved in general health and functional capacity, being able to manage all activities with greater confidence and ease. He was not relying on his parents as much to assist during his self-care routine. He could manage accessing all areas of the home that were modified with safety and ease. The home modifications were installed as per the original occupational therapy report. The products and finishes appeared to be coping with wear and tear and were reported to suit the needs of all the family.

Since this post modification visit, the therapist has kept in contact with family members who report that Dave continues to manage his activities in the bathroom confidently and independently, and he uses the ramp with ease.

CASE STUDY 2: A YOUNG ADULT WITH A SPINAL INJURY

Client Interests and Daily Activities

Emily is a 26-year-old who lives with her partner in a detached house in a suburban area of a large city. She is currently attending university. Outside of her university routine, she enjoys socializing with her family and friends, and her partner. She hopes to get married to her partner soon.

Table 15-1. Dave's Canadian Occupational Performance Measure Rating

| Performance: 1 = Not able to do it at all; 10 = Able to do extremely well | | | | | |
| Satisfaction: 1 = Not satisfied at all; 10 = Extremely satisfied | | | | | |
OCCUPATIONAL PERFORMANCE PROBLEMS	IMPORTANCE	PERFORMANCE T1	SATISFACTION T1	PERFORMANCE T2	SATISFACTION T2
1 Unable to independently access the home	10	1	1	10	10
2 Difficulty completing self-care	10	1	1	10	10
3					
4					
5					
		Total Performance T1	Total Satisfaction T1	Total Performance T2	Total Satisfaction T2
Total Scores		2	2	20	20
		Average Performance T1	Average Satisfaction T1	Average Performance T2	Average Satisfaction T2
Average Scores		1	1	10	10
				Change in Performance	Change in Satisfaction
Change in Scores (T2 – T1)				9	9

Health Condition and Functional Performance

Emily sustained a spinal injury because of a motor vehicle accident 3 years ago.

She has a T1-T4 spinal injury resulting in complete paralysis of the lower body, has full function of her upper limbs but reports having "poor feeling down the sides" of her arms. Emily has full neck and head movement but reported experiencing fluctuating blood pressure that is worse in the mornings compared to the afternoons. This has been caused by a compromise of her sympathetic nervous system function resulting in autonomic dysreflexia, a condition where there is over activity of the autonomic nervous system. She experiences severe spasms, neuropathic pain around the injury levels, hypersensitivity below the injury level, and generalized pain. She has had cortisone injections to her shoulders due to bursitis and tendonitis in both shoulders. Emily also experiences significant illness because of ongoing urinary tract infections. She has a suprapubic in dwelling catheter that is changed once per month by a registered nurse; she can manage her colostomy bag independently.

Over the long term, there may be bone, soft tissue, and joint changes in the upper and lower limb joints and spine. Emily may be at risk of developing a syrinx, a fluid-filled cavity that develops in the spinal cord causing altered sensation, spasm, and weakness depending on the area affected. This may impact on her physical and functional capacity. Her equipment such as her wheelchair, and mobile shower commode, might change over time and she may need additional equipment such as a hoist, as she ages further into disability and develops greater functional limitations.

Location and Description of the House

Emily was provided with finance from her insurance claim to purchase a home and complete minor and major modifications to meet her needs. She recently signed a contract for the purchase of a house.

The occupational therapist visited the home with Emily. The home is a slab on ground house situated on a large block of land that is level. The home is located on a busy main road. There are fences around the side and rear of the house, and no fence at the front of the property.

The house has one step entry at the front, rear, side, and garage entries.

The house has:

+ Four bedrooms

+ Living room at the front of the house

+ En suite bathroom off the master bedroom

+ Main bathroom and separate toilet

+ Laundry adjacent to the main bathroom

+ Combined standard kitchen and dining room

+ Double garage with panel lift door– internal access through a doorway into the home

+ Outdoor patio at the rear

+ Clothesline at the side of the house off the laundry

The house is of brick construction with tiled floors in the living room, dining room, kitchen, laundry and bathroom areas, carpet on the bedroom floors, and vinyl in the kitchen and dining room areas. There are small changes in floor levels in the main areas of the home.

Client Goals

A home visit referral requested an occupational therapist visit to make home modification recommendations to ensure that Emily would be able to live in the home without having to rely on her partner or paid caregiver services to assist her with transfers, mobility, self-care, and household tasks.

Emily indicated that her goals included the following:

+ To have safe and independent access into the home.

+ To be able to use specific areas for self-care and household tasks, without relying on others to do most of the tasks.

Specifically, she wanted to achieve safety and independence completing the following activities:

+ Park under cover and being able to gain aceess to the front entry of the property in all weather conditions, with sufficient lighting.

+ Access to and through the front door.

+ Access from the front master bedroom into the en suite and second bedroom to enable completion of self-care activities; access to the

wardrobe areas for access to and storage of, clothing.

+ Use of the kitchen to prepare all meals including hot and cold meals.

+ Use of the laundry and capacity to get to the rear yard for access to the clothesline for laundry activities.

+ Access through the rear sliding glass door out onto the patio for outdoor dining, social activities and to hang clothes on a small airer in all weather conditions.

+ Use of all door handles and locks to ensure the safety and security of the home and to facilitate access.

+ Use of light switches to light all areas of the home for activities, safety, and to switch off to save power, saving money.

+ Use of power points for charging of or use of appliances for household and self-care activities.

Evaluating Occupational Performance and Identifying Needs

Prior to the home visit, the therapist reviewed Emily's health information and interviewed the treating rehabilitation staff to establish Emily's current physical and functional status.

During the home visit, the therapist interviewed Emily using the COPM to identify her goals and to ascertain her capacity to function in the home. She was observed undertaking transfers, wheeling herself around in her manual wheelchair, and completing various activities in areas such as the entries, garage, master bedroom, en suite bathroom, main bathroom, living room, dining room, laundry, kitchen, and rear patio.

Mobility and Transfers

Emily reported that she uses her manual wheelchair to propel himself short and long distances. She stated that she can negotiate curbs and steep inclines but needed assistance to manage the step in and out of the entries and she was parking her car, with the wheelchair hoist, in front of the garage on the driveway. She struggles to wheel over uneven ground. She could wheel within the home but could not use the facilities due to their lack of access. She reported that she could not use the en suite or laundry and she was struggling to manage in the kitchen and at the entries because of the inaccessible environment. Emily was also observed to transfer in and

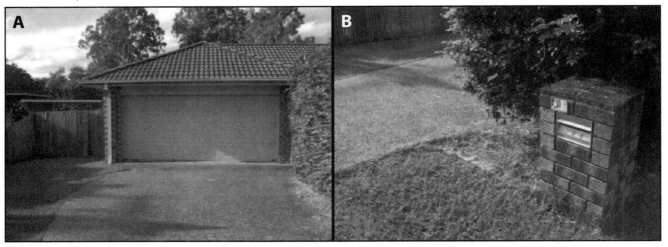

Figure 15-5. Before home modifications. (A) Parking. (B) Mailbox.

out of her wheelchair at the car. She didn't have her mobile shower commode with her at the time of the home visit.

Self-Care and Household Activities

Emily indicated that she could manage some of her self-care activities independently, including dressing, bathing, and basic grooming in an accessible environment. Emily anticipated that she would not be able to move into the home until home modifications could be done to enable her to toilet and shower herself using her equipment; and to make meals for herself and her partner. She stated that she could not access the different areas in the kitchen as it was not accessible. She would have to rely on her partner to prepare the main meals at night when he returned home from work. She would need assistance to complete basic cleaning tasks and rely on her partner to wash up. He would also need to complete heavier tasks such as gardening and doing the laundry. She has a routine of ordering the groceries online and organizing home delivery using the online shopping service, and hoped to do this when in her new home.

Anthropometric Measurements and Equipment

At the first visit, Emily's anthropometric measurements, including her reach range, eye height, and turning circle dimensions, were taken of her in the manual wheelchair.

A second visit was organized to see Emily at the home where she was living while waiting for modifications to be done to the new property. It was at this visit that further anthropometric measurements were taken of Emily while she was seated in her mobile shower commode, and tub transfer bench. This included her reach ranges and eye height while seated on the various pieces of equipment in the bathroom and in the kitchen. The environment was observed and checked against her measurements, to plan the ideal layout for her new home. She was living in a social housing unit that was accessible and discussion occurred about what worked well and what didn't, from a design perspective.

Environmental Issues and Intervention Options

Various environmental issues and intervention options were discussed during the initial walk-through of the home with Emily at the time of the first visit.

Car Parking Under Cover

The home had a driveway leading to a double garage (Figure 15-5). Emily required a covered area in which to park her vehicle which was a car with space behind the driver's side to place her wheelchair. Emily indicated that she intended to get a van in the future, to reduce the strain on her shoulders of lifting her wheelchair frame and wheels in and out of her current car. She has shoulder injuries from overuse and strain on the muscles and ligaments.

The underside of the panel lift roller door on the garage measured 2,100 mm above finished floor level. While she was not clear on the type of van she was going to purchase, discussion occurred about the problem with some vans not fitting under this height garage door. Further, the ceiling height had the potential to limit the lifting of a rear door on the van if a van reversed into the garage. The header above the door opening could not be lifted as it is the main support beam for the roof and the door could not be raised due to the length of the runners and the size of the panels on the opening.

The solution chosen included the provision of a carport at the front of the garage with access to the front entry that would ensure Emily had some degree of protection in all weather conditions when transferring in and out of her car (Figure 15-6). An additional piece of concrete was needed to the side of the carport closest to the front entry so that the van or car could park on the front door side of the carport if there is a second vehicle parked underneath. She required a sensor light to provide illumination to the area in all weather conditions or at night for safety.

Access to the Mailbox

Emily could wheel to the mailbox but had to wheel on grass to access this area. The mailbox had a rear opening door and a garden bed has been planted directly behind the area. She could not reach into the current mailbox without displacing her center of balance and placing undue stress on her shoulders. She holds onto one wheel with one hand when reaching with the other to maintain her trunk stability.

The solution chosen included the provision of a concrete slab that was next to the driveway to ensure she could remain on a firm level surface when getting the mail.

Wheelchair Access Into the Home

Level Access and Ramp to Front Door

There is a small step at the front door that Emily had difficulty negotiating in her manual wheelchair (Figure 15-7). She also experienced shoulder pain when having to reach high to access the door handle and lock with both upper limbs. There were also two doors that she needs to manage on entry and exit— a swing security screen door and a main door.

A portable ramp was considered; however, this would mean Emily would have had to sit on a slope to manage the doors on entry and exit.

The provision of the ramp and landing, a level entry with a combined main door and security screen door as one door, and locks and handles within her reach range, were chosen as solutions to ensure she can wheel onto a level platform to open one door and wheel into the home without fear of displacing her center of balance, and falling out of the wheelchair (Figure 15-8). She could also carry items on her lap without them falling off as she had

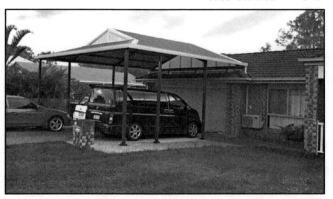

Figure 15-6. After home modifications—parking and mailbox.

an easier area to negotiate and a flat area to sit on at the door.

Level Access and Ramp to Garage Door

There was a step at the doorway leading from the kitchen into the garage. One option considered included the use of a portable ramp but Emily would have had to sit on a slope to manage the doors on entry and exit. She would not be sitting on the level, which is the safest position for door access while reaching forward to access door handles.

She was provided with a ramp and landing that included a level access entry to ensure she could wheel onto a level platform to open one door and wheel into the home without fear of displacing her center of balance and falling out of the wheelchair. She could then carry items on her lap without them falling off as she will have an easier area to negotiate and a flat area to sit on at the door.

Small Threshold Ramp to Rear Patio

Emily requested access through the sliding glass door out onto the covered rear patio as she wanted to have meals outdoors, hang washing undercover, complete gardening activities in the shade and entertain in this area (Figure 15-9). Options considered included the use of a portable ramp or a landing and ramp. The portable ramp would not allow easy and safe access for Emily as she would still need to open and close the security screen door and the sliding glass door. Further, she would have to negotiate the still at the top of the ramp and this is potentially very unsafe. A landing that leads to the rear door and it level with the sill height, and ramp leading off this landing, was considered a viable option but it would take up a significant amount of space on the rear patio, providing limited options with respect to placement of furniture and direction of travel for approach to the door opening.

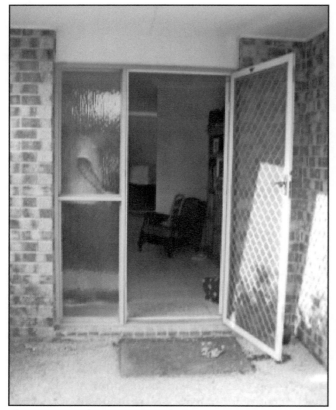

Figure 15-7. Before home modifications—front door.

A small threshold ramp was installed on the inside of the sliding glass door sill to provide access from inside the home, onto a false timber floor that is level with the top of the sill and provides level access at the rear of the home (Figure 15-10). The false timber floor was installed over the rear patio. This level floor provides flexibility and space to fit furniture and for wheelchair approach to the doorway. It is also a very safe option as Emily could sit on the level at the doorway.

Safe Flooring

Emily requested the removal of the carpet in the bedrooms and the installation of floating timber flooring. Options considered included the client not using the bedrooms or leaving the flooring in place but risking further damage to her shoulders. The client indicated that she wanted to use the bedrooms as she will use at least one area as a study space for her higher education courses and the others will accommodate children in the future.

The carpet flooring was worn and had a "pull effect" on equipment being used by Emily and her caregivers. It was replaced with floating timber flooring as requested

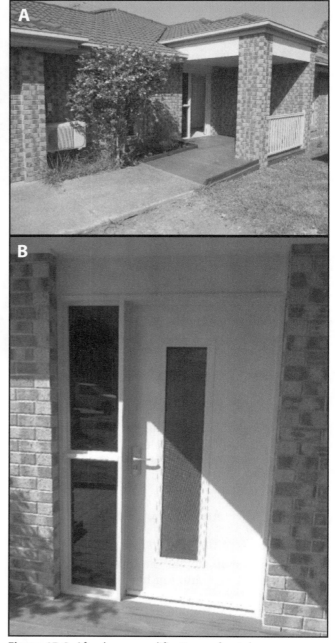

Figure 15-8. After home modifications—front door

Wheelchair Access to Bedroom and En Suite Bathroom

The master bedroom had an inaccessible en suite containing a shower, vanity, and toilet area. This is located next to the walk-in wardrobe (Figure 15-11). There is a second bedroom located on the other side of the en suite that is accessed off a short hallway.

Emily stated that she would like to do her self-care activities in an accessible bathroom on her mobile shower commode and then move into an area that

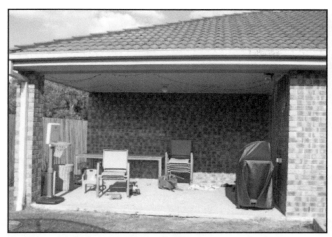

Figure 15-9. Before home modifications—rear patio.

can fit a plinth for her to do her dressing. She also needed a cupboard within the bathroom to store her toiletries and equipment for her colostomy.

Ideas discussed included combining the main bathroom with the toilet area and creating a wheelchair accessible bathroom. Discussion occurred about placing the shower, toilet and vanity in their current positions and providing ramped access rather than level access into the area to keep the cost of the works low. The client requested a doorway through the adjacent laundry wall into the adjacent bedroom rather than her needing to wheel along the hallway to a bedroom to change on the plinth. The modification of the laundry would have resulted in the need to remove the linen cupboard. This option was discounted as it would not provide a cost-effective option compared to the final option.

The solution chosen was that the master bedroom en suite bathroom be renovated to create a wheelchair accessible area suitable for wheelchair and mobile shower commode access (Figure 15-12). This area could accommodate a wheelchair accessible shower, vanity, and toilet with a storage cupboard with above bench door and under bench drawers. A wardrobe was installed, opening into the bedroom, to retain some storage and this is to have open shelving, a pull-down clothes rack and sliding doors with mirrors on a low-profile sill. A second opening was created from the en suite into the second bedroom that is to fit the plinth and another storage cupboard with sliding mirrored doors and height adjustable shelving (Figure 15-13). The flooring was changed from carpet in the second bedroom, to floating timber, for ease of wheeling and to sustain wear and tear over time.

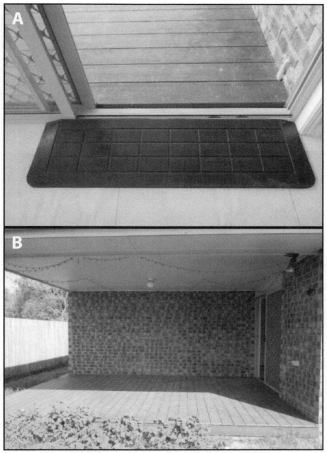

Figure 15-10. After home modifications—rear patio.

Enhanced Space and Design of the Kitchen

The kitchen had a standard layout and did not provide wheelchair accessible features (Figure 15-14). It had benches that were high with limited space between the two sets of parallel benches. There were doors with cupboards, and some drawers, a below bench oven (below the hotplates) and below bench dishwasher. There was a deep double bowl sink and large high corner pantry with narrow door entry. The door leading to the garage was positioned between the two benches, resulting in a lack of continuous bench space.

Ideas considered but discounted included the partial modification of the kitchen to include a breakfast bar with power points for appliances, such as a convection microwave oven; lower area for a sink but leaving the section with the below bench over and hotplates, and the client using her own microwave convection oven only. A second idea included non-use of the kitchen but reliance on her partner and caregivers, and possible preparation of cold foods only at the kitchen table. Both options were not

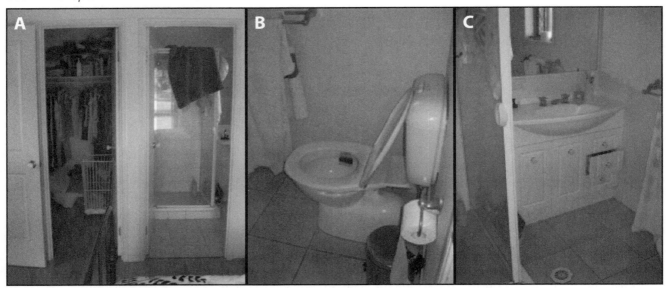

Figure 15-11. Before home modifications—master bedroom wardrobe and en suite area

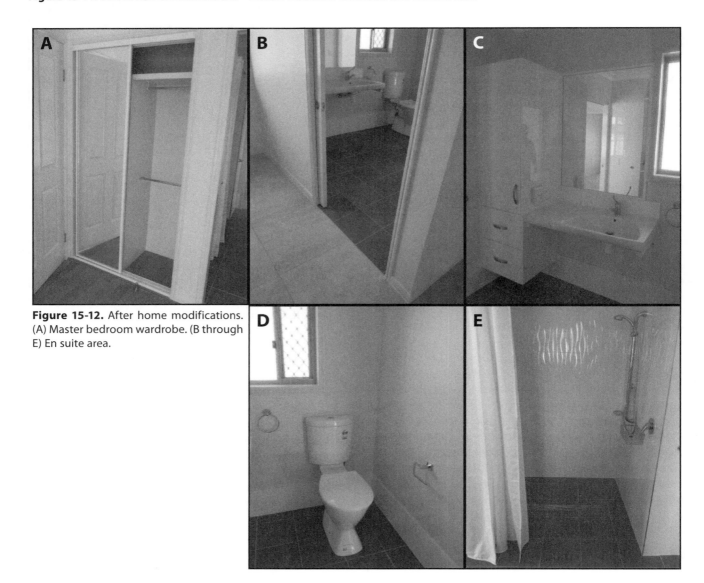

Figure 15-12. After home modifications. (A) Master bedroom wardrobe. (B through E) En suite area.

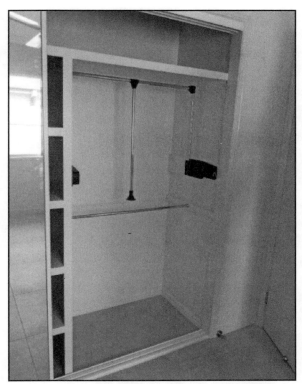

Figure 15-13. After home modifications—second bedroom wardrobe.

considered suitable as the client wanted to be fully independent and capable of accessing all areas of the kitchen.

The kitchen was remodeled (Figure 15-15) to include wheelchair accessible features such as:

✦ Lower benches with wheel under access under the sink and hotplates, with the option to put the doors, mid and bottom shelves in to retain storage as needed; clearance for wheel under access

✦ Wall oven with side opening door and adjacent level hotplates and range hood above; pull out shelf with steel finish on the surface and pot drawer underneath

✦ Dishwasher—drawers style

✦ Shallow double bowl sink with drainer; lever tap with long lever handle and movable spout; central drain; insulation on the underside

✦ Pantry with doors above bench and drawers below bench; height adjustable shelving above bench behind the doors

✦ D-shaped handles on cupboard doors and drawers

✦ High and deep toe recess

✦ Drawers on easy glide runners with stops

✦ Doors to have 180-degree hinges

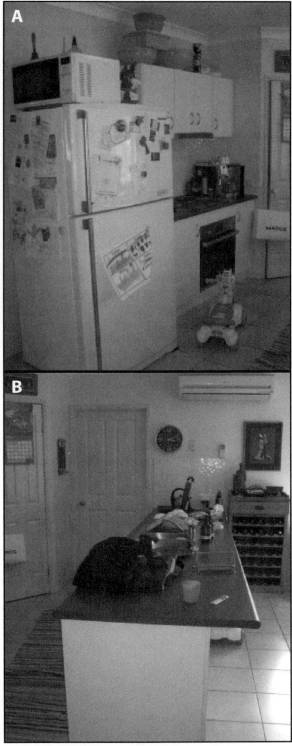

Figure 15-14. Before home modifications—kitchen area.

✦ Space for a refrigerator (door is hinged on the right when facing)

✦ Breakfast bar with wheel under access

✦ Bench space for microwave, kettle

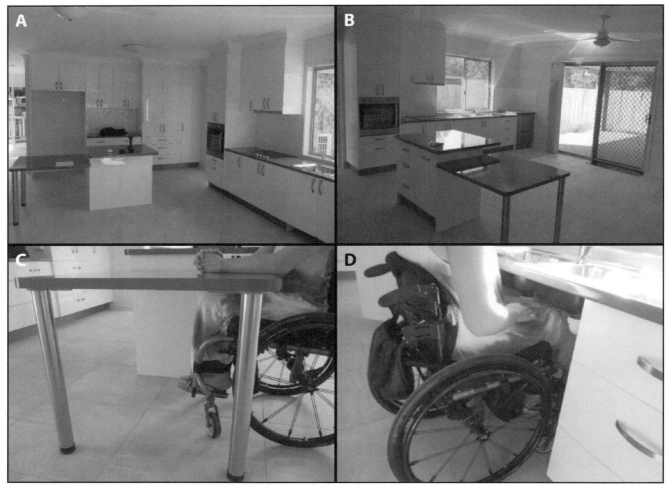

Figure 15-15. After home modifications—kitchen area.

The previously mentioned features aimed to prevent overreach and displacement of the client's center of balance. The design has continuous benches to ensure the client can prepare hot food or liquids in specific areas without needing to place items on her lap when moving between appliances. The well-designed kitchen also enabled her to rely less on caregivers to assist during her routine.

Relocation of Laundry Area

The laundry that is located off the hallway adjacent to the main toilet and main bathroom was not accessible due to the small room size (Figure 15-16). The clothesline was located on the side of the home and was accessed via the laundry door with a step onto the grass. There was no path to the clothesline.

One option considered included not modifying the laundry and the client relying on the caregiver to do all laundry activities. This would involve an ongoing cost relating to funding caregiver hours rather than the client doing some of these activities.

Emily stated that she wanted the laundry installed in the garage rather than undertaking expensive modifications to the existing laundry that is not accessible. The laundry was relocated to the garage and the existing paraline was relocated to the external garage wall in the backyard for ease of access (Figures 15-17 through 15-19). Emily could then wheel through the door at the end of the garage, out onto the concrete slab that sits under the clothesline. The relocation of the laundry and the clothesline provided easier access with fewer obstacles.

Modified Height of Electrical Fittings

The power points and light switches throughout the home needed to be altered and placed in a different location for ease of reach by the client. The light switches were high, and the power points were low– out of comfortable reach from the wheelchair. One option considered include relying on others to operate the switches or not using the switches, but Emily wanted to be independent managing these

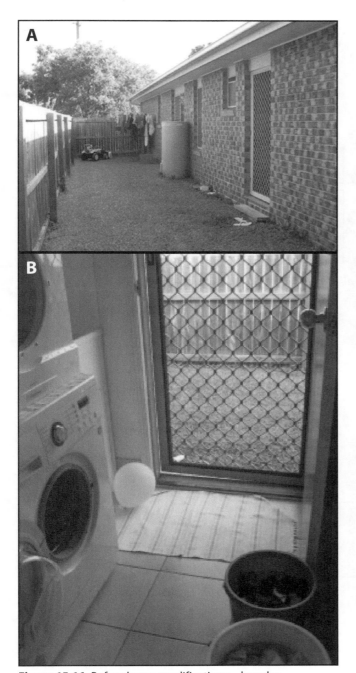

Figure 15-16. Before home modifications—laundry.

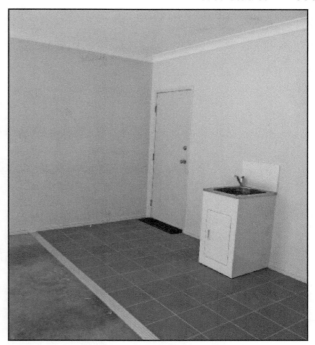

Figure 15-17. After home modifications—laundry.

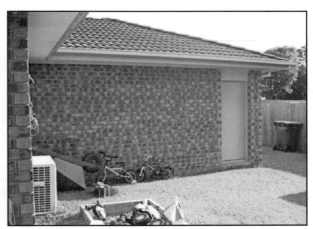

Figure 15-18. Before home modifications—adjacent to rear patio at rear of garage.

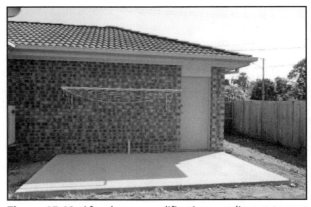

Figure 15-19. After home modifications—adjacent to rear patio, new clothesline area.

fittings. She was using two hands to plug items into power points, depending on their height and this results in her being unsteady with her balance. She also experienced weakness in the upper limbs on occasions, which made putting plugs in and out difficult at times.

The electrical fittings were modified in relation to height to allow Emily to manage her reach with greater safety and ease and to ensure she did not have to rely on others to operate the switches.

Figure 15-20. After home modifications—diagram of layout of home with modified areas (not to scale).

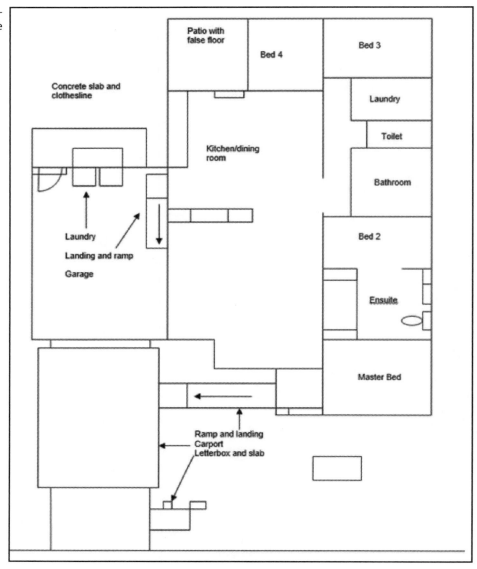

Additional Factors Considered for Final Home Modification Solution

Funding for the home modifications had become available through an insurance claim and, though limited, it was allocated based on her housing needs for the rest of her life. Emily was conscious of the need to have modifications that were considered "reasonable and necessary" in accordance with the requirements of the insurance company, but were of good quality to ensure they lasted for many years without the need for ongoing expenditure of her insurance funds on maintenance and repair.

The choice of materials was considered. For example, an external timber ramp and timber patio was selected because it was considered a reasonable cost compared with hiring a portable ramp

for the short- to medium-term for use at front and rear entries. The timber ramp and patio areas also matched the look of the home and did not appear out of place in the design of the property. Anthropometric and equipment measurements were considered in planning clearances and circulation space and for positioning fittings and fixtures in all areas of the home.

The technical advisor provided samples of products and finishes and sketched preliminary designs to be discussed with Emily and her partner. After concluding the home visit, the therapist and builder, over a period of several weeks, developed design options for the her to consider. The therapist visited the home for a third time to show Emily a finalized concept option (Figure 15-20) and to trial the layouts drawn. This option was finalized, and the final

Table 15-2. Emily's Canadian Occupational Performance Measure Rating

Performance: 1 = Not able to do it at all; 10 = Able to do extremely well					
Satisfaction: 1 = Not satisfied at all; 10 = Extremely satisfied					
OCCUPATIONAL PERFORMANCE PROBLEMS	*IMPORTANCE*	*PERFORMANCE T1*	*SATISFACTION T1*	*PERFORMANCE T2*	*SATISFACTION T2*
1 Unable to independently access the home	10	5	1	9	10
2 Difficulty completing self-care	10	1	1	8	10
3 Difficulty completing household tasks	10	4	1	9	10
4					
5					
		Total Performance T1	Total Satisfaction T1	Total Performance T2	Total Satisfaction T2
Total Scores		10	3	26	30
		Average Performance T1	Average Satisfaction T1	Average Performance T2	Average Satisfaction T2
Average Scores		3.3	1	8.6	10
				Change in Performance	Change in Satisfaction
Change in Scores (T2 – T1)				5.3	9

therapy report, including the builder's plans and specifications, was forwarded to Emily to approve.

Outcomes

Quotes were obtained from builder who was engaged by the insurance company, to assist the client and occupational therapist plan the home modifications. The modifications were installed, and the therapist visited Emily in her home to complete a post modification evaluation. The therapist conducted an interview using the COPM and undertook structured observation of Emily in the various areas of the home. The interview included the review of the original occupational therapy report to determine whether there had been any changes in Emily's capacity to manage the various activities in the home and community. The COPM scores indicated that there had been an improvement in performance and satisfaction in the three general areas of concern (Table 15-2).

The therapist observed that Emily had improved in general health and functional capacity, being able to manage all activities with greater confidence. She could manage accessing all areas of the home that were modified with safety and ease. The home modifications were installed as per the original occupational therapy report. The products and finishes appeared to be coping with wear and tear and were reported to suit the needs of all Emily and her partner.

Since this post modification visit, the therapist has kept in contact with Emily who reported that she continues to make progress with respect to her day to day routines and managing her shoulder pain.

CASE STUDY 3: ELDERLY MAN WITH A NEUROLOGICAL CONDITION

Client Interests and Daily Activities

Bill is an older man aged in his 60s who lives with his wife in a detached house in a quiet suburban area of a regional city. He is a retired builder who enjoys socializing with friends and his children and grandchildren. He enjoyed his work life and continues to have an interest in renovation projects. His wife has been in good health until recently when she was diagnosed with arthritis.

Health Condition and Functional Performance

Bill has inclusion body myositis, an inflammatory condition within the muscle that causes the body's immune system to attack and destroy muscle cells. Myositis is a rare disease that occurs mainly in adults which results in weakening of the thigh, hip, and shoulder muscles, making it difficult to walk distances, particularly up and down stairs; standing up from a chair; rising from the floor; raising the arms above the head; rolling over in bed; lifting the head from the pillow. It can also affect the heart, lungs, swallowing, hands and fingers, and lower legs causing foot drop. Over time there is a reduction in strength, dexterity, and mobility, and in extreme cases the heart and lung muscles may be affected-the impact can be fatal.

Bill was diagnosed with myositis approximately 10 years ago. His lower limbs have been affected more than the upper limbs, and his left side has been affected more than the right side. He has experienced a gradual deterioration in his muscle function and is currently having trouble swallowing. He can flex and extend at the elbows but lacks capacity to do full range of motion at the shoulders and has reduced grip in his hands. He has weakening of the legs which impacts on his capacity to walk and complete transfers. Bill is currently 172 pounds (78 kg) and when standing, he is approximately 6-ft (182-cm) tall. He has lost weight over time.

Bill's past medical history includes having cancer of the bowel at 45 years of age and he had an operation to remove the cancer. He had a fall 2 years ago which resulted in a fracture to the left shoulder. Since this fall, he has had regular falls in the home.

At the time of the first visit, Bill was using a manual wheelchair, with assistance from his wife to propel distances, and over carpet and uneven surfaces, and learning to operate his new powerchair. He had a seat to lift him on and off the toilet but the treating therapist had scripted a mobile shower commode to enable him to be wheeled in and out of the bathroom and on and off the toilet without needing to do multiple transfers. He relied on his wife to assist him with all transfers and she was starting to experience significant back pain. His equipment will continue to change over time as he develops greater functional limitations associated with his health condition.

Location and Description of the House

Bill lives in a slab on ground brick home that has already had modifications completed at the front and rear entries and within the home to provide wheelchair access. There was one step at the front and rear entries that has had platforms and ramps installed to assist his wife push Bill in his manual wheelchair in and out of the home. He has also had a step ramp installed within the home as it is split level between the kitchen and living room area and the dining room and rumpus room. The home is set on a large block of land. There are four bedrooms, a living room, combined dining room and kitchen area, large rear rumpus room, a main bathroom with toilet and a separate toilet located near the kitchen. The flooring consists of carpet in all areas except the kitchen, dining room, toilets, and rear rumpus room where there is tile. Bill has a large shed at the back of the block where he stores his tools. The family have a double garage that store that family car and a boat that Bill had been using for fishing. A beautifully manicured lawn and gardens surround the house. There are no fences at the front of the property but has fencing at the side and rear.

Client Goals

His long-term goals included the following:

+ Setting up the home for floor based hoist transfers

+ To maintain his ability to do as much as possible for himself with respect to self-care and household routines, to enable his wife to have a break and enjoy community activities with her friends

Bill indicated that his short-term goals included the following:

+ Gaining confidence and skill using his newly acquired powerchair

+ Changing his showering routine with his caregivers once his new mobile shower commode arrived

The occupational therapist and Bill and his wife decided to focus on his self-care routine and the need to provide an accessible area for the completion of this routine, as a priority.

Evaluating Occupational Performance and Identifying Needs

A home visit referral requested an occupational therapist visit to make home modification recommendations to ensure that Bill would be able to live in the home with his wife for as long as possible. The referral stated that he was having difficulty managing in the bathroom that was not wheelchair accessible and that he was about to receive a new mobile shower commode that would likely not fit in this area.

Prior to the home visit, the therapist reviewed Bill's health information and interviewed the visiting physiotherapist and nursing staff from a non-government organization to establish Bill's current physical and functional status.

During the home visit, the therapist interviewed Bill and his wife using the COPM to identify their goals and to ascertain Bill's capacity to function in the home. He was observed wheeling himself around in his wheelchair with some assistance from his wife. He did not want to complete any transfers at the time of the visit. He discussed the various tasks he could manage in the bathroom and kitchen, and showed the therapist each of these areas. Bill decided to leave the modification of the kitchen for a later date, indicating that the bathroom was the priority with respect to his home modification requirements.

Mobility and Transfers

Bill stated that he had poor static and dynamic sitting and standing balance. He needs a back support in his wheelchair to maintain his sitting posture. He needed assistance from his wife to be wheeled in his manual wheelchair on carpet, up and down the ramps located around the home, and long distances. He used his feet to self-propel himself in his manual wheelchair on tile floors a short distance in the home. He was learning how to use the powerchair and was worried about managing the controls and driving the equipment within the home.

He reported that although he could manage a pivot transfer on and off the toilet, and the mobile shower commode when hospitalized recently after a fall, he was struggling at home because of the inaccessible environment. He was standing and holding onto horizontal grab rails to side step into the small shower. The shower had the glass doors removed but still had a hob that he had to negotiate, before he could stand or sit on the height adjustable shower chair. He could not sit right under the sink at the vanity bench and he was using the second toilet in the house that was close to the kitchen as it was easier to approach and use. This second toilet had been fitted out with a spring-loaded seat that could lift him into standing. He also had similar seats fitted to the wheelchair and to the dining room chair. He required occasional assistance from his wife to move from sitting to standing such as in the bedroom, when moving on and off the bed. Bill also stated that he was having trouble managing transfers in and out of the car due to the lack of a spring-loaded seat to move him from sitting into standing.

Self-Care and Household Activities

Bill stated that he could manage some of his self-care activities independently, including standing and sitting to shower, dressing, apart from managing zippers and buttons and other activities requiring fine motor control, and basic grooming such as shaving and doing his teeth. He showed the therapist where he was undertaking his self-care routine and explained the steps involved in this process.

He was having difficulty with swallowing and he was relying on his wife to cut up his food. He used a fork and spoon to feed himself independently and he could use a mug and glass.

Bill and his wife used on an online shopping service to order their groceries that were delivered to the home. His wife did the cooking though Bill could make light meals and cups of hot tea when his wife was out. He could do this in the seated position. Bill stated that the counters, oven, and sink areas were inaccessible. He and his wife relied on community services to provide cleaning once per fortnight for one and a half hours. Bill's wife did the laundry tasks and some of the gardening. A local government funded maintenance service visits to do repairs around the home. The couple also received support from their four adult sons who live locally and visit regularly. They assisted with gardening and transport.

Anthropometric Measurements and Equipment

Bill's anthropometric measurements were taken while seated in his manual wheelchair. This included his reach ranges and eye height. The treating therapist was contacted about the brand, size and dimensions of the mobile shower commode that was on order. Discussion also occurred about the need for a hoist and the fit of this equipment in the home in the future.

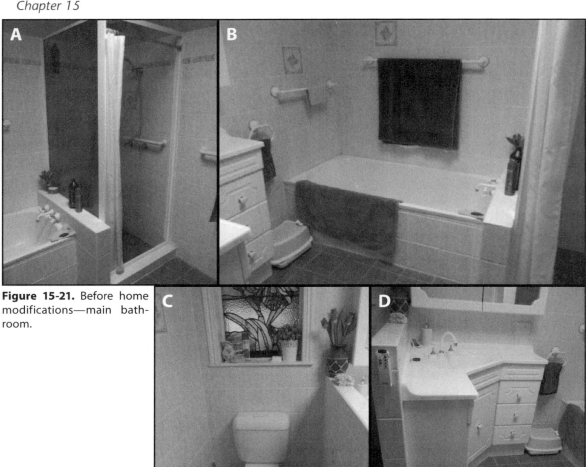

Figure 15-21. Before home modifications—main bathroom.

Environmental Issues and Intervention Options

During the interview and the process of observing Bill in his wheelchair negotiating spaces and environmental features, he and his wife discussed the layout of their existing home and the possible changes required to enable him to manage the built environment with ease. This discussion included the look and the possible cost of various modifications, given Bill's current and future physical and functional status, and the structure of the home. Consideration was also given to the changing nature of his disability over time and his current and future equipment needs.

Various environmental issues and intervention options were discussed during the walk-through of the home with Bill and his wife.

Access Within the Bathroom

Wheelchair Access

Because of the presence of a narrow doorway with a small step at the threshold, the low bath, small shower enclosure, inaccessible vanity, high mirror and storage cupboard, and a step into the bathroom, Bill experienced difficulty in the bathroom (Figure 15-21). He had trouble getting into the bathroom and positioning himself to the side or in front of various features. He could not reach to access the sink, he was not using the toilet within the room, and he has struggling to step over the shower hob. The mobile over-toilet shower chair could not fit in the area or be used in the shower.

Options considered included leaving the features with their current location and design, resulting in Bill having limited use of the facilities, or redesigning

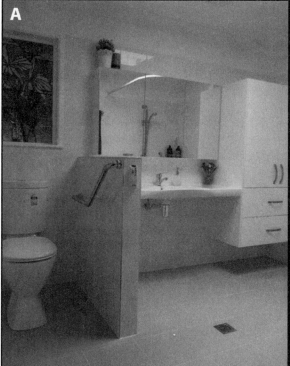

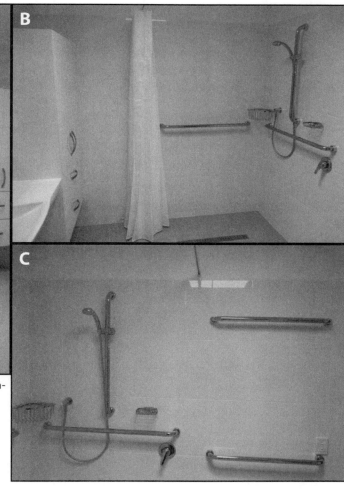

Figure 15-22. After home modifications—main bathroom.

the area to include an accessible vanity, larger and lower mirror to suit the needs of the whole family, an accessible shower, a large waterproof storage cupboard with shelves at various heights and drawers below bench level, and eliminating the step at the entry to the bathroom.

The final recommendation included the redesign of the area to ensure that Bill had better wheelchair access (Figure 15-22). This included the removal of all existing features, bath, and the redesign to include the installation of a wheel-in shower, hand-held shower, lever taps in the shower and sink areas, soap basket and a larger basket for bottles in the shower; a shallow basin set into a vanity counter with storage above and below the counter level; a new mirrored cabinet above the bench, with a power point; new slip-resistant-when-wet flooring with no step at the doorway; and provision of a new accessible toilet suite.

Outcomes

Quotes were obtained from two building firms who specialized in home modification installations (including the builder who visited with the occupational therapist), and a builder was chosen to proceed with the work. The modifications were installed, and the therapist visited Bill and his wife in their home to complete a post modification evaluation. The therapist conducted an interview and structured observation of Bill in the bathroom. The interview included the review of the original occupational therapy report to determine whether there had been any change in Bill's capacity to manage the various activities in this area. The COPM was readministered to determine if there were any changes in the scores because of the home modifications. He rated higher scores for performance and satisfaction post modification, compared to pre-modification (Table 15-3). He was still concerned that he continued to need his wife's assistance during his self-care routine but this was due to his limited reach range.

Table 15-3. Bill's Canadian Occupational Performance Measure Rating

| Performance: 1 = Not able to do it at all; 10 = Able to do extremely well | | | | | |
| Satisfaction: 1 = Not satisfied at all; 10 = Extremely satisfied | | | | | |
OCCUPATIONAL PERFORMANCE PROBLEMS	IMPORTANCE	PERFORMANCE T1	SATISFACTION T1	PERFORMANCE T2	SATISFACTION T2
1 Unable to independently access the home	9	3	2	10	10
2 Difficulty completing self-care	9	2	3	8	8
3					
4					
5					
		Total Performance T1	Total Satisfaction T1	Total Performance T2	Total Satisfaction T2
Total Scores		5	5	18	18
		Average Performance T1	Average Satisfaction T1	Average Performance T2	Average Satisfaction T2
Average Scores		2.5	2.5	9	9
				Change in Performance	Change in Satisfaction
Change in Scores (T2 – T1)				6.5	6.5

The therapist observed that he could move into the bathroom and access the different features with confidence in his manual wheelchair. He reported that he had driven the powered wheelchair into the room and was able to maneuver around and access each area. He had not received his mobile shower commode at the time of the last visit but was hopeful the environment would suit the equipment. The home modifications were installed as per the original occupational therapy report. The products and finishes appeared to be coping with wear and tear and were reported to suit the needs of both Bill and his wife.

Since this post modification visit, the therapist has kept in contact with family members who report that Bill now needs paid caregivers to assist him with his routine. They have given Bill feedback to indicate that they loved the layout, and how easy his self-care routine is to manage in the accessible environment. He has also received the mobile shower commode and this fits over the toilet, under the vanity sink, and in the shower.

CASE STUDY 4: TWO MEN WITH INTELLECTUAL AND PHYSICAL DISABILITIES SHARING A HOME

Client Interests and Daily Activities

Tony and Dean are 31-year-old men who have lived together in a house with 24-hour support for the past 11 years. Prior to living together, the two men lived with three other people in a shared housing arrangement in the same city suburb. They receive an additional 5 hours of support funding to enable them to access the community.

Tony enjoys going to the local park and the beach. His family members live on the opposite side of the city from him, but they visit monthly. Tony's mother assists him as his informal decision maker in relation to lifestyle and financial matters.

Dean enjoys drives in the country and visiting his family. His family members live locally, and he sees them on a regular basis. Dean's father acts as Dean's informal decision maker on matters relating to his lifestyle. A government service acts as the administrator of finances for Dean.

Both clients rely on support staff to drive them to facilities in the community.

Health Condition and Functional Performance

Both men have an intellectual disability. Tony has:

+ Epilepsy, controlled by medication

+ Urinary incontinence, particularly at night

+ Flexion deformity of the spine (a significant static scoliosis)

+ Internal rotation of hips secondary to cerebral palsy

Tony tends to be impulsive and likes to climb fences or benches and grab at items during meal preparation and other activities in the home. He has had a history of falls both inside and outside of the home, and he has damaged the walls inside of the home by chipping away at the sheeting. He also tends to fiddle with taps if left alone in the bathroom and has been known to drink the hot tap water from the bath spout when bathing unsupervised.

Dean has:

+ Autism

+ Temporal lobe epilepsy, controlled by medication

+ Occasional incontinence

He demonstrated difficulty with fine motor control in the upper limbs.

Over the long term, both clients might require more equipment as they age. This could include a mobile shower commode, particularly to suit Tony's needs.

Location and Description of the House

The two men live in a standard three-bedroom brick home that is slab on ground (one step into the property) in a quiet city suburban area. There are detached houses located on either side of the property, in close proximity. Their house was purchased specifically for Tony and Dean, and it is typical of other detached houses in their city suburb. It has not been built specifically for people who use mobility equipment, such as wheelchairs.

The garage is located at the front of the property, and the front entry is at the side of the home. This entry is accessed by a path that has gardens planted on either side. There is a step at the front door. The spacious backyard is enclosed by a 3-ft (1,000-mm) high timber fence. The rear yard contains a rotary clothesline. The rear entry includes a sliding glass door that leads in from a covered patio area. There is a step up into the house from this area.

The three bedrooms are located at the front of the dwelling. The kitchen is U-shaped and located to the side of the combined kitchen and living room area at the rear of the home. The laundry is located at the side of the home. The bathroom is separate from the toilet, and both areas are located along a hallway toward the front of the home. The bathroom includes a bath, vanity bench, and shower with a shallow tray floor. The home is carpeted throughout the living room, dining room, hallway, and bedrooms. The bathroom and laundry are tiled, and the kitchen area has vinyl flooring.

Client Goals

When Tony and Dean moved into their new home, their long-term goals, established with their parents as informal decision makers and staff helpers, were to enable them to:

+ Become familiar with the neighborhood and its residents

+ Participate in local community activities

+ They also wanted to have home modifications that would accommodate the changing activity and access and mobility requirements of the two men, and their caregivers, as they aged.

Their short-term goals included:

+ Establishing a familiar routine of daily activities with staff in their new home

+ Managing the new environment during these daily activities

At the time of interview, the men had established their routine of household activities, undertaking their self-care routines in the morning and hobbies or resting at the house during the day. They also had a well-established routine for participating in activities in the community on a regular basis. Some features in the home were presenting as barriers to Tony and Dean.

Evaluating Occupational Performance and Identifying Needs

A home visit referral requested home modification recommendations to ensure that Tony and Dean would be able to use the bathroom and other areas of the home with greater safety.

Prior to the home visit, the therapist reviewed the medical information available to establish Tony and Dean's functional statuses prior to being housed and their current abilities.

During the home visit, the therapist interviewed staff and family representatives using the COPM to identify the goals that they felt were important for the men to achieve within the home and to ascertain their capacity to manage safely in the home. The therapist also observed the two men as they moved around the various areas of the home and interacted with staff and visitors.

Mobility and Transfers

Tony was observed to walk short distances independently; staff reported that he relied on the use of an attendant-propelled manual wheelchair to manage long distances, particularly outdoors. He demonstrated that he could manage transfers on and off the bed, a chair, and the toilet by himself without assistance. He was reported to have had falls in the past, both indoors and outdoors, because of his unsteady gait and tripping over uneven surfaces or small steps. He frequently moved from standing to sitting on the floor during the visit, and staff helped him to move up from the floor into the standing position. Despite such mobility difficulties, he could scale the rear fence.

Dean was observed to have difficulty managing transfers in and out of the bath and shower because of his reduced balance. He, too, was tripping in areas where there were small changes in floor levels. Staff provided physical assistance during these activities.

Self-Care and Household Activities

Staff reported that both men relied on them for assistance during self-care activities. During dressing activities, Tony requires full assistance, whereas Dean relies on verbal prompting. Staff indicated that they wanted to leave the men unsupervised during some activities to ensure that they maintained their dignity and to enhance their independence. This has resulted in Tony damaging the built environment or injuring himself through fiddling with the taps, drinking the scalding hot water, and hitting the toilet cistern with his back. Tony's urinary incontinence resulted in ongoing spillage on the carpet in his bedroom, which was creating an unhealthy environment.

Staff also reported that they complete all household tasks for the two men, because they are not able to participate safely in these activities. They indicated that they have been experiencing difficulty managing the two men when preparing meals because Tony and Dean tend to interrupt the activities by grabbing at the various cooking items and accessing the kitchen cupboards. This is of concern to the staff, who indicated that only one member of their team works in the household at any one time.

Anthropometric Measurements and Equipment

Tony and Dean's physical stature and reach ranges were reviewed as well as the wheelchair that Tony uses. There was no need to take measurements of the wheelchair because it is not being used indoors at present. Thought was given to the future use of a mobile over-toilet shower chair in the bathroom, and measurements for this equipment were considered when planning various modifications.

Environmental Issues and Intervention Options

External Access

Safe Fenced Area

Tony could scale the 39.25-in (1,000-mm) high fence easily. Options discussed included increasing the current level of supervision while the men were using the yard or changing the style of fence to ensure that if Tony attempted to climb the structure, he would be slowed down by its height and style of construction. Extra funding from the support service was not available to provide more hours of support staff supervision. The final recommendation included the construction of a 70.75-in (1,800-mm) high fence that had no gaps in the palings or horizontal support beams on the inside of the fence that would act as footholds.

Safe Surface on the Rear Concrete Patio

Staff reported that Tony was having falls on the rear concrete patio and injuring himself. Options discussed included limiting the time Tony spent outdoors, restricting his access to the rear patio, laying carpet, or installing a more permanent outdoor ground cover that was cushioned. The final recommendation included installing the cushioned cover, which was funded by Tony's family. This was considered the best option rather than restricting Tony's use of the area and laying carpet that would not suit the outdoor conditions.

Internal Access

Easy-to-Grasp Door Handles

Dean was experiencing difficulty using the door handles and accessing the various areas of the home. The main recommendation considered was removing the existing door handles and replacing them with lever handles. This modification would enhance Dean's level of independence in the home.

Durable and Safe Flooring

Tony had urinary incontinence, and the ongoing spillage on the carpet in his bedroom was creating an unhealthy environment. The options considered included trialing medication with him, new continence products to be worn under his clothes, and removing the existing carpet and replacing it with a vinyl that was slip-resistant-when-wet and did not absorb the spillages so readily. All three options were recommended to enhance Tony's current health status and to ensure a clean environment for him and others in the household. Vinyl in other areas of the home, such as the kitchen and hallway, had holes and were slippery when wet. It was recommended that these areas be laid with new vinyl that was also slip-resistant-when-wet.

Safe Access to the Outdoors

Tony was having difficulty stepping over the sill of the rear sliding glass door and down onto the patio unsupported. Staff reported that he had fallen on this patio. Options considered included restricting Tony's access to the rear patio, allowing him access only with staff supervision, installing a grab rail on the inside and outside of the door wall for him to hold onto when stepping in and out of the area, and raising the level of the outside patio to the level of the sill. Restricting Tony's access to the outdoor area was considered inappropriate, because it did not encourage ongoing independence and monitoring and helping Tony was time consuming for staff. Raising the level of the outside patio was considered too costly. The recommended option included installing grab bars on either side of the door entry to encourage the client to manage this area with greater safety and independence.

Kitchen

Switch Control Safety at the Stove

Both men tended to fiddle with switches. It was recommended that the stove be connected to an isolation switch that allowed it to be deactivated. This switch needed to be in an inaccessible area.

This modification was recommended to enhance the men's safety in the kitchen area.

Easy-to-Use Tap Handles

Dean was having trouble managing the taps in the various areas of the home. The main option considered was to remove the existing tap handles and replace them with short lever handles. This was recommended to enhance Dean's current level of independence in the home.

Fixed Kitchen Sink Spout

The spout over the kitchen sink tended to rotate and hit the splash back and spray water onto the counter and over the drainage area when turned by the men, who enjoy the activity. The recommendation made by the therapist included installing a fixed spout to direct the water flow into the sink.

Bathroom and Toilet

Circulation Space in the Bathroom and Toilet Areas for Future Wheelchair Access

The separation of the two areas did not allow future ease of access to a mobile over-toilet shower chair. It was also perceived to be undignified to be wheeled between the two rooms during their self-care routines. Further, the men appeared agitated when in the bathroom, and there was little space to move between the shower, bath and vanity, and caregivers. Options considered included leaving the current layout and relocating the men to another home in the future or combining the toilet and bathroom into one room to create more space. Relocating the men was considered disruptive and costly, and there might not be a suitable home available in the short or medium term. Combining the two rooms was recommended, because it was a home modification that could be done quickly and address immediate behavioral concerns.

Safe Flooring in Bathroom and Toilet Areas

The men and the caregivers alike experienced difficulty negotiating the flooring in the toilet and bathroom because it was not slip-resistant-when-wet. Options included either applying a slip-resistant coating or etching to the floor or replacing the existing floor covering with a better-quality product. The preferred option was to remove the existing flooring and replace it with a product that was slip-resistant in wet areas, as indicated in the access standards. The etching or coating of the floor would need ongoing maintenance over time; and the finish might ruin the look of the existing tiles and not provide as much grip.

Level Access Into the New Bathroom

There is a small step leading into the toilet and bathroom areas, which the men were tending to trip over. It was determined that this could be eliminated by combining the bathroom and toilet into one area rather than installing a small ramp, ensuring that the entry had a neat, level finish. The presence of a small ramp intruding into the hallway could still create a trip hazard.

Grab Rails for Transfers on and off the Toilet or in and out of the Shower Recess

Options included the men using a toilet surround frame or over-toilet frame in the toilet area and shower chair in the shower or the use of a drop-down shower seat in the shower combined with the installation of grab bars. The use of freestanding equipment was discounted, being considered less stable and safe than the grab bars and a drop-down shower seat as permanent fixtures.

Safe Style of Toilet Roll Holder

The current toilet roll holder protruded from the wall and was a hazard, particularly if the men had falls in the toilet area. Options considered included removing this feature completely or installing a semi-recessed toilet roll holder. The final recommendation included installing the semi-recessed toilet roll holder to enhance the men's safety, especially in the event of a fall in the area.

Safe Style of Soap Holder

The soap holder in the shower recess protruded and could cause an injury if one of the men fell in this area. Options considered included removing of this feature completely or installing a semi-recessed soap holder. The final recommendation included installing the semi-recessed soap holder to enhance the men's safety, especially in the event of a fall in the area.

Presence of Grab Bars

The men tended to lean heavily on the towel rails on the bathroom wall. They are not designed to take the weight of a person and are a hazard. Options considered included removing the rails completely or installing grab bars that could act as towel rails and support the clients as they completed their self-care routine. The final recommendation included installing grab bars to enhance the men's safety, especially in the event of a fall in the area.

Robust Toilet Cistern and Toilet Seat

The toilet cistern and toilet seat were broken repeatedly by the rocking motion of Tony when he was seated on the toilet. Options included applying rubber foam on the existing cistern or removing the existing cistern and pan and installing an in-wall concealed cistern and new heavy-duty pan.

Various options were considered, including implementing various behavior modification strategies and the partial modification and full modification of the bathroom and toilet areas. Given the future access requirements of the men and the time taken and varying success of the behavior modification strategies, it was recommended that the bathroom be redesigned to include the toilet area and to enable full wheelchair access. It was also proposed that the toilet be removed and replaced with a concealed cistern and a heavy-duty bowl that matched the color of the rest of the room.

Bedrooms

Easy-to-Grasp Wardrobe Handles

Dean was having trouble managing the wardrobe handles in the various areas of the home. The main option considered included removing the existing wardrobe handles and installing D-shaped handles. This was recommended to enhance Dean's current level of independence in the home.

Electrical

Larger Light Switches

Dean was having trouble managing the small light switches in the various areas of the home. The main option considered included removing the existing small light switches and installing large rocker switches. This was recommended to enhance Dean's current level of independence in the home.

Other

Water Temperature Control

Options considered included staff providing constant supervision of the men around water or providing a thermostatic control device. The latter option was recommended to ensure the safety of the two men at all times, regardless of the level of supervision they were receiving around water.

Table 15-4. Tony's Canadian Occupational Performance Measure Rating

Performance: 1 = Not able to do it at all; 10 = Able to do extremely well					
Satisfaction: 1 = Not satisfied at all; 10 = Extremely satisfied					
OCCUPATIONAL PERFORMANCE PROBLEMS	IMPORTANCE	PERFORMANCE T1	SATISFACTION T1	PERFORMANCE T2	SATISFACTION T2
1 Difficulty using rear yard, patio, and entries with safety	10	3	2	8	9
2 Lack of safety when using switches	10	1	2	8	8
3 Poor hygienic area within bedroom	10	1	2	10	8
4 Safety at toilet area	10	4	3	8	9
5 Difficulty completing self-care routine	10	4	2	8	9
		Total Performance T1	Total Satisfaction T1	Total Performance T2	Total Satisfaction T2
Total Scores		13	11	42	43
		Average Performance T1	Average Satisfaction T1	Average Performance T2	Average Satisfaction T2
Average Scores		2.6	2.2	8.4	8.6
				Change in Performance	Change in Satisfaction
Change in Scores (T2 – T1)				5.8	6.4

Outcomes

Quotes were obtained from three building firms that specialize in home modification installations, and a builder was chosen to proceed with the work. The modifications were installed over a period of several weeks, and the therapist visited the two men in their home to complete a post modification evaluation. Staff members were interviewed, and structured observation of the two men in the various areas of the home was conducted. The interview included the review of the original occupational therapy report to determine whether there had been any changes in the clients' capacities to manage the various activities in the home and community.

Feedback from support staff indicated that both clients had learned to manage their self-care routines with assistance in the modified bathroom. They reported that both men were not as agitated in the bathroom area, possibly because the combined bathroom and toilet provided greater space for movement and activities with the caregivers. The combined bathroom and toilet area had fewer fittings and fixtures that is, the bath was removed, and the shower cubicle opened to become wheelchair accessible, and there was greater light in the area.

Other outcomes included the clients experiencing fewer falls at the doorways and greater independence managing doors, taps, and light switches.

The COPM was reviewed (Tables 15-4 and 15-5) and scored with input from the clients' family and the support staff and there was a noticeable difference in scores for both men regarding their performance and satisfaction with tasks.

The home modifications were installed per the original occupational therapy report. The products and finishes appeared to be coping with wear and tear and were reported to suit the needs of the two men.

Table 15-5. Dean's Canadian Occupational Performance Measure Rating

| Performance: 1 = Not able to do it at all; 10 = Able to do extremely well | | | | | |
| Satisfaction: 1 = Not satisfied at all; 10 = Extremely satisfied | | | | | |
OCCUPATIONAL PERFORMANCE PROBLEMS	IMPORTANCE	PERFORMANCE T1	SATISFACTION T1	PERFORMANCE T2	SATISFACTION T2
1 Difficulty accessing door handles	10	1	2	9	9
2 Lack of safety when using switches	10	1	2	8	9
3 Difficulty completing self-care routine	10	3	2	8	8
4 Difficulty managing taps and spout	10	2	2	7	8
5					
		Total Performance T1	Total Satisfaction T1	Total Performance T2	Total Satisfaction T2
Total Scores		7	8	32	34
		Average Performance T1	Average Satisfaction T1	Average Performance T2	Average Satisfaction T2
Average Scores		1.7	2	8	8.5
				Change in Performance	Change in Satisfaction
Change in Scores (T2 – T1)				6.3	6.5

CASE STUDY 5: AN ELDERLY WOMAN WITH A VISION IMPAIRMENT

Client Interests and Daily Activities

Olive is a 69-year-old woman who lives alone in a one-bedroom ground-floor apartment in a beachside suburb of a regional city. Olive has a daughter, living approximately 2 miles (4 km) away, who assists as necessary with some transport and general support. Olive walks along the beach promenade using a long white cane and often uses the bus to return home. When accessing the shopping precinct, she uses local council-subsidized taxicabs or the cab-charge subsidy vouchers supported by the state government. Twice monthly, Olive has access to a community transport service to attend medical appointments anywhere in the city. She states that she goes to the movies twice per month using public transport.

Olive likes to maintain her apartment independently as much as she is able, doing her own cooking, light household cleaning, and laundry tasks. She spends most of the time in her bedroom, especially in the winter months, because this room receives the most sunlight, which helps her limited sight and minimizes heating costs. In the evenings, she watches television in the lounge room. She has a large-screen television, which compensates for her limited sight.

Health Condition and Functional Performance

In 2005, Olive was traveling in California when she had a cerebral hemorrhage. She was hospitalized in Los Angeles for 2 months, and her family was advised that she was critically ill. However, she recovered to be well enough to be flown back home to begin rehabilitation. Prior to this event, Olive experienced good health.

Because of the cerebral hemorrhage, Olive has significant visual field loss, with vision in the upper left quadrant only, but has enough vision not to be declared legally blind. To be legally blind, a person must have visual acuity of 20/200 or less or a visual field of 20 degrees or less. Wearing glasses will not improve Olive's vision.

Physically, Olive recovered well, experiencing some balance problems when she moves quickly, which may be more related to the vision loss, and having a slow deliberate speech pattern. Olive showed no significant cognitive impairment. Other than the white cane to assist mobility, it is anticipated she would not need any other equipment in the future.

During her rehabilitation, Olive was taught how to adapt to her limited visual field by moving her head to scan the environment to avoid bumping into people and objects. Olive can read large print; however, her reading time is limited to a maximum of 15 minutes because of the concentrated effort required.

Olive states she is managing well with all activities of daily living, but adds she does not feel as confident when walking alone as she used to, especially in crowded areas. She states she is not "as sure on my feet, as if I might stumble." Olive is proficient at using the long white cane for mobility and orientation and turning her head to scan the entire surrounding environment, but states she has an intangible uncertainty in recent months. She prefers to use buses rather than taxis to access community facilities, stating that the bus drivers are more helpful than the taxi drivers.

Olive was concerned that she may have further neurological problems and has been regularly monitored by a neurologist.

Location and Description of the Home

Olive's apartment is one of 18 in a complex of brick construction situated on a busy four-lane arterial road. There is a bus stop outside of the complex and a pedestrian crossing with audible traffic light controls that enable her to cross the road safely to access the beach promenade.

The apartment has one step at the entry and one step from the lounge area to the outdoor patio at the rear of the apartment. A previous tenant had installed a timber wedge and handrail at this entry. There is a small combined lounge and dining area, a separate kitchen, one bedroom large enough to accommodate a queen-sized bed, and a closet-style laundry. The bathroom has a toilet, vanity unit, and shower recess with a curb. There was originally a bath with a shower over it, but this was removed by a previous tenant, and a shower recess was installed. There is a shower curtain around the perimeter of the recess.

There is a small fenced private courtyard outside of the lounge room. Unfortunately, given the position of the apartment in the middle of an L-shaped block, there is very little sunlight in the courtyard or lounge area of the apartment. Some western sun filters into the bedroom on the opposite side of the unit. This influences the luminance in all rooms of the apartment.

Client Goals

Olive's primary goal is to live safely and independently in her own home for as long as possible. She has concern about having to move into an aged residential care facility if she cannot manage at home.

Olive's short-term goals are to:

+ Improve her independence within the home
+ Improve her safety by increasing the lighting and modifying the step access to the apartment

Olive's daughter would like her mother to maintain her independence living alone and to improve her safety by minimizing the risk of falls.

Evaluating Occupational Performance and Identifying Needs

The referral for occupational therapy intervention from the orientation and mobility officer was supported by health reports from the local doctor and Olive's neurologist updating Olive's health status and functional ability. The occupational therapy referral requested an assessment of the home environment to minimize possible safety risks so Olive could maintain her independence with minimal reliance on her daughter. Falls prevention was the primary concern. Since her cerebral hemorrhage, Olive has experienced significant vision loss, causing limitations in negotiating the general environment and increasing her risk of falls. Olive had recently moved to her apartment and was unfamiliar with the new surroundings and was having trouble with access into the apartment and the shower.

The therapist conducted a home visit and interviewed Olive to ascertain her goals. The therapist observed her doing tasks in various areas of her apartment to determine her functional limitations.

Mobility and Transfers

Indoors, Olive does not use any mobility aid, and she was observed to be independent in transfers to

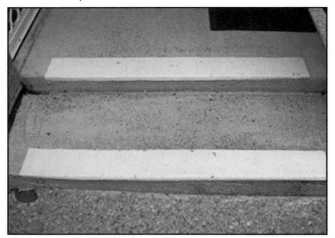

Figure 15-23. After home modifications—concrete landing and highlighted strip on each tread.

and from the chair and bed and to move independently around the apartment.

Olive reported that she uses a long white cane to assist outdoor mobility. She was instructed in its use during her rehabilitation by an orientation and mobility trainer from a community agency specializing in training people in mobility activities.

Olive leaves the lights on in all rooms of her apartment to compensate for her poor vision and to assist her in daily activities.

Self-Care and Household Activities

Olive is fully independent in all personal care activities. She does her own shopping, cooking, and laundry activities, and she has help once a fortnight with the heavier household cleaning, such as vacuuming and washing the floors.

Environmental Issues and Intervention Options

External Areas

Access to the Front of the Unit

Olive stated that she found the height of the front step (5.5 in/140 mm) very difficult to negotiate. Options considered included the installation of a ramp and landing or a half-step and landing at the entry. There was inadequate space to install an appropriate ramp and landing without impeding the public walk space.

The final recommendation was to provide a concrete landing at the height of the step and then a half-step (Figure 15-23). This provided two 2.75-in

(70-mm) steps, which had a 2-in (50-mm) wide highlighted strip on each tread, and a handrail on the left side ascending. This modification enabled the client to safely negotiate the smaller step risers and use the handrails for extra support.

Highlighted Strips on Ramp at Doorway From the Lounge Onto Patio

The condition of the timber ramp was excellent and not assessed as needing replacement. The timber surface was coated with a slip-resistant paint, and a handrail was in place on the right side descending from the lounge door. The paint surface was a dark green and blended with the shadows of the patio overhang. The outer edges were not clearly distinguishable.

Options considered were to install an extra handrail on the left side to match that on the right or highlight the outer edges of the ramp. The position of the glass sliding patio door prevented installation of the rail in an appropriate position.

The final recommendation was to paint a contrasting highlighted strip on the outer edges of the ramp. Because the concrete and the timber wedge were a dark green, yellow was chosen as the most appropriate color.

Bathroom

Modified Curb Step for Safety in Shower

The corner of the existing curb step into the shower had a sharp tiled corner and had caused Olive to trip on many occasions. The floor tiles and those of the curb step were the same pastel color so there was little distinction to highlight the hazard.

Options considered included complete removal of the curb step or modification to the curb. The entire bathroom floor would need to be removed and relaid to track to the shower waste if the curb step was eliminated. This was considered a complex and costly modification that would result in Olive needing to move out of the unit for several days until the work was completed. Olive was not willing to relocate to enable this work to be completed.

The modification to the curb was considered the most appropriate option. This included work to bevel the corner of the shower curb near the vanity and retile the entire curb step in a contrasting color (Figure 15-24). A dark tile color was requested so it could be distinguished against the lighter toned floor tiles. This would ensure that the edge would not be a trip hazard and the contrasting color would provide a visual highlight to the area, ensuring that the edges could be seen. An additional handgrip in the shower and a handheld shower were also recommended to improve Olive's general safety and independence when she was showering.

Internal Areas

Improved Lighting Throughout the Apartment

The therapist observed that the lighting in the apartment was very dim. Except in the bedroom, there was no sunlight entering the apartment because of the overhang from the apartments above. Olive had no task lighting in the kitchen or bathroom but did have direction lamps in the lounge and bedroom to assist reading. When asked if she considered the lighting poor, she stated she was unaware it could be improved. All lighting in the apartment was incandescent globes providing a maximum of 60 lux (100-watt incandescent standard bulb). The client reported that she had difficulty with her personal grooming activities in the bathroom and difficulty seeing to prepare meals at night in the kitchen.

Small halogen spotlights can be used for task lighting when placed in strategic positions, but they must be inserted into the ceiling space or alternatively as track lighting. Because Olive's apartment was on the ground level with a solid concrete slab as the ceiling, it was difficult to install inset lighting. Track lighting can be expensive and unsuitable to achieve light in specific positions. Another less expensive option is the use of fluorescent lighting with triphosphor tubes. Triphosphor fluorescent tubes, often called daylight tubes, provide a clear white light similar to the daylight on a clear day and cast a softer shadow than incandescent globes or halogen lighting.

The final recommendation was to install a circular fluorescent light fitting (60 lux) to improve luminance at the front entry and 47.25-in (1,200-mm) long double fluorescent light fittings in the bathroom and kitchen (240 lux with standard 36-watt tubes) because these were the areas where Olive needed light to assist in her daily activities, such as personal grooming and meal preparation. A double fluorescent light fitting was also recommended for the lounge/dining area to help Olive see better when eating her meals or reading. Triphosphor fluorescent tubes were requested because these increased the luminance to 320 lux.

Additional Factors Considered for Final Home Modification Solution

To understand Olive's functional vision, the therapist asked her to explain the limitations of her vision and how it affected her day-to-day tasks and mobility. She explained that she had vision on her left side only and that she had to be aware of her environment

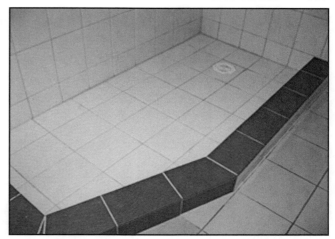

Figure 15-24. After home modifications—contrasting tiled shower curb.

to avoid bumping into objects or people. She reported that lighting was important so she could better determine the outline of objects within the environment and that, even though she kept the lights on in the apartment, they did not seem to give enough light to complete her tasks to her satisfaction. Olive indicated that contrast was important for her to distinguish one object from another or changes in the environment (e.g., distinguishing steps or changes in ground level). In the kitchen, she stated that she had difficulty distinguishing the control knobs on the stove because the dim lighting did not allow her to distinguish the white knobs against the white enamel of the stovetop, saying, "It all looks the same."

Olive indicated that she could see better on a clear sunny day than she could on a dull, cloudy day. Although she was unaware of the various lighting options and modifications to the environment available to assist her, she was open to suggestions that helped guide the decision-making process during the home visit.

The therapist had a comprehensive knowledge of environmental issues relevant to people with vision impairment to apply to this scenario. For example, sufficient lighting and contrast are two important elements in the environment of a client who has significant vision loss. Each client has individual needs concerning the extent of lighting improvement, so it is important to allow the client to explain how he or she sees his or her environment and how light and glare impacts his or her vision. In select instances, "more lighting is better than less lighting" but glare from bright light will lessen contrast and cause difficulty in distinguishing colors of similar tones or hues. Contrast can be improved by reducing glare and improving luminance. The color spectrum can

Table 15-6. Olive's Canadian Occupational Performance Measure Rating

Performance: 1 = Not able to do it at all; 10 = Able to do extremely well

Satisfaction: 1 = Not satisfied at all; 10 = Extremely satisfied

OCCUPATIONAL PERFORMANCE PROBLEMS	IMPORTANCE	PERFORMANCE T1	SATISFACTION T1	PERFORMANCE T2	SATISFACTION T2
1 Lack of safety—bathroom	10	1	2	10	10
2 Lack of safety—front entry	10	1	2	8	9
3 Lack of safety—general access within the home	10	3	2	9	8
4					
5					
		Total Performance T1	Total Satisfaction T1	Total Performance T2	Total Satisfaction T2
Total Scores		5	6	27	27
		Average Performance T1	Average Satisfaction T1	Average Performance T2	Average Satisfaction T2
Average Scores		1.6	2	9	9
				Change in Performance	Change in Satisfaction
Change in Scores (T2 – T1)				7.4	7

be used to create contrast or improve luminance. Light pastel colors will reflect light and help improve the ambient luminance in a room, whereas dark colors absorb light. White or yellow are often used to highlight step edges or indicate changes in ground level because these reflect light well and provide an exaggeration of contrast against most other colors.

Outcomes

Quotes were obtained from three building firms that specialize in home modification installations, and a builder was chosen to proceed with the work. The modifications were installed, and the therapist visited Olive in her home to complete a post modification evaluation including the administration of the COPM (Table 15-6). Olive was observed in her home environment and an interview was conducted, which included the review of the original occupational therapy report to determine whether there had been any changes in the client's capacity to manage the various activities in the home and community.

Olive was enthusiastic in her appreciation of the improvements in the environment. She reported that the bathroom was a major improvement with better lighting and the installation of the contrast shower curb step. She was observed in the bathroom using the new grab bar in the shower and stepping over the curb step without hesitation. She reported that she has not had a fall since the modifications were installed and, subsequently, is less fearful in the shower.

Olive was observed going in and out of the front entry using the handrail and negotiating the smaller steps. It was noted she could find the key in the door lock more easily. She stated that the front entry was easier to access, and she no longer feared falling while entering her apartment. She also stated that the improved lighting generally enabled her to see, especially on cloudy days when the apartment was very dim. It is now only on these days that she leaves the lights on all day.

It is anticipated that Olive might require future intervention as her health status changes or if she has any deterioration in her mobility. Olive is cognizant of the services available and indicated that she would contact the occupational therapist when she requires further assistance.

CASE STUDY 6: A YOUNG MAN WITH A PSYCHIATRIC DISABILITY

Client Interests and Daily Activities

Chris is a 31-year-old man who shares a three-bedroom detached house with another young man. His mother, who is his formal adult guardian, lives 5 miles (approximately 8 km) away but visits three to four times per week to ensure that her son is managing with daily activities. Chris's main interest is watching television or DVDs and listening to music. He is not involved in community groups or activities. His support worker takes him shopping, or his mother drives him to community facilities as required.

Health Condition and Functional Performance

In 1998, at the age of 22, Chris was diagnosed with schizophrenia and spent many months in the psychiatric ward of the local hospital. His behavior was aggressive, and he exhibited significant symptoms of his schizophrenic illness, such as constant voices in his head, a delusive state of mind, and antisocial behaviors. His mother was unable to care for him in her home.

He applied to a social housing provider for a one-bedroom apartment. In the ensuing 6 years, Chris was relocated three times before being housed in his current accommodation. In each of the three locations, Chris had difficulty maintaining his tenancy because of his overt unacceptable behavior, constant loud music, and offensive language. Chris stated that he needed the music to drown out the voices in his head.

Attempts to encourage him to use earphones or to govern the volume of the stereo failed. Other residents in the apartment complexes made many complaints about the music and his antisocial behavior.

In each of these properties, Chris lived alone, with his mother visiting daily to try to keep the peace and to support her son. There were other supports provided for Chris: a case manager from the community mental health unit visited twice weekly, and he had daily visits from the mental health intervention team to provide daily medications. Additionally, a worker from the community home care service visited fortnightly to assist with household cleaning.

Five years after his application for housing, the social housing provider decided to provide a detached house for Chris. At that time, he had a friend, who also had a diagnosis of schizophrenia, staying in his apartment from time to time. The two men decided to try a shared accommodation arrangement. It was anticipated that the house would provide space away from neighbors so the music and behaviors would not have as great of an impact.

Location and Description of the Home

The detached house is situated in a densely populated suburb with older couples and families. There are neighbors on two sides of the home and a park area at the rear boundary. The neighbor on one side is separated by a driveway between the homes.

The house has five steps at the front and eight at the back. There is a small bathroom consisting of a shower over the bath and a vanity. The toilet is separate and adjacent to the bathroom. There is a large backyard and several feet from the house to each side boundary. The front entry faces the street. There is a 6-ft (1,830-mm) high fence on three boundaries but no fencing at the front of the property.

Client Goals

Chris's primary goal is to live safely and independently in his own home and to be able to live in harmony with his community.

His long-term goal is to remain living in his own home, using community services to support him and minimize his admissions to hospital.

His short-term goals are to have safety and privacy in his home and not feel as if others are always watching him.

Chris's mother would like her son to maintain his tenancy and increase his independence so she can reduce her visits to once-weekly and limit her involvement in his day-to-day life.

Evaluating Occupational Performance and Identifying Needs

The referral for occupational therapy intervention was the result of a case conference with the mental health community workers, Chris's mother, and staff of the social housing provider. It was felt that the house required some modifications to enable Chris to feel comfortable, safe, and secure.

During a home visit from the therapist, where Chris, his mother, and case manager were present, Chris was observed doing tasks in the home and was asked how the home environment affected symptoms of his illness. The therapist discussed all issues

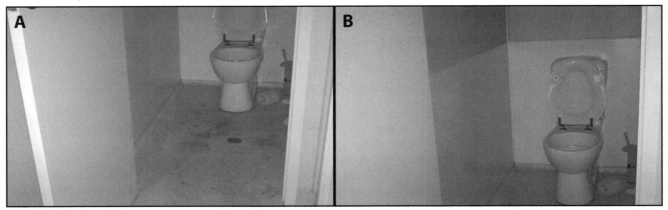

Figure 15-25. (A) Before and (B) after home modifications—toilet area.

with the case manager and Chris's mother, who could provide insight into the issues and difficulties experienced by Chris and the community workers.

Mobility and Transfers

Chris does not have any mobility problems. He is a tall man, about 6 ft, 2 in (1,880 mm) in height and weighing 196 pounds (approximately 89 kg, or 14 stone).

Self-Care and Household Activities

Chris is independent in all personal care activities but needs prompting to bathe and groom himself regularly. He uses water, either in the shower or bath, to reduce his anxiety and symptoms of his illness.

He relies on help for cooking and shopping, household cleaning, and laundry. His mother or case-worker provides transport to community facilities.

Purpose of Occupational Therapy Involvement

The occupational therapy referral requested an assessment of the home environment to provide privacy from the neighbors and to improve hygiene in the home. The community home care workers had complained that the habits of the two men in the home were such that workers were at risk. The toilet was always in an unclean state with urine all over the floor and around the crevices of the toilet pan.

During the assessment, interview, and observation process, the caseworker and Chris's mother raised their concerns that the home care workers had refused to clean the home until the bathroom and toilet areas were improved. The other area of concern was the front entry being open to the street and having limited privacy from the neighbors opposite.

It was particularly important to discuss with Chris's mother and the caseworker the options to modify behaviors and interventions attempted in the past.

Environmental Issues and Intervention Options

External Areas

Privacy Fence at the Front of the Home

The front door was exposed to the neighbors' opposite, causing Chris to feel that he was being watched constantly. Neighbors also needed privacy from Chris's overt behaviors.

A lattice screen had been installed across the front entry but Chris still felt that he was being watched. Several other homes on the street had fences and gates across the front boundary, so a similar installation would be in keeping with the streetscape and look to fit in.

The final recommendation was to provide a 6-ft (1,830-mm) high timber fence across the front boundary.

Toilet Area

Improved Cleanliness in Toilet Area

The problem arose because both men have difficulty urinating into the toilet bowl, causing urine to contaminate the floor and risking it being walked throughout the house (Figure 15-25A).

The options considered included modifying the behavior by providing a target, such as a ping-pong ball, in the toilet pan. However, other such devices had been tried several times without success.

Although the vinyl floor covering had been changed to tiles at the case manager's request, because it was felt that the tiles were easier to scrub, it was also unsuccessful.

The final recommendation was to install a toilet pan with fully enclosed plumbing to minimize areas in which the urine could collect. It was also recommended that Lamipanel (Laminex) sheeting be installed around the walls of the toilet to provide a water-resistant surface to clean or scrub (Figure 15-25B) and to install vinyl flooring cover 4 in (100 mm) up the wall to provide a water-impervious seal. A floor waste drainage was also installed so the floor could be sluiced with water and contaminated water could be washed away. Chris and his co-tenant were happy to use a portable toilet during the time the work was in progress and tolerated the inconvenience for that short time.

Bathroom Area

Improved Flow of Water on Bathroom Floor

Because Chris showers for a long time, is a big man, and does not use a shower curtain, excess water flows onto the bathroom floor. The floor is not profiled to drain the water away and so the water pools, causing a slip hazard.

Options considered included installing a shower screen on the bath edge, but this suggestion was rejected because it could be broken easily if Chris became aggressive. A shower curtain was also refused because of Chris's intolerance to using one. Floor mats posed another hazard as well as creating added laundry.

The final recommendation was to remove the existing flooring in the bathroom and profile the floor so that the water would drain to the floor waste and not pool into the center of the floor.

The modifications enabled Chris to feel in control of his environment and enabled the caregivers to feel safe when having to clean a contaminated area.

Outcomes

A technical adviser visited the home with the therapist to determine the exact floor specifications so that the contracted builder could understand the unusual request for the floor drainage in the toilet area and the need for drainage in the bathroom.

Quotes were obtained from three building firms that specialize in home modification installations, and a builder was chosen to proceed with the work. The modifications were installed, and the therapist visited Chris in his home to complete a post modification evaluation. The therapist observed Chris in his home environment and conducted an interview with him, which included a review of the original occupational therapy report and rescoring of the COPM (Table 15-7), to determine if there had been any changes in Chris's capacity to manage the various activities in the home and community.

Chris enthusiastically showed the therapist the improvements in the environment. He reported that the bathroom was a major improvement with the floor being much safer and the cleaners happier being able to sluice the toilet floor.

Chris was also appreciative of the privacy at the front of the home, which he stated gave him a greater feeling of security.

His caseworker reported that the home care workers were much happier now that the modifications were completed. Chris's mother also reported that she is not visiting as often to supplement the cleaning when the community agency does not visit.

It is anticipated that Chris might require future intervention as his symptoms change. The community mental health service continues a close liaison with the occupational therapist and the property owner to ensure that Chris can maintain his tenancy with minimal impact on his surrounding community into the future.

CASE STUDY 7: SPOUSE SUPPORTING A PERSON WITH DEMENTIA

Client Interests and Daily Activities

Eighty-two-year-old Alan and his 80-year-old wife Doris live in a house in a regional city suburb. The house has been Alan and Doris's home for the past 50 years, where they raised two sons and a daughter. Their daughter Jenny lives with her family in the local community and their sons live in nearby suburbs. One grandson also lives nearby. Alan and Doris's daughter, son-in-law, or grandson visits them 4 to 5 days per week, providing them with ongoing emotional and physical support.

Alan was a mechanic by trade prior to his retirement and was the main provider for the family. He continues to enjoy reading automobile magazines, as well as helping his son-in-law to restore an old car. Alan and Doris played lawn bowls together for years but, since the onset of her dementia, Doris is no longer able to participate in this activity. She has spent most of her married life as a homemaker, raising the children, and looking after the home. Her hobbies included gardening, knitting, and crocheting.

Table 15-7. Chris's Canadian Occupational Performance Measure Rating

OCCUPATIONAL PERFORMANCE PROBLEMS	IMPORTANCE	PERFORMANCE T1	SATISFACTION T1	PERFORMANCE T2	SATISFACTION T2
Performance: 1 = Not able to do it at all; 10 = Able to do extremely well					
Satisfaction: 1 = Not satisfied at all; 10 = Extremely satisfied					
1 Sense of privacy in relation to neighbors	10	5	1	9	8
2 Safety and cleanliness during and after routines in the toilet	10	6	4	9	9
3 Safety and cleanliness during and after routines in the bathroom	10	6	3	9	8
4					
5					
		Total Performance T1	Total Satisfaction T1	Total Performance T2	Total Satisfaction T2
Total Scores		17	18	27	25
		Average Performance T1	Average Satisfaction T1	Average Performance T2	Average Satisfaction T2
Average Scores		5.6	2.6	9	8.3
				Change in Performance	Change in Satisfaction
Change in Scores (T2 – T1)				3.4	5.7

Health Condition and Functional Performance

Doris was diagnosed with dementia 2 years ago. Since then, she has shown increased symptoms of the disease, including memory loss and repeated questioning, wandering at night, pacing, decreased visual perception, incontinence, poor sleep routine, disorientation, confusion, and agitation.

She can complete her daily living activities of showering, dressing, and toileting with assistance and prompting but has been susceptible to falls in the home because of her reduced visual perception and loss of good dynamic balance when standing and walking. Doris also has a medical history of osteoporosis. She is currently on medication for this condition and experiences occasional back pain. Doris is no longer capable of independently completing household tasks or activities previously of interest to her, such as gardening, knitting, and crocheting.

Alan has a medical history of arthritis, particularly affecting his knees and shoulders; reduced vision because of his poorly controlled diabetes; and clinical depression. He has experienced increased physical and emotional distress over the past 2 years as the symptoms of Doris's dementia have worsened and as he has had to take on the role of caregiver. He regularly consults his local doctor, who has prescribed medication for his depression.

Location and Description of the Home

Alan and Doris's home is a four-bedroom detached brick house, located on level land on a quiet suburban street. The house is high set with external staircases of 12 stairs at both front and back entrances. All living areas of the house are located upstairs. Downstairs houses a double garage, the laundry, and storage and work areas Alan uses to store car components and workshop tools and materials. There is a pathway leading from the base of the external stairs to the driveway. The backyard has a well-established lawn with garden beds and a 4-ft (1,200-mm) high wooden paling fence around the perimeter. There is a path at the rear of the building, as well as a pathway leading from the laundry door to the clothesline located in the middle of the backyard.

The home has a living room, dining room, and kitchen located at front of the house and a narrow hallway leading to the bathrooms and bedrooms at the rear. There is low-pile carpet on the floor in the living areas, linoleum on the floor in the kitchen, and tiles on the floor in the bathroom and toilet. The bathroom contains a bath, separate shower, and a vanity basin with a mirror and towel rails. The shower recess has a 60-mm–high curb and is enclosed by a shower screen that has a pivoting door. The toilet is in a separate room adjacent to the bathroom.

With Alan and Doris having lived in the home for 50 years, the living room has become cluttered with personal items and furniture to accommodate family who visit frequently. The home is fitted with smoke detectors. The interior of the home is dim during the day.

Client Goals

A home visit referral from Alan and Doris's local doctor indicated the need for the occupational therapist to review the existing home environment. The referral indicated a need for equipment, home modification, support service recommendations, and practical advice to enable Alan to provide Doris with ongoing support.

The couple has lived in the same home for 50 years and, despite increasing stress, Alan wished to continue supporting Doris there for as long as possible. He acknowledged Doris's deteriorating function and indicated that he continued to struggle with the personal loss of relationship and intimacy with his wife and his changing role and routines.

Alan stated that his long-term goals included the following:

+ Maintaining his own physical and emotional health in his role as a caregiver
+ Safely and effectively assisting his wife in her daily self-care activities and supporting her for as long as possible in the family home

Alan indicated that his short-term goals included the following:

+ Gaining increased understanding and acceptance of his wife's dementia and developing strategies to better manage her symptoms,

including her incontinence, poor sleep routine, disorientation, confusion, and agitation
+ Improving the safety of both himself and his wife when assisting her with transfers, mobility in and around the home, and her showering and toileting routine
+ Managing his increased anxiety and stress associated with ensuring his wife's safety in the home day and night

Evaluating Occupational Performance and Identifying Needs

The occupational therapist had reviewed Alan and Doris's health information prior to the visit to establish Doris's current physical, emotional, cognitive, and functional status. Because of Alan's overwhelming sense of loss, change in lifestyle and roles in the home, and feelings of anxiety about how he would manage in the future, the therapist conducted a series of four visits spread over 1 month. During the home visits, the therapist interviewed Alan to gather information on the functional status and daily routines of both Alan and Doris. They were also observed walking in and around the home environment and demonstrating how they managed Doris's self-care activities. The therapist interviewed the clients identify the couple's goals and to ascertain their capacity to function in the home.

Doris and Alan's daughter was present during some of the home visits. She reported that she and her family provided regular assistance with tasks such as shopping, meal preparation, caring for the yard, and driving Alan and Doris to community facilities. Alan reported that he no longer drives because of his poor vision. The daughter indicated that the extended family provided emotional support and cared for Doris 1 day per week to enable Alan to have a break and go shopping or visit the doctor.

Mobility and Transfers

Doris walked around independently both in- and outdoors. The therapist noted that Doris tended to lean on Alan or on nearby walls and furniture to maintain her balance, particularly when negotiating a change in level or when moving from sitting into the standing position. Doris was also observed to lean heavily on Alan when transferring on and off the toilet.

Alan indicated that Doris required increasing physical support when negotiating the front and back stairs. The stairs at the back and front entrances have one handrail on the left side when ascending. The handrail at the back stairs has deteriorated and is an unstable support. Doris experiences decreased visual perception, and Alan indicated that she frequently "catches" her foot on the nosing when ascending the stairs. She supports herself using the handrail and holds onto Alan for support. Alan has reduced vision and balance; consequently, the couple is at risk of falling on the stairs.

Alan indicated safety concerns when assisting Doris to transfer in and out of the shower recess and when helping her with showering, particularly because she tends to become agitated and move around unpredictably. Doris stands as she showers. Alan stated that Doris clings to him during showering because of a fear of falling and that she strikes out at him when agitated. The physical space available to allow the caregiver to access the shower recess to assist Doris during her showering routine was observed to be limited by the fixed shower screen and the pivoting door. There were no grab bars in the recess, and Alan indicated that Doris frequently leaned on him or used the taps for support when transferring in and out of the area and when standing in the shower. The shower recess had a fixed shower head limiting the control of the water flow. The shower curb is white, providing little differentiation between the white shower tray and white floor tiles. This raised step is a trip hazard for both Alan and Doris.

Alan reported that Doris spends many hours of the day and night pacing and wandering around the house. He stated that his wife also liked to wander around the backyard and look at the garden; however, he keeps external entrances locked because he is anxious about Doris's safety should she attempt to negotiate the back stairs independently. The backyard has uneven areas between the pathways, landings, and the turf. Alan noted that Doris frequently stumbles when stepping off the pathways onto the turf because of the change in surface heights. He expressed concern that she may fall if this were not rectified. Alan reported that, if he felt confident that Doris was safe in the yard, he would be able to sit down on the back landing and look through his magazines, allowing time for relaxation.

Alan walked independently around the house but used a single-point stick to assist with maintaining his balance when mobilizing outdoors. In addition to the arthritic pain in his knees, Alan indicated that his mobility has been affected by his lack of confidence walking over uneven terrain or negotiating change in levels and surfaces. He stated that his vision had deteriorated over time and that he had nearly fallen a few times. Alan indicated that neither he nor his wife had fallen in the home. He is independent with transfers; however, he reported increased difficulty transferring from low-seated surfaces, particularly when tired or experiencing knee pain.

Self-Care and Household Activities

Alan reported that Doris can undertake her daily living activities of showering, dressing, and toileting with prompting and assistance but that she required an increasing amount of attention and monitoring.

Alan indicated that he organizes Doris's clothes for her and that she sits on the bed to dress. He must prompt and assist Doris to orient her clothing during the dressing routine.

Doris is no longer capable of completing household tasks; however, she wanders into the kitchen and rummages through doors and cupboards, turns on the stove and other switches, and fills the sink to wash the dishes. At times, she wanders off, leaving the stove or oven on or the water overflowing from the sink onto the floor.

Alan stated that he does the laundry, vacuuming, and mopping and cleans the bathroom and toilet on a regular basis. His family assists with preparing meals that the couple freezes until required. Their daughter does most of the shopping, and their grandson mows the lawn and maintains the yard.

Alan reported difficulty coping with household tasks, which were always completed by Doris previously. He stated that a combination of emotional and physical stress, as well as reduced sleep, contributes to his diminishing capacity to cope with these tasks as well as monitor and care for his wife.

Anthropometric Measurements and Equipment

Alan and Doris's anthropometric measurements were taken in the seated and standing positions, including reach range. It was important that both clients' measurements were taken because they both use the same areas of the home and will both use specific interventions, such as grab bars and handrails, as they continue to age.

Environmental Issues and Intervention Options

External Access

Improved Handrail Support at Front and Back Entrances

Relocation to ground-level accommodation was not considered a viable option for Alan and Doris because it would be expensive. Alan indicated that he wished to remain in the family home because they were both familiar with the environment and it contained a lot of memories associated with them raising their family.

Options of installing a lift or stair-lift were considered; however, Doris would not be able to independently operate these devices. They were also considered too costly for Alan and his wife.

The final recommendations included the following:

+ Repairing the existing handrail at the back stairs. The handrail had deteriorated with the weather and was no longer stable.

+ Providing an additional handrail on the right side ascending at both the front and back stairs, so that the clients could use the bilateral rails. This would also eliminate the need for Alan to support Doris when she ascends and descends the stairs.

+ Providing strips of contrasting color to the edge of each stair tread to improve visibility. Because the stair treads were dark brown, a contrasting white strip was an appropriate application for the tread of each step.

Level Adjacent Surface Areas in the Backyard to Eliminate Trip Hazards

The option of fencing off a large section of even yard to allow Doris to safely wander was discussed; however, Alan indicated a preference to allow as much access for Doris to available yard space. The recommendation made was to raise the turf and soil adjacent to all the paths and landings around the home to ensure smooth transitions between the lawn and paths and reduce trip or fall hazards.

Bathroom

Enhanced Space and Design of the Shower Recess

Options reviewed included remodeling the bathroom to reprofile the bathroom floor to allow installation of a curb-free shower recess, providing color-contrasting strips to the existing curb to improve visibility, and installing grab bars to provide the couple with support as they stepped over the curb. The installation of a fixed shower seat or a freestanding chair was also discussed.

In making final recommendations, the cost of the changes, the potential disruption to routines, and the impact of works completion on Alan's stress levels were considered.

The final recommendations included:

+ Removing the existing shower screen with its pivot door and replacing it with a rod and shower curtain to open the area and provide more space for Doris and her caregiver

+ Applying color-contrasting strips to the curb at the entrance of the shower to highlight the edges and to reduce the trip hazard

+ Installing a vertical and horizontal grab bar on the tap wall of the shower recess to provide Doris with support when she stands in the shower and transfers in and out of the area. It was recommended that the vertical grab rail be fitted with a friction-sliding mount on which the handheld shower could be positioned, to enable the caregivers to better direct water flow. A handheld shower was a safer alternative to retaining the shower head.

+ Installing a temperature-control device for the hot water to reduce the risk of Doris burning herself if left unsupervised in the shower

+ Providing a freestanding shower chair for trial to allow Doris to sit during her showering routine

Enhanced Safety of the Towel Rail Fittings

The towel rail in the bathroom area has come loose, and Alan indicated that Doris supported herself on the rail when moving around the bathroom. It was recommended that the towel rail be replaced with a grab bar that could be used as a towel rail but that could also take her weight if she leaned on it for support.

Enhanced Safety in Toilet Area During Transfers

Doris tends to lean heavily on her husband when moving from sitting to standing in the toilet area. Options considered included Doris using an over-toilet frame or a toilet raiser and grab bars. Due to the potential trip hazard presented by the legs of an over-toilet frame in the confined toilet area, installing grab bars and a toilet raiser were selected as the most appropriate options. Alan indicated a preference to initially trial grab bars only, because of concerns about Doris potentially becoming confused about the change to the toilet setup and the general aesthetics of a raised toilet seat.

The final recommendation was to install vertical and horizontal grab bars on both sides of the toilet, because this configuration would ensure that Doris would not hold onto Alan for support and she could complete transfers safely and independently.

Kitchen

Risk Reduction of Injury, Electrocution, Water Damage, or Fire

Because Doris tends to wander and turn switches and taps on and off, various options were considered for the kitchen area. These included closing off the kitchen with a lockable door to restrict Doris from accessing the kitchen or installing locks on cupboards, removable tap heads on taps, and isolating switches linked to the stove, oven, and refrigerator.

Because Doris previously completed household tasks in the kitchen, Alan felt reluctant to completely restrict her from there.

The final recommendations included the following:

+ Installing an isolation switch to the oven, stove, and refrigerator

+ Removing appliances, such as the toaster and electric jug, from the kitchen countertops and placing them in lockable cupboards

+ Installing a lock on one kitchen cupboard in which to store knives, medications, cleaning fluids, and electrical devices. Sink plugs are to be stored in the cupboard also to reduce the risk of flooding the kitchen

Bedroom

Reduced Visual Cues That May Stimulate Activity During Sleeping Hours

Alan noted that Doris frequently gets up during the night and tends to undertake activities such as dressing, toileting, or wandering to the kitchen to turn on taps and switches. These activities tend to be triggered by visual cues, such as leaving clothing at the end of the bed or a cup being left on the bedside table. Alan continues to sleep in the same room as Doris because of the need to monitor her movements and activities. He indicated that, although he is frequently awakened during the night, he wants to continue sharing a room with Doris.

It was recommended that Alan remove distracting items in the bedroom, particularly at night, to reduce visual cues that may stimulate activity. It was also recommended that nightlights be installed in the hallway and toilet to assist Doris with finding the toilet at night.

Internal Access

Improved Lighting Throughout the Home to Reduce Risk of Tripping and Falling

The therapist observed that the lighting in the home was very dim, causing concern for client safety in high-risk areas, including the bathroom, hallway, bedroom, and kitchen.

Installing daylight tone fluorescent lighting with diffuser shields was recommended in these areas to improve illumination and minimize glare and a shadowing effect.

Added Security on External Doors

Alan indicated increasing anxiety that Doris might wander outdoors, particularly at night. The use of various alarms that could alert Alan to Doris's movements through one of the external doorways was discussed. Alan expressed concern that an alarm may agitate and upset Doris.

The final recommendation was that a deadbolt lock be installed on both the front and back doors and for Alan to keep the keys on him always, especially in the event of the couple needing to make a quick exit from the home.

Improved Safety When Pacing and Wandering

The living room was cluttered with personal items, including photographs of Alan and Doris's extended family and additional furniture items to accommodate the increasing size of family that visited over the years. Doris frequently paced within the living room, and it was recommended that a glass table within the room and two lounge chairs that are rarely used be removed. Alan was also encouraged to consider reducing clutter within the room by hanging some of the family photos on a wall or asking his daughter to place the photos in a memory album for him and his wife.

The therapist also made referrals to various services to ensure that Alan would receive adequate support in the home. This included referral to:

+ An incontinence specialist for education about night toileting and incontinence

+ The nursing service to recommence assistance with self-care activities

+ Physical therapy regarding mobility device options and to provide a freestanding height-adjustable shower chair

+ A rheumatologist to monitor the current integrity of Alan's joints and effectiveness of pain control measures

+ An ophthalmologist for an assessment of Alan's vision

+ A respite service for regular respite care

Additional Factors Considered for Final Home Modification Solution

Various recommendations were made at the end of each visit. In addition to environmental modifications, Alan and his wife were referred to the local Alzheimer's Association Support Group and to other community services for respite, nursing and social work support, and caregiver assistance with domestic tasks. Given the nature of Doris's dementia, a team approach and ongoing support were fundamental to the intervention planning process.

The recommendations were discussed with Alan and his family and were presented in writing to ensure that they had a record of the discussion and proposed actions arising out of each visit. This considered and paced approach allowed Alan and his family time to review and discuss the proposals and to prioritize recommendations in collaboration with the various stakeholders, including staff from community agencies. It was envisioned that this process would provide Alan with a reasonable sense of control over the intervention planning process and would ensure that he would not become overwhelmed by the number of recommendations or the effort involved in coordinating the introduction of further changes into their lifestyle.

When making the recommendations about interventions, it was important to allow Alan and his family to prioritize the suggestions. It was recognized that Alan was seeking to exert some level of control over his immediate environment and over the process of introducing changes into the home. His aim was to keep things "normal" and to maximize quality of life for both Doris and himself. It was acknowledged that Alan struggled with continually adjusting his personal goals and daily routines, coping with the profound personal loss of relationship with his wife, and recognizing and adapting to what Doris was no longer able to do.

Outcomes

Following several visits and discussions on the range of suitable interventions, Alan was provided with a written list of identified environmental issues and final recommendations. Once these were prioritized and Alan felt comfortable that the recommendations would assist him to better manage his wife within the home, he arranged quotes from building firms specializing in the installation of home modifications. Doris was placed in respite for a 2-week period while the environmental modifications were completed.

Referrals to other services were initiated by the occupational therapist, in consultation with the doctor. Support services were introduced, including cleaning and respite services.

The therapist visited Alan and Doris to complete a post modification evaluation in the form of an interview and structured observation. The COPM was also completed (Table 15-8).

The home modifications and changes were completed as per the final recommendations, with Alan reporting increased ease in assisting his wife and decreased anxiety over safety. He continued to experience sleepless nights and concern about his wife's safety around the home but reported that she had not had any falls or accidents. He indicated that he has felt less overwhelmed with the housekeeping activities since the introduction of support services.

Because of the ongoing decline of Doris's health because of her dementia and Alan's ongoing physical and mental health issues, the therapist has kept in regular contact with the couple. It is anticipated that the environment will need to be modified again in the future because of the ongoing changes in the couple's health conditions. It is also likely that their support and equipment needs will change periodically. Intersectoral collaboration with a range of services will be required to ensure that the clients can remain at home for as long as possible.

CONCLUSION

Each scenario in this chapter has highlighted the difference that occupational therapy-based home modification practice can make in the lives of a range of people encountering barriers to occupational performance in the home environment. The case studies have demonstrated that much information can be gained from undertaking a home visit to hear the client's story and observe his or her ability to manage in the home. The therapist can then use this information and use the clinical reasoning process to plan and negotiate interventions. This includes the therapist engaging in professional reasoning, using knowledge of the functional impacts of health conditions (scientific reasoning), the understanding of the client's life story and his or her perspective as an "expert" in his or her own life (narrative reasoning), and assessment of the practical limitations and ethical considerations of the situation (pragmatic and ethical reasoning) to determine the best outcome for a client.

This chapter has shown that an occupational therapist can introduce the client to a range of interventions, in addition to home modifications, including providing equipment, finding alternative ways of undertaking activities, and referring to service providers who can provide a further support and advice. Further, the therapist has a role in working with design and construction professionals to evaluate proposed home modification designs to ensure that alterations meet the client's needs effectively.

Table 15-8. Doris's Canadian Occupational Performance Measure Rating

Performance: 1 = Not able to do it at all; 10 = Able to do extremely well					
Satisfaction: 1 = Not satisfied at all; 10 = Extremely satisfied					
OCCUPATIONAL PERFORMANCE PROBLEMS	IMPORTANCE	PERFORMANCE T1	SATISFACTION T1	PERFORMANCE T2	SATISFACTION T2
1 Understanding Doris's dementia	10	5	1	7	8
2 Safety during transfers and mobility	10	3	4	9	9
3 Safety during showering and toileting routines	10	3	3	9	8
4 Coping as a carer	10	2	2	6	8
5					
		Total Performance T1	Total Satisfaction T1	Total Performance T2	Total Satisfaction T2
Total Scores		13	10	31	33
		Average Performance T1	Average Satisfaction T1	Average Performance T2	Average Satisfaction T2
Average Scores		3.2	2.5	7.7	8.2
				Change in Performance	Change in Satisfaction
Change in Scores (T2 – T1)				4.5	5.7

The case studies have emphasized that clients may present with a range of occupational performance issues at the time of the home visit. Issues discussed in this chapter include ensuring physical access to the home, completing self-care and household tasks, ensuring safe performance of caregiving, maintaining tenancy and neighborhood relationships, establishing community integration, and being able to age in place.

Further, a range of types of interventions have been showcased to help maintain or improve the person's occupational performance, including relocating, refitting or replacing fittings and fixtures, redesigning spaces, and ensuring adjustability and usability of the home modifications by a range of users. The types of interventions elected in these case studies included products and designs that would suit the current and long-term needs of the client and the household, including changes in equipment and caregiver support over time.

While this case study information can guide future occupational therapy practice, it is important that occupational therapists not overgeneralize this information when dealing with other clients but continue to take an individualized approach to evaluating the needs of individuals and the effectiveness of home modification interventions. This will ensure that solutions are tailored to achieve the best possible outcomes for each person, his or her family, caregivers, the various roles and activities he or she undertakes, and the home environment in which he or she lives.

Minor Modifications
It's Not as Simple as "Do It Yourself" (DIY)

THE PROBLEM

Minor and major home modifications have not been clearly or comprehensively defined in much of the international legislation informing policy and service development. This has resulted in a divergence of opinion about how home modification services should be defined and delivered, and who needs to be involved in recommending and installing these alterations. There is a limited understanding outside the profession of the value of minor home modifications. Further, there is ongoing debate both outside and within the profession about the role of occupational therapists in working with consumers to make minor home modifications. Naive understandings of the home modification practice result in the perception that minor modifications are simple and able to be undertaken by anyone. This approach can be problematic, especially considering the complexity associated with the process of determining the most appropriate solution. When the complexity of the process is not acknowledged and addressed, and an occupational therapist is not considered or included in this process, poor home modification outcomes may result.

The following discussion provides definitions of minor and major home modifications that could be considered in practice and policy development, details about the complexity of decision making that is highlighted by a framework for home modification service delivery, and information on why occupational therapists need to be involved in the minor modification process. Client scenarios are also described to enable the reader to understand the complexity associated with the minor modification process despite the simplicity of the chosen solution.

DEFINITIONS OF MINOR AND MAJOR MODIFICATIONS

There is a difference between minor and major modifications as per the following definitions:

+ Minor modifications: Nonstructural modifications, including the installation or alteration of fittings and fixtures (e.g., grab rails, shower seats, and other assistive devices; Jones, de Jonge, & Phillips, 2008). These modifications may be installed at minimal cost by unskilled labor and do not trigger the need for building or plumbing code or local planning compliance in local jurisdictions.

+ Major modifications: Structural modifications involving changes to the fabric of the home (e.g., widening doorways, moving plumbing, installing ramps; Jones et al., 2008). These modifications may be costly and require suitably qualified/registered staff to install. Their installation may require compliance with building or plumbing code requirements, depending on the requirements of local, state, or federal building, plumbing, or planning codes or legislation.

This is one set of definitions of minor and major home modifications within a broad range that are being discussed in literature around the world.

Ainsworth, E., & de Jonge, D. *An Occupational Therapist's Guide to Home Modification Practice, Second Edition (pp. 381-388).*

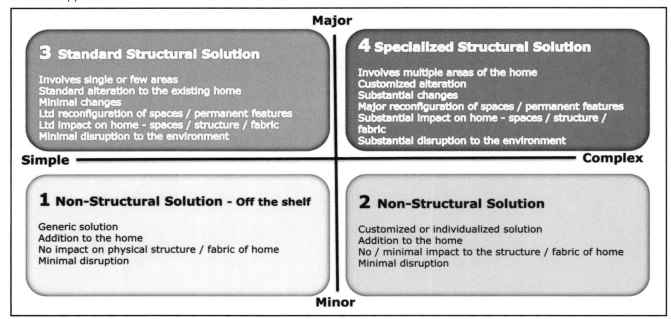

Figure A-1. Framework for home modification service delivery.

Determining the Need for Occupational Therapy Input

The need for a framework for modification service delivery has emerged because of a lack of clarity and consistency around home modification definitions in the international context, and the assumption that occupational therapists need not be involved with people who can adopt their own "do it yourself" (DIY) approach to minor modifications.

Figure A-1 depicts the four types of modifications, which are placed on a vertical and horizontal axis. The vertical axis differentiates between minor (nonstructural) modifications and major (structural) modifications. The horizontal axis differentiates between simple situations, where the person, occupation, and/or environment are uncomplicated, and complex situations, where the person, occupation, and/or environment provide challenges to developing an effective modification. Simple situations can generally be addressed by nonstructural "off the shelf" solutions and be undertaken without the assistance of an occupational therapist. Similarly, structural modifications common in renovations undertaken by the householders at times of transition do not require an occupational therapist when the person, occupation, and environment are not complex. However, complex situations benefit from the input of an occupational therapist when developing structural and nonstructural solutions. This framework provides a consistent international perspective in relation to defining minor and major home modifications, conceptualizing the role and contribution of the occupational therapist, and acknowledging the complexities associated with determining the most appropriate solutions.

Why Occupational Therapists Are Needed in the Minor Modification Process

Occupational therapists are best suited to undertake the process for determining the best solution, rather than leaving people to adopt a DIY approach. They possess the knowledge and skills necessary to determine the most appropriate solution for a person.

Their areas of expertise to assist with planning minor modifications include:

+ Knowledge of health conditions and disabilities, how people may present over time physically and functionally, and how this affects their equipment and care needs

+ Knowledge of evidence of efficacy of alternative products and design solutions

+ Knowledge of universal, accessible, adaptable, and purpose-built design principles to guide product selection and development of solutions

✦ Knowledge of the intent and application of legislation, including disability discrimination and/or antidiscrimination legislation and the national construction code

✦ Knowledge of the relevance, intent, and application of access standards

✦ Knowledge and skills in measuring to gather information on the anthropometrics of the person for the choice and placement of products and design features

✦ Knowledge and skills in measuring the built environment to gather information on the space and layout of features

✦ Knowledge and application of ergonomics and biomechanics to the selection of products and design of the home environment

Occupational therapists contribute to the home modification process by examining:

✦ Factors associated with the person

✦ How people complete activities

✦ The environments in which people operate

✦ Alternatives such as:

+ A different way to complete an activity

+ Equipment and/or technology options

+ Carer support

+ Home modifications

THE ROLE OF COMPLEXITY IN HOME MODIFICATION DECISION MAKING

The simplicity of a home modification does not always reflect the simplicity of the situation it is addressing. Figure A-1 presents a framework for differentiating between the simplicity and complexity of the solution versus the simplicity and complexity of the situation.

A minor modification may be considered a simple solution, but the process used to determine this minor modification can be complex. Complexity may arise from factors associated with the person, their occupation, and/or how the environment presents. The complexity of the situation—the person's circumstances, the way in which they undertake activities in the home, and the immediate and broader socioeconomic/legislative environment—affect home modification decisions and outcomes. Achieving good outcomes requires a well-considered

home modification approach that includes a clear understanding of products and design solutions so they can be matched to the needs of the consumer and the household. Occupational therapists possess the knowledge and skills necessary to assist people in identifying the best home modification solution.

The considerations that occupational therapists work through to identify suitable options for discussion with clients are detailed next.

Dimensions of Complexity

Table A-1 details the differences between simple and complex situations with specific reference to considerations related to the person, occupation, and environment. In addition, it describes considerations related to the home modification solution that differentiate between simple and complex options.

CLIENT EXAMPLES

Person: Unwell elderly person with arthritis, rents the property, has limited money, and requires grab rails for access in and out of the shower

Mrs. Smith is a pensioner who is 80 years of age with a history of arthritis and heart disease. She walks short distances around the home with a wheelie walker and relies on community services to assist with meal delivery, cleaning, and gardening in the home. She is having difficulty stepping in and out of her shower over the bath in her small rental property. She has been living in the property for years, originally as an owner but having sold it after her husband died. The new landlord is allowing her to remain in the property but only wants modifications that don't ruin the look of the home. She feels she really needs a grab rail to help her manage. Her son has called and he doesn't know what to buy, how to install it so that it is secure and won't crack the tiles, and where to place it so that she is safe during transfers.

Contribution of the occupational therapist to the problem-solving process:

✦ Interview with Mrs. Smith to gather background information

✦ Discussion with Mrs. Smith about her rights under the antidiscrimination act for home modification installation in a rental property

✦ Observation of mobility and transfers and discussion about how she completes activities

✦ Discussion about alternative ways of doing the showering, equipment options, and minor modifications

Table A-1. Considerations Differentiating Simple and Complex Home Modifications

PERSON

Simple	Complex
Experience With Condition/Impairment	
• Health condition stable/predictable • Experienced in own condition • No further growth (child to adult) • Diagnosed some time ago • Awareness of short-/long-term needs • Minimal impact on identity and roles	• Recent onset of condition, comorbidities • Health condition unpredictable, deteriorating, variable, or changeable • Growth continuing (child to adult) • Recent diagnosis • Limited awareness of short-/long-term needs • Substantial impact on identity and roles
Nature of Need	
• Not urgent • Modification to address quality-of-life issues • No need for equipment in the immediate short or long term	• Urgent • Health, independence, and safety issues of concern • Need to accommodate equipment short or long term
Capacity to Undertake a Home Modification	
• Person has had previous awareness and experience doing home modifications • Skills and resources to access home modifications • Effective literacy • Independent communicating needs and making decisions • Independent funds • Open to suggestions and ideas	• Person has had no previous awareness or experience of doing home modifications • Limited skills and access to resources • Low literacy • Support required communicating needs and making decisions • Requires financial support • Well-established ideas about what he or she will or won't have as a home modification
Lifestyle and Preferences	
• Stable lifestyle • No concern about aesthetics • No concern about resale • No concern about visitors/friends using area	• Imminent life transition • Concern about aesthetics • Concern about resale • Concern about visitors/friends using area

TASKS, ACTIVITIES, OCCUPATIONS

Simple	Complex
• Low-risk activity • Carer not required during activity • No equipment required/in use	• High-risk activity • Carer required during activity/inconsistent or compromised care support • Range of equipment in use/required during activity

ENVIRONMENT

Simple	Complex
Physical	
• Location of studs/reinforcement known • Substantial size of area for fit • Environment new and not needing maintenance	• Location of studs/reinforcement unknown • Lack of size for fit • Environment deteriorating and needing maintenance

(continued)

Table A-1. Considerations Differentiating Simple and Complex Home Modifications (continued)

ENVIRONMENT	
Simple	**Complex**
Social	
• Supportive family, community • Acceptance by family/other stakeholders • No diversity of need by others	• Nonsupportive family, community • Nonacceptance by family and other stakeholders • Diversity of need by others in household
Societal	
• Home owned by the person • No building and planning approvals required • Retirement village/landlord approvals not required	• Landlord's viewpoint on modifications: acceptability and willingness to allow installation • Building and planning approvals required • Retirement village/landlord approvals required

SOLUTION	
Simple	**Complex**
Characteristics of the Intervention	
• Home modification only required • Products well known on the market • Products readily available • Materials known and information targeted and available • Evidence about effectiveness in research • Follow-up not required • Minimal cost to purchase • Not a specialized solution • Simple componentry • Quality of material established and tested • Warranty	• Provision of home modification in combination with other interventions • Products new/changing on the market • Products not readily available • Materials not known and information not targeted and available • Lack of evidence about effectiveness in evidence-based practice • Follow-up required • Expensive: costly to purchase, service, and repair • Highly specialized solution • Complex componentry • Quality of material unknown • No or short-term warranty period
Usability and Accessibility	
• Simple • Intuitive • Minimal physical effort required • Adjustable • Accommodates diverse methods, preferences, and approaches • Clear information regarding use • High tolerance for error • No impact on layout and space in environment	• Complex, unfamiliar, and requires training/supervision • Instructions needed • Physical effort required • Fixed, inflexible, and not able to be changed as person's needs change over time • Only supports restricted methods, preferences, and approaches • Information difficult to interpret • Low tolerance for error • Impact on layout and space in environment
Maintenance and Care Requirements	
• No risk of breakdown • Needing no or minimal care • No maintenance and/or servicing required • Solution not requiring expertise for installation and maintenance	• High risk of breakdown • Needing care • Regular/costly maintenance and servicing required • Solution requiring expertise for installation and maintenance

✦ Demonstration of alternative ways of doing the transfers

✦ Discussion and demonstration and trial of alternative equipment options

✦ Discussion about minor modification options

✦ Provision of photos of grab rails

✦ Measurement of the environment for fit of equipment and grab rails

✦ Observation of transfer technique and measurement of reach for correct placement of grab rails

✦ Provision of information about funding options to assist with the chosen solution

✦ Provision of information on services that can assist with the installation of the grab rails in the correct position for safe transfers and to ensure the tiles on the wall don't crack on installation

✦ Fitting and trial of equipment and review of Mrs. Smith's capacity to manage the equipment

✦ Solution determined: Mrs. Smith decided to trial a tub transfer bench with handheld shower and have carers visit to supervise her as she completed her routine. She decided not to arrange for the installation of the grab rails despite being aware of her rights under the legislation. The occupational therapist visited after the equipment was delivered to fit it to the bathtub and train Mrs. Smith in the use of the equipment. The occupational therapist also provided an information sheet with photos and written instructions on how to use the equipment. She checked to make sure Mrs. Smith had been given information from the supplier on how to care for the equipment.

Consequence of not involving an occupational therapist in the problem-solving process:

✦ No solution provided and potential for Mrs. Smith to have ongoing falls, be hospitalized

✦ Mrs. Smith relocates from her residence

Occupation: Middle-aged person with arthritis, owns the home, has limited funds, needs a bath for pain relief but is struggling to get in and out of the bathtub

Mr. Jones is a middle-aged man living in his own home with his wife. They have limited funds, as they have only recently paid off their home and completed renovations, including changes to the bathroom. He says that he requires a soak in the bath for pain relief, as he has arthritis affecting his joints, but he is struggling to get in and out. He has only recently been provided with pain medication. He has a new shower that is located over the bath and does not want to spend more money on changes. He said that he just needs a grab rail to help get in and out of the bath. He admitted that he did get "stuck" in the bath recently and had to get his wife to help him out, and he wasn't sure how they would manage if this happened again.

Contribution of the occupational therapist to the problem-solving process:

✦ Interview with Mr. and Mrs. Jones to gather background information

✦ Observation of mobility and transfers and discussion about how Mr. Jones completes activities

✦ Discussion about and demonstration of alternative ways of doing the showering, equipment options, and minor modifications

✦ Measurement of environment for potential future equipment

✦ Observation of transfer technique and measurement of reach for possible future provision of equipment

✦ Provision of information about services and funding options to assist with sourcing equipment

✦ Provision of assistance sourcing a tub transfer bench and bath seat and handheld shower to trial while waiting for medication to take effect

✦ Fitting of equipment and observation of use

✦ Review of satisfaction with respect to using equipment

✦ Provision of information about services and funding to assist with future funding of bath lift

✦ Solution determined: Mr. Jones decided to trial the equipment, as he acknowledged that getting in and out of the bath was getting harder and that the grab rail may not be the best solution.

Consequence of not involving an occupational therapist in the problem-solving process:

✦ Grab rail installed and Mr. Jones has ongoing difficulty getting in and out of the bath

✦ No grab rail installed and Mr. Jones may have a fall

✦ Abandonment of bathing routine

✦ Ongoing assistance required from Mrs. Jones, who may hurt herself

✦ Money spent on renovating bath area without consideration of alternatives

Environment: Elderly person living in a new retirement village, needs rails for showering, limitations on location of nogging for installation of grab rails

Mr. and Mrs. Archer have just moved into a two-bedroom, two-bathroom unit in a relatively new retirement village. Mr. Archer stated that he requires grab rails, as he has Parkinson's disease. He had just recently discharged himself from hospital due to progressive weight loss and poor nursing care. He was having falls in the new home, and his wife was struggling to cope. She felt that he needed to go back to hospital if something could not be done urgently. She did not know if the walls were reinforced or who to contact for help to sort out their needs. They stated that they were happy to pay for whatever services were needed.

Contribution of the occupational therapist to the problem-solving process:

+ Interview with Mr. and Mrs. Archer to gather background information

+ Observation of mobility and transfers and discussion about how Mr. Archer completes activities in the bathroom

+ Discussion about alternative ways of doing the showering, equipment options, and minor modifications

+ Discussion and demonstration and trial of alternative equipment options to fit into space

+ Discussion about minor modification options

+ Provision of photos of grab rails, discussion about range, suppliers, and cost

+ Liaison (or making client aware of need to liaise) with retirement village about location of nogging, paperwork required for installation of grab rails by occupants, policies regarding insurance requirements for building and deactivating smoke alarms during installation of grab rails by builder

+ Measurement of the environment for fit of equipment and grab rails

+ Measurement of reach for correct placement of grab rails

+ Provision of information on services that can assist with the installation of the grab rail in the correct position for safe transfers and to ensure the tiles on the wall don't crack on installation. Liaison with services regarding availability to do the work urgently.

+ Provision of information about services that can provide hire and sale of equipment and liaison with services to order the equipment on behalf of the clients

+ Fitting of equipment after delivery and training Mr. Archer in its use

+ Observation of use of equipment and grab rails and review of satisfaction with respect to using equipment

+ Solution determined: Mr. and Mrs. Archer agreed that a combination of equipment and grab rails was required due to the complexity of not having wall space for grab rails to be installed in the en suite bathroom off the master bedroom. Main bathroom rather than the en suite to be fitted out with a rail near the toilet. Equipment to be used in en suite. Both showers to be fitted out with rails and the towel rails to be replaced with grab rails.

Consequence of not involving an occupational therapist in the problem-solving process:

+ Grab rail installed and not in correct location, causing injury or accident

+ No grab rail installed and Mr. Archer may have a fall

+ Abandonment of showering routine

+ Ongoing assistance required from Mrs. Archer, who may hurt herself

+ Payment for care services

Environment: Young girl with physical disability, family has no money, renting with a view to purchasing. Needs a rail beside the toilet for balance as she transfers with assistance, growth to be considered.

Tammy and her family have just moved into a four-bedroom, two-bathroom house in a new city. Tammy's mother stated that Tammy requires grab rails, as she can sit on the toilet and hold on, so her mother would like to give her more independence. She said that Tammy is growing quickly. She is not sure what rails are on the market. The toilet is a distance from the wall.

Contribution of the occupational therapist to the problem-solving process:

+ Interview with Tammy and her mother to gather background information

+ Observation of mobility and transfers and discussion about how Tammy completes activities in the bathroom

+ Discussion about minor modification options

+ Provision of photos of grab rails, discussion about range, suppliers, and cost

+ Measurement of the environment for fit of grab rails

+ Measurement of reach for correct initial placement of grab rails

+ Provision of information on services that can assist with the installation of the grab rail in the correct position for safe transfers and to ensure the tiles on the wall don't crack on installation. Liaison with services regarding availability to do the work.

+ Observation of use of grab rails and review of satisfaction after installation

+ Solution determined: Tammy's mother stated that she would like the fold-down rail that is height adjustable so that it can fold away for others using the toilet but fold down for Tammy. It can also be moved up over time as Tammy grows, saving the need to remove and reinstall the rail at different heights, and saving the cost of hiring a tradesman.

Consequence of not involving an occupational therapist in the problem-solving process:

+ Incorrect grab rail chosen

+ Grab rail installed and not in correct location, causing injury or accident

+ No grab rail installed and Tammy may have a fall

+ Ongoing assistance required from Tammy's mother

+ Payment for care services

SUMMARY

A minor modification is sometimes considered a simple solution that can be implemented through a DIY approach, but many situations are more complex than is immediately apparent. Consequently, a systematic and deliberate process is required to examine factors associated with the person; the devices they rely on; the activities being undertaken; and the physical, social, temporal, personal, occupational, and societal dimensions of the home environment.

Achieving good outcomes requires a well-considered home modification approach that includes a clear understanding of products and design solutions so they can be matched to the needs of the consumer and the household. Rather than occupational therapists, consumers, and other stakeholders seeing all minor modifications as a simple DIY solution, it is far better for staff to identify the potential complexities associated with this type of intervention and support people to understand the range of options that need to be considered. This will assist in building people's capacity to make informed decisions about the best solution for their circumstances.

REFERENCE

Jones, A., de Jonge, D., & Phillips, R. (2008). *The impact of home maintenance and modification services on health, community care and housing outcomes in later life*. Queensland, Australia: Australian Housing and Urban Research Institute Queensland Research Centre. Retrieved from https://www.ahuri.edu.au/__data/assets/pdf_file/0022/2893/AHURI_Positioning_Paper_No103-The-impact-of-home-maintenance-and-modification-services-on-health.pdf

Outline of Shapes and Occupied Wheelchairs

✦ Edges of spaces traversed by turning wheelchairs are inscribed by key outermost points (most salient points [MSPs]). The locations of the points is not invariant for all turns: the points may be located at different locations on the outline of the wheelchair, depending upon the wheelchair shape and degree of asymmetry, the direction of turn (clockwise or counterclockwise) and the location of the center of rotation.

✦ For a wheelchair performing the eight turns shown here, five MSPs inscribe its paths. Only one MSP inscribes Turn 2 and almost only one for Turn 1; two MSPs inscribe Turns 3, 6, 7 and 8; three MSPs inscribe Turn 5, although one of these (MSP3) inscribes only a very short initial length of the turn path.

✦ There is no MSP that inscribes the path for all turns.

✦ With decreasing diameter of turning circles, the MSPs tend to occur at the ends of the wheelchair; with increasing diameter, they tend to occur at the sides (Figure B-1).

Ainsworth, E., & de Jonge, D. *An Occupational Therapist's Guide to Home Modification Practice, Second Edition (pp. 389-390.*
© 2019 SLACK Incorporated.

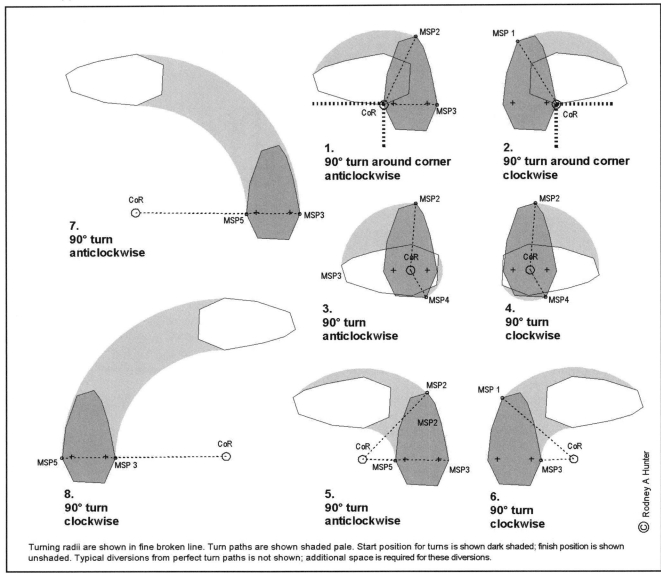

Turning radii are shown in fine broken line. Turn paths are shown shaded pale. Start position for turns is shown dark shaded; finish position is shown unshaded. Typical diversions from perfect turn paths is not shown; additional space is required for these diversions.

Figure B-1. Outline shapes of occupied wheelchairs, MSPs, and turn paths. (Reprinted with permission from Rodney A. Hunter.)

APPENDIX C

Fundamental Types of Compact Turns

Notes on Fundamental Types of Compact Turns

Wheelchairs and scooters turn around a center of rotation located on the axis through their drive wheels. The distance of the center of rotation from the mid-point between the drive wheels of the wheelchair or scooter corresponds with the size of the turning circle determines: the further away, the large the turning circle.

The center of rotation can occur between the drive wheels for wheelchairs but typically not for scooters. In other words, wheelchairs are pivotable, scooters are typically not.

Wheelchairs are steered by exerting force individually to each of the drive wheels, the difference between the amount and direction of force accounting for the potential complexity (intended and unintended) of wheelchair motion. For scooters, force is applied to both drive wheels equally and steering is by control of one or two pivot wheels located usually at the front and operated by steering handlebars (tiller).

Castor wheels have no direct role in the steering of wheelchairs. A Segway mobility device is kinematically the same as a mid-wheel drive wheelchair without castor wheels.

Scooters with only one pivot wheel (three-wheeled scooters) typically enable smaller turning circles than scooters with two pivot wheels (four-wheeled scooters). This is because the connection with the tiller of the single pivot wheel is simpler and more direct than the connection of the two pivot wheels; the single pivot wheel can therefore be rotated further than each pivot wheel of a four-wheel scooter.

Wheelchairs are typically available as rear-, mid- and front-wheel drives. The distinction relates to the relative portion of the appliance (and occupant) in front and behind the drive wheel axis and therefore the size and shape of the space used by the appliance as it turns.

Outlines (in plan view) of occupied wheelchairs and scooters are typically complex and asymmetrical. Shape contributes to turning space requirements; hence, two wheelchairs of the same drive type and overall length and width, and performing the same turn, can occupy different turning space.

Two types of turns can be distinguished: circular (see Diagrams 1 through 17) and noncircular (Diagram 18). Noncircular turns can be parabolic, hyperbolic, ellipsoidal, and splinal. A circular turn is achieved by maintaining constant force on (and therefore revolution of) each drive wheel or, for scooters, maintaining the same steering angle throughout the turning motion. Noncircular motion is achieved for wheelchairs by successively varying the force during the turn to (and therefore successively varying the revolutions of) each wheel. For scooters, noncircular turns are achieved by varying the steering angle during the turning motion.

The most compact turning circle of scooters is larger than the most compact turning circle of wheelchairs.

Ainsworth, E., & de Jonge, D. *An Occupational Therapist's Guide to Home Modification Practice, Second Edition (pp. 391–393).*
© 2019 SLACK Incorporated.

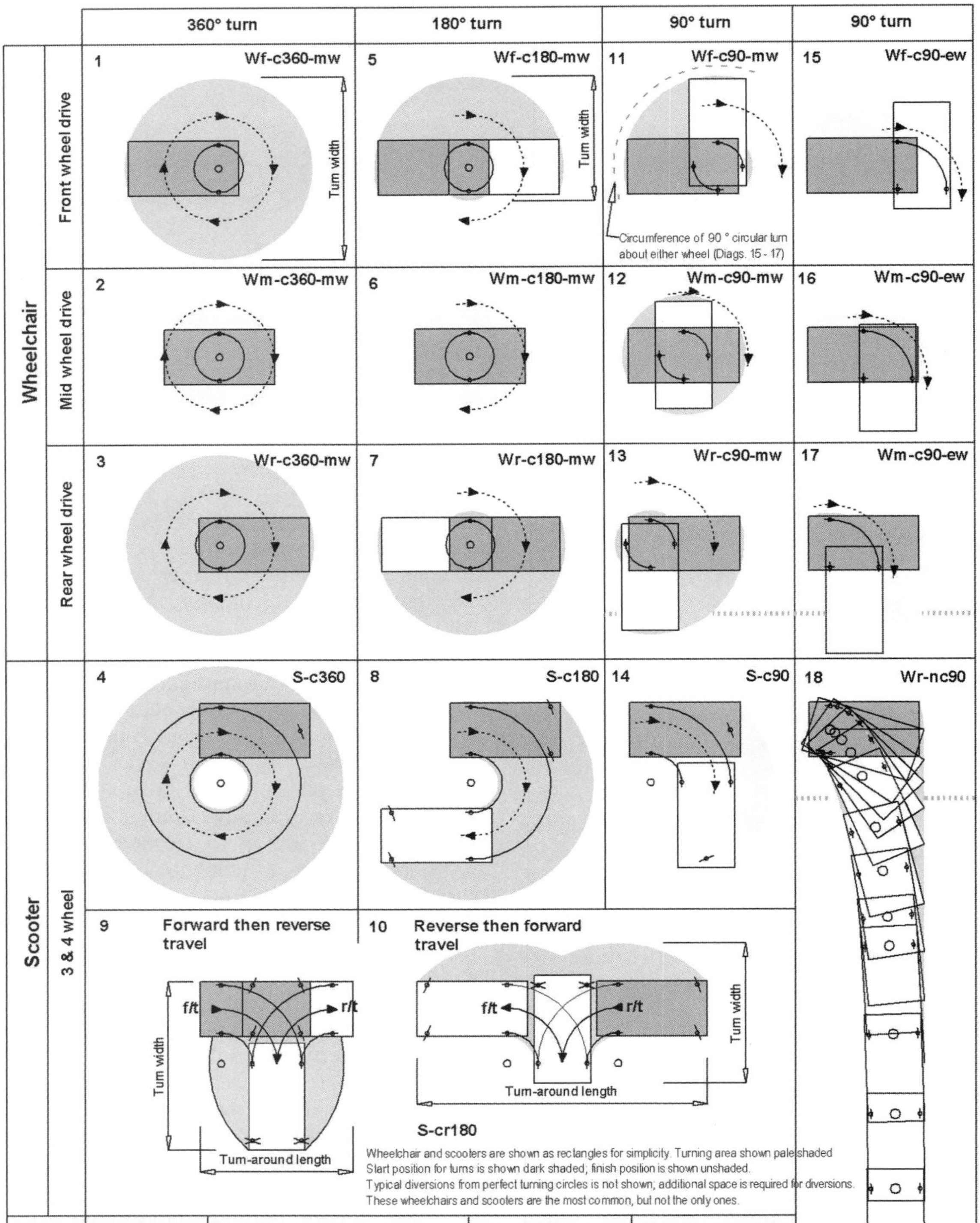

Turn type	Center of rotation at:	Example of application	Uni-directional turn (clockwise or anti-clockwise)	Reversing turn (clockwise and anticlockwise)
Circular	Mid-wheel	Turn between two or more walls	Yes	Yes
	Either wheel	Turn around outside of a corner	Yes	Yes
Non-circular		Turn around inside of a corner	Yes	Yes

Figure C-1. Fundamental types of compact turns. (Reprinted with permission from Rodney A. Hunter.)

For wheelchairs of the same size and shape, the turning circle of mid-wheel–drive wheelchairs is smaller than for rear- and front-wheel–drive wheelchairs.

The turnaround width for a 360-degree turn is less than that for a 180-degree turn (see Diagrams 1 and 5).

The turning circle diameter about either wheel is larger than for a turn about the mid-point between the drive wheels (see Diagrams 11 and 15).

The circulation space shape for a turn is comprised of the principal turn and its approach and departure travel. Diagram 8 illustrates this: if the approach and departure paths are required to converge, a funnel shaped path would need to be added to the principal turn shape.

Reversing turns are an alternative to simple 180-degree turns. They are comprised of circular turns (see Diagram 9 and 10), noncircular turns, or both.

Two principal types of reversing turns can be distinguished: a reversing turn followed by a forward turn (see Diagram 9), and a forward turn followed by a reversing turn (Diagram 10). The turnaround width of the forward-turn–first maneuver is greater than that for the reversing-turn–first maneuver, but its length is less.

The relevance or choice of a turning maneuver is with respect to obstacles, such as walls and doorways. For example, the circular 90-degree turn by the rear-wheel–drive wheelchair in Diagram 13 snugly enables the wheelchair to turn through an opening in a wall (shown in thick broken lines) whereas the noncircular 90-degree turn in Diagram 18 is amply accommodated by the opening.

Ramp Installation Considerations

Ramps are often provided as an alternative to stairs and can be permanent or temporary installations. Permanent installations are those that are fixed in place; temporary ramps are usually modular and adjustable. Ramps are suitable for people who use wheeled mobility equipment, such as wheelchairs or wheeled walkers, but they also have practical applications for a range of people. For example, they help where access to the home is needed for pushing shopping carts or prams or people moving furniture on wheels (Alderson, 2010). Because some older people and people with disabilities can find ramps difficult to use, they should always be in close proximity to steps where possible (Alderson, 2010; Center for Universal Design, 2004).

The following discussion provides broad design principles in relation to the design of ramps and detail about tailoring ramps to suit the needs of individuals, their equipment, and caregivers. There are also practical instructions on how to design an external ramp for a home.

BUILDING ADVICE AND ACCESS STANDARDS

To ensure the most appropriate ramp design for a home, occupational therapists might need to consult with companies that manufacture or supply ramps or seek advice from builders or design professionals

who have experience installing them. Information discussed among therapists and the ramp company representatives and/or builders can include the following:

+ Ramp design and construction requirements as indicated in local planning schemes, local building codes, and the relevance and application of access standards

+ Alternative ramp configurations to suit the space available, the desired direction of travel, and the slope of the land (i.e., whether the ramp needs to be straight, L-shaped, U-shaped, switchback, or curved)

+ Types of building materials suitable for construction

+ The appearance of the ramp in relation to the home, garden, fencing, and other features in the yard

+ The cost of ramp design options and associated works, such as paths leading to the bottom of the ramp

+ Product warranty

+ The source and level of availability of technical assistance for repairs and maintenance over time

+ The cost of alternative ramp configurations and associated building works in relation to the cost of other building solutions such as vertical lifts

Ainsworth, E., & de Jonge, D. *An Occupational Therapist's*
Guide to Home Modification Practice, Second Edition (pp. 395–413).
© 2019 SLACK Incorporated.

Local building codes and access standards are used to guide the design of public buildings and spaces. Therapists can also make use of the standards when designing domestic ramps, and they may be a mandatory requirement for ramp design and construction by local councils. The public access standards provide important measurements and detail on essential features and design elements to ensure ramps are safe to use by people who can walk unaided or those who use mobility equipment. Such information includes, for example, detail on the minimum and maximum gradients, ramp width, ramp length dimensions between landings, and rail and curb height.

Occupational therapists need to ensure that the dimensions in the access standards suit the relevant client's measurements, his or her equipment, and other people who might assist the client with their equipment, including caregivers or other household members. If the dimensions that are listed in access standards do not suit the measurements and function of the person and his or her equipment and caregivers, they will need to be altered. This might include, for example, decreasing the ramp gradient (to make it less steep), increasing the ramp width (to make it wider), or altering the size of the landing at the turns (to make it longer and wider).

Local building codes and access standards can serve as ramp design guides where there is little or no information on the characteristics and requirements of the ramp user or if there is likely to be a range of ramp users (Hunter, 1992).

The quality and structural integrity of the ramp will be guided by compliance with industry standards and local building code requirements. There might be a range of design or manufacturing standards existing in various countries that relate to the construction of ramps (e.g., standards relating to slip resistance, loads, the construction of aluminum and steel structures, and the construction of fixed platforms and walkways).

People, Their Mobility, and Their Equipment

A ramp might suit someone who uses a manual wheelchair and has sufficient upper-limb strength and endurance to push the equipment along a gradual slope, or it might suit an individual using a powered wheelchair or scooter to travel distances. It can also prove a more appropriate alternative to stairs for a client who uses a wheelie walker or walking aid, or who can walk without a mobility device. In these instances, the client needs to demonstrate the required endurance and capacity to manage the gradient and walk the length of a ramp without adversely affecting his or her health, safety, and independence.

Therapists need to observe and measure the person with the disability and his or her equipment and caregivers to ensure the correct design of the ramp. If a person with a disability is to walk along a similar ramp, with or without mobility equipment, to trial it, therapists should observe the person's capacity to negotiate distances on a slope, noting whether he or she has a safe stride and good balance and endurance. Therapists should also note whether the person needs to hold on to the rail for support and whether he or she requires frequent level landings to rest. Further, all ramp users, especially people who have a vision impairment, might need enhanced lighting at the entry and exit to the ramp and along its length. People with a vision impairment might benefit from the curb that can act as a guide during wayfinding.

Clients might use a ramp in a range of ways, and hence the design can vary to suit its use (Goldsmith, 2000). For example, a client may wheel along the ramp in his or her wheelchair or scooter and use the rails more as a physical barrier to prevent the equipment from rolling off the edge of the structure, rather than holding onto them or pulling on them for support. Other clients might use both handrails to pull themselves up the ramp run and as an alternative to pushing themselves in the wheelchair.

The types of measurements relating to the clients, their equipment, and their caregivers that determine the design of the ramp and whether the access standards are applicable include the following:

+ The overall occupied length and width of the equipment, influencing the length and width of the level landings and the width of the ramp

+ The turning space of the equipment (90, 180, or 360 degrees), which affects the length and width of the landings on entry and exit and the width of entry landings

+ The reach range of the person, influencing the height of the rails

+ The hand size of the person, influencing the shape of the rails

+ Space for the caregiver standing behind or beside the client and his or her equipment, determining the width of the ramp and the width and length of landings

Therapists can establish these measurements by using a large indoor or outdoor area to mark out the space required, or they can set up obstacle courses to test their final dimensions. For example, chalk or adhesive tape can be used on a level surface to set out the diameter measurement of a turning circle of a person in a wheelchair or scooter.

Therapists will also need to check the weights of clients and their wheelchairs or scooters to ensure that the builder constructs ramps that are able to withstand the load. Further, therapists might need to contact the manufacturers or suppliers of scooters and wheelchairs to determine the maximum safe gradient that the equipment can negotiate. Consideration needs to be given to the alternative uses of the ramp, particularly if it is installed at the main entry that is also used for the fit of furniture and other items through the doorway. The weight of furniture and any other items that may be transported along the ramp need to be considered in the design of the structure.

SUITABILITY OF THE HOME

Ramp design and materials need to reflect the overall look of the dwelling rather than appear as an addition that stands out from the rest of the home (Center for Universal Design, 2004). Therapists should give consideration to the type of materials used and choose colors that make the ramp design blend with the home and its surrounding garden area. For example, if there is a wooden house requiring modification, the therapist might consider recommending the installation of a wooden ramp painted in the same colors as the home.

Using a screen, such as a decorative wall or foliage, can serve to disguise the area and prevent highlighting that a person with a disability lives in the home (Center for Universal Design, 2004). In other cases, it might be more aesthetically pleasing to place the ramp at the side or rear of the premises.

The homeowner will also need to consider whether expenditure on the ramp is cost-effective, given the age and condition of the home. Further, the location and size of the ramp might affect the use of yard area and how the client, other members of the household, and visitors use the various entries of the home. Other factors that might influence the final design of the ramp are permanent structures, such as car parking facilities; the location of outdoor sheds, meters, hot water units, or tanks; or the style of windows near the proposed ramp location. Extra expenditure might be required to change some of the permanent fittings and fixtures to accommodate the ramp. If there is an extreme level change that requires a long, circuitous ramp or, if space is limited, a vertical lift may be a more appropriate design solution.

RAMP DESIGN FEATURES AND ELEMENTS

The following features and design elements are important for occupational therapists to consider when designing a ramp.

Length

The ramp run is the horizontal distance the ramp must travel from entrance threshold to the surface or level of the ground (also called *grade*; NAHB Research Center, 2006).

If a short and long ramp are placed on the same height step or rise (the vertical distance the ramp must rise from the grade to the entrance threshold; NAHB Research Center, 2006), the quicker the wheelchair ramp will increase in steepness, whereas a longer wheelchair ramp will be less steep. Ramps with long runs might be fatiguing for people to negotiate and more hazardous to descend compared with shorter ramps (Hunter, 1992). It is best to design a ramp that will result in the shortest length possible by taking advantage of the high points on the existing site grade (Center for Universal Design, 2004).

Gradient or Running Slope

The ramp gradient or running slope is the rate of incline expressed in a ratio or in degrees (NAHB Research Center, 2006). Ramp gradient should be constant between landings or changes in direction. If the characteristics and requirements of the ramp user are not known or if the ramp is to be used by a range of people, the gradients recommended in the access standards should be used as a guide (Hunter, 1992).

A ramp gradient of 1:3 is steeper than a ramp gradient of 1:12. The steeper the gradient, the harder to wheel up and down the slope. A shallow ramp gradient might be suitable for people who push themselves in their wheelchair. A steeper gradient might be more appropriate for someone who uses a scooter or electric wheelchair manufactured to suit steeper inclines and long distances. Further, there might be space restrictions limiting the run length of the ramp, resulting in the need for a short, steep ramp, but this would only be provided if the client is able to safely manage this type of design. As indicated earlier, therapists will need to consider manufacturers' information regarding the maximum safe gradient that the equipment can negotiate. The shallower the gradient, the more likely it will suit a large range of people with different disabilities and equipment (Hunter, 1992).

The therapist will also need to consider the age- and disease-related deterioration of the person over time, because the gradient can become one of the most significant features of the ramp, influencing a person's mobility over time. For example, a person in a wheelchair might experience upper-limb joint deterioration and pain over time, affecting his or her capacity to wheel up and down a ramp. Older people and people with a disability who are ambulant may experience fatigue as they ascend a ramp and joint pain in the lower limbs on descent, depending on their heath condition or disability.

The transition between a ramp and landing needs to be smooth to ensure that wheelchairs do not have to negotiate changes in surface levels. The gradients of the two surfaces that are transitioning should be shallow enough to ensure that wheelchair foot-plates do not catch when moving from one surface to another (e.g., from the landing onto the ramp). Further, the angle of the transition from the ramp to the landing and vice versa needs to be such that the four wheels on a wheelchair are always on a surface. This is important to ensure that there is no twist or instability or displacement of the person's center of gravity, which can result in the individual falling out of his or her equipment as the equipment transitions across the surfaces.

When compared with curved ramps, straight runs are preferred for easier maneuverability and landing construction (NAHB Research Center, 2006). On a curved ramp, the gradient might need to be shallower than that of a straight ramp to ensure the equipment does not roll off of the ramp edge on the turns. There will need to be a reduction in the curved ramp gradient in proportion to the decreasing radii of the curvature so that a ramp with a smaller curve has a shallower gradient than a ramp with a larger curve (Hunter, 1992).

Ramps can be L-shaped, switchback, or U-shaped, with landings at the changes in direction (Center for Universal Design, 2004). Ramps can be configured in these arrangements as a result of limitations of space and the presence of permanent structures (Center for Universal Design, 2004).

Cross-Slope or Cross-Fall

The slope perpendicular to the direction of travel is the cross-slope (NAHB Research Center, 2006). A shallow slope, rather than a flat surface, is required on the ramp to ensure water drains away or small particles or loose objects run off the area. If the cross-slope is too steep, it is difficult to control the direction of the wheelchair or scooter, and the person may tip over in his or her equipment. On curved ramps, the cross-slope should fall toward the center of the curvature of the ramp (Hunter, 1992).

Vertical and Horizontal Clearance

The ramp width provides horizontal clearance for the person and his or her equipment. The ramp might need to be wider than the measurements in the access standards along its run or at the landings where the wheelchair turns to ensure that long and wide equipment can fit on the turns and through doorways that open onto landings.

The space above the ramp surface provides vertical clearance, and it is to be free of obstructions to ensure people who might vary in height and who might use a range of equipment are safe mobilizing along the ramp. For example, windowsills, windows, window shades, light fittings, or trees might need to be altered to ensure that the necessary vertical clearance is attained. Occupational therapists need to check with design/construction professionals about building code requirements regarding the minimum height for vertical clearance above the surface of the ramp.

Landings

Landings are the intermediate platforms between sloped segments of a ramp (NAHB Research Center, 2006). They are also required at the top and bottom of the ramp run and at any point where there is a change in direction.

Landings should be level or have a very shallow gradient and be large enough to accommodate the length of the person using his or her mobility equipment. Landings provide a flat surface on which people can rest. If designed wide enough and long enough, landings can provide a surface on which wheelchairs and other equipment can change direction safely without any wheels leaving the ramp surface.

The interim landing should be as wide as the widest ramp run leading to this landing. The length dimension may vary, depending on the turning space requirements of the person with a disability and his or her equipment.

Therapists will need to examine the path of travel leading up to and away from the landing areas to ensure that the ramp is suitably positioned for ease of access from other areas of the yard. Landings should not intrude or terminate in areas that do not provide sufficient space for the person and his or her equipment to exit or enter the ramp.

The door circulation space on landings needs to be considered where a ramp leads to a landing that has a doorway. A door might swing inward or outward, which can influence the size of the landing required near this area. It is useful to refer to access standards and observe the movement of the person with their equipment and carer at the doorway to guide the design of the landing in relation to the door clearance, the direction of door swing, and approach.

Rails

Rails are the horizontal member supported by vertical posts and include top, mid-rails, and curbs; the mid-rail is a rail positioned midway between the top railing member and the deck of the ramp or the ramp surface, and the curb is positioned near the decking at the edge of the ramp (NAHB Research Center, 2006).

Rails act as a barrier to prevent individuals and their equipment from falling off the edge of the ramp. They are also used as a support to help people maintain their balance as they ascend or descend the ramp. Clients who might benefit from the use of rails on ramps include people with sensory impairment or those who lack stamina.

Rails should begin in the ramp approach and departure zones to act as an indicator of the start and finish of the ramp. They should be located on both sides of a ramp and be continuous. They should not, however, protrude into a person's path of travel, particularly when there is a 90-degree approach to a ramp. The ends of the rails should turn to the side or down, close to the final balustrade. These types of terminations to the rails will ensure that people are not injured when approaching or passing the landing area at the top or bottom of the ramp.

Rails can provide support for people making the transition onto or from a level landing area (Hunter, 1992). Bilateral rails provide better support than just one rail, especially if people have the use of only one arm when ascending and descending the ramp or if a person needs support on both sides of the ramp.

Clients might not use the rail or they might use it only as a guide, without holding onto it firmly. But if clients hold the rails for support, they should be rounded or elliptical in shape to ensure their hand can grasp them easily, with clearance above and below the rail. They can be made of wood, metal, or polyvinyl chloride (PVC) supported at intervals by brackets (NAHB Research Center, 2006). Clearance is required to the side of handrails to ensure the hand is able to run along the rail without getting caught or fingers getting injured.

Rails with a round or elliptical shape should have fittings attached to the underside with finger clearance so the hand can run freely along the rail length. The fixture adjoining the rail to a wall or a support post should be supportive enough to allow the rail to take significant body weight in any direction as indicated in the access standards.

Any bends in the rails need to have a smooth finish to ensure there are no sharp edges on which people can hurt themselves if they run their hands along the surface.

Balustrades may be required by the national construction code, where the surface of the ramp sits high above the adjacent ground. This feature is required to ensure the safety of children and is designed to prevent them gaining access through the railings and being at risk of having a fall. If a balustrade needs to be provided, it is usually a requirement that a handrail is installed to enable the person to hold onto a support.

Curb or Edge Protection

In some countries, curbs are required on ramps and are installed directly underneath rails or set back from the inner edge of the rails to ensure the wheels on mobility equipment do not roll off the edge of the ramp. Curbs should be installed on each side of ramp runs and at each side of ramp landings. They might not be required if there is a wall adjacent to the ramp that can act as a curb, or if the landing adjacent and extending out for a distance is level with the ramp edges. This level edge ensures that if someone rolls off of the edge of the ramp, he or she is still on a safe, flat surface.

Curbs can aid people who are blind or who have a vision impairment and who use a cane to guide their mobility. This edge protection provides a surface along which the cane can run for wayfinding as the person walks along the ramp, or to allow a wheelchair to turn into the curb and use its front caster to stop on the slope.

Curbs should be installed so that they are flush with the inside face of the rail and should not intrude into the horizontal circulation space of the ramp. They are to be high enough to prevent footplates catching on them or riding over the top of them.

Construction Materials

A range of materials can be used to construct a ramp, and the materials selected might depend on a client's budget and the type of finish he or she wishes to achieve. The choice of ramp material might be determined by maintenance requirements and how well it can withstand weather conditions and manage loads. Further, it is important that the ramp can be used in all weather conditions, so chosen materials should guarantee traction and slip resistance when wet. National construction codes might have a mandatory requirement that the surface of the ramp provide slip resistance.

Additionally, ramps might require specific materials and finishes to prevent termite damage. This is an issue that will need to be discussed with the builder, particularly if termites are prevalent in the client's residential area.

Weight Limit

Lightweight materials make the ramp easier to transport and for builders to install, although the final construction will need to take the weight of a range of loads. The supplier or builder of any ramp should state the maximum load limit for the structure.

Therapists working with a designer or builder of a ramp will need to consider, for example, the following:

+ The weight of the client in the wheelchair or scooter

+ The weight of the person's caregiver, if the client requires assistance to wheel up and down ramps

+ The weight of a number of people standing on the ramp

+ The weight being taken by the ramp if it is used during the process of moving furniture or other items in and out of the home

Adaptability

It is useful to question whether the ramp can be installed in such a way as to allow it to be dismantled and removed or modified in the future (e.g., if the ramp is to be stored and reconstructed at a later date or at an alternative location, or if the landings and ramp surfaces need to be widened to accommodate larger equipment). The ramp might need to be dismantled, stored, and reconstructed again in an alternative location. Simple and easy assembly and installation can contribute to reduced transport and building labor costs and increased adaptability.

In situations where a permanent ramp cannot be installed, a temporary ramp might be the preferred solution. The longer the temporary ramp, the heavier and more awkward it might be to manage, depending on the materials used for its construction. Further, the temporary ramp needs to be installed in such a way that ensures that it is positioned firmly and securely on two surfaces.

Lighting

Adequate lighting of an external ramp is required to ensure that the features of the ramp are easily distinguished day or night in varying weather conditions. A sensor light at the door to activate the outdoor lighting prevents having to consider the location of switches along the path leading to the ramp.

Obstacles

The ramp should extend into areas where there are no obstacles (e.g., clotheslines, garden sheds, driveways, garages or carports, garden beds, push-out windows, or brick sills on windows). If there are obstacles in the area of the proposed ramp, these will need to be removed or modified or the ramp designed to accommodate the obstructions.

When planning the ramp design and location, therapists will also need to consider the location of in-ground drainage or sewer pipes for easy access by tradesmen. A ramp should not sit over ground pipes because it will be difficult for plumbers to gain access to undertake repair work.

Local Building Codes and Permit Issues

In the United States, local building codes might have requirements for ramps based on safety, health, and welfare rather than access. Safety issues might include information about the slope of the ramp, the amount of weight that the rail has to withstand, landing size, and the distance between the balusters on a ramp railing. Local code and permit requirements might need to be considered and federal codes consulted for guidance or for compliance information (Center for Universal Design, 2004; NAHB Research Center, 2006). The therapist might need to consult with the builder or local inspection or planning office for advice regarding planning or legislative requirements regarding the design or construction (Center for Universal Design, 2004).

Other countries, such as Australia, have a national construction code as well as a range of design or manufacturing standards relating to the construction of permanent or temporary ramps, including standards for slip resistance of surfaces, loads, the construction of aluminum and steel structures, and the construction of fixed platforms and walkways. This information can be used in discussions with design and building professionals on the design of ramps.

Cost of Installation

It is important to compare the cost-effectiveness of providing a ramp in relation to the installation of a stair lift, lift, or relocation of the client to an alternative accommodation. The longer the ramp, the more expensive it will be and the greater the area it will occupy. It might be more expensive than a lift or stair lift, which can be more aesthetically pleasing, easier to manage, and take up less space. A lift or stair lift can be removed and sold or relocated, and the external area of the home restored to its original design.

CONSIDERATIONS WHEN LOCATING AN EXTERNAL RAMP

Location of the Ramp

A home may have one step up from ground level or a set of stairs. There could be one or several entries into the home. When siting a ramp, all access points to the home and access areas around the home, including the slope of the land, need to be investigated. It is important to determine where the person enters the property (e.g., through the front gate and path or always through the garage or carport). Ramps might be installed to provide access to and from the house to the area where the car might be parked, or they can run to and from a path that leads out of the property and onto the street.

Establishing the Ramp Design

Rise of the Ramp

The first step to determining the length of a ramp in a specific location is to measure the rise, or the vertical distance from the ground level to the height of the landing. The height of the landing at the door is usually the starting point for measuring the ramp.

The end point of the ramp will be the grade or ground where the features of a landing are needed. There might already be a path or concreted area at the end of the ramp that can act as the landing; consequently, a separate landing might not need to be installed.

Ramp Gradient, Length, and Direction

The measurement of the rise and information about the slope direction of the land will influence the run length and the direction of the ramp. If the land slopes up away from the home, running the ramp away from the house will result in a short ramp (Figure D-1). If land slopes down away from the home, running the ramp away from the house will result in a very long ramp (Figure D-2).

Essential Measurements that Guide the Design

As indicated previously, important measurements for the ramp design include the following:

- The overall occupied length and width of the equipment, influencing the length and width of the level landings and the width of the ramp
- The turning space of the equipment (from 90 to 360 degrees), affecting the length and width of the landings on entry and exit and the width of entry landings
- The reach range of the person, influencing the height of rails
- Space for the caregiver standing behind or beside the client and his or her equipment, determining the width of the ramp, and the width and length of landings

Equipment and Resources

The equipment required to measure up for a ramp includes the following:

- Tape measure (at least 16-ft/5,000-mm long) to measure dimensions
- Small spirit level that can hang on string or a clinometer
- String to use to show the length of the ramp from the start of the ramp to the point of termination
- Tent pegs for tying the string to at ground level
- Access standards and design guides to direct the design of the ramp

Builders and other design/construction professionals may possess more sophisticated electronic equipment to measure up for a ramp, such as a laser level.

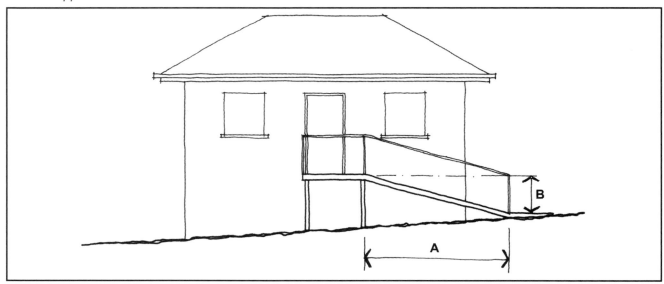

Figure D-1. Land sloping up away from the home and running a ramp toward the slope. (Reprinted with permission from Paul Coonan.)

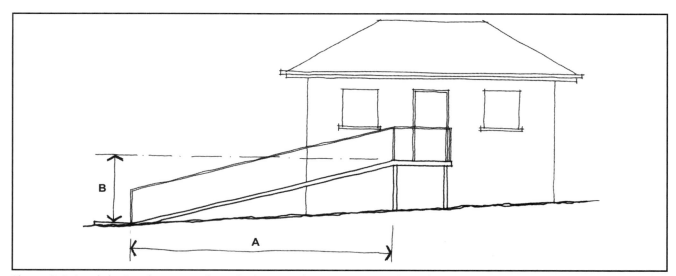

Figure D-2. Land sloping down away from the home and running a ramp along the slope. (Reprinted with permission from Paul Coonan.)

Measuring the Gradient of the Land

The therapist can measure the gradient of land with a spirit level or two uprights placed a distance apart and a horizontal line to measure the distance between them (Figure D-3). The bubble in the spirit level is to be located centrally to denote a horizontal position. The gradient in the diagram is the X measurement in relation to the Y measurement. Alternatively, Figure D-4 shows the rise in relation to the length and the resulting gradient. Units are usually expressed in inches or in metric measurement (Tables D-1 and D-2).

Calculating the Length of a Straight Ramp in Relation to the Gradient of the Ramp and the Fall of the Land—Level Land

✦ Identify the height, length, and width dimensions of the landing required at the entrance to the home.

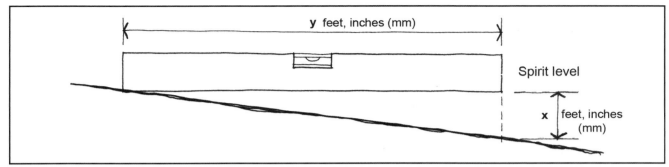

Figure D-3. Measuring the gradient of the land with a spirit level. (Reprinted with permission from Paul Coonan.)

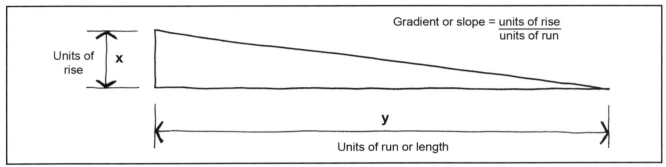

Figure D-4. The rise in relation to length. (Reprinted with permission from Paul Coonan.)

Table D-1. Gradient Table for 1:12 Gradient

	X:Y	*GRADIENT*
Imperial	3 7/8 in:47 1/4 in	1:12
Metric	100 mm:1,200 mm	

Table D-2. Gradient Table for 1:14 Gradient

	X:Y	*GRADIENT*
Imperial	3 7/8 in:55 1/4 in	1:14
Metric	100 mm:1,400 mm	

✦ Fix the end of the string to the outer edge of the proposed landing where the ramp will start (Figure D-5).

✦ Extend the string to the proposed point of termination of the ramp and place the spirit level in the middle of the extended string line.

✦ At the point of the proposed termination of the ramp, pull the string tight and ensure that it is level by checking the small spirit level. The most accurate reading will be achieved by placing the spirit level in the middle of the total length of the string. The bubble needs to be located at the center of the spirit level to indicate that the string is level. Alternatively, the clinometer can be held on the string to judge whether it is level.

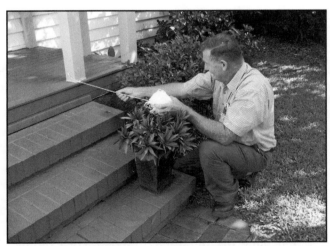

Figure D-5. Fixing the string to the outer edge of the proposed landing.

Table D-3. Examples of Gradient Calculation

| | GRADIENT – 1:12 | | GRADIENT – 1:14 | |
	Imperial	Metric	Imperial	Metric
A	168 3/4 in	4,286 mm	196 7/8 in	5,000 mm
B	14 3/16 in	360 mm	14 3/16 in	360 mm

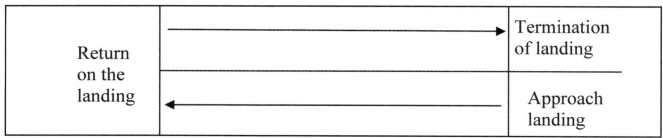

Figure D-6. Site plan view of a ramp with a switchback or turn that has a level landing.

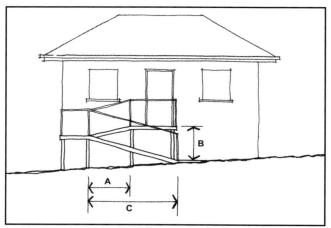

Figure D-7. Ramp with a switchback or turn that has a level landing (refer to Table D-5). (Reprinted with permission from Paul Coonan.)

✦ At the point of proposed start of the ramp, measure the distance from the landing to the ground. Multiply this measurement by the gradient you wish to achieve (e.g., 1:12 or 1:14) to determine the required length of the ramp. Once you know the length needed to cover the fall, measure the length of the string and extend it to the required ramp length. Then remeasure the drop from the string to the ground and calculate the ramp length again. For example, if the landing height is 24 in, or 2 ft (600 mm), multiply this figure by 12 to get the estimated length of the ramp. The length will be 288 in, or 24 ft (7.2 m) for a 1:12 ramp (on level land).

Alternatively, divide the measurement of the string to the ground into the length dimension of the string line to determine the gradient of the ramp and whether ending the ramp at this point would result in it being shallower or steeper than the desired gradient. For example, for a 1:12 gradient, the string should be dropped 1 in per ft length toward the ground. If the distance from the string to the ground is 14.1875 in (360 mm) and the length of the string from the starting point of the ramp is 168.75 in (4,286 mm), the gradient of the ramp will be 1:12 (Table D-3).

Calculating the Length of a Straight Ramp With a Switchback or Return in Relation to the Gradient of the Ramp and the Fall of the Land—Level Land or Land Running Away From the House

If there is insufficient room for a straight ramp or if the ground falls away from the home, increasing the fall and the length of the ramp, it may be necessary to incorporate a switchback or turn that has a level landing to have a more appropriate length and endpoint (Figures D-6 and D-7). Installing a ramp on land that slopes away from the home may be problematic, as the ramp may be quite long or not touch the ground within the confines of the area, even with the desired gradient.

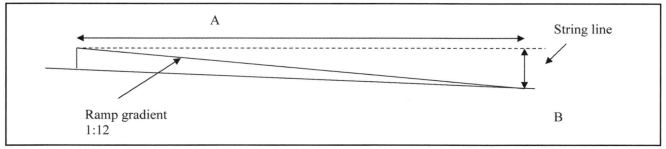

Figure D-8. Land sloping away from the home for a longer ramp. Extending a string line level (A) and measuring the distance from the horizontal line to the ground (B) to establish the gradient.

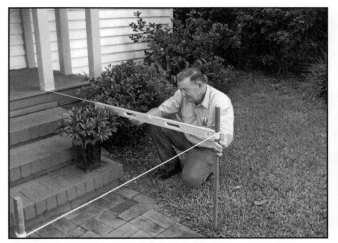

Figure D-9. Checking the level of the landing section.

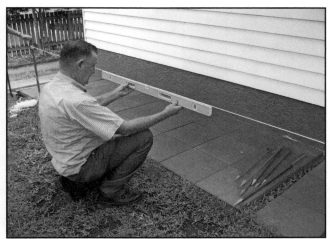

Figure D-10. Measuring the level of the line.

✦ Identify the height, length, and width dimensions of the landing required at the entrance to the home.

✦ Fix the end of string to the outer edge of the proposed landing where the ramp will start.

✦ Extend the string, pull it tight, and ensure that it is level by checking the small string level that is hung centrally on the string or using a spirit level to measure the level (Figures D-8 through D-11).

✦ Divide the calculated ramp length and add the landing dimension to determine where the ramp would be located as it turns. Adjust the ramp length to suit the location of the landing but maintain a consistent gradient on the slope (Figures D-7; D-12 through D-14).

✦ Pull the string level to the point where the interim landing would start, and measure from this point back to the edge of the first landing. Measure the distance of the string to the ground, and lower the string the required distance to achieve the desired gradient. For example, if there is a 15.75-in (400-mm) high landing and there is a need to install a 1:12

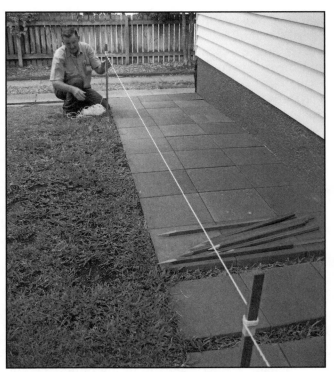

Figure D-11. Determining the size and position of the middle landing.

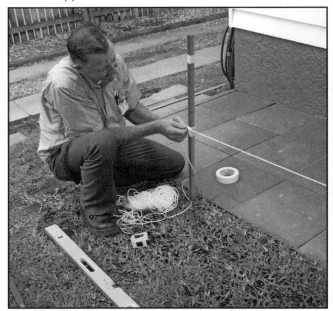

Figure D-12. Lowering the string to the landing level.

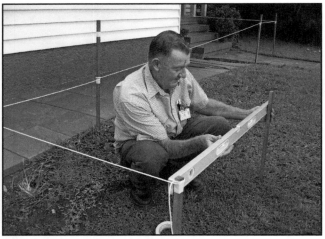

Figure D-13. Measuring the level of the landing.

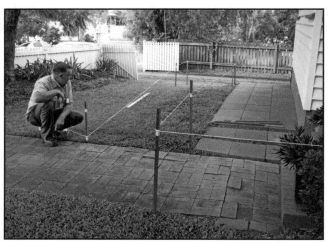

Figure D-14. The final proposed ramp set out with string.

gradient ramp, this measurement of the landing is multiplied by 12. The total length of the ramp will then be 189 in (4,800 mm). Divide the 189-in (4,800-mm) measurement and have the ramp-run sections sit between the location of the three sets of landings.

When dividing the ramp, it is not necessary to split the measurement for the ramp length evenly between the landings. Rather, the location of the interim landing is dependent on how the client wants the landing to look in relation to the rest of the home and the presence of available space and permanent structures (Tables D-4 and D-5).

Ramps may be designed in a range of configurations as illustrated in Figures D-15 through D-17.

Calculating the Length of a Straight Ramp in Relation to the Gradient of the Ramp and the Fall of the Land—Land Sloping Up Away From (or Toward) the House

Installing a straight ramp on land that slopes up away from the home (or toward the home as in Figure D-1) may be to the person's advantage even if the landing is positioned quite high above the ground. It may be possible to achieve the desired gradient despite the height of the landing. The focus for calculating where the end of the ramp will land on the ground in relation to the gradient is not the

landing height, but the gradient of the ramp, which can be replicated through the use of two pieces of string, a spirit level, and stakes.

✦ Fix the end of the first piece of string to the outer edge of the proposed landing where the ramp will start (Figure D-18).

✦ Extend the first piece of string, pull it tight, and ensure that it is level by checking the small string level that is hung centrally on the string or using a spirit level to measure the level. Attach the level string to a stake or tent peg (Figures D-18 through D-23).

✦ Fix a second piece of string to the outer edge of the proposed landing where the ramp will start. This string will be pulled out at an angle to match the proposed gradient of the ramp (Figures D-24 through D-28). To calculate a 1:12 gradient for the second string:

Table D-4. Examples of Gradient Calculation

	GRADIENT – 1:12		GRADIENT – 1:14	
	Imperial	**Metric**	**Imperial**	**Metric**
A	234 1/4 in	5,952 mm	275 5/8 in	7,000 mm
B	19 3/4 in	500 mm	19 3/4 in	500 mm

Table D-5. Example of Calculations for a Ramp With a Switchback or Turn That Has a Level Landing

	GRADIENT – 1:12		GRADIENT – 1:14	
	Imperial	**Metric**	**Imperial**	**Metric**
A	78 3/4 in	2,000 mm	78 3/4 in	2,000 mm
B	15 3/4 in	400 mm	15 3/4 in	400 mm
C	110 1/4 in	2,800 mm	141 3/4 in	3,600 mm

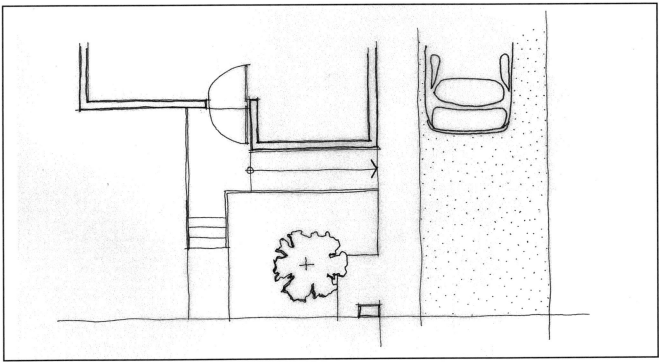

Figure D-15. Example of a part of a site plan showing a ramp location option for vehicle and house access. (Reprinted with permission from Paul Coonan.)

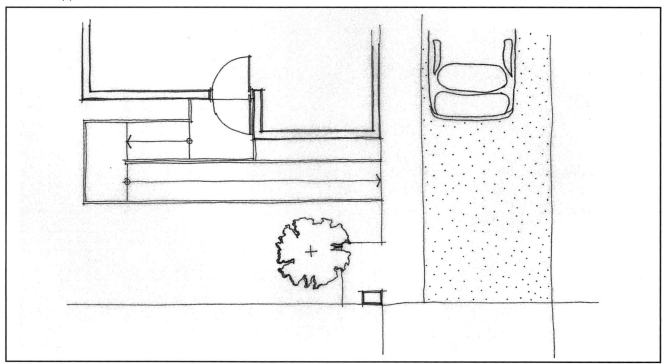

Figure D-16. Example of a part of a site plan showing a ramp location option for vehicle and house access. (Reprinted with permission from Paul Coonan.)

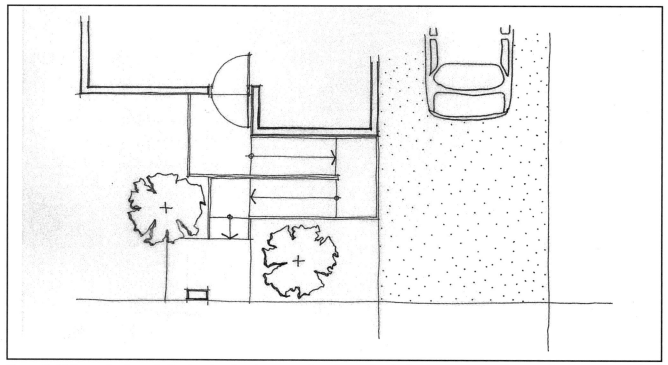

Figure D-17. Example of a part of a site plan showing a ramp location option for front entry access. (Reprinted with permission from Paul Coonan.)

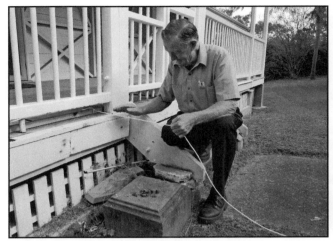

Figure D-18. Attaching the string to the landing.

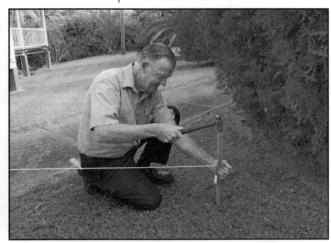

Figure D-19. Fastening the string to a stake.

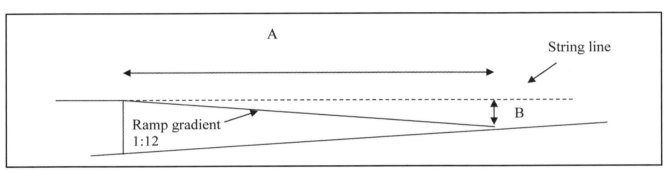

Figure D-20. Landing sloping toward the home for a shorter ramp. Extending a string line level (A) and measuring the distance from the horizontal line to the ground (B) to establish the gradient.

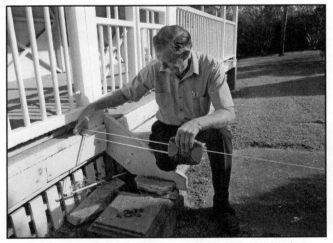

Figure D-21. Pulling the tape measure out from the landing.

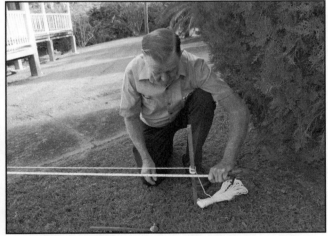

Figure D-22. Measuring the distance of the stake from the landing.

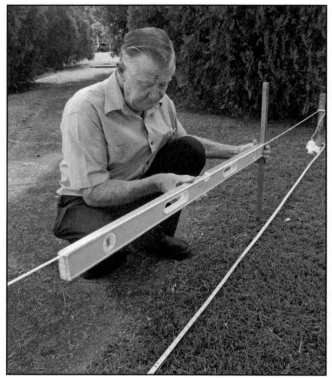

Figure D-23. Checking to ensure the string is level.

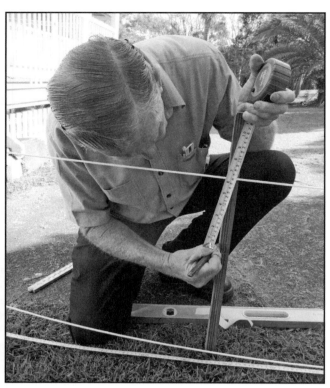

Figure D-24. Measuring the drop of the second string from the horizontal that will show the gradient of the ramp.

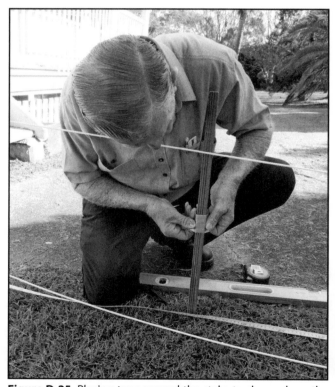

Figure D-25. Placing tape around the stake to show where the string will sit on an angle.

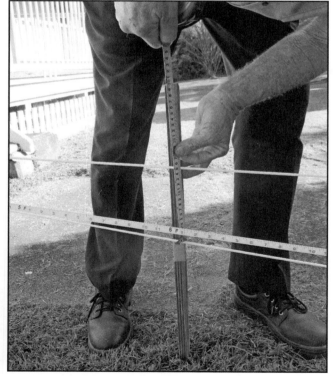

Figure D-26. Double checking measurements of distance from horizontal. Top string = horizontal; bottom string = showing the slope of the ramp surface.

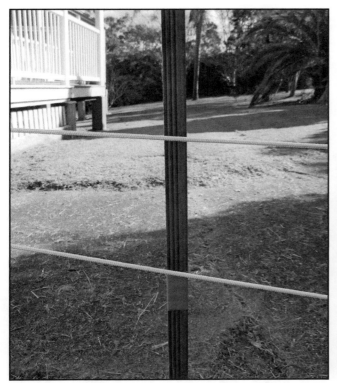

Figure D-27. Top string = horizontal; bottom string = showing the slope of the ramp surface.

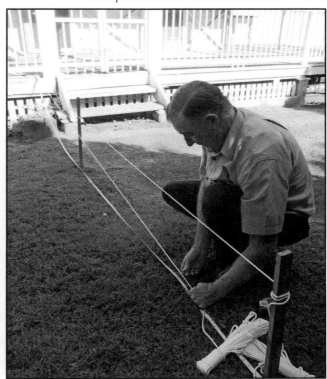

Figure D-28. Estimating where the string (ramp) will land on the ground.

✦ In imperial: Measure 3 ft along the horizontal string that extends out from the landing. At this point, measure down from the horizontal string a distance of 3 in and pull the string along to this point to create the 1:12 gradient. At 6 ft from the landing edge measure down from the horizontal string 6 in and adjust the second string to this endpoint; at 9 ft, measure down 9 in, etc (see Figures D-25 and D-26). By following this calculation, this second piece of string will slope toward the land at 1:12. Continue to measure along the horizontal string at set locations and down to the second string until the second string touches the land (see Figure D-28).

✦ In metric: Measure 1,000 mm along the horizontal string that extends out from the landing. At this point, measure down from the horizontal string a distance of 83 mm and pull the string along to this point to create the 1:12 gradient. At 2,000 mm from the landing edge, measure down from the horizontal string 166 mm and adjust the second string to this endpoint; at 3,000 mm, measure down 249 mm, etc (see Figure D-26). By following this calculation, this second piece of string

will slope toward the land at 1:12. Continue to measure along the horizontal string at set locations and down to the second string until the second string touches the land (see Figure D-28).

The figures for measurement are calculated as follows:

✦ For a 1:12 gradient calculation:

   ✦ 3 ft divided by 12 (for the 1:12 gradient) equates to 3 in, or 1,000 mm, divided by 12 (for 1:12 gradient) equates to approximately 83 mm

✦ For a 1:14 gradient calculation:

   ✦ 3 ft divided by 14 (for the 1:14 gradient) equates to 2.57 in, or 1,000 mm, divided by 14 (for 1:14 gradient) equates to approximately 72 mm

The ramp could be made shallower than the gradient if there is opportunity to do so, depending on the height and location of the sloped land opposite the landing.

Figures D-29 through D-31 illustrate the full stringing out of the ramp once the gradient of the string has been established.

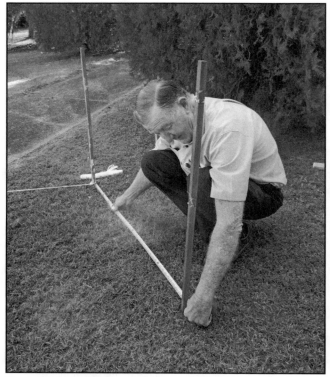

Figure D-29. Measuring out the width of the ramp.

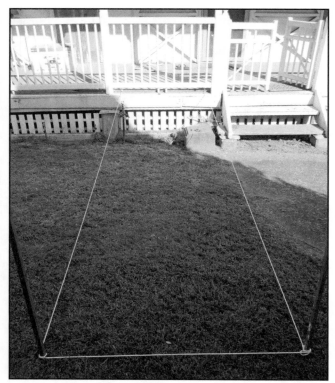

Figure D-30. Final ramp configuration.

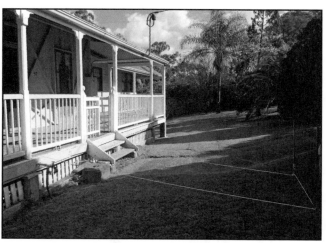

Figure D-31. Final ramp configuration, side view.

Alternative Options to Ramps

A ramp might not suit someone who cannot manage the gradient and length of the ramp or who requires stairs to ensure intentional foot lift and placement on a surface. In these instances, other cost-effective solutions might be available. For example, a no-step entry or zero-level entry can be created that allows a person to enter the home without negotiating steps. This type of entry may be created by regrading the yard and landscaping and adding a path or new landing over the existing level area at the bottom of the step at the entry (Center for Universal Design, 2004; NAHB Research Center, 2006). Landscaped options can be expensive but can have a longer lifespan and need less maintenance than ramps (Center for Universal Design, 2004).

If a house is high-set and located on flat land, it may be more appropriate to install a lift or stair lift than an excessively long ramp with many turns, which could be difficult to negotiate and expensive to install (Center for Universal Design, 2004). The choice of lift or stair lift will depend on the client's budget, the availability of space and vertical height for travel of the device, and the person's capacity to use the device, including operating the controls and maintaining a safe body position during its use.

Lifts vary in style and finishes and features, such as single or double entries, laminated mirrors, rails, an intercom, forced ventilation, and a fold-down chair. Lifts have rated weight loads, and cabin and landing doors can be automatically or manually operated.

Safety devices might also be fit to lifts. These can include safety switches, automatic return of the car to the ground floor, followed by automatic door opening in the event of power failure, accurate leveling at the floor, door protection devices, and an auto-call emergency communicator (for a bidirectional communication between the assistance center and the passengers in an emergency).

Stair lifts can be installed on internal or external stairs, depending on the type and style of construction of the stairs and the clearance along the length and top and bottom of the stairs for egress. Features include remote control or switch operation, swivel seats, armrests, seat belts, battery backup in the event of power failure, automatic shutoff if there is a collision with an obstruction, and the capacity to pace the rate of travel. They might have a platform design rather than a fold-down seat to accommodate a wheelchair.

Both vertical lifts and stair lifts are required to comply with industry standards in a range of countries, which ensures the quality of the manufactured item and the safety of the client using the equipment.

Occupational therapists need to consider whether one option is more suitable than the other by examining the ramp, stair lift, or lift in relation to various factors, including the following:

+ The client's capacity to manage each of these alternatives

+ How his or her mobility equipment will be accommodated by each option

+ The access needs of other household members

+ Whether each option suits the style and condition of the home

+ The cost of installing each option, as well as the associated building works

+ Whether there is sufficient space to incorporate each of the options

+ The appearance of the home from the street with respect to each option

+ Local building code and fire regulations for installation

To assist therapists in the assessment process, manufacturers and suppliers of stair lifts and lifts can provide advice on client factors and the possible structural changes to the home when incorporating the item as a home modification.

REFERENCES

Alderson, A. (2010). *Stairs, ramps, and escalators: Inclusive design guidance*. London, UK: RIBA Publishing.

Center for Universal Design. (2004). Wood ramp design: How to add a ramp that looks good and works too. Retrieved from https://www.ncsu.edu/ncsu/design/cud/pubs_p/docs/ramp-booklet296final.pdf

Goldsmith, S. (2000). *Universal design: A manual of practical guidance for architects*. Woburn, MA: Architectural Press.

Hunter, R. A. (1992). *More accessible housing for independent living: A guide to designing and adapting dwellings for the aged and people with disabilities*. City of Sale, Australia: McPherson's Printing.

NAHB Research Center. (2006). *Safety first: A technical approach to home modifications*. Washington, DC: Author.

Home Modification Practice Resources

This appendix has been generated as a starting point for occupational therapists to expand their resources to support their knowledge, skill development, and clinical application in the area of home modifications and design. It is important to note that it is not an exhaustive list of all of the available resources, but instead a guide for the types of information that are available to assist in learning, practice, and research in this area. Please note that resources, particularly those based on the internet, are subject to frequent change.

DEDICATED ORGANIZATIONS, RESOURCE SITES, AND GUIDES TO AGING, DISABILITY, HOME MODIFICATION, AND REMODELING

The following list contains information on organizations (profit and nonprofit), resource sites and guides that are generally relevant to home modification practice. The list is organized by region; however, many resources may be useful to clinicians who practice in different locations.

Asia

+ Center For Housing Renovation and Dispute Settlement Support: www.chord.or.jp/foundation/index.html

+ Hong Kong Housing Society: www.hkhs.com/eng/wnew/udg.asp

+ Japanese Society for Wellbeing Science and Assistive Technology: www.jswsat.org/index.html

+ Rehabilitation Engineering Society of Japan (RESJA): www.resja.or.jp/eng/index.html

Australia/New Zealand

+ Australian Housing and Urban Research Institute: www.ahuri.edu.au

+ Australian Network for Universal Housing Design: www.anuhd.org

+ Australian Rehabilitation and Assistive Technology Association: www.arata.org.au

+ Home Design for Living: http://homedesignfor-living.com

+ Home Modifications Australia: www.moda.org.au

+ Home Modification Information Clearinghouse (University of New South Wales, Australia): www.homemods.info

+ Independent Living Centres Australia: http://ilcaustralia.org.au

+ Lifemark: www.lifemark.co.nz

+ Livable Housing Australia: www.livablehousingaustralia.org.au

Ainsworth, E., & de Jonge, D. *An Occupational Therapist's Guide to Home Modification Practice, Second Edition (pp. 415–418).*

- ✦ New Zealand Ministry of Health: www.health. govt.nz/your-health/services-and-support/ disability-services/types-disability-support/ equipment-and-modifications-disabled-people/ housing-modifications-disabled-people
- ✦ Queensland Action for Universal Housing Design: www.qauhd.org
- ✦ Scope Home Access: www.scopehomeaccess. com.au
- ✦ Summer Foundation: www.summerfoundation. org.au
- ✦ Technical Aid to the Disabled Australia Inc.: www.tadaustralia.org.au

Canada

- ✦ Canadian Mortgage and Housing Corporation: www.cmhc-schl.gc.ca/en
- ✦ iDAPT—Toronto Rehabilitation Institute: www. idapt.org
- ✦ March of Dimes Canada: www.marchofdimes.ca/ EN/programs/hvmp/Pages/HomeandVehicle. aspx

Europe

- ✦ Handisam (Sweden): www.mfd.se

International

- ✦ HOUZZ: www.houzz.com

United Kingdom

- ✦ Care and Repair Cymru: www.careandrepair. org.uk/en
- ✦ Care and Repair England: www.careandrepair-england.org.uk
- ✦ Care and Repair Ireland: www.ageaction.ie/ how-we-can-help/care-and-repair
- ✦ Care and Repair Scotland: www.careandre-pairscotland.co.uk
- ✦ Centre for Accessible Environments: www.cae. org.uk
- ✦ Centre for Ageing Better: www.ageing-better. org.uk
- ✦ Habinteg: www.habinteg.org.uk
- ✦ Helen Hamlyn Centre for Design, Royal College of Art: www.rca.ac.uk/research-innovation/ helen-hamlyn-centre

- ✦ Home Adaptations Consortium: www.homead-aptationsconsortium.wordpress.com
- ✦ Housing Learning and Improvement Network (Housing LIN): www.housinglin.org.uk
- ✦ Joseph Rowntree Foundation: www.jrf.org.uk
- ✦ Lifetime Homes: www.lifetimehomes.org.uk
- ✦ Royal College of Occupational Therapists, United Kingdom—genHOME: www.rcot.co.uk/ about-us/specialist-sections/housing-rcot-ss/ genhome

United States of America

- ✦ American Association of Retired Persons (AARP) Livable Communities: http://www.aarp. org/livable-communities
- ✦ Better Living Design: www.betterlivingdesign. org
- ✦ Department of Housing and Urban Development (HUD): https://www.hud.gov/ topics/information_for_disabled_persons
- ✦ National Council on Independent Living, Visitability: www.visitability.org
- ✦ National Directory of Home Modification and Repair Resources: https://homemods.org/ national-directory
- ✦ National Kitchen+Bathroom Association: https://nkba.org
- ✦ National Resource Center on Supportive Housing and Home Modifications at the University of Southern California, Leonard Davis School of Gerontology: www.homemods.org

ORGANIZATIONS AND RESOURCE SITES FOR HOME MODIFICATION AND REMODELING RELATED TO SPECIFIC AREAS OF CLINICAL PRACTICE

The following list contains examples of organization and resource sites that include information that pertains to home modification and remodeling related to specific populations or areas of clinical practice. This is once again not intended as an exhaustive list but provides evidence of the types of information that can be found that may be specific to an area of clinical practice or expertise. Some of the examples listed have been included in the general list provided earlier but include specific information relevant to a specific population or clinical area, so they have been listed here again.

Aging

United States of America

✦ American Association of Retired Persons (AARP) Policy and Research: www.aarp.org

Autism

United Kingdom

✦ Helen Hamlyn Centre for Design, Royal College of Art: www.rca.ac.uk/research-innovation/helen-hamlyn-centre

Bariatrics

Australia

✦ Australasian Bariatric Innovations Group (AUSBIG): www.ausbig.com.au

Dementia

Australia

✦ HammondCare: www.hammond.com.au

United Kingdom

✦ Centre for Excellence in Universal Design: http://universaldesign.ie/Built-Environment/Housing
✦ Dementia Services Development Centre (DSDC): http://dementia.stir.ac.uk

Keeping Populations Healthy

United States of America

✦ Center for Active Design: https://centerforactivedesign.org

Minor Modifications

Australia

✦ Queensland Department of Public Works and Housing: www.redcliffetpi.com/uploads/1/2/3/3/12330600/100_ways_to_improve_home_access.pdf

United Kingdom

✦ Housing Executive: www.nihe.gov.uk

Pediatrics

United Kingdom

✦ Joseph Rowntree Foundation: www.jrf.org.uk
✦ Professor Rob Imrie, London University: www.universalisingdesign.info

United States of America

✦ My Child at Cerebral Palsy: www.mychildatcerebralpalsy.org

Vision Impairment

Australia

✦ Vision Australia: https://visionaustralia.org/community/news/20-06-2017/household-modifications-how-older-people-can-enjoy-the-comfort-of-their-own-home-for-longer

United States of America

✦ American Foundation for the Blind: www.afb.org/info/low-vision/living-with-low-vision/creating-a-comfortable-environment-for-people-with-low-vision/235

EDUCATION OPPORTUNITIES VIA HOME MODIFICATION WEBINARS/WEBCASTS

The following two organizations are examples of groups that provide online educational opportunities for occupational therapists who are interested in developing their knowledge and skills in home modification practice through further professional development.

Australia

✦ Home Design for Living: http://homedesignforliving.com/blog

United States of America

✦ American Occupational Therapy Association: www.aota.org/webcasts

DEDICATED ORGANIZATIONS, RESOURCE SITES, AND GUIDES RELEVANT TO DESIGN

The following list contains information on organizations, resource sites, and guides that are available and discuss design in a more general sense. These resources often contain information that is relevant to universal design, design for all, and inclusive design, which are concepts that apply to environments beyond just the home. The list is organized again by region, but resources will frequently be applicable and of interest to clinicians who practice in different locations.

Asia

✦ International Association for Universal Design (Japan): www.iaud.net/global

Australia/New Zealand

✦ Centre for Universal Design Australia: www.universaldesignaustralia.net.au

Europe

✦ European Design for All e-Accessibility Network (EDeAN): https://tecnoaccesible.net/node/779

✦ EIDD—Design for All Europe: http://dfaeurope.eu

✦ iF World Design Guide (Germany): www.ifworld-designguide.com

United Kingdom

✦ Centre for Excellence in Universal Design: www.universaldesign.ie

✦ Design Council: www.designcouncil.org.uk

✦ Inclusive Design Toolkit, University of Cambridge, UK: www.inclusivedesigntoolkit.com/whatis/whatis.html

✦ OPENspace: www.openspace.eca.ed.ac.uk

✦ Professor Rob Imrie, London University: http://universalisingdesign.info

✦ The Institute for Design and Disability: www.idd.ie

United States of America

✦ Center for Active Design: https://centerforactivedesign.org

✦ Center for Inclusive Design and Environmental Access (IDEA), Buffalo: http://idea.ap.buffalo.edu

✦ Center for Universal Design, College of Design, North Carolina State University: https://projects.ncsu.edu/design/cud/

✦ Early Childhood Technical Assistance Center (ECTAC): http://ectacenter.org/topics/atech/udl.asp

✦ The RL Mace Universal Design Institute: www.udinstitute.org

SOCIAL NETWORKING OPPORTUNITIES RELATED TO HOME MODIFICATIONS AND DESIGN

Social media and social networking are currently being used widely in order to share and disseminate information that is relevant to home modifications and design. Social networking sites (e.g., Facebook, Twitter, LinkedIn) are frequently established and used by professional groups and organizations as a way to provide information and support for therapists and professionals working in applicable fields. The following is a list of some organizations and professional groups who provide social networking opportunities that are relevant to areas of home modification and design.

✦ Association of Consultants in Access Australia: Available via Facebook and Twitter

✦ Australian Network for Universal Housing Design: Available via Facebook and Twitter

✦ Centre for Universal Design Australia: Available via Facebook, Twitter, and LinkedIn

✦ HomeMods4OT: Available via Facebook

✦ Home Design for Living: Available via Facebook, Twitter, and LinkedIn

Access Standards Resources

Australia

✦ Standards Australia (SA): www.standards.org.au

Canada

✦ Canadian Standards Association (CSA): www.csagroup.org

China

✦ Standardization Administration of the People's Republic of China (SAC): www.sac.gov.cn/sacen

Japan

✦ Japanese Standards Association (JSA): www.jsa.or.jp/en

Korea

✦ Korean Standards Association (KSA): http://eng.ksa.or.kr/ksa_english/index.do

New Zealand

✦ Standards New Zealand: www.standards.govt.nz

Norway

✦ Standards Norway: www.standard.no/en

Sweden

✦ Swedish Standards Institute (SSI): www.sis.se/en

Ainsworth, E., & de Jonge, D. *An Occupational Therapist's Guide to Home Modification Practice, Second Edition (pp. 419-420).*
© 2019 SLACK Incorporated.

UNITED KINGDOM

+ British Standards Institution (BSI): www.bsigroup.com
+ National Standards Authority of Ireland (NSAI): www.nsai.ie

UNITED STATES OF AMERICA

+ American National Standards Institute (ANSI): www.ansi.org
+ ADA Accessibility Guidelines (ADAAG; as amended through September 2002): www.access-board.gov/guidelines-and-standards/buildings-and-sites/about-the-ada-standards/background/adaag

+ Uniform Federal Accessibility Standards (UFAS; 1984): www.access-board.gov/guidelines-and-standards/buildings-and-sites/about-the-aba-standards/ufas
+ Revised ADA-ABA Guidelines (2004): www.access-board.gov/attachments/article/412/ada-aba.pdf

OTHER INTERNATIONAL RESOURCE

+ International Organization for Standardization (ISO): www.iso.org/iso/about.htm

APPENDIX G

Home Visit Checklist

Ainsworth, E., & de Jonge, D. *An Occupational Therapist's Guide to Home Modification Practice, Second Edition* (pp. 421-432).
© 2019 SLACK Incorporated.

HOME VISIT CHECKLIST

MAY BE PHOTOCOPIED AND USED ON HOME VISIT

Confidential

Name:

Address:

Phone Number:

Date of Birth:

File Number:

Source of Request:

Date of Request:

Documentation on File:

Consent to contact others	YES	NO
Permission to take images	YES	NO
Health information	YES	NO

Appointment Made:

Date of Visit:

Present at Visit:

Occupational Therapist:

Health Condition/Disability-Specific Information (relevant to housing/home modification needs only):

Level of Mobility (include community access):
_____   Independently mobile—no assistive devices
_____   Independently mobile using a single-point walking stick
_____   Independently mobile using a four-point walking stick
_____   Independently mobile using a walking frame
_____   Independently mobile using a wheeled walking frame
_____   Independently mobile using a manual wheelchair

CLIENT: FILE NUMBER:

Page 1 of 11

_____   Uses a manual wheelchair—dependent on others to push
_____   Independently mobile using a powered wheelchair
_____   Dependent for mobility
_____   Mobilizes on floor
_____   Other

Static/dynamic sitting balance: _____
_____

Static/dynamic standing balance: _____
_____

Level of coordination: _____
_____

Physical endurance: _____

Ability to manage stairs: _____

Ability to manage ramp: _____

Ability to manage hills: _____

Ability to manage uneven ground: _____

Access to community (including use of public transport—bus, train, cab): _____

Other: _____

Transfers

Bed
_____   Independent rolling
_____   Assistance required to roll
_____   Independent on and off the bed
_____   Managing transfers on and off the bed with difficulty
_____   Requires assistance from one person to transfer on and off the bed
_____   Requires hoist transfers on and off the bed
_____   Other

Chair
_____   Independent moving from sitting to standing
_____   Managing transfers with difficulty
_____   Requires assistance from one person to transfer

CLIENT: **FILE NUMBER:**

Page 2 of 11

<u>Toilet</u>

_____	Independent
_____	Managing transfers with difficulty—benefit from grab bars
_____	Uses over-toilet frame
_____	Uses mobile shower commode—self-propelled
_____	Uses mobile shower commode—attendant-propelled
_____	Requires assistance from one person to transfer
_____	Other

<u>Shower</u>

_____	Independent transferring in/out of bath to access shower
_____	Managing to transfer in/out of bath/shower with difficulty
_____	Has/requires grab bars
_____	Has/requires bath board
_____	Has/requires shower hose
_____	Has/requires folding shower seat
_____	Uses/needs shower recess
_____	Can manage hob
_____	Needs hob-free or level access
_____	Requires assistance from one person to transfer
_____	Other

<u>Bath</u>

_____	Independent
_____	Problems getting in/out of bath
_____	Has/requires grab bars
_____	Has/requires handheld shower
_____	Has/requires bath board
_____	Has/requires tub transfer bench
_____	Requires assistance from one person to transfer
_____	Other

<u>Car</u>

_____	Independent
_____	Problems getting in/out of car
_____	Has/requires handle on doorway
_____	Has/requires car hoist
_____	Requires assistance from one person to transfer
_____	Other

CLIENT: **FILE NUMBER:**

Page 3 of 11

Household Duties:

Heavy duties: _____

_____

Light duties: _____

_____

Shopping: _____

_____

Meal preparation: _____

_____

Laundry: _____

_____

Cleaning: _____

_____

Mowing and gardening: _____

_____

Household maintenance: _____

_____

Other: _____

_____

Use of Equipment—Current:

_____	Walking stick	_____	Bath trolley
_____	Walking frame	_____	Mobile shower commode (self-propelled)
_____	Wheeled walking frame	_____	Mobile shower commode (attendant-propelled)
_____	Crutches	_____	Scooter
_____	Manual wheelchair	_____	Perching stool
_____	Powered wheelchair	_____	Bed
_____	Over-toilet frame	_____	Floor-based hoist
_____	Toilet surround	_____	Tub transfer bench
_____	Shower chair (static)	_____	Other
_____	Bath board		

CLIENT: FILE NUMBER:

Page 4 of 11

<u>Use of Equipment – Future:</u>

<u>Measurements:</u>

Measurements—Client: Anthropometrics (sitting/standing; eye height; reach range):

Measurements—Client: Turning circle with equipment:

Measurements—Client's equipment:

Measurements—Carer's anthropometrics:

Other:

<u>Support Services:</u>

<u>Current Housing Situation—Description and Measurements of Existing Environment:</u>

1. Age, size, layout, and construction of accommodation:

2. Details of existing tenants/occupants and the relationship between them (is the accommodation underoccupied?):

3. External access:

Size of land: _____

Slope of land: _____

Access to street: _____

Access to yard areas (front, side, and rear): _____

Paths: _____

Vehicle access: _____

Carport/garage, door type, and access to home: _____

Mailbox: _____

Rubbish bin: _____

Clothesline: _____

Garden shed: _____

Type of fencing: _____

Height of fencing: _____

Location and type of gates: _____

Obstacles: _____

CLIENT: **FILE NUMBER:**

Page 5 of 11

Other comments:

Front Door Access:

Description: _____

Stairs: Measurements _____ Number _____ Rails _____ R _____ L _____

Landing: _____

Door: _____

Ramps: _____

Obstacles: _____

Other comments:

Rear Door Access:

Description: _____

Stairs: Number _____ Rails _____ R _____ L _____

Landings: _____

Ramps: _____

Obstacles: _____

Other comments:

Side Door Access:

Description: _____

Stairs: Number _____ Rails _____ R _____ L _____

Landings: _____

Ramps: _____

Obstacles: _____

Other comments:

CLIENT: **FILE NUMBER:**

4. Internal Access:

Hallway width: _____

Door entry: _____

Door widths: _____

Floor levels (changes in level, location, heights): _____

Room positions (e.g., right-angled off hall): _____

Other comments:

5. Bathroom: (separate diagrams required giving measurements)

Location and description: _____

Door type: _____

Door width: _____

Door handle type: _____

Door handle height: _____

Floor covering: _____

Wall surface: _____

Light switch: _____

Power point: _____

Other comments:

Bath:

Location and description: _____

Bath type: _____

Bath edge height: _____

Length: _____

Width: _____

Screen/curtain: _____

Tap(s) type: _____

Tap(s) height: _____

CLIENT: **FILE NUMBER:**

Outlet height: _____

Grab bars in situation: _____

Grab bars required: _____

Other comments:

Shower:

Shower type: _____

Location and description: _____

Shower cubicle: _____ Hob height: _____

Shower over bath: _____

Types of screening: _____

Door clearance: _____

Dimensions: _____

Taps: Double: _____ Single: _____

Shower hose: _____

Grab bars in situation: _____

Grab bars required: _____

Other comments:

Basin:

Basin type: _____

Location and description: _____

Taps: _____

Spout: _____

Height: _____

Mirror: _____

Storage: _____

Power point: _____

Other comments:

CLIENT: **FILE NUMBER:**

Page 8 of 11

Toilet:

Toilet type: _____

Location and description: _____

Dimensions of room: _____

Door width: _____

Door opening: _____

Toilet heights in situation: _____

Grab bars in situation: _____

Grab bars required: _____

Floor covering: _____

Access to toilet paper: _____

Other comments:

6. Kitchen:

Location and description: _____

Counter height: _____

Counter width: _____

Counter depth: _____

Space between benches: _____

Sink access: _____

Sink style: _____

Sink depth: _____

Insulation under sink: _____

Tap style: _____

Spout style: _____

Stove/oven type: _____

Hotplate type: _____

Storage type: _____

Floor covering: _____

Pantry size and type: _____

Dishwasher type and access: _____

Other comments:

CLIENT: **FILE NUMBER:**

7. Laundry:

Location and description: _____

Type of appliances: _____

Sink height: _____

Sink depth: _____

Sink width: _____

Location of tap(s): _____

Location of spout: _____

Counter height: _____

Counter width: _____

Counter depth: _____

Storage type: _____

Location of power point: _____

Location of clothesline: _____

Height of clothesline: _____

Other comments:

8. Miscellaneous:

<u>Details of Home Modification Request:</u>

CLIENT: **FILE NUMBER:**

<u>Proposals discussed including:</u>

Options considered: _____

_____

Reasons for not recommending options: _____

_____

Reasons for recommending final option: _____

_____

Consequence of not providing the recommended home modification: _____

_____

Occupational Therapist _____

Address _____

Hours of work _____

Phone number _____

Date _____

CLIENT: **FILE NUMBER:**

Page 11 of 11

Home Modification Report Template

Ainsworth, E., & de Jonge, D. *An Occupational Therapist's Guide to Home Modification Practice, Second Edition (pp. 433–441).*
© 2019 SLACK Incorporated.

OCCUPATIONAL THERAPY HOME MODIFICATION REPORT

Client Information—Confidential

<u>Name:</u>

<u>Address:</u>

<u>Contact Phone Number:</u>

<u>File Number:</u>

<u>Date of Birth/Age:</u>

<u>Date of Occupational Therapist Visit:</u>

<u>Present at Visit:</u>   Client,   Occupational Therapist (include name of organization and phone #)

<u>Client Profile:</u>

Health Condition or Disability-Specific Information

Brief detail, including the following:

+ Health condition and/or disability that affects his or her daily function and associated issues with physical and functional status (e.g., presence of pain, issues with endurance)
+ Quality of vision and hearing and aids used
+ Handedness for activities
+ Capacity to manage medications
+ Past health history (e.g., illnesses, operations, diseases)

Level of Mobility

Brief detail, including the following:

+ Primary method of mobility (e.g., walking, wheeling)
+ Sitting, standing, and walking tolerances
+ Static and dynamic sitting and standing balance
+ Capacity to bear weight in standing and for transfers
+ Transfer ability/technique—on/off bed, chair, toilet; in/out bath, shower
+ Ability to use stairs, how many, reliance on use of handrail
+ Ability to manage ramps and hills
+ Community access—public transport options used, private vehicle use

CLIENT:

Level of Independence

Brief detail, including the following:

+ Roles and occupations
+ Self-care activities: toileting, showering, drying, dressing, grooming, feeding
+ Household activities: shopping, cooking, cleaning, laundry, gardening, mowing, maintenance, banking
+ Work activities
+ School activities
+ Daily routine
+ Weekly routine

Use of Equipment

Brief detail, including the following:

+ List of current equipment used
+ List of anticipated future equipment

Measurements for occupied and unoccupied equipment (include product information sheets if available), for example:

Wheelchair—note if occupied/unoccupied/both

+ Length
+ Width
+ Floor to top of toe with foot on footplate
+ Floor to top of knee with foot on footplate
+ Floor to armrest
+ Floor to hand on top of hand control on armrest
+ Turning circles—90, 180, 360 degrees
+ Reach ranges in seated position with right and left upper limbs
+ Eye height in seated position

Hoist—unoccupied

+ Width
+ Length
+ Height of feet above floor level
+ Turning circles—90, 180, 360 degrees

Other equipment—note if occupied/unoccupied/both

+ Length
+ Width
+ Turning circles—90, 180, 360 degrees

CLIENT:

Anthropometric measurements of client, for example:

✦ Person seated—floor to popliteal crease

<u>Support Services:</u>

✦ Type of support services being used—health and community services
✦ Frequency of service
✦ Informal and family support being provided

<u>Brief Description of Property:</u>

Note the following:

✦ Age, style, materials, condition, and location of the home in the community
✦ Slope and size of the land on which the home is located
✦ Fencing style and height; type and location of access gates
✦ Lawn and gardens

Car Parking

✦ Type (car parking bay, carport, garage)
✦ Size
✦ Location in relation to home
✦ Presence and type of storage facilities
✦ Electricity
✦ Presence and type of lighting
✦ Type of access to the internal area of the home
✦ Existing modifications

External Access

✦ Paths/driveways—type, location, material, and condition
✦ Step/stairs—location and number of risers; location and type of handrails; presence and size of landing(s) at top and bottom, type of path to access step/stairs
✦ Security screens—location (windows, doors) and type
✦ Mailbox, trash cans, garden shed, and clothesline—location and type, type of path to access these features
✦ Existing modifications

CLIENT:

Internal Access

✦ Flooring type and condition

✦ Presence of changes in floor levels (bathroom, toilet, laundry)

✦ Presence of internal stairs—location and number of risers; location and type of handrails; presence and size of landing(s) at top and bottom, type of path to access step/stairs

✦ Corridor widths

✦ Doors—location, type, clearance, style, and height of handles and locks

✦ Existing modifications

✦ Lighting—style, location, and location and style of switches

Bathroom

✦ Location

✦ Overall room size

✦ Features within the area, including existing modifications

✦ Step at door threshold

✦ Flooring type and condition

✦ Door(s)—location, type, clearance, style, and height of handles and locks

✦ Window(s)—location, type, glass type, style, and height of handles and locks

✦ Vanity area

  + location

  + style

  + height

  + width

  + length

  + tap(s)—type and size

  + toe recess height

  + storage above and/or below—type, dimensions

✦ Bath/shower over the bath

  + location

  + style and shape

  + height of side

  + width

  + length

  + tap(s)—location and type

CLIENT:

- ✦ Shower recess
  - ✦ location
  - ✦ style and shape
  - ✦ height of hob
  - ✦ width
  - ✦ length
  - ✦ tap(s)—location and type
  - ✦ outlet—location
  - ✦ accessories/grab bars—location and type
- ✦ Toilet
  - ✦ location
  - ✦ style and shape
  - ✦ height of datum point (or top of pan)
  - ✦ location, height, and style of buttons
  - ✦ location, height, and style of toilet roll holder
  - ✦ centerline measurement
  - ✦ front tip of pan from rear cistern wall measurement
- ✦ Storage
  - ✦ location and type
  - ✦ dimensions
  - ✦ type and size of handles
- ✦ Mirror
  - ✦ location and type
  - ✦ dimensions
- ✦ Towel rails
  - ✦ location and type
  - ✦ dimensions
- ✦ Lighting, heat, exhaust—style, location; style and location of switches
- ✦ Separate toilet
  - ✦ as per earlier

Kitchen

- ✦ Location
- ✦ Overall room size
- ✦ Style, shape, materials
- ✦ Windows—location, sill height, width, presence of curtains/blinds
- ✦ Benches—height, width, length

CLIENT:

+ Above and below bench storage—location and type
+ Appliances—type, condition, location
+ Sink—style, condition, location
+ Hotplates—style, condition, location
+ Oven—style, condition, location
+ Flooring—type and condition
+ Lighting—style and location of switches

Laundry
+ Location
+ Overall room size
+ Door style
+ Door handle type and height
+ Door clearance
+ Windows—location, sill height, width, presence of curtains/blinds
+ Benches—height, width, length
+ Above and below bench storage—location and type
+ Appliances—type, condition, location
+ Sink—style, condition, location
+ Flooring type and condition
+ Lighting—style and location of switches

Bedroom(s)
+ Location
+ Overall room size
+ Door style
+ Door handle type and height
+ Door clearance
+ Windows—location, sill height, width, presence of curtains/blinds
+ Wardrobe/storage—location and type
+ Flooring type and condition
+ Lighting—style and location of switches
+ Existing modifications

CLIENT:

Other electrical arrangements in the home

- ✦ Lighting—style and location
- ✦ Switches—style and location
- ✦ Air conditioning—type and location
- ✦ Fans—type and location
- ✦ Existing modifications

Recommendations:

Proposals	Environmental barriers, interventions considered, and clinical reasoning

The client(s) agreed with the recommendations listed here at the time of the interview.

Signed: Approved by:

_____   _____

Occupational Therapist   *Program Manager*

Date: _____   Date: _____

CLIENT:

SCOPE OF WORK FOR BUILDING SERVICES PROVIDER

<u>Name:</u>

<u>Address:</u>

<u>Contact Phone Number:</u>

<u>File Number:</u>

<u>Modifications:</u>
- ✦ Eternal Access
- ✦ Internal Access
- ✦ Bathroom
- ✦ Toilet
- ✦ Bedroom
- ✦ Kitchen
- ✦ Laundry
- ✦ Electrical
- ✦ Other
- ✦ Paint/repair all areas disturbed

<u>Note:</u>

1. Modifications are based on specific client requirements. Any alteration to the items listed on this scope of work should be checked with the occupational therapist, _____ .
   Phone: _____ Hours of work: _____

2. Concept drawings (where provided) are/are not to scale and should be read in conjunction with the written scope of work.

3. Please refer to the attached photographs for information about the existing environment to be modified.

Signed: Approved by:

_____   _____
Occupational Therapist   *Program Manager*

Date: _____   Date: _____

APPENDIX I

Example of an
Occupational Therapy Report

Ainsworth, E., & de Jonge, D. *An Occupational Therapist's*
Guide to Home Modification Practice, Second Edition (pp. 443–454).
© 2019 SLACK Incorporated.

Section 1

Susan Taylor
Occupational Therapist
Central Home Modifications Program
PO Box 12AA
New York
Phone: (212) 925-2742
Fax: (212) 925-2745

OCCUPATIONAL THERAPY
HOME MODIFICATION REPORT

Client Information—Confidential

Name: Mr. and Mrs. Alan Gray

Address: 8 Lakeside Close
                                     New York, NY, 10012

Contact Phone Number: (212) 925-2742

File Number: AKH 13222555

Date of Birth/Age: Mrs. Doris Gray: January 3, 1938 (80 years old)
                                     Mr. Alan Gray: April 11, 1936 (82 years old)

Date of Occupational   June 6, 2018
Therapist Visit:

Present at Visit: Mr. and Mrs. Gray, their daughter Mrs. April Jones, Miss Susan Taylor
                                     (Occupational Therapist, Central Home Modification Program)

Source and Reason for Referral:

Peter Jones from Jones, Light, and O'Brien Attorneys provided a referral to the occupational therapist requesting a home assessment for Mr. and Mrs. Gray, with a view to making recommendations for home modifications. This information is to form part of Mrs. Gray's claim for damages following a motor vehicle accident on January 1, 2018. The referral was received on May 5, 2018.

Client Profile:

Information about Health Conditions or Disabilities:

Health information reviewed prior to the home visit included the following:

A letter from Doctor Barrington dated May 5, 2018. This documentation states that the client was in her car, stopped at a traffic light, and was run into by a truck on January 1, 2018. Her car was described to

© SLACK Incorporated, 2019. Ainsworth, E., & De Jonge, D. (2019).
An Occupational Therapist's Guide to Home Modification Practice (2nd ed.). Thorofare, NJ: SLACK Incorporated.

have been pushed into an electric pole (light pole), and as a result, she sustained a traumatic brain injury and multiple orthopedic and neurological injuries. The injuries reported in this documentation include the following:

+ Fractured right humerus
+ Fractured left tibia
+ Acquired brain injury (diffuse axonal injury, subarachnoid and subdural hemorrhage) resulting in left-sided hemiplegia with fluctuating upper limb and lower limb tone
+ Aphasia

She was observed to be wearing a second skin-pressure garment on her left upper limb to reduce the tone in this arm. Mr. Gray indicated that he uses a communication board with his wife.

The medical documentation indicates that prior to her accident she had the following conditions:

+ Urinary incontinence
+ Urinary tract infections June 2002, May 2003, May 2004

At the time of interview with this couple, Mr. Gray indicated that he is the main caregiver for his wife.

Mr. Gray reported that he has been diagnosed with the following conditions:

+ Rheumatoid arthritis affecting the knees and shoulders: the client has pain, stiffness, and swelling of the joints, limiting his capacity to walk long distances and bend
+ Non–insulin-dependent diabetes: poorly controlled; currently experiencing difficulty with his vision
+ Clinical depression: managed by medication administered by Mr. Gray

Level of Mobility:

Mr. Gray stated that his wife relies on the use of a manual wheelchair to wheel short and long distances. He indicated that her fractures have healed but that she is not able to bear weight on her lower limbs and relies on the use of a floor-based electric hoist for all transfers. Mr. Gray reported that he has used the hoist with occasional caregiver assistance when transferring her on and off the bed, chair, and in and out of the mobile over-toilet shower chair.

At the time of the home visit, the occupational therapist observed Mr. Gray wheeling his wife around the home in her attendant-propelled wheelchair and attendant-propelled mobile over-toilet shower chair. He also demonstrated the various transfers on and off this equipment using the hoist. He indicated that he experiences joint pain as he undertakes this activity by himself without caregiver assistance due to the need to bend and reach to fit the sling around his wife and maneuver the hoist into position over the bed or other piece of equipment on carpet in the bedroom.

Mr. Gray reported that his wife is mainly confined to the upstairs area of the home because of the presence of the external stairs that she is unable to negotiate.

Mr. Gray reported that he is experiencing joint pain and finds his own transfers on and off low seats, such as the toilet, quite difficult. He indicated that he is able to walk short distances indoors and uses a single-point stick when walking outdoors. Mr. Gray stated that his mobility has been affected his arthritis and by his lack of confidence when walking over uneven terrain or when negotiating changes in levels. He indicated that his vision has deteriorated and that he has nearly had falls in outdoor areas.

<u>Self-Care and Household Tasks:</u>

Mr. Gray indicated that the doctor had arranged for a nursing service to visit once a day to assist his wife as she was showered, but this service discontinued after a few months when she returned home from rehabilitation.

Mr. Gray indicated that he completes all household tasks, such as shopping, cooking, cleaning, and laundry, although his daughter has been providing meals for the freezer and his grandson has been mowing the yard and maintaining the garden. He demonstrated how he experiences difficulty reaching and bending during his own and his wife's showering activities and while in the kitchen undertaking meal preparation.

<u>Community Access:</u>

Mrs. Jones stated that she and her husband take her parents on drives and to appointments when required since her father no longer drives because of his diminishing eyesight. She indicated that both she and her husband physically lift Mrs. Gray down the stairs and into the vehicle. Mrs. Jones indicated that she worries that these transfers are often unsafe.

<u>Equipment Dimensions:</u>

Attendant-Propelled Wheelchair

Occupied length:	43 1/4 in (1,100 mm)
Occupied width:	26 1/2 in (670 mm)
Floor to top of toe with foot on footplate:	8 in (200 mm) above floor level (AFL)
Floor to top of seat cushion:	23 1/2 in (600 mm) AFL
Floor to top of knee with foot on footplate:	25 1/2 in (650 mm) AFL
Floor to top of armrest:	28 1/2 in (720 mm) AFL
Turning circle:	59 in (1,500 mm) diameter
Turning capacity:	Can fit through a 33 1/2-in (850-mm) clear doorway and turn 90 degrees in a 47 1/4-in (1,200-mm) wide corridor

Mobile Over-Toilet Shower Chair

Occupied length:	43 1/4 in (1,100 mm)
Occupied width:	23 3/4 in (600 mm)
Floor to top of toe with foot on footplate:	9 3/4 in (250 mm) AFL
Floor to top of knee with foot on footplate:	25 1/2 in (650 mm) AFL
Floor to top of armrest:	31 1/2 in (800 mm) AFL
Turning circle:	59 in (1,500 mm) diameter
Turning capacity:	Can fit through a 33 1/2-in (850-mm) clear door and turn 90 degrees in a 47 1/4-in (1,200-mm) wide corridor

Mr. and Mrs. Gray
8 Lakeside Close
New York, NY 10012

Floor-Based Electric Hoist

Unoccupied width:	27 1/2 in (700 mm)
Unoccupied length:	43 1/4 in (1,100 mm)
Floor to top of legs:	4 3/4 in (120 mm)
Turning capacity:	Can fit through a 30 3/4-in (780-mm) clear door but needs 51 1/4-in (1,300-mm) clearance in front of the door for turning 90 or 180 degrees

Bed (hospital style, height adjustable)

Width:	41 1/4 in (1,050 mm)
Length:	82 3/4 in (2,100 mm)

Other Issues:

Mr. Gray indicated that his wife is now no longer able to undertake any of her hobbies (gardening, knitting, and sewing). He stated that he is finding it increasingly difficult to care for his wife and he feels that his own mental and physical health is declining. He indicated that he used to be a motor mechanic but is now retired and enjoys reading his automobile magazines and helping his grandson restore an old car. He reported that he barely has time to engage in these leisure activities due to his need to monitor his wife all day. Mr. Gray indicated that he and his wife do not want to move out of their home because they have lived there for more than 50 years, raising their family and enjoying the relationships they have established in the neighborhood. Mr. Gray stated that his wife was very unsettled when in rehabilitation after her accident, and he reported that she showed an improvement in her mood when she returned home.

Assessment Tools:

A combination of interview and observation was used during the assessment phase. In addition, the *Canadian Occupational Performance Measure* was used with Mr. Gray to establish outcomes to be measured after the interventions were introduced. Mr. Gray rated all of his daily activities as to importance. The five top-rated activities are listed here, with ratings of performance ("how well I do this activity") and satisfaction ("how satisfied I am with this activity.") All ratings are on a scale of 1 (lowest rating) to 10 (highest rating).

Occupation	Importance (1-10)	Performance (1-10)	Satisfaction (1-10)
Caring for his wife: showering, dressing, toileting, transfers	10	4	4
Household tasks	10	6	3
Self-care routine	10	5	5
Going shopping at least once a week	8	10	10
Reading	7	10	10
Restoring the car with his grandson	8	5	10

Mr. Gray indicated that his short-term goals included:

- ✦ Gaining an increased understanding and acceptance of his wife's condition and developing strategies to better manage her symptoms, including her ongoing incontinence
- ✦ Improving the safety of both he and his wife when providing her with assistance with her transfers and mobility in and around the home, and during her showering and toileting routine
- ✦ Managing his increasing anxiety and stress associated with ensuring his wife's health and well-being

Mr. Gray stated that his long-term goals included:

- ✦ Maintaining his own physical and emotional health in his role as a caregiver
- ✦ Safely and effectively assisting his wife in her daily self-care activities and supporting her for as long as possible in the family home

<u>Brief Description of Property:</u>

Mr. and Mrs. Gray live in a four-bedroom detached brick house that is high-set with the following features:

- ✦ Twelve brick stairs at the front and rear of the home with a wooden handrail on the left side ascending
- ✦ Living and dining room, kitchen, four bedrooms, bathroom, and separate toilet located on the first level of the home
- ✦ Double garage, laundry, and storage areas located on the ground level of the home
- ✦ Pathway leading from the base of the external front stairs to the driveway
- ✦ 47 1/4-in (1,200-mm) high wooden paling fence around the perimeter of the yard
- ✦ Pathway along the rear wall of the home
- ✦ Pathway leading from the laundry to the clothesline
- ✦ Flooring: low-pile carpet in the living and dining rooms and bedrooms; linoleum in the kitchen; and tiles in the bathroom, toilet, and laundry areas
- ✦ Bathroom upstairs: vanity with mirror above; bath; separate shower with a fixed shower screen and pivoting door and a curb; and towel rails.

The client's movements and capacity to access various features of the home was assessed at the time of the visit, and the following home modification items are recommended to suit the client. These recommendations take into consideration the client's current health status and their present level of safety, independence, and quality of life. The features are relevant for the client's current and future physical status. This report concentrates on the most essential home modification features required by the client, the options considered (if any), and the reasoning for the home modification recommendations. The performance criteria of the various features have been described rather than specific brands of products.

Mr. and Mrs. Gray
8 Lakeside Close
New York, NY 10012

Proposals	Environmental barriers, interventions considered, and clinical reasoning
Provide a wheelchair-accessible lift from the ground level to the first level of the home at the rear of the home. Lift to be installed at the rear of the home and a wheelchair-accessible path that is at least 47 1/4-in (1,200-mm) wide to be installed from the rear garage door to the lift. The path that is to adjoin the garage door is to have no step at the entry. The consequence of not providing these modifications are that Mrs. Gray will be confined to the upstairs area of the home and someone will need to physically carry her when she needs to leave the home for medical and other appointments.	The house is too high to ramp from the ground level to the first level, and Mrs. Gray would not be able to maintain safe static balance perched on a stair lift. The couple are not willing to relocate to ground-level accommodation, despite their deteriorating mobility. There is also insufficient area under the home to create a living, bedroom, and bathroom area for Mrs. Gray to prevent the need for her to go upstairs. The lift is recommended to enable the client to move between the two levels with ease in her wheelchair. The pathway is also recommended to ensure the clients have a level path of travel from the garage door area to the lift in all weather conditions.
Extend the width of the pathways around the home so that they are at least 47-in (1,200-mm) wide. Raise the turf and soil by all the paths and landings around the home to ensure that the various surfaces are level. The consequence of not widening the paths around the home is that Mr. Gray may have an accident wheeling his wife along the narrow paths and over uneven terrain, or they may need to seek assistance to wheel her.	Mr. Gray reported that he is experiencing difficulty wheeling his wife on the narrow paths and uneven terrain. Installing wider paths and leveling the turf and soil with the paths will eliminate any hazards and improve their current level of safety.
Remove the bath, shower, vanity, and toilet in the upstairs bathroom and re-lay the floor to remove the step at the door and install wheelchair-accessible shower, vanity, and toilet areas and slip-resistive flooring. The consequence of not creating a wheelchair-accessible bathroom is that Mr. Gray will likely continue to shower his wife over the floor waste and damage the surrounding bathroom fittings such as cupboards due to the splash during the routine. He is at risk of falling and he may injure himself (and his wife) as he continues to push equipment over the threshold step, in and out and around the bathroom. Extra time and effort will continue to be needed to complete the routine.	The current bathroom is not wheelchair accessible. Mr. Gray is showering his wife over the floor waste and experiencing difficulty positioning the mobile over-toilet shower chair over the toilet. There is limited space, and the floor appeared slippery when wet. The installation of a wheelchair-accessible bathroom with no step at the door and slip-resistive flooring will ensure a more spacious layout that suits the size of the equipment, the client, and Mr. Gray as they use the area during Mrs. Gray's self-care routine.

(continued)

Mr. and Mrs. Gray
8 Lakeside Close
New York, NY 10012

Proposals (continued)	Environmental barriers, interventions considered, and clinical reasoning (continued)
Remove the existing carpet in the main bedroom and replace with vinyl. The consequence of not removing the carpet and replacing it with vinyl is that Mr. Gray may injure himself as he pushes the equipment over the carpet. Further, extra time and effort will be required to clean the carpet after accidents.	Mr. Gray indicated that his wife continues to experience incontinence and that there have been "accidents" in the bedroom on occasions. He also reported that the hoist and other equipment are difficult to maneuver on the carpet. The removal of the carpet and replacement is recommended to enable Mr. Gray to clean the floor and move the equipment with greater ease and safety.
Remove the rear entry, main bedroom and bathroom doors, and door frames. Install sliding doors that achieve 33 1/2-in (850-mm) clearance. Relocate light switches to adjacent wall at standard height to suit location of new doors. The consequence of not installing the wider doorways is that the equipment will continue to damage the door frames. These frames will likely require repair and replacement over time, at a cost to the client.	Mr. Gray stated that the entries into the rear door, main bedroom, and bathroom are narrow and that the mobility equipment is scraping the door frames. The door clearances are approximately 30 1/4 in (770 mm). It is recommended to provide wider door clearance and changing the style of the doors from swing doors to sliding doors to give more space through which the equipment can safely move. The wider doorways will also accommodate wider equipment if this is required in the future.
Install a vertical grab bar on the tap wall of the shower recess. Vertical grab bar to be fitted with a friction-sliding mount. Remove and replace shower rose with handheld shower that is to attach to the friction sliding mount. The consequence of not installing the vertical grab bar is that the water may flow outside of the shower area, and the area will need to be mopped.	The vertical grab bar that is to be fitted with a friction-sliding mount on which the handheld shower could be positioned will enable Mr. Gray to better control water flow. A handheld shower was a safer alternative than retaining the shower rose.
Install daylight tone fluorescent lighting with diffuser shields in the kitchen, living room, dining room, and corridor areas. The consequence of not installing the enhanced lighting is that the paths of travel within the home will not be well lit to ensure safe wheeling of the client, and safe activity completion.	At the time of the home visit, the occupational therapist noted that the interior of the home required enhanced lighting because it was quite dark. The installation of stronger lighting is required to ensure the safety of the clients as they wheel through the various areas of the home and undertake activities. It will also improve illumination and minimize glare and a shadowing effect in the home.

(continued)

Mr. and Mrs. Gray
8 Lakeside Close
New York, NY 10012

Additional Recommendations:

Mr. Gray to:

✦ Reduce the clutter within the various rooms by hanging some of the family photos on a wall or asking his daughter to create a memory album he and his wife can use

Services required:

✦ Referral to incontinence specialist for education about toileting/incontinence

✦ Referral to the nursing service to recommence immediate assistance with self-care activities

✦ Referral to rheumatologist to monitor the current integrity of Mr. Gray's joints and effectiveness of pain control measures

✦ Referral to ophthalmologist for an assessment of Mr. Gray's vision

✦ Referral to a social worker for assessment for regular respite care

Mr. Gray agreed with the previously mentioned recommendations at the time of the home visit.

Signed:

_____

Occupational Therapist

Date: _____

Approved by:

_____

Program Manager

Date: _____

Mr. and Mrs. Gray
8 Lakeside Close
New York, NY 10012

Section 2

OCCUPATIONAL THERAPY REPORT FOR BUILDING SERVICES PROVIDER

Name: Mr. and Mrs. Allan Gray

Address: 8 Lakeside Close
                               New York, NY, 10012

Contact Phone Number: (212) 925-2742

File Number: AKH 13222555

Modifications

External Access:

+ Extend the rear landing on the first level of the home to suit the installation of a wheelchair-accessible lift with outward swinging doors with 33 1/2-in (850-mm) clearance.

+ Landing dimension to be 98 1/2-in (2,500-mm) long × 78 3/4-in (2,000-mm) wide.

+ Widen rear entry door to achieve 33 1/2-in (850-mm) clearance and ensure there is no change in level between the landing and the internal floor greater than 1/4 in (6 mm).

+ Install wheelchair-accessible lift with wheelchair carriage size to accommodate standard wheelchair and caregiver.

+ Install a wheelchair-accessible path that is at least 48-in (1,200-mm) wide and extend from the rear garage door to the lift. The path that is to adjoin the garage door is to have no step at the entry.

+ All paths to be 48-in (1,200-mm) wide (excluding obstacles) with a slip-resistive finish.

+ Abutting surfaces to have a smooth transition with maximum tolerance of 1/4 in (6 mm) with the protruding surface having a rounded end.

+ Paths level with adjoining turfed edges and turfed edges to extend horizontally for at least 23 1/2 in (600 mm) before ramping away due to a slight gradient in the land.

+ Vertical clearance of 78 3/4 in (2,000 mm) required along full length of path.

+ Maximum cross fall of 1:40.

+ Paths adjoining grass: no abutments between the two surfaces greater than 1/4 in (5 mm).

Internal Access:

+ Remove the main bedroom and bathroom doors and door frames.

+ Install sliding doors that achieve 33 1/2-in (850-mm) clearance.

+ Relocate light switches to adjacent wall at standard height to suit location of new doors.

Mr. and Mrs. Gray
8 Lakeside Close
New York, NY 10012

Bathroom/Toilet

+ Remove the flooring, fittings, and fixtures in the existing bathroom.
+ Remove the existing sliding door and install a face of wall-sliding door that achieves 33 1/2-in (850-mm) clearance.
+ Door to have 2 1/2-in (60-mm) clearance on either side of D-shaped handles.
+ Flooring to be "slip resistant when wet."
+ Install 2 × 23 1/2-in (600-mm) long towel rails at standard height on the walls of the bathroom.

Wheel-in shower with no hob

+ Install large shower recess with continuous curtain track that is located 71 in (1,800 mm) to the underside and weighted shower curtain that extends to the floor: shower recess size to be 47 1/4 in (1,200 mm) × 59 in (1,500 mm).
+ Install handheld shower on a friction slide mount on a vertical grab rail: base of the rail to be located 35 1/2 in (900 mm) AFL.
+ Fall in bathroom floor to drain to the shower: 1:50 to 1:60 fall within the shower and 1:70 to 1:80 fall from the door to the shower edge.
+ Shower fixtures configuration to include handheld shower on a friction-sliding mount on a vertical grab rail, recessed soap holder, and lever tap.
+ Recessed soap holder and lever tap to be located between 35 1/2 in (900 mm) and 43 1/4 in (1,100 mm) AFL and to be positioned so that the tap is on the open side of the shower and the soap holder is on the other side of the grab bar that is located centrally on the wall.
+ Shower hose to be nonheat conducting.

Vanity

+ Vanity unit to have a bench top and drawers located in the corner area; to be on easy-glide runners with stops; and to have D-shaped handles.
+ Bench width to be 13 3/4 in (350 mm).
+ Clearance under bench at least 32 1/4-in (820-mm) wide; pipe work not to intrude into knee space.
+ Datum point of semi-recessed basin in the vanity to be 33 1/2 in (850 mm) AFL.
+ Corners of vanity to be rounded and ends truncated.
+ Large mirror to be installed above the vanity, to start 2 in (50 mm) above the level of the bench.

Toilet

+ Center line of toilet to be located 17 3/4 in (450 mm) to 18 in (460 mm) from adjacent wall.
+ 450-mm clearance required from the center line of the toilet to the open side.
+ Toilet height to be 18 in (460 mm) to 18 3/4 in (480 mm) AFL including solid seat but not lid.
+ Front of toilet to be located 31 in (790 mm) to 31 3/4 in (810 mm) distance from cistern wall.
+ Toilet roll holder to be recessed in style and to be located 27 1/2 in (700 mm) AFL and 33 1/2 in (850 mm) from the rear cistern wall.
+ Solid toilet seat and lid with metal hinges to be installed.

Temperature Control:

✦ Install a temperature-control device to be on line to the bathroom, kitchen, and laundry.

Lighting:

✦ Remove existing lighting in the kitchen, living room, dining room, and corridor areas and install daylight tone fluorescent lighting with diffuser shields.

Other:

✦ Please paint/repair all areas disturbed.

✦ Please note that measurements have been undertaken as per the following technique:

   + Horizontal grab bar—floor to top of grab bar

   + Vertical grab bar—corner to inside edge of grab bar

Please note that the proposed home modifications are based on specific client requirements. Any alteration to this scope of works should be checked with the occupational therapist.

Signed:

_____

Occupational Therapist

Date: _____

Approved by:

_____

Program Manager

Date: _____

Mr. and Mrs. Gray
8 Lakeside Close
New York, NY 10012

Financial Disclosures

Elizabeth Ainsworth has no financial or proprietary interest in the materials presented herein.

Dr. Tammy Aplin has no financial or proprietary interest in the materials presented herein.

Kathleen Baigent has no financial or proprietary interest in the materials presented herein.

Ruth Cordiner has no financial or proprietary interest in the materials presented herein.

Shirley Darlison has no financial or proprietary interest in the materials presented herein.

Desleigh de Jonge has no financial or proprietary interest in the materials presented herein.

May Eade has no financial or proprietary interest in the materials presented herein.

Dr. Louise Gustafsson has no financial or proprietary interest in the materials presented herein.

Melanie Hoyle has no financial or proprietary interest in the materials presented herein.

Andrew Jones has no financial or proprietary interest in the materials presented herein.

Barbara Kornblau has no financial or proprietary interest in the materials presented herein.

Rhonda Phillips has no financial or proprietary interest in the materials presented herein.

Dr. Jon Pynoos has no financial or proprietary interest in the materials presented herein.

Jon Sanford has no financial or proprietary interest in the materials presented herein.

Bronwyn Tanner has no financial or proprietary interest in the materials presented herein.

Dr. Merrill Turpin has no financial or proprietary interest in the materials presented herein.

Index